NCLEX-RN®
PREMIER

2014–2015

with 2 Practice Tests

NCLEX-RN® PREMIER

2014-2015

with 2 Practice Tests

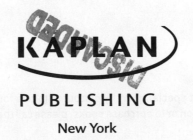

KAPLAN PUBLISHING

New York

© 2014 by Kaplan, Inc.

Published by Kaplan Publishing, a division of Kaplan, Inc.
395 Hudson Street
New York, NY 10014

Printed in the United States of America

10 9 8 7 6 5 4 3 2 1

ISBN-13: 978-1-61865-499-1

Kaplan Publishing books are available at special quantity discounts to use for sales promotions, employee premiums, or educational purposes. For more information or to purchase books, please call the Simon & Schuster special sales department at 866-506-1949.

CONTENTS

KAPLAN) NURSING

KAPLAN) NURSING

KAPLAN) NURSING

ABOUT THE AUTHORS

BARBARA J. IRWIN, MSN, RN

Barbara J. Irwin is Executive Director of Nursing for Kaplan Nursing. She supervises development of the Kaplan course for preparation for the NCLEX-RN® examination for U.S. nursing students and international nurses, as well as integrated testing programs implemented by nursing schools. Ms. Irwin developed a critical thinking framework to answer higher-level test questions that has helped students achieve success on this high-stakes test. She developed and presents seminars to student nurses on how to study effectively to achieve deep learning and improve critical thinking. She has presented seminars to nursing faculty about the NCLEX-RN® and NCLEX-PN® examinations and how to overcome the challenge of non-self-efficacious nursing students. Ms. Irwin holds a bachelor of science degree in nursing from the University of Oklahoma and a master of science degree in nursing and nursing education from Kaplan University.

JUDITH A. BURCKHARDT, PhD, RN

Dr. Judith Burckhardt is Vice President of Strategic Development for the Kaplan University School of Nursing. With senior leadership she coordinates activities to promote excellence in the Kaplan School of Nursing. She interacts with health care organizations and systems to develop strategic partnerships that advance the mission of the health care organization and the Kaplan University School of Nursing. She holds a bachelor of science in nursing from Loyola University in Chicago, a master's in education from Washington University, a master of science in nursing degree from Kaplan University, and a doctorate in educational administration from the University of Nebraska, Lincoln. Her professional background includes many years of experience as an educator in diploma, ADN, and BSN nursing programs. She works with schools of nursing to develop curriculum and testing programs. She has developed programs and materials to prepare students for the NCLEX-RN® exam and has presented NCLEX-RN® exam preparation and career development seminars to students, nurses, and health care professionals in the United States and abroad. Ms. Burckhardt has also given item-writing workshops to nursing school faculties. She writes articles for nursing publications and has developed instructor-led continuing education programs for online delivery.

Kaplan thanks the following nursing professionals for their contributions to this book:

Barbara Arnoldussen, RN, MBA, CPHQ
Shawna M. Butler, RN, BSN, JD
Tamara Dolan, RN, MSN, OCN
Terri Forehand, RN
Constance Krueger, RN
Rene Jackson, MS, BSN, RN, LHRM, CPHRM

FOR ANY TEST CHANGES OR LATE-BREAKING DEVELOPMENTS

kaptest.com/publishing

The material in this book is up-to-date at the time of publication. However, the National Council of State Boards of Nursing may have instituted changes in the test after this book was published. Be sure to carefully read the materials you receive when you register for the test. If there are any important late-breaking developments—or any changes or corrections to the Kaplan test preparation materials in this book—we will post that information online at *kaptest.com/publishing*.

READERS' COMMENTS

Here's what our readers have to say about Kaplan's NCLEX-RN® exam guide:

"I was the classic unsuccessful test taker when I started your book. When I was done, I had become a successful test taker. I took my NCLEX-RN® exam and passed on the first attempt. I credit Kaplan with that." —A. Duane Deyo, Stafford, VA

"The questions in the review book were just like the ones on the test. The tips on how to take the exam really helped me. I took my NCLEX-RN® exam and passed the first time!" —Heather G. Sabott, Egg Harbor Township, NJ

"Thank you, Kaplan. This book, test, and strategies really helped me get through my boards. I passed on my first attempt with only 75 questions. Your program definitely prepares the student for success." —Deirdre A. Beasley, Rancho Cucamonga, CA

"The book is very user-friendly, well organized, and very comprehensive. It…gave me more self-confidence in answering NCLEX-RN® exam questions.…Two thumbs up!" —G. B. Perdigones, Chicago, IL

"After doing all my reviews, I read this book twice and I went to take the test with confidence. I did it—thank you!" —Elisabeth Boursiquot, Spring Valley, NY

"Out of the 15 NCLEX-RN® books I bought, this Kaplan book was the only one that helped. The critical thinking and test taking skills were very useful in studying for the NCLEX-RN® exam. Thank you so much!" —Sherrie Corcuera, Barnegat, NJ

"I had taken the NCLEX-RN® exam twice and failed, I'd taken courses, etc. I didn't need another study book—I needed a book that emphasizes test taking skills for NCLEX-RN® exam and test anxiety reduction. I took the test for the third time and passed!" —Beatrice Ordoñez, O'Fallon, MO

"I am a foreign-educated nurse…On my exam day I was so confident and passed the first time. Thank you." —Nimfa C. Garrison, Raritan, NJ

"Before I started to prepare for the NCLEX-RN® exam, I started with this book (I'm a foreign nurse from Switzerland), and it really helps me to have a critical thinking strategy and to answer the NCLEX-RN® exam question types. The practice test and the answer key are extremely helpful, the way it explains every single answer. So now, I think I'm ready to start the Kaplan course book. Thank you."

—Celine Cucchia, San Jose, CA

"Special thanks to the creators of this wonderful book and others related to NCLEX-RN® exam. It was the best I could ever have gotten. I just feel sorry I didn't take your review class due to [the fact that] I didn't know about you guys until after I took another review class. But I was lucky to find this wonderful book. Thanks! I will recommend this book or anything related to Kaplan to the future generations of my nursing school. You guys are the best! Thank you and keep up with the good work."

—Elvia Manrique, Port Jefferson Station, NY

"My husband gave me this book for Christmas and it was one of the best gifts I ever received. By reading your book cover to cover, I gained some confidence, learned how to reword questions, how to correctly read a question, and how to decrease some of my anxiety....Thank you for a great book that I will definitely recommend to anyone taking the boards."

—Nancy D. Zimmerman, South Windsor, CT

"This book was a blueprint to the NCLEX-RN® exam. I passed the test on the first try. Everything that was explained in the book was actually on the test."

—Jacquelyn Claude, Suffolk, VA

"I plan to call my school and recommend this book!"

—Nicole Sary, East Peoria, IL

"Reading the book was like an instructor talking....The book is absolutely GREAT!"

—Lianna Williams, Bronx, NY

"Very easy to understand—MADE SENSE. Everything about this book was exceptional. After my self-esteem dropped when I found out I failed the first time, I didn't know what to do....This book, I felt, was easy to understand, and when I went to take my test a second time, I walked out with confidence. The strategies in this book are why I am an RN today. Thank you so much!"

—Dana Adams, Fort Worth, TX

"Truly an indispensable review...for every internationally educated nurse!"

—Lamberto F. Valera, RN, MAN, Jordan Valley, Israel

"Thank you, Kaplan, for this book!"

—Dawn Nicole Lake Prince, Van Nuys, CA

"I bought [the] Kaplan textbook when I was preparing for [the] NCLEX-RN® exam last month. I was a foreign-trained nurse so I was finding it hard to answer NCLEX-RN® exam questions. The book helped me a lot....I recommend this Kaplan study guide to everybody preparing for the NCLEX-RN® exam."

—Ngozi Uketui, AR

HOW TO USE THIS BOOK

STEP 1: Access Your Online Companion

Log on to *kaptest.com/booksonline* to access your online companion. You will be asked for a password derived from the text to access the online companion, so have your book available.

Your online companion resources include the following:

- **The computer-based practice test.** This full-length, timed practice test comes complete with detailed answer explanations and a personalized performance analysis.
- **A 20-question sample of Kaplan's NCLEX-RN® Question Bank.** For more information and to order the full version of more than 1,300 questions, please visit *kaplannursing.com*.
- **A timed 27-item practice sample of alternate format questions.** Practice answering the Select All that Apply, Hot Spot, Fill-in-the-Blank, and Ordered Response question types.
- **Online Classroom Events schedule and sign-up instructions.** See "Sign up for an Online Classroom Event" in this book for more details and to register.

STEP 2: View the DVD

In our exclusive DVD, renowned NCLEX® preparation expert Barbara Irwin, MSN, RN, presents two video lessons to help you master the exam:

- Test-Taking Workshop: Answering Application-Level Test Questions
- Rules of the NCLEX-RN®: Living in NCLEX®-Land

STEP 3: Read and Complete Part 1

Part 1, NCLEX-RN® Exam Overview and Test Taking Strategies, is a comprehensive, detailed strategy guide for each type of question on the NCLEX-RN® exam. This information will teach you how to analyze each question and use your nursing knowledge to select the correct answer choice.

STEP 4: Read and Complete Part 2

Part 2, NCLEX-RN® Exam Content Review and Practice, contains an essential review of all subject areas that appear on the exam, designed to help you master NCLEX-RN® exam questions. In the quiz at the end of each chapter, practice using the strategies you have learned and check your work against the detailed answer explanations provided.

STEP 5: Take the Practice Tests

Kaplan has prepared two different practice tests for you: the paper-and-pencil test in Part 3 and the computer-based practice test provided in your online companion. You may benefit from taking the computer-based practice test first. When the test is completed, you will receive immediate feedback on your performance, as the software analyzes your strengths and weaknesses in various content areas. You can then review the areas in which your performance was weak before you tackle the paper-and-pencil test.

STEP 6: Register for the Exam

When you are prepared to take the NCLEX-RN® exam, use the contact information and licensure requirements provided in Appendix D, State Licensing Requirements, to initiate the registration process. All of the steps you'll need to follow are contained in Part 4, The Licensure Process.

SIGN UP FOR AN ONLINE CLASSROOM EVENT

Kaplan's NCLEX-RN® online classroom sessions are interactive, instructor-led NCLEX-RN® prep lessons that you can participate in from anywhere you can access the Internet.

The online sessions are held in a state-of-the-art virtual classroom—actual lessons in real time, just like a physical classroom experience. Interact with your teacher and other classmates using audio, instant chat, whiteboard, polling, and screen-sharing functionality. And just like courses at Kaplan centers, a NCLEX-RN® online classroom session is led by an experienced Kaplan instructor.

To register for your NCLEX-RN® online classroom session:

1. Go to *kaptest.com/booksonline* and sign up for the online companion. See "How to Use This Book" for more information on how to sign up.

2. Once you've signed up for the online companion, sign in to "My Student Homepage" and go to "My Courses and Services."

3. Click on "Live Online Event" to see the dates and times of upcoming NCLEX-RN® online classroom events.

4. Select a date for your live classroom event by clicking on it. A separate window will appear with registration instructions.

Please note: Registration begins one month before the session date. Be sure to sign up early, since spaces are reserved on a first-come, first-served basis.

PART 1

NCLEX-RN® EXAM OVERVIEW AND TEST TAKING STRATEGIES

CHAPTER 1

OVERVIEW OF THE NCLEX-RN® EXAM

The NCLEX-RN® exam is, among other things, an endurance test, like a marathon. If you don't prepare properly, or approach it with confidence and rigor, you'll quickly lose your composure. Here is a sample, test-like question:

> A man had a permanent pacemaker implanted one year ago. He returns to the outpatient clinic because he thinks the pacemaker battery is malfunctioning. It is MOST important for the nurse to assess which of the following?
>
> 1. Abdominal pain, nausea, and vomiting
> 2. Wheezing on exertion, cyanosis, and orthopnea
> 3. Peripheral edema, shortness of breath, and dizziness
> 4. Chest pain radiating to the right arm, headache, and diaphoresis

As you can see, the style and content of the NCLEX-RN® exam is unique. It's not like any other exam you've ever taken, even in nursing school!

The content in this book was prepared by the experts on Kaplan's Nursing team, the world's largest provider of test prep courses for the NCLEX-RN® exam. By using Kaplan's proven methods and strategies, you will be able to take control of the exam, just as you have taken control of your nursing education and other preparations for your career in this incredibly challenging and rewarding field. The first step is to learn everything you can about the exam.

WHAT IS THE NCLEX-RN® EXAM?

NCLEX-RN® stands for *National Council Licensure Examination-Registered Nurse*. The NCLEX-RN® examination is administered by the National Council of State Boards of Nursing (NCSBN), whose members include the boards of nursing in each of the 50 states in the United States, the District of Columbia, and four U.S. territories: American Samoa, Guam, the Northern Mariana Islands, and the Virgin Islands. These boards have a mandate to protect the public from unsafe and ineffective nursing care, and each board has been given responsibility to regulate the practice of nursing in its respective state. In fact, the NCLEX-RN® exam is often referred to as "the Boards" or "State Boards."

The NCLEX-RN® exam has only one purpose: to determine if it is safe for you to begin practice as an entry-level nurse.

Why Must You Take the NCLEX-RN® Exam?

The NCLEX-RN® exam is prepared by the NCSBN. Each state requires that you pass this exam to obtain a license to practice as a registered nurse. The designation *registered nurse* or *RN* indicates that you have proven to your state board of nursing that you can deliver safe and effective nursing care. The NCLEX-RN® exam is a test of minimum competency and is based on the knowledge and behaviors that are needed for the entry-level practice of nursing. This exam tests not only your knowledge, but also your ability to make competent nursing judgments.

What Is Entry-Level Practice of Nursing?

In order to define *entry-level* practice of nursing, the National Council conducts a job analysis study every three years to determine what entry-level nurses do on the job. The kinds of questions they investigate include: In which clinical settings does the beginning nurse work? What types of care do beginning nurses provide to their clients? What are their primary duties and responsibilities? Based on the results of this study, the National Council adjusts the content and level of difficulty of the test to accurately reflect what is happening in the workplace.

What the NCLEX-RN® Exam Is *NOT*

It is not a test of achievement or intelligence. It is not designed for nurses who have years of experience. The questions do not involve high-tech clinical nursing or equipment. It is not predictive of your eventual success in the career of nursing. You will not be tested on all the content that you were taught in nursing school.

What Is a CAT?

CAT stands for *Computer Adaptive Test*. Each test is assembled interactively based on the accuracy of the candidate's response to the questions. This ensures that the questions you are answering are not "too hard" or "too easy" for your skill level. Your first question will be relatively easy; that is, below the level of minimum competency. If you answer that question correctly, the computer selects a slightly more difficult question. If you answer the first question incorrectly, the computer selects a slightly easier question (Figure 1). By continuing to do this as you answer questions, the computer is able to calculate your level of competence.

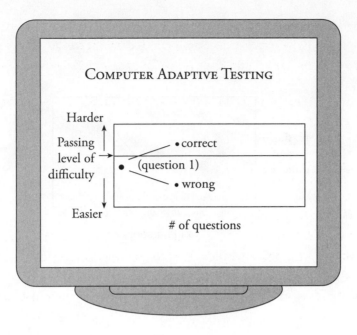

Figure 1

In a CAT, the questions are adapted to your ability level. The computer selects questions that represent all areas of nursing, as defined by the NCLEX-RN® detailed test plan and by the level of item difficulty. Each question is self-contained, so that all of the information you need to answer a question is presented on the computer screen.

Taking the Exam

There is no time limit for each individual question. You have a maximum of six hours to complete the exam, but that includes the beginning tutorial, an optional 10-minute break after the first two hours of testing, and an optional break after an additional 90 minutes of testing. Everyone answers a minimum of 75 questions to a maximum of 265 questions. Regardless of the number of questions you answer, you are given 15 questions that are experimental. These questions, which are indistinguishable from the other questions on the test, are being tested for future use in NCLEX-RN® exams, and your answers do not count for or against you. Your test ends when one of the following occurs:

- You have demonstrated minimum competency and answered the minimum number of questions (75) (Figure 2)
- You have demonstrated a lack of minimum competency and answered the minimum number of questions (75) (Figure 3)
- You have answered the maximum number of questions (265)
- You have used the maximum time allowed (six hours)

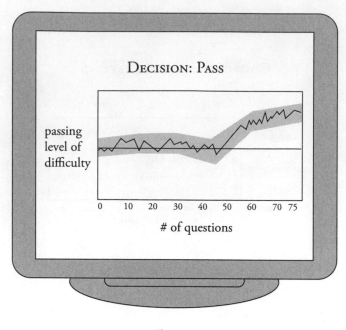

Figure 2

Try not to be concerned with the length of your test. In fact, you should plan on testing for six hours and seeing 265 questions. You are still in the game as long as the computer continues to give you test questions, so focus on answering them to the best of your ability.

Remember, every question counts. There is no warm-up time, so it is important for you to be ready to answer questions correctly from the very beginning. Concentration is also key. You need to give your best to each question because you do not know which one will put you over the top.

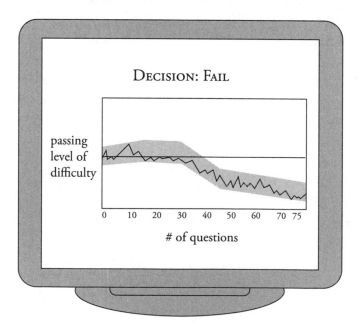

Figure 3

 NURSING

CONTENT OF THE NCLEX-RN® EXAM

The NCLEX-RN® exam is not divided into separate content areas. It tests integrated nursing content. Many nursing programs are based on the medical model. Students take separate medical, surgical, pediatric, psychiatric, and obstetric classes. On the NCLEX-RN® exam, all content is integrated.

Look at the following question.

> A woman with type 1 diabetes is returned to the recovery room one hour after an uneventful delivery of a 9 lb., 8 oz., baby boy. The nurse would expect the woman's blood sugar to do which of the following?
>
> 1. Change from 220 to 180 mg/dL.
> 2. Change from 110 to 80 mg/dL.
> 3. Change from 90 to 120 mg/dL.
> 4. Change from 100 to 140 mg/dL.

Is this an obstetrical question or a medical/surgical question? In order to select the correct answer, (2), you must consider the pathophysiology of diabetes along with the principles of labor and delivery. This is an example of an integrated question.

The NCLEX-RN® Exam Blueprint

The NCLEX-RN® exam is organized according to the framework "Client Needs." There are four major categories of client needs; two of the major categories are further divided for a total of six subcategories. This information is distributed by NCSBN, the developer of the NCLEX-RN® exam.

Client Need #1: Safe and Effective Care Environment

The first subcategory for this client need is **Management of Care**, which accounts for **20** percent of the questions on the exam. Nursing actions that are covered in this subcategory include:

- Advance directives
- Advocacy
- Case management
- Client rights
- Collaboration with interdisciplinary team
- Concepts of management
- Confidentiality/information security
- Consultation

- Continuity of care
- Delegation
- Establishing priorities
- Ethical practice
- Information technology
- Informed consent
- Legal rights and responsibilities
- Performance improvement (quality improvement)
- Referrals
- Supervision

Here is an example of a typical question from the Management of Care subcategory:

> Which of the following assignments by the RN would be appropriate for an LPN/LVN?
>
> 1. A 34-year-old woman with low back pain scheduled for a myelogram in the afternoon
> 2. A 41-year-old woman in traction with a fractured femur
> 3. A 43-year-old woman newly diagnosed with type 1 diabetes mellitus
> 4. A 56-year-old man with emphysema scheduled to be discharged later today

The correct answer is (2). This client is in stable condition and can be cared for by an LPN/LVN with supervision of an RN.

Here is another example of a Management of Care question:

> After receiving a report from the night nurse, which of the following clients should the nurse see *FIRST?*
>
> 1. A 31-year-old woman refusing sucralfate (Carafate) before breakfast
> 2. A 40-year-old man with left-sided weakness asking for assistance to the commode
> 3. A 52-year-old woman complaining of chills who is scheduled for a cholecystectomy
> 4. A 65-year-old man with a nasogastric tube who had a bowel resection yesterday

The correct answer is (3). This is the least stable client.

You will learn more about the content covered by the Safe and Effective Care Environment: Management of Care subcategory in Chapter 4.

The second subcategory for this client need is **Safety and Infection Control**, which accounts for **12** percent of the questions on the exam. Nursing actions that are covered in this subcategory include:

- Accident/injury prevention
- Emergency response plan
- Ergonomic principles
- Error prevention
- Handling hazardous and infectious materials
- Home safety
- Reporting of incident/event/irregular occurrence/variance
- Safe use of equipment
- Security plan
- Standard precautions/transmission-based precautions/surgical asepsis
- Use of restraints/safety devices

Here is an example of a question from the Safety and Infection Control subcategory:

> The physician orders tobramycin sulfate (Nebcin) 3 mg/kg IV every 8 hours for a 3-year-old boy. The nurse enters the client's room to administer the medication and discovers that the boy does not have an identification bracelet. Which of the following should the nurse do?
>
> 1. Ask the parents at the child's bedside to state their child's name.
> 2. Ask the child to say his first and last name.
> 3. Have a coworker identify the child before giving the medication.
> 4. Hold the medication until an identification bracelet can be obtained.

The correct answer is (1). This action will allow the nurse to correctly identify the child and enable the nurse to give the medication on time.

You will learn more about the content covered by the Safe and Effective Care Environment: Safety and Infection Control subcategory in Chapter 5.

Client Need #2: Health Promotion and Maintenance

This client need accounts for **9** percent of the questions on the exam. Nursing actions that are covered in this category include:

- Aging process
- Ante/intra/postpartum and newborn care
- Developmental stages and transitions

- Health and wellness
- Heath promotion/disease prevention
- Health screening
- High-risk behaviors
- Lifestyle choices
- Principles of teaching/learning
- Self-care
- Techniques of physical assessment

It is important to understand that not everyone described in the questions will be sick or hospitalized. Some clients may be in a clinic or home-care setting. Some clients may not be sick at all. Wellness is an important concept on the NCLEX-RN® exam. It is necessary for a safe and effective nurse to know how to promote health and prevent disease.

This is an example of a typical question from the Health Promotion and Maintenance category:

A 21-year-old woman in active labor is admitted to the labor suite. An hour later, the membranes rupture spontaneously. The nurse observes a glistening white cord protruding from the vagina. Which of the following actions should the nurse take *FIRST*?

1. Return to the nurses' station and place an emergency call to the physician.
2. Administer oxygen by mask at 10–12 L/min and assess the mother's vital signs.
3. Place a clean towel over the cord and wet it with sterile normal saline.
4. Apply manual pressure to the presenting part and have the mother assume a knee-chest position.

The correct answer is (4). A prolapsed cord is an emergency situation. The nurse must relieve pressure on the cord to prevent fetal anoxia.

You will learn more about the content covered by the Health Promotion and Maintenance category in Chapter 6.

Client Need #3: Psychosocial Integrity

This client need accounts for **9** percent of the questions on the exam. Nursing actions that are covered in this category include:

- Abuse/neglect
- Behavioral interventions
- Chemical and other dependencies

- Coping mechanisms
- Crisis intervention
- Cultural diversity
- End of life care
- Family dynamics
- Grief and loss
- Mental health concepts
- Religious and spiritual influences on health
- Sensory/perceptual alterations
- Stress management
- Support systems
- Therapeutic communication
- Therapeutic environment

This is an example of a typical question from the Psychosocial Integrity category:

A 50-year-old male client comes to the nurses' station and asks the nurse if he can go to the cafeteria to get something to eat. When told that his privileges do not include visiting the cafeteria, the client becomes verbally abusive. Which of the following approaches by the nurse would be *MOST* effective?

1. Tell the client to lower his voice, because he is disturbing the other clients.
2. Ask the client what he wants from the cafeteria and have it delivered to his room.
3. Calmly but firmly escort the client back to his room.
4. Assign the nursing assistive personnel (NAP) to accompany the client to the cafeteria.

The correct answer is (3). The nurse should not reinforce abusive behavior. Clients need consistent and clearly defined expectations and limits.

You will learn more about the content covered in the Psychosocial Integrity category in Chapter 5.

Client Need #4: Physiological Integrity

The first subcategory for this client need is **Basic Care and Comfort**, which accounts for **9** percent of the questions on the exam. Nursing actions that are covered in this subcategory include:

- Assistive devices
- Elimination

- Mobility/immobility
- Non-pharmacological comfort interventions
- Nutrition and oral hydration
- Personal hygiene
- Rest and sleep

The following question is representative of the Basic Care and Comfort subcategory:

> A cast is applied to a 9-month-old girl for the treatment of talipes equinovarus. Which of the following instructions is *MOST* essential for the nurse to give to the child's mother regarding her care?
>
> 1. Offer appropriate toys for her age.
> 2. Make frequent clinic visits for cast adjustment.
> 3. Provide an analgesic as needed.
> 4. Do circulatory checks of the casted extremity.

The correct answer is (4). A possible complication that can occur after cast application is impaired circulation. All of these answer choices might be included in family teaching, but checking the child's circulation is the highest priority.

You will learn more about the content covered in the Physiological Integrity: Basic Care and Comfort category in Chapter 8.

The second subcategory for this client need is **Pharmacological and Parenteral Therapies**, which accounts for **15** percent of the questions on the exam. Nursing actions that are covered in this subcategory include:

- Adverse effects/contraindications/side effects/interactions
- Blood and blood products
- Central venous access devices
- Dosage calculation
- Expected actions/outcomes
- Medication administration
- Parenteral/intravenous therapies
- Pharmacological pain management
- Total parenteral nutrition

Try this question from the Pharmacological and Parenteral Therapies subcategory:

> The home health nurse is going to start an IV with 5% dextrose in water (D_5W) for a 76-year-old woman. To perform the venipuncture, the nurse should start the IV with which of the following?
>
> 1. The veins of the client's wrist on the nondominant side
> 2. The veins of the leg so it will not interfere with the client's ability to feed herself
> 3. The dorsal veins of the client's forearm on the nondominant side
> 4. The dorsal surface of the client's hand on the nondominant side

The correct answer is (3). This is the best site for the nurse to use for the IV because of its ease of access, availability of elastic veins, and limited use by the client.

You will learn more about the content covered in the Physiological Integrity: Pharmacological and Parenteral Therapies category in Chapter 9.

The third subcategory for this client need is **Reduction of Risk Potential**, which accounts for **12** percent of the questions on the exam. Nursing actions that are covered in this subcategory include:

- Changes/abnormalities in vital signs
- Diagnostic tests
- Laboratory values
- Potential for alterations in body systems
- Potential for complications of diagnostic tests/treatments/procedures
- Potential for complications from surgical procedures and health alterations
- System specific assessments
- Therapeutic procedures

This is an example of a question from the Reduction of Risk Potential subcategory:

> A 7-year-old girl with type 1 insulin-dependent diabetes mellitus (IDDM) has been home sick for several days and is brought to the Emergency Department by her parents. If the child is experiencing ketoacidosis, the nurse would expect to see which of the following lab results?
>
> 1. Serum glucose 140 mg/dL
> 2. Serum creatine 5.2 mg/dL
> 3. Blood pH 7.28
> 4. Hematocrit 38%

The correct answer is (3). Normal blood pH is 7.35–7.45. A blood pH of 7.28 indicates diabetic ketoacidosis.

You will learn more about the content covered in the Physiological Integrity: Reduction of Risk Potential category in Chapter 8.

The fourth subcategory for this client need is **Physiological Adaptation**, which accounts for **13** percent of the questions on the exam. Nursing actions that are covered in this subcategory include:

- Alterations in body systems
- Fluid and electrolyte imbalances
- Hemodynamics
- Illness management
- Medical emergencies
- Pathophysiology
- Unexpected response to therapies

The following question is an example of the Physiological Adaptation subcategory:

> The nurse delivers external cardiac compressions to a client while performing cardiopulmonary resuscitation (CPR). Which of the following actions by the nurse is *BEST*?
>
> 1. Maintain a position close to the client's side with the nurse's knees apart.
> 2. Maintain vertical pressure on the client's chest through the heel of the nurse's hand.
> 3. Re-check the nurse's hand position after every 10 chest compressions.
> 4. Check for a return of the client's pulse after every 8 breaths by the nurse.

The correct answer is (2). The nurse's elbows should be locked, arms straight, with shoulders directly over hands. Incorrect pressure or improperly placed hands could cause injury to the client.

You will learn more about the content covered in the Physiological Integrity: Physiological Adaptation category in Chapter 9.

The Nursing Process

Several processes are integrated throughout the NCLEX-RN® exam. The most important of these is *the nursing process.*

The nursing process involves the *assessment*, *analysis*, *planning*, *implementation*, and *evaluation* of nursing care. As a graduate nurse, you are very familiar with each step of the nursing process and how to write a care plan using this process. Knowledge of the nursing process is essential to the performance of safe and effective care. It is also essential to answering questions correctly on the NCLEX-RN® exam.

Now we are going to review the steps of the nursing process and show you how each step is incorporated into test questions. The nursing process is a way of thinking. Using it will help you select correct answers.

Assessment. Assessment is the first step in the nursing process. It involves establishing and verifying a database of information about the client, so you can identify actual and/or potential health problems. The nurse obtains subjective data (information given to you by the client that can't be observed or measured by others), and objective data (information that is observable and measurable by others). This data is collected by interviewing and observing the client and/or significant others, reviewing the health history, performing a physical examination, evaluating lab results, and interacting with members of the health care team.

An example of an assessment test question is:

> The nurse obtains a health history from a client admitted with acute glomerulonephritis that is associated with beta-hemolytic *Streptococcus*. The nurse expects which of the following to be significant in the health history?
>
> 1. The client had a sore throat 3 weeks earlier.
> 2. There is a family history of glomerulonephritis.
> 3. The client had a renal calculus 2 years earlier.
> 4. The client had an accident involving renal trauma several years ago.

The correct answer is (1). Glomerulonephritis is an immunologic disorder that is caused by beta-hemolytic Streptococcus. *It occurs 21 days after a respiratory or skin infection.*

Analysis. During the analysis phase of the nursing process, you examine the data that you obtained during the assessment phase. This allows you to analyze and draw conclusions about health problems. During analysis, you should compare the client's findings with what is normal. From the analysis, you establish nursing diagnoses. A nursing diagnosis is an actual or potential health problem that the nurse is licensed to manage.

Here is an analysis question:

> The nurse plans care for a client diagnosed with an acute myocardial infarction (MI). An appropriate nursing diagnosis is decreased cardiac output secondary to which of the following?
>
> 1. Ventricular dysrhythmias
> 2. Congestive heart failure
> 3. Recurrent myocardial infarction
> 4. Hypertensive crisis

The correct answer is (1). Ventricular dysrhythmias are common after an MI and reduce the efficiency of the heart.

Planning. During the planning phase of the nursing process, the nursing care plan is formulated. Steps in planning include:

- Assigning priorities to nursing diagnosis
- Specifying goals
- Identifying interventions
- Specifying expected outcomes
- Documenting the nursing care plan

Goals are anticipated responses and client behaviors that result from nursing care. Nursing goals are client-centered and measurable, and they have an established time frame. *Expected outcomes* are the interim steps needed to reach a goal and the resolution of a nursing diagnosis. There will be multiple expected outcomes for each goal. Expected outcomes guide the nurse in planning interventions.

This is an example of a planning question:

> A client comes to the emergency room complaining of nausea, vomiting, and severe right upper quadrant pain. His temperature is 101.3° F (38.5° C), and an abdominal x-ray reveals an enlarged gallbladder. He is scheduled for surgery. Which of the following actions should the nurse take *FIRST*?
>
> 1. Assess the client's need for dietary teaching.
> 2. Evaluate the client's fluid and electrolyte status.
> 3. Examine the client's health history for allergies to antibiotics.
> 4. Determine whether the client has signed consent for surgery.

The correct answer is (2). Hypokalemia and hypomagnesemia commonly occur after repeated vomiting.

Implementation. Implementation is the term used to describe the actions that you take in the care of your clients. Implementation includes:

- Assisting in the performance of activities of daily living (ADL)
- Counseling and educating the client and family
- Giving care to clients
- Supervising and evaluating the work of other members of the health care team

It is important for you to remember that nursing interventions may be:

- *Independent* actions that are within the scope of nursing practice and do not require supervision by others.
- *Dependent* actions based on the written orders of a physician.
- *Interdependent* actions shared with other members of the health care team.

The NCLEX-RN® exam includes questions that involve all three types of nursing interventions.

Here is an example of an implementation question:

> A client is being treated in the burn unit for second- and third-degree burns over 45% of his body. The physician's orders include the application of silver sulfadiazine (Silvadene cream). The *BEST* way for the nurse to apply this medication is to use which of the following?
>
> 1. Sterile 4 × 4 dressings soaked in saline
> 2. Sterile tongue depressor
> 3. Sterile gloved hand
> 4. Sterile cotton-tipped applicator

The correct answer is (3). A sterile, gloved hand will cause the least amount of trauma to tissues and will decrease the chances of breaking blisters.

Evaluation. Evaluation measures the client's response to nursing interventions and indicates the client's progress toward achieving the goals established in the care plan. You compare the observed results to expected outcomes.

This is an evaluation question:

> When caring for a client with anorexia nervosa, which of the following observations indicates to the nurse that the client's condition is improving?
>
> 1. The client eats all the food on her meal tray.
> 2. The client asks friends to bring her special foods.
> 3. The client weighs herself daily.
> 4. The client's weight has increased.

The correct response is (4). The client's weight is the most objective outcome measure in the evaluation of this client's problem.

Integrated Processes

Several other important processes are integrated throughout the NCLEX-RN® exam. They are:

Caring. As you take the NCLEX-RN® exam, remember that the test is about caring for people, not working with high-tech equipment or analyzing lab results.

Communication and Documentation. For this exam, you are required to understand and utilize therapeutic communication skills with all professional contacts, including clients, their families, and other members of the health care team. Charting or documenting your care and the client's response is both a legal requirement and an essential method of communication in nursing. On this exam, you may be asked to identify appropriate documentation of a client behavior or nursing action.

Teaching/Learning Principles. Nursing frequently involves sharing information with clients so optimal functioning can be achieved. You may see questions that focus on teaching a client about his or her diet and/or medications.

You might see some questions on the NCLEX-RN® exam that contain graphics (pictures). These questions may include the picture of a client in traction or the abdomen of a woman who is pregnant. These questions do count, so take them seriously. We have included several questions with graphics in the practice questions and test found in this book, and others can be found online at *kaptest.com/booksonline*.

Knowledge Is Power

The more knowledgeable you are about the NCLEX-RN® exam, the more effective your study will be. As you prepare for the exam, keep the content of the test in mind. Thinking like the test maker will enhance your chance of success on the exam.

Are you still thinking about that pacemaker battery from page 3? What do you think the correct answer is?

A man had a permanent pacemaker implanted one year ago. He returns to the outpatient clinic because he thinks the pacemaker battery is malfunctioning. It is important for the nurse to assess for which of the following?

1. Abdominal pain, nausea, and vomiting
2. Wheezing on exertion, cyanosis, and orthopnea
3. Peripheral edema, shortness of breath, and dizziness
4. Chest pain radiating to the right arm, headache, and diaphoresis

The correct answer is (3). These are symptoms of decreased cardiac output. These symptoms occur with pacemaker battery failure. Other symptoms include changes in pulse rate, irregular pulse, and palpitations.

Gastrointestinal symptoms (1) are not found with pacemaker malfunction. The items listed in (2) are not symptoms of pacemaker failure. And although chest pain may occur with decreased output (4), chest pain that radiates to the right arm is suggestive of angina. Headache and diaphoresis are not seen with pacemaker failure.

CHAPTER 2

GENERAL AND COMPUTER ADAPTIVE TEST STRATEGIES

As a nursing student, you are used to taking multiple-choice tests. In fact, you've taken so many tests by the time you graduate from nursing school, you probably believe that there won't be any more surprises on any nursing test, including the NCLEX-RN® exam.

But if you've ever talked to graduate nurses about their experiences taking the NCLEX-RN® exam, they probably told you that the test wasn't like *any* nursing test they had ever taken. How can that be? How can the NCLEX-RN® exam seem like a nursing school test, but be so different? The reason is that the NCLEX-RN® exam is a standardized test that analyzes a different set of behaviors from those tested in nursing school.

STANDARDIZED EXAMS

Many of you have some experience with standardized exams. You may have been required to take the SAT or ACT to get into nursing school. Remember taking that exam? Was your experience positive or negative?

All standardized exams share the same characteristics:

- Tests are written by content specialists and test construction experts.
- The content of the exam is researched and planned.
- The questions are designed according to test construction methodology (all answer choices are about the same length, the verb tenses all agree, etc.).
- All the questions are tested before use on the actual exam.

The NCLEX-RN® exam is similar to other standardized exams in some ways, yet different in others:

- The NCLEX-RN® exam is written by nurse specialists who are experts in a content area of nursing.

- All content is selected to allow the beginning practitioner to prove minimum competency on all areas of the test plan.
- Minimum-competency questions are most frequently asked at the application level, not the recognition or recall level. All the responses to a question are similar in length and subject matter, and are grammatically correct.
- All test items have been extensively tested by NCSBN. The questions are valid; all correct responses are documented by two different sources.

What does this mean for you?

- NCSBN has defined what is minimum-competency, entry-level nursing.
- Questions and answers are written in such a way that you cannot, in most cases, predict or recognize the correct answer.
- NCSBN is knowledgeable about strategies regarding length of answers, grammar, and so on. It makes sure you can't use these strategies in order to select correct answers. English majors have no advantage!
- The answer choices have been extensively tested. The people who write the test questions make the incorrect answer choices look attractive to the unwary test taker.

WHAT BEHAVIORS DOES THE NCLEX-RN® EXAM TEST?

The NCLEX-RN® exam does *not* just test your nursing knowledge: It assumes that you have a body of knowledge and that you understand the material because you have graduated from nursing school. So what does the NCLEX-RN® exam test? Primarily, it tests your nursing judgment and discretion. It tests your ability to think critically and solve problems. The NCLEX-RN® exam recognizes that as a beginning practitioner, you will be managing LPN/LVNs and NAPs providing care to a group of clients. As the leader of the nursing team, you are expected to make safe and competent judgments about client care.

Critical Thinking

What does the term *critical thinking* mean? Critical thinking is problem solving that involves thinking creatively. It requires that the nurse do the following:

- Observe.
- Decide what is important.
- Look for patterns and relationships.
- Identify the problem.
- Transfer knowledge from one situation to another.
- Apply knowledge.
- Evaluate according to criteria established.

You successfully solve problems every day in the clinical area. You are probably comfortable with this concept when actually caring for clients. Although you've had lots of practice critically thinking in the clinical area, you may have had less practice critically thinking your way through test questions. Why is that?

During nursing school, you take exams developed by nursing instructors to test a specific body of content. Many of these questions are at the knowledge level. This involves recognition and recall of ideas or material that you read in your nursing textbooks and discussed in class. This is the most basic level of testing. Figure 1 illustrates the different levels of questions on nursing exams.

The following is an example of a knowledge-based question you might have seen in nursing school.

> Which of the following is a complication that occurs during the first 24 hours after a percutaneous liver biopsy?
>
> (1) Nausea and vomiting
>
> (2) Constipation
>
> (3) Hemorrhage
>
> (4) Pain at the biopsy site

The question restated is, "What is a common complication of a liver biopsy?" You may or may not remember the answer. So, as you look at the answer choices, you hope to see an item that looks familiar. You do see something that looks familiar: "Hemorrhage." You select the correct answer based on recall or recognition. The NCLEX-RN® exam rarely asks passing questions at the recall/recognition level.

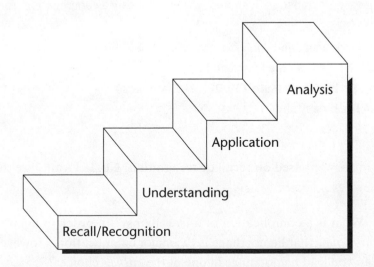

Figure 1: Levels of Questions in Nursing Tests

In nursing school, you are also given test questions written at the comprehension level. These questions require you to understand the meaning of the material. Let's look at this same question written at the comprehension level.

> The nurse understands that hemorrhage is a complication of a liver biopsy due to which of the following reasons?
>
> (1) There are several large blood vessels near the liver.
> (2) The liver cells are bathed with a mixture of venous and arterial blood.
> (3) The test is performed on clients with elevated enzymes.
> (4) The procedure requires a large piece of tissue to be removed.

The question restated is, "Why does hemorrhage occur after a liver biopsy?" In order to answer this question, the nurse must understand that the liver is a highly vascular organ. The portal vein and the hepatic artery join in the liver to form the sinusoids that bathe the liver in a mixture of venous and arterial blood.

The NCLEX-RN® exam asks few minimum-competency questions at the comprehension level. It assumes you know and understand the facts you learned in nursing school.

Minimum-competency NCLEX-RN® exam questions are written at the application and/or analysis level. Remember, the NCLEX-RN® exam tests your ability to make safe judgments about client care. Your ability to solve problems is not tested with questions at the recall/recognition or comprehension level.

Let's look at this same question written at the application level.

> Which of the following symptoms observed by the nurse during the first 24 hours after a percutaneous liver biopsy would indicate a complication from the procedure?
>
> 1. Anorexia, nausea, and vomiting
> 2. Abdominal distention and discomfort
> 3. Pulse 112, blood pressure 100/60, respirations 20
> 4. Pain at the biopsy site

Can you select an answer based on recall or recognition? No. Let's analyze the question and answer choices.

The question is: What is a complication of a liver biopsy? In order to begin to analyze this question, you must *know* that hemorrhage is the major complication. However, it's not listed as an answer. Can you find hemorrhage in one of the answer choices?

ANSWERS:

(1) "Anorexia, nausea, and vomiting." Does this indicate that the client is hemorrhaging? No, these are not symptoms of hemorrhage.

(2) "Abdominal distention and discomfort." Does this indicate that the client is hemorrhaging? Perhaps. Abdominal distention could indicate internal bleeding.

(3) "Pulse 112, blood pressure 100/60, respirations 20." Does this indicate that the client is hemorrhaging? Yes. An increased pulse, a decreased blood pressure, and increased respirations indicate shock. Shock is a result of hemorrhage.

(4) "Pain at the biopsy site." Does this indicate the client is hemorrhaging? No. Pain at the biopsy site is expected due to the procedure.

Ask yourself, "Which is the best indicator of hemorrhage?" Abdominal distention or a change in vital signs? Abdominal distention can be caused by liver disease. The correct answer is (3).

This question tests you at the application level. You were not able to answer the question by recalling or recognizing the word *hemorrhage*. You had to take information you learned (hemorrhage is the major complication of a liver biopsy) and select the answer that best indicates hemorrhage. Application involves taking the facts that you know, and using them to make a nursing judgment. You must be able to answer questions at the application level in order to prove your competence on the NCLEX-RN® exam.

Let's look at a question that is written at the analysis level.

> The nurse is caring for a 56-year-old man receiving haloperidol (Haldol) 2 mg PO bid. The nurse assists the client to choose which of the following menus?
>
> 1. 3 oz. roast beef, baked potato, salad with dressing, dill pickle, baked apple pie, and milk
> 2. 3 oz. baked chicken, green beans, steamed rice, 1 slice of bread, banana, and milk
> 3. Cheeseburger on a bun, french fries with catsup, chocolate chip cookie, apple, and milk
> 4. 3 oz. baked fish, slice of bread, broccoli, ice cream, and pineapple drink taken 30–60 minutes after the meal

Many students panic when they read this question because they can't immediately recall any diet restriction required by a client taking Haldol. Because students can't recall the information, they assume that they didn't learn enough information. Analysis questions are often written so that a familiar piece of information is put in an unfamiliar setting. Let's think about this question.

What type of diet do you choose for a client receiving Haldol? In order to begin analyzing this question, you must first recall that Haldol is an antipsychotic medication used to treat psychotic disorders. There are no diet restrictions for clients taking Haldol. Because there are no diet restrictions, you must problem-solve to determine what this question is *really* asking. Based on the answer choices, it is obviously a diet question. What kind of diet should you choose for this client? Because you have been given no other information, there is only one type of diet that can be considered: a regular balanced diet. This is an example of taking the familiar (a regular balanced diet) and putting it into the unfamiliar (a client receiving Haldol). In this question, the critical thinking is deciding what this question is *really* asking.

QUESTION: "What is the most balanced regular diet?"

ANSWERS:

(1) "3 oz. roast beef, baked potato, salad with dressing, dill pickle, baked apple pie, and milk." Is this a balanced diet? Yes, it certainly has possibilities.

(2) "3 oz. baked chicken, green beans, steamed rice, 1 slice of bread, banana, and milk." Is this a balanced diet? Yes, this is also a good answer because it contains foods from each of the food groups.

(3) "Cheeseburger on a bun, french fries with catsup, chocolate chip cookie, apple, and milk." Is this a balanced diet? No. This diet is high in fat and does not contain all of the food groups. Eliminate this answer.

(4) "3 oz. baked fish, slice of bread, broccoli, ice cream, and pineapple drink taken 30–60 minutes after the meal." Does this sound like a balanced diet? The choice of foods isn't bad, but why would the intake of fluids be delayed? This sounds like a menu to prevent dumping syndrome. Eliminate this answer.

Which is the better answer choice: (1) or (2)? Dill pickles are high in sodium, so the correct answer is (2).

Choosing the menu that best represents a balanced diet is not a difficult question to answer. The challenge lies in determining that a balanced diet is the topic of the question. Note that answer choices (1) and (2) are very similar. Because the NCLEX-RN® exam is testing your discretion, you will be making a decision between answer choices that are very close in meaning. Don't expect obvious answer choices.

These questions highlight the difference between the knowledge/comprehension-based questions that you may have seen in nursing school, and the application/analysis-based questions that you will see on the NCLEX-RN® exam.

STRATEGIES THAT DON'T WORK ON THE NCLEX-RN® EXAM

Whether you realize it or not, you developed a set of strategies in nursing school to answer teacher-generated test questions that are written at the knowledge/comprehension level. These strategies include the following:

- "Cramming" in hundreds of facts about disease processes and nursing care
- Recognizing and recalling facts rather than understanding the pathophysiology and the needs of a client with an illness
- Knowing who wrote the question and what is important to that instructor
- Predicting answers based on what you remember or who wrote the test question
- Selecting the response that is a different length compared to the other choices
- Selecting the answer choice that is grammatically correct
- When in doubt, choosing answer choice (C)

These strategies will not work on the NCLEX-RN® exam. Remember, the NCLEX-RN® exam is testing your ability to make safe, competent decisions.

BECOMING A BETTER TEST TAKER

The first step to becoming a better test taker is to assess and identify the following:

- The kind of test taker you are
- The kind of learner you are

Successful NCLEX-RN® Exam Test Takers

- Have a good understanding of nursing content.
- Have the ability to tackle each test question with a lot of confidence because they assume that they can figure out the right answer.
- Don't give up if they are unsure of the answer. They are not afraid to think about the question, and the possible choices, in order to select the correct answer.
- Possess the know-how to correctly identify the question.
- Stay focused on the question.

Unsuccessful NCLEX-RN® Exam Test Takers

- Assume that they either know or don't know the answer to the question.
- Memorize facts to answer questions by recall or recognition.

- Read the question, read the answers, read the question again, and pick an answer.
- Choose answer choices based on a hunch or a feeling instead of thinking carefully.
- Answer questions based on personal experience rather than nursing theory.
- Give up too soon, because they aren't willing to think hard about questions and answers.
- Don't stay focused on the question.

If you are a successful test taker, congratulations! This book will reinforce your test-taking skills. If you have many of the characteristics of an unsuccessful test taker, don't despair! You can change. If you follow the strategies in this book, you will become a successful test taker.

What Kind of Learner Are You?

It is important for you to identify whether you think predominantly in images or words. Why? This will assist you in developing a study plan that is specific for your learning style. Read the following statement:

> A nurse walks into a room and finds the client lying on the floor.

As you read those words, did you hear yourself reading the words? Or did you see a nurse walking into a room, and see the client lying on the floor? If you heard yourself reading the sentence, you think in words. If you formed a mental image (saw a picture), you think in images.

Students who think in images sometimes have a difficult time answering nursing test questions. These students say things like:

> *"I have to study harder than the other students."*
>
> *"I have to look up the same information over and over again."*
>
> *"Once I see the procedure (or client), I don't have any difficulty understanding or remembering the content."*
>
> *"I have trouble understanding procedures from reading the book. I have to see the procedure to understand it."*
>
> *"I have trouble answering test questions about clients or procedures I've never seen."*

Why is that? For some people, imagery is necessary to understand ideas and concepts. If this is true for you, you need to visualize information that you are learning. As you prepare for the NCLEX-RN® exam, try to form mental images of terminology, procedures, and diseases. For example, if you're reviewing information about traction but you have never seen traction, it would be ideal for you to see a client in traction. If that isn't possible, find a picture of traction and rig up a traction setup with whatever material you have available. As you read about traction, use the photo or model to visualize care of the client. If you can visualize the theory that you are trying to learn, it will make recall and understanding of concepts much easier for you.

It is also important that you visualize test questions. As you read the question and possible answer choices, picture yourself going through each suggested action. This will increase your chances of selecting correct answer choices.

Let's look at a test question that requires imagery.

> An adolescent is seen in the emergency room for a fracture of the left femur sustained in a sledding accident. The fracture is reduced and a cast is applied. The client is taught how to use crutches for ambulating without bearing weight on the left leg. The nurse would expect the client to learn which of the following crutch-walking gaits?
>
> 1. Two-point gait
> 2. Three-point gait
> 3. Four-point gait
> 4. Swing-through gait

Don't panic if you can't remember crutch-walking gaits. Instead, visualize!

Step 1. "See" a person (or yourself) walking normally. First the right leg and left arm are extended, and then the left leg and right arm are extended.

Step 2. Put crutches in your hands. Now walk. Each foot and each crutch is a point.

Step 3. "See" a person (or yourself) with a full cast on the left leg, with the foot never touching the ground.

Step 4. Visualize the answers.

(1) Two-point gait. One leg and one crutch would be touching the ground at the same time. Sounds like normal walking. Eliminate this choice because the client is non-weight-bearing.

(2) Three-point gait. Both crutches and one foot are on the ground. This would be appropriate for a non-weight-bearing client.

(3) Four-point gait. This would require both legs and crutches to touch the ground. However, in this question the client is non-weight-bearing. Eliminate this option.

(4) Swing-through gait. This gait means advancing both crutches, then both legs, and requires weight-bearing. The gait is not as stable as the other gaits. Eliminate this option: the client in this question is non-weight-bearing.

The correct answer is (2). Even if you are unsure of crutch-walking gaits, imaging and thinking through the answer choices will enable you to select the correct answer.

NCLEX-RN® EXAM QUESTION TYPES

The NCLEX-RN® exam is composed of primarily multiple-choice, four-option, text-based questions written at the application/analysis level of difficulty. These questions may include charts, tables, or graphic images.

Your NCLEX-RN® exam may also contain questions in a format other than traditional four-option, text-based, multiple-choice questions. These other types of questions, called *alternate questions*, are part of the test pool of questions for the NCLEX-RN® exam. These alternate question types include:

- Multiple response questions that require you to select all answer choices that apply from among five or six answer options
- "Hot spot" questions that require you to identify a "hot spot" or specific area on a graphic image by clicking on the correct area with the mouse
- Fill-in-the-blank questions that require you to calculate a number and then type it into a blank space provided after the question
- Drag-and-drop/ordered-response questions that ask you to place answers in a specific order

There are also three types of alternate questions that are variations on the traditional four-option multiple-choice question. These include:

- Chart/exhibit questions that require you to click an Exhibit button to display charts and/or exhibits that provide information needed to answer the question. Once you have done so, you then select the correct choice from among four multiple-choice answer options.
- Audio item questions that present you with an audio clip that you listen to on head-phones. After listening to the clip, you then select the correct choice from among four multiple-choice answer options.
- Graphics questions that present you with graphics instead of text as the four multiple-choice answer options.

These questions are either counted toward your NCLEX-RN® exam results or they are experimental questions for future exams that are not counted.

The following sections contain strategies that will help you correctly answer both alternate questions and traditional four-option, text-based, multiple-choice questions.

ALTERNATE TEST QUESTIONS

Let's first look at the individual alternate question types and the strategies that will help you correctly answer these questions.

Select All That Apply—Click on all appropriate answer choices

Take a look at the following question.

The nurse cares for a client diagnosed with a right-sided cerebrovascular accident (CVA) with dysphagia. Which of the following actions by the nurse reflects appropriate care for the client? **Select all that apply.**

☐ 1. The nurse assesses the client's ability to swallow.

☐ 2. The nurse offers the client apple juice.

☐ 3. The nurse positions the client at a 45-degree angle.

☐ 4. The nurse offers the client scrambled eggs.

☐ 5. The nurse instructs the client to place food on the left side of the mouth.

☐ 6. The nurse turns off the television.

You will know that the question is a "Select all that apply" alternate question because after the question stem and before the answer choices you will be instructed to "**Select all that apply.**" You will note that there are more than four possible answer choices; usually five or six are provided. Also, there is a box in front of each answer choice rather than the radio button you see with multiple-choice, four-option, text-based questions.

To answer this type of question, determine which of the answer choices provided are correct. It is important to remember that in order for the question to be scored as correct, you must select *all* of the answer choices that apply, not just the *best* response. You will not receive any partial credit if you do not. Left-click on the box in front of each answer choice that you think is correct. A small check mark appears in the box indicating that you selected that answer. If you change your mind about a particular answer choice, just click on the box again: the check mark disappears and the answer choice is no longer selected.

How should you approach this type of question? What doesn't work is to compare and contrast the individual answer choices. For a "Select all that apply" question, any number of answer choices may be correct. Instead, consider each answer choice a True/False question. Reword this question to ask, "What is appropriate care for a client with a right-sided CVA who has dysphagia?" Dysphagia means the client is having difficulty swallowing; if the CVA is in the right hemisphere, the client's left side is affected.

Let's look at the answers. The strategy is to change each answer choice into a statement, and then determine if the statement is true or false.

(1) "I should assess the client's ability to swallow." Is this true for a client with dysphagia? Yes. This is a correct response because the nurse needs to make sure that the client can swallow food before giving him anything to eat. Select this answer choice.

(2) "I should offer the client apple juice." Is this an appropriate fluid for a client with dysphagia? Yes. Although the client may have some difficulty taking oral fluids, it is important to offer them slowly. Select this answer choice.

(3) "I should position the client at a 45-degree angle." Is this the correct position for a client with dysphagia? No. The client should be sitting upright in a chair or the bed. Eliminate this answer choice.

(4) "I should offer the client scrambled eggs." Is this an appropriate food for a client with dysphagia? Yes. Soft or semi-soft foods are more easily tolerated than a regular diet. Select this answer choice.

(5) "I should instruct the client to place food on the left side of his mouth." Is this what should be done? If the client has a right-sided CVA, that means the left side of the client's body is affected. The food should be placed on the unaffected side—the right side of the mouth for this client. Eliminate this answer.

(6) "I should turn off the television." What are they getting at with this statement? Many clients are easily distracted after a CVA. If the client has dysphagia, you don't want him to aspirate because he is distracted by the television. It is best to turn off the TV during meals. Select this answer choice.

So, which answers should be checked as correct? For this question, choices (1), (2), (4), and (6) are correct. Left-click on the boxes in front of each of these answer choices to select them. When you have selected all the responses you believe to be correct, click on the NEXT (N) button in the bottom left of the screen or press the Enter key on the keyboard to lock in your answer and go on to the next question. Remember, once you click on the NEXT (N) button or press the Enter key, you have entered your answer to the question and you cannot return to the question.

> The nurse cares for a client diagnosed with a right-sided cerebrovascular accident (CVA) with dysphagia. Which of the following actions by the nurse reflects appropriate care for the client? **Select all that apply.**
>
> ☐ 1. The nurse assesses the client's ability to swallow.
> ☐ 2. The nurse offers the client apple juice.
> ☐ 3. The nurse positions the client at a 45-degree angle.
> ☐ 4. The nurse offers the client scrambled eggs.
> ☐ 5. The nurse instructs the client to place food on the left side of the mouth.
> ☐ 6. The nurse turns off the television.

Hot Spot—Select the correct area and click the mouse

This type of alternate question asks you to identify a location on a graphic or table. It is important to understand that this is not a test of your fine motor skills but is designed to evaluate your knowledge of nursing content, anatomy, and physiology and pathophysiology.

Let's take a look at a question that involves a hot spot.

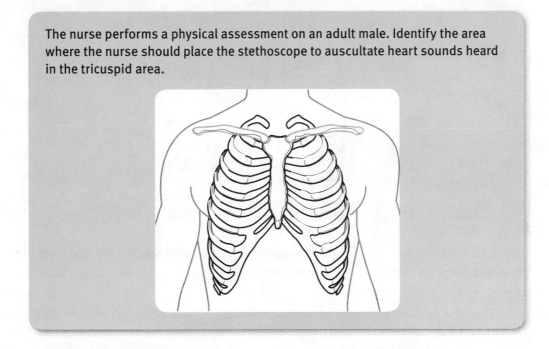

The nurse performs a physical assessment on an adult male. Identify the area where the nurse should place the stethoscope to auscultate heart sounds heard in the tricuspid area.

This question asks you to identify where you would listen to heart sounds in the tricuspid area. The strategy you should use is to locate anatomical landmarks. You need to know that the tricuspid area is located on the client's left side. It is found in the space between ribs, two ribs up from the bottom of the seven true ribs. The tricuspid area is located in the fourth and fifth intercostal spaces at the lower left of the sternal border.

Using the computer's mouse, move the cursor to the location you think is correct. Then, left-click the mouse. Check to make sure that you have selected the location you wanted. Then enter your answer by clicking on the NEXT (N) button or pressing the Enter key. If you click on the right side of the chest, or four ribs up from the bottom, or at the midclavicular area instead of the sternal border, the location would be inaccurate for the tricuspid area and the question would be counted as incorrect. Just do your best and use anatomical landmarks to get your bearings and select the location.

Here's the answer to this hot spot question.

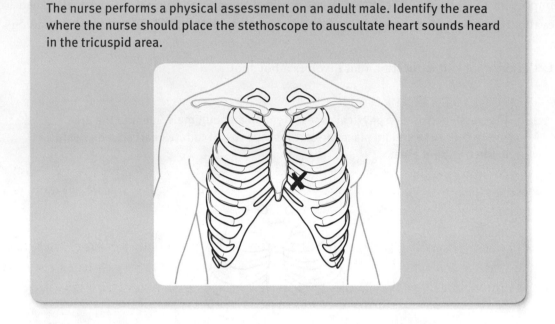

The nurse performs a physical assessment on an adult male. Identify the area where the nurse should place the stethoscope to auscultate heart sounds heard in the tricuspid area.

It is important for you to know where to listen to specific heart sounds. In addition to the tricuspid area, you should be able to locate other anatomical landmarks to evaluate heart sounds:

- Angle of Louis—manubrial sternal junction at the second rib
- Aortic area—second intercostal space to the *right* of the sternum
- Pulmonic area—second intercostal space to the *left* of the sternum
- Erb's point—third intercostal space to the *left* of the sternum
- Mitral area—fifth intercostal space at the *left* midclavicular line

In the mitral area of an adult is the *apical impulse*, also known the point of maximal impulse (PMI), where the impulse of the left ventricle is felt most strongly; on an infant, the apical impulse is lateral to the left nipple.

Fill-in-the-Blank—Enter the answer

This type of alternate question asks you to fill in the blank with a number based on a calculation.

The following is an example of a fill-in-the-blank question.

> The nurse cares for a client receiving hourly peritoneal dialysis exchanges. During a one-hour exchange, the nurse infuses 2,000 mL of dialysate and 1,900 mL of outflow is returned. During the exchange, the client drinks 8 oz. of apple juice, 2 cups of water, and voids 150 mL of urine. Calculate and record the client's intake in milliliters.
>
> _____ mL

To answer this question, calculate the client's intake from the information provided. **Note: Pay close attention to the unit of measure you need for your final answer.** In this situation, you are asked for the client's intake in milliliters, not cups or ounces.

You can use the drop-down calculator provided on the computer to do the math. The button that displays the calculator is on the bottom of the right side of the computer screen. Use your mouse to click on the numbers or functions you want. Remember, the slash (/) is used for division.

To answer this question you need to know that intake includes what the client drinks along with the amount of dialysate that is retained after the one-hour exchange of solution.

First, convert cups into ounces. One cup of fluid = 8 oz. Then convert ounces into milliliters. One ounce = 30 milliliters.

The client's intake is:

    8 oz. apple juice = 240 mL
    2 cups = 16 oz. water = 480 mL
    100 mL = retained dialysate

Use the computer mouse to move the cursor inside the text box. Left-click on the cursor. Type in the correct intake using the number keys on the keyboard. The correct answer is 820. Do not put mL or any unit of measure after the number. Only the number goes into the box. Rules for rounding are typically provided with the question.

The nurse cares for a client receiving hourly peritoneal dialysis exchanges. During a one-hour exchange, the nurse infuses 2,000 mL of dialysate and 1,900 mL of outflow is returned. During the exchange, the client drinks 8 oz. of apple juice, 2 cups of water, and voids 150 mL of urine. Calculate and record the client's intake in milliliters.

| 820 | mL |

Drag and Drop/Ordered Response—Arrange the answers in the correct order

This is one of the newer alternate question types introduced by NCSBN. These questions ask you to place answers in a specific order.

Take a look at the following question.

The nurse prepares to insert an indwelling Foley catheter in an elderly female client. Arrange the following steps in the order the nurse should perform them. **All options must be used.**

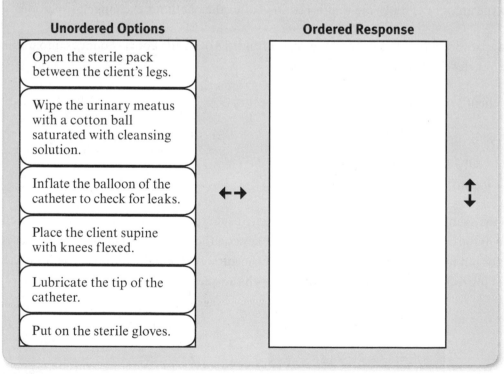

Unordered Options

Open the sterile pack between the client's legs.

Wipe the urinary meatus with a cotton ball saturated with cleansing solution.

Inflate the balloon of the catheter to check for leaks.

Place the client supine with knees flexed.

Lubricate the tip of the catheter.

Put on the sterile gloves.

Ordered Response

The strategy to use in answering this kind of question is to picture yourself performing the procedure. First, prepare the client. Next, prepare the equipment in the correct order, using sterile technique. Open the sterile pack between the client's legs. Next, put on the sterile gloves. Inflate the balloon of the catheter to check for leaks. Lubricate the tip of the catheter. Once the equipment is ready, prepare the client for the insertion of the catheter. The last step from those provided is to wipe the urinary meatus with a cotton ball saturated with cleansing solution.

To place the options in the correct order, click on an option and drag it to the box on the right. You can also move an answer from the left column to the right column by highlighting the option and clicking the arrow key that points to the column on the right. You may also rearrange the order of the options in the right column using the arrow keys pointing up and down.

Here's the answer to this question.

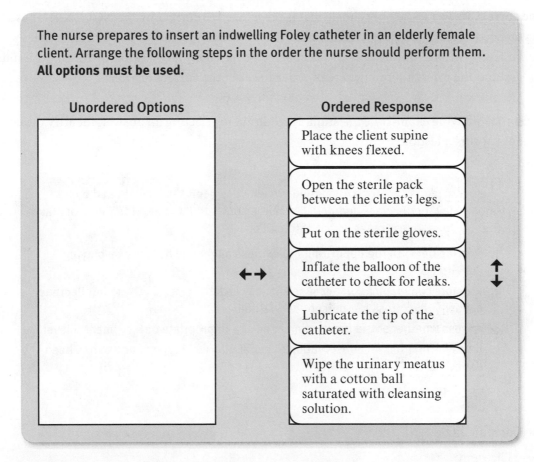

The nurse prepares to insert an indwelling Foley catheter in an elderly female client. Arrange the following steps in the order the nurse should perform them. **All options must be used.**

Unordered Options | **Ordered Response**

Place the client supine with knees flexed.

Open the sterile pack between the client's legs.

Put on the sterile gloves.

Inflate the balloon of the catheter to check for leaks.

Lubricate the tip of the catheter.

Wipe the urinary meatus with a cotton ball saturated with cleansing solution.

MULTIPLE-CHOICE TEST QUESTIONS

Multiple-choice questions with four answer options may take the form of a traditional text-based question, or may be in the form of an alternate question that includes an exhibit/chart, is based on an audio clip, or contains graphics in place of some of the text. No matter the form, to effectively apply the strategies discussed in this book, you need to understand the components of an NCLEX-RN® exam multiple-choice question. They are as follows:

- The *stem* of the question. The stem includes the situation that describes the client, his or her problems or health care needs, and other relevant information. It also includes a question or an incomplete statement. This is the question that you must answer.
- Three incorrect answers, referred to here as *distracters*.
- The correct answer.

The three distracters will probably sound logical to you. They may even be based on information provided in the stem, but they don't really answer the question. Other incorrect answers may be actions that are common nursing practice but not ideal nursing practice.

The correct answer is the only choice that is recognized as correct by the NCLEX-RN® exam, so you need to learn to select it. Remember that most answer choices are written at the application level: you will not be able to select answers based on recognition or recall. You must understand the *whys* of nursing care in order to select the correct response.

Read the following exam-style question. In addition to selecting an answer, identify the components of this question.

> The nurse plans care for a 4-year-old girl who has been sexually abused by her father. Play therapy is scheduled. The nurse knows that the *PRIMARY* goal of play therapy for a 4-year-old is which of the following?
>
> 1. Provide her with the opportunity to express anger and hostility by playing with dolls.
> 2. Promote communication because she may lack the emotional and intellectual capacity to express her perceptions verbally.
> 3. Assess whether she is functioning at an age-appropriate developmental level.
> 4. Reveal through direct observation of her at play what type of abuse has been experienced.

The Components

- The stem:
  - 4-year-old girl
  - Sexually abused by her father
  - Play therapy is scheduled
  - What is the primary goal of play therapy for a 4-year-old?
- The answer choices:

(1) Provide opportunity to express anger and hostility. Play therapy will allow children to express anger and hostility if that's what they want to communicate. Some students select this answer because they focus on the treatment of sexual abuse mentioned in the situation. This is a distracter.

(2) Promote communication. Play is the universal language of children. The purpose of play therapy is to give children the opportunity to communicate using their own "language." This is the correct answer.

(3) Assess her developmental level. The nurse might be able to assess whether a child is functioning at an age-appropriate level, but this is not the primary purpose of play therapy. This is a distracter.

(4) Find out what type of abuse she has experienced. The child might communicate the type of abuse she has experienced if that is what she chooses to communicate. The nurse should focus on the purpose of play therapy, not the type of abuse. This is a distracter.

Let's try another question.

> A client is being treated for heart failure with diuretic therapy. Which of the following assessments *BEST* indicates to the nurse that the client's condition is improving?
>
> 1. The client's weight has remained stable since admission.
> 2. The client's systolic blood pressure has decreased.
> 3. There are fewer crackles heard when auscultating the client's lungs.
> 4. The client's urinary output is 1,500 mL per day.

The Components

- The stem:
  - Heart failure
  - Treatment is diuretic therapy
  - How do you know the client's condition is improving?

- The answer choices:
  (1) Weight has remained stable. The client's weight should decrease because he is taking a diuretic. Weight addresses issues involved with diuretic therapy. However, it is not the best indication of improvement in a client with heart failure. This is a distracter.
  (2) The systolic blood pressure has decreased. Decreased blood pressure may be the result of diuretic therapy, but the reduction could also be due to other causes (change of position, calm rather than in an excited state, etc.). This is not the best indication of an improvement in a client with heart failure. This is a distracter.

(3) There are fewer crackles. A client with heart failure has crackles due to pulmonary edema. Diuretics are given to promote excretion of sodium and water through the kidneys. Decreased crackles would indicate that the pulmonary edema is improving. This is the correct answer.

(4) Urinary output of 1,500 mL in 24 hours. This is within normal limits. Although a normal output addresses diuretic therapy, it is not the best indication of improvement of heart failure. This is a distracter.

CRITICAL THINKING STRATEGIES

- The NCLEX-RN® exam is not a test about recognizing facts.
- You must be able to correctly identify what the question is asking.
- Do not focus on background information that is not needed to answer the question.
- The NCLEX-RN® exam focuses on thinking through a problem or situation.

Now that you are more knowledgeable about the components of a multiple-choice test question, let's talk about specific strategies that you can use to problem-solve your way to correct answers on the NCLEX-RN® exam.

Remember, the NCLEX-RN® exam is testing your ability to think critically. Critical thinking for the nurse involves the following:

- Observation
- Deciding what is important
- Looking for patterns and relationships
- Identifying the problem
- Transferring knowledge from one situation to another
- Applying knowledge
- Discriminating between possible choices and/or courses of action
- Evaluating according to criteria established

Are you feeling overwhelmed as you read these words? Don't be! We are going teach you a step-by-step method to choose the appropriate path. The Kaplan Nursing team has developed a decision tree that shows you how to approach every NCLEX-RN® exam question. In this book, these strategies appear as 10 critical thinking paths.

There are some strategies that you must follow on *every* NCLEX-RN® exam test question. You must *always* figure out what the question is asking, and you must *always* eliminate answer choices.

Choosing the right answer often involves choosing the best of several answers that have correct information. This may entail your correct analysis and interpretation of what the question is really asking. So let's talk about how to figure out what the question is asking.

REWORD THE QUESTION

The first step to correctly answering NCLEX-RN® exam questions is to find out what each question is *really* asking.

Step 1. Read each question carefully from the first word to the last word. Do not skim over the words or read them too quickly.

Step 2. Look for hints in the wording of the question stem. The adjectives *most, first, best, primary,* and *initial* indicate that you must establish priorities. The phrase *further teaching is necessary* indicates that the answer will contain incorrect information. The phrase *client understands the teaching* indicates that the answer will be correct information.

Step 3. Reword the question stem in your own words so that it can be answered with a *yes* or a *no,* or with a specific bit of information. Begin your questions with *what, when,* or *why.* We will refer to this reworded version as THE REWORDED QUESTION in the examples that follow.

Step 4. If you can't complete step 3, read the answer choices for clues.

Let's practice rewording a question.

A preschooler with a fractured femur is brought to the emergency room by her parents. When asked how the injury occurred, the child's parents state that she fell off the sofa. On examination, the nurse finds old and new lesions on the child's buttocks. Which of the following statements *MOST* appropriately reflects how the nurse should document these findings?

1.

2.

3.

4.

We omitted the answer choices to make you focus on the question stem this time. The answer choices will be provided and discussed later in this chapter.

Step 1. Read the question stem carefully.

Step 2. Pay attention to the adjectives. *Most appropriately* tells you that you need to select the best answer.

Step 3. Reword the question stem in your own words. In this case, it is, "What is the best charting for this situation?"

Step 4. Because you were able to reword the question, the fourth step is unnecessary. You didn't need to read the answer choices for clues.

We have all missed questions on a test because we didn't read accurately. The following question illustrates this point.

> A construction worker is admitted to the hospital for treatment of active tuberculosis (TB). The nurse teaches the client about TB. Which of the following statements by the client indicates to the nurse that further teaching is necessary?
>
> 1.
> 2.
> 3.
> 4.

Again, just the question stem is given to encourage you to focus on rewording the question. We will discuss the answer choices for this question later in this chapter.

Step 1. Read the question stem carefully.

Step 2. Look for hints. Pay particular attention to the statement "further teaching is necessary." You are looking for negative information.

Step 3. Reword the question stem in your own words. In this case, it is, "What is incorrect information about TB?"

Step 4. Because you were able to reword the question, the fourth step is unnecessary. You didn't need to read the answer choices for clues to determine what the question is asking.

Try rewording this test question.

> A woman admitted to the hospital in premature labor has been treated successfully. The client is to be sent home on an oral regimen of terbutaline (Brethine). Which of the following statements by the client indicates to the nurse that the client understands the discharge teaching about the medication?
>
> 1.
> 2.
> 3.
> 4.

Again, just the question stem is given to encourage you to focus on rewording the question. We will discuss the answer choices for this question later in this chapter.

Step 1. Read the question stem carefully.

Step 2. Look for hints. Pay attention to the words *client understands*. You are looking for true information.

Step 3. Reword the question stem. This question is asking, "What is true about Brethine?"

Step 4. Because you were able to reword this question, the fourth step is unnecessary. You didn't need to obtain clues about what the question is asking from the answer choices.

ELIMINATE INCORRECT ANSWER CHOICES

Now that you've mastered rewording the question, let's examine how to select the correct answer.

Remember the characteristics of unsuccessful test takers? One of their major problems is that they do not thoughtfully consider each answer choice. They react to questions using feelings and hunches. Unsuccessful test takers look for a specific answer choice. The following strategy will enable you to consider each answer choice in a thoughtful way.

Step 1. Do not look at any of the answer choices except answer choice (1).

Step 2. Read answer choice (1). Then repeat THE REWORDED QUESTION after reading the answer choice. Ask yourself, "Does this answer THE REWORDED QUESTION?" If you know the answer choice is wrong, eliminate it. If you aren't sure, leave the answer choice in for consideration.

Step 3. Repeat the above process with each remaining answer choice.

Step 4. Note which answer choices remain.

Step 5. Reread the question to make sure you have correctly identified THE REWORDED QUESTION.

Step 6. Ask yourself, "Which answer choice best answers the question?" That is your answer.

Let's practice the elimination strategy using the same questions.

> A preschooler with a fractured femur is brought to the emergency room by her parents. When asked how the injury occurred, the child's parents state that she fell off the sofa. On examination, the nurse finds old and new lesions on the child's buttocks. Which of the following statements *MOST* appropriately reflects how the nurse should document these findings?
>
> 1. "Six lesions noted on buttocks at various stages of healing."
> 2. "Multiple lesions on buttocks due to child abuse."
> 3. "Lesions on buttocks due to unknown causes."
> 4. "Several lesions on buttocks caused by cigarettes."

THE REWORDED QUESTION: What is the best charting for this situation?

Step 1. Do not look at any of the answer choices except for answer choice (1). Thoughtfully consider each answer choice individually.

Step 2. Read answer choice (1). Does it answer the question, "What is the best charting for this situation?"

(1) "Six lesions noted on buttocks at various stages of healing." Is this good charting? Maybe. Leave it in for consideration.

Step 3. Repeat the process with each remaining answer choice.

(2) "Multiple lesions on buttocks due to child abuse." Is this good charting? No, because the nurse is making a judgment about child abuse.

(3) "Lesions on buttocks due to unknown causes." Is this good charting? Maybe. Leave it in for consideration.

(4) "Several lesions on buttocks caused by cigarettes." Is this good charting? No. The question does not include information about how the lesions occurred.

Step 4. Answer choices (1) and (3) remain.

Step 5. Reread the question to make sure you have correctly identified THE REWORDED QUESTION. This question asks you to identify good charting.

Step 6. Which is better charting? "Six lesions noted on buttocks at various stages of healing," or "Lesions due to unknown causes"? Good charting is accurate, objective, concise, and complete. It must reflect the client's current status. The correct answer is (1).

Some students will select answer (3), thinking, "How can I be sure about the stages of healing?" But the purpose of this question is to test your ability to select good charting.

Select the answer choice that shows you are a safe and effective nurse. Remember, questions on the NCLEX-RN® exam are not designed to trick you. Stay focused on the question.

Let's select the correct answer for the second question.

> A construction worker is admitted to the hospital for treatment of active tuberculosis (TB). The nurse teaches the client about TB. Which of the following statements by the client indicates to the nurse that further teaching is necessary?
>
> 1. "I will have to take medication for 6 months."
> 2. "I should cover my nose and mouth when coughing or sneezing."
> 3. "I will remain in isolation for at least 6 weeks."
> 4. "I will always have a positive skin test for TB."

THE REWORDED QUESTION: What is incorrect information about TB?

Step 1. Do not look at any of the answer choices except answer choice (1).

Step 2. Read answer choice (1). Does it answer THE REWORDED QUESTION, "What is incorrect (or wrong) information about TB?"

(1) "I will have to take medication for 6 months." Is this wrong information? No, it is a true statement. The client will need to take a medication, such as isonicotinyl hydrazine (INH), for 6 months or longer. Eliminate this choice.

Step 3. Repeat the process with each remaining answer choice.

(2) "I should cover my nose and mouth when coughing or sneezing." Is this wrong information about TB? No, this is a true statement. TB is transmitted by droplet contamination. Eliminate it.

(3) "I will remain in isolation for at least 6 weeks." Is this wrong information about TB? Maybe. Leave it in for consideration.

(4) "I will always have a positive skin test for TB." Is this a wrong statement about TB? No, this is true. A positive skin test indicates that the client has developed antibodies to the tuberculosis bacillus. Eliminate this choice.

Step 4. Only answer choice (3) remains.

Step 5. Reread the question to make sure you have correctly identified THE REWORDED QUESTION. The question is, "What is incorrect information about TB?"

Step 6. The correct answer is (3). You "know" this is the correct answer because you've eliminated the other three answer choices. The client does not need to be isolated for 6 weeks. The client's activities will be restricted for about 2–3 weeks after medication therapy is initiated.

A few things to remember when using this strategy:

- Eliminate only what you know is wrong. However, once you eliminate an answer choice, do not retrieve it for consideration. You may be tempted to do this if you do not feel comfortable with the one answer choice that is left. Resist the impulse!
- Stay focused on THE REWORDED QUESTION. How many times have you missed a question that asked for negative information because you selected the answer choice that contained correct information?

Here's another question.

> A woman admitted to the hospital in premature labor has been treated successfully. The client is to be sent home on an oral regimen of terbutaline (Brethine). Which of the following statements by the client indicates to the nurse that the client understands the discharge teaching about the medication?
>
> 1. "As long as I take my medication, I can be sure I will not deliver prematurely."
> 2. "It is important that I count the fetal movements for one hour, twice a day."
> 3. "I may feel a rapid heartbeat and some muscle tremors while on this medication."
> 4. "Bed rest is necessary in order for the medication to work properly."

THE REWORDED QUESTION: What is true about Brethine?

Step 1. Do not look at any of the answer choices except answer choice (1).

Step 2. Read answer choice (1). Does it answer the question, "What is true about Brethine?"

(1) "As long as I take my medication, I won't deliver prematurely." Is this true about Brethine? No. Brethine will inhibit uterine contractions, but there is no guarantee that there won't be a premature delivery. Eliminate it.

Step 3. Repeat the process with each remaining answer choice.

(2) "It is important that I count the fetal movements for one hour, twice a day." Is this true about Brethine? Maybe. Clients are told to be aware of fetal movement. Keep it as a possibility.

(3) "I may feel a rapid heartbeat and some muscle tremors while on this medication." Is this true of Brethine? Yes. Brethine is a smooth-muscle relaxant. Side effects include increased maternal heart rate, palpitations, and muscle tremors. Leave this choice in for consideration.

(4) "Bed rest is necessary in order for the medication to work properly." Is this true about Brethine? No. Brethine will work whether the client is on bed rest or not. Eliminate it.

Step 4. Note that only answer choices (2) and (3) remain.

Step 5. Reread the question to make sure you have correctly identified THE REWORDED QUESTION. The reworded question is, "What is true about Brethine?"

Step 6. Which choice best answers the question, (2) or (3)? If you are focused on the question, you will select (3). Some students focus on the background information (pregnancy). This question has nothing to do with pregnancy. If you chose (2), you fell for a distracter.

Remember: Focus on the question, and not the background information. If you can answer the question—"What is true about Brethine?"—without considering the background information (pregnancy), do it. Many students answer a question incorrectly because they don't focus on THE REWORDED QUESTION. Don't fall for the distracters.

At this point you're probably thinking, "Will I have enough time to finish the test using these strategies?" or "How will I ever remember how to answer questions using these steps?" Yes, you will have time to finish the test. Unsuccessful test takers spend time agonizing over test questions. By using these strategies, you will be using your time productively. You will remember the steps because you are going to practice, practice, practice with test questions. You will not be able to absorb this strategy by osmosis; the process must be practiced repeatedly.

DON'T PREDICT ANSWERS

On the NCLEX-RN® exam, you are asked to select the best answer from the four choices that you are given. Many times, the "ideal" answer choice is not there. Don't sit and moan because the answer that you think should be there isn't provided. Remember:

- Identify THE REWORDED QUESTION.
- Select the best answer *from the choices given.*

Look at this question.

> The nurse describes the procedure to a male client for collecting a clean-catch urine specimen for culture and sensitivity testing. Which of the following explanations by the nurse would be MOST accurate?
>
> 1. "The urinary meatus is cleansed with an iodine solution and then a urinary drainage catheter is inserted to obtain urine."
> 2. "You will be asked to empty your bladder one-half hour before the test; you will then be asked to void into a container."
> 3. "Before voiding, the urinary meatus is cleansed with an iodine solution and urine is voided into a sterile container; the container must not touch the penis."
> 4. "You must void a few drops of urine, then stop; then void the remaining urine into a clean container, which should be immediately covered."

Step 1. Read the question stem.

Step 2. Focus on the adjectives. *"Most accurate"* tells you that more than one answer may seem correct.

Step 3. Reword the question stem. What is true about a clean-catch urine specimen for culture and sensitivity?

Step 4. Read each answer choice and ask yourself, "Is this true about a clean-catch urine specimen for culture and sensitivity?"

(1) This choice describes how to obtain a catheterized urine specimen. Urine isn't usually collected by catheterization due to the increased risk of infection. This answer does not answer the question about a clean-catch urine specimen. Eliminate.

(2) This describes a double-voided specimen. This action is usually done when testing urine for glucose and ketones. It is not relevant to a clean-catch urine specimen. Eliminate.

(3) This is true of a clean-catch urine specimen for culture and sensitivity. The urinary meatus is cleansed, a sterile container is used, and the penis must not touch the container. Leave it in for consideration.

(4) This does describe a clean-catch urine specimen. The client does void a few drops of urine, stops, and then continues voiding into the container. There is only one problem. For a culture and sensitivity, the container must be sterile. Eliminate.

The correct answer is (3). Many students will select answer choice (4) because they see the expected words: "Void a few drops, then stop; continue voiding." Be careful. This question is a good example of why scanning for expected words could get you into trouble. You may see expected words in an answer choice that is not correct.

OK. You've practiced how to identify the topic of the question and how to eliminate answer choices. You know that predicting answers does not work on the NCLEX-RN® exam. You are well on your way to correctly answering NCLEX-RN® exam test questions. Unfortunately, this is just the starting point. Let's talk about specific paths and how you can correctly decide which paths to use on the NCLEX-RN® exam. Remember, the correct answer is at the end of the path!

RECOGNIZE EXPECTED OUTCOMES

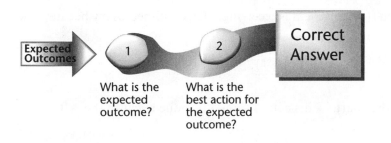

You spent much of your time in nursing school learning about what might go wrong with clients and their care. This makes sense; after all, nurses need to deal with problems and illnesses. Many test questions that your nursing school faculty wrote focused on what was wrong with clients and their care. In order to prove minimum competence, the beginning practitioner must demonstrate the ability to make appropriate nursing judgments. Competent nursing judgments include recognizing both expected and unexpected behaviors, so it is important for you to recognize expected outcomes on the NCLEX-RN® exam. Expected outcomes are the behaviors and changes you think are going to occur as a result of nursing care. These outcomes allow the nurse to evaluate whether goals have been met.

Look at the following question.

> The physician orders an arterial blood gas (ABG) for a client receiving oxygen at 6 L/min. Results show pH 7.37, HCO_3 26 mm Hg, pCO_2 42 mm Hg, pO_2 90 mm Hg. Which of the following should the nurse do *FIRST*?
>
> 1. Increase the rate of oxygen flow the client is receiving.
> 2. Elevate the head of the bed.
> 3. Document the results in the chart.
> 4. Instruct the client to cough and deep-breathe.

If this question were included on one of your medical/surgical tests, you would assume that a problem was being described. So you would choose an answer choice that involves "fixing" the problem. Let's look at this question.

THE REWORDED QUESTION: What should you do with a client with these ABGs?

Step 1. Recognize normal. Interpret the ABGs. All are within normal limits.

Step 2. Decide how you should use this information. Because they are all normal, let's reword the question again using this information.

Now **THE REWORDED QUESTION** is: What should you do for a client with normal ABGs?

ANSWERS:

(1) "Increase the rate of oxygen flow the client is receiving." This is unnecessary because his O_2 is within normal limits. Eliminate.

(2) "Elevate the head of the bed." This is unnecessary because the ABGs are within normal limits. Eliminate.

(3) "Document the results in the chart." This action should be done because the ABGs are normal.

(4) "Instruct the client to cough and deep-breathe." This is usually recommended in a situation in which there is some limitation of respiratory function, due to immobility or post-operative conditions, for example. The only information you are given in this question is the client's ABGs, which are within normal limits. Although this could be done, you are given no indication that it is necessary. Eliminate.

The correct answer is (3). The ABGs are within normal limits. Some students select answer choice (2) because they think there's something they missed, or it must be a trick question. The "trick" is deciding whether the information that you are given is normal or abnormal, and then answering the question accordingly.

Try this question.

> A client is brought to the emergency room complaining of pressure in her chest. Her blood pressure is 150/90, pulse 88, respirations 20. The nurse administers nitroglycerin 0.4 mg sublingually as ordered. After five minutes her blood pressure is 100/60, pulse 96, respirations 20. Which of the following should the nurse do next?
>
> 1. Notify the physician that the client has become hypotensive, and obtain an order to administer IV fluids.
> 2. Place the client in semi-Fowler's position, and administer O_2 at 4 L.
> 3. Administer a second dose of nitroglycerin.
> 4. Document the results, and continue to monitor the client.

THE REWORDED QUESTION: What should you do for this client? To answer this question you need to know what these vital signs indicate.

Step 1. Recognize normal. Nitroglycerin is a potent vasodilator with anti-anginal, anti-ischemic, and antihypertensive actions. It increases blood flow through the coronary arteries. Side effects include orthostatic hypotension, tachycardia, dizziness, and palpitations. A decreased blood pressure, increased pulse, and stable respirations after administration of a potent vasodilator are normal and expected.

Step 2. Decide how you should use this information. The question should be reworded as, "What should you do for a client who has responded as expected to a dose of nitroglycerin?"

ANSWERS:

(1) "Notify the physician that the client has become hypotensive and obtain an order to administer IV fluids." The blood pressure has decreased due to vasodilatation. Decreased blood pressure is expected. Eliminate.

(2) "Place the client in semi-Fowler's position and administer O_2 at 4 L." Respirations are stable and there is no indication of respiratory distress. Eliminate.

(3) "Administer a second dose of nitroglycerin." The nurse should assess the client for chest pain first, and administer a second dose of the medication only if the client continues to complain of chest pain. Eliminate.

(4) "Document the results and continue to monitor the client." This is the correct choice because you recognized the client's response as normal, thus eliminating the other three answer choices.

The correct answer is (4). You would expect a client's blood pressure to decrease after administration of nitroglycerin. The key to this question is understanding how the medication works, and correctly identifying the expected outcome.

READ ANSWER CHOICES TO OBTAIN CLUES

Because the NCLEX-RN® exam is testing your critical thinking, the topic of the questions may be unstated. You may see a question that concerns a disease process or procedure with which you are unfamiliar. Most test takers who are "clueless" about a question will read the question and answer choices over and over again. They do this because they hope that:

- They will remember seeing the topic in their notes or on a textbook page.
- The light will dawn and they will remember something about the topic.
- They believe there is some clue in the question that will point them toward the correct answer.

What usually happens? Absolutely nothing! The student then randomly selects an answer choice. When you randomly select an answer, you have 1 chance in 4 of getting it right. You can better those odds, and here's how: When you encounter a question that deals with unfamiliar nursing content, look for clues in the answer choices instead of in the question stem.

If you find yourself "clueless" after you carefully read a question, follow these steps:

Step 1. Resist the impulse to read and reread the question. Read the question only once. Identify the topic of the question. It is often unstated.

Step 2. Read the answer choices, not to select the correct answer but to figure out, "What is the topic of the question?" or "What should I be thinking?" You are looking for clues from the answer choices.

Step 3. After reading the answer choices, reword the question using the clues that you have obtained.

Step 4. Then use the strategies previously discussed to answer the question you have formulated.

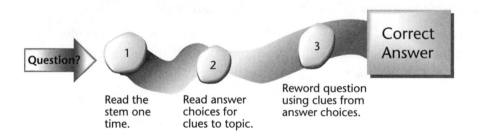

Let's try this strategy with a question.

> A client contacts his home care nurse with complaints of nausea and abdominal pain. He has type 1 diabetes. The nurse should advise the client to do which of the following?
>
> 1. "Hold your regular dose of insulin."
> 2. "Check your blood glucose level every 3–4 hours."
> 3. "Increase your consumption of foods containing simple sugars."
> 4. "Increase your activity level."

Step 1. Read the stem of the question. Can you identify the topic of the question? No, you can't. The nurse is telling the client to do something, but about what topic? The topic is unstated in the question.

Step 2. Read the answer choices to obtain clues about the topic of the question. Each answer choice deals with ways to maintain a normal blood sugar.

Step 3. Reword the question: "What does the nurse tell the client about 'sick day rules'?"

ANSWERS:

(1) "Hold your regular dose of insulin." This is an implementation that would increase the blood glucose level. The nurse should assess first. Eliminate.

(2) "Check your blood glucose level every 3–4 hours." This is an assessment. Before you can advise the client, you must identify whether the client is hypoglycemic or hyperglycemic. Keep this answer for consideration.

(3) "Increase your consumption of foods containing simple sugars." This is an implementation and would increase the client's blood glucose level. The nurse should assess first. Eliminate.

(4) "Increase your activity level." This is an implementation that would decrease the client's blood glucose level. The nurse should assess first. Eliminate.

The nurse should always assess before implementing nursing care. The correct answer is (2).

No matter how much you prepare for the NCLEX-RN® exam, there may be topics you see on your test with which you are unfamiliar. Reading the answer choices for clues will increase your chances of selecting a correct answer. Remember, you do have a body of knowledge. You just have to be calm and access this knowledge.

Read this question.

> A client is being treated for Addison's disease. The physician orders cortisone 25 mg PO daily. The nurse should explain to the client that adjustment of the dosage may be required in which of the following situations?
>
> 1. Dosage is increased when the blood glucose level increases.
> 2. Dosage is decreased when dietary intake is increased.
> 3. Dosage is decreased when infection stimulates endogenous steroid secretion.
> 4. Dosage is increased relative to an increase in the level of stress.

Not sure what Addison's disease is? Not sure how to adjust the dose of cortisone?

Step 1. Read the question once. Resist the impulse to reread the question.

Step 2. Read the answer choices. What should you be thinking? The question concerns cortisone. If the client is receiving cortisone, Addison's disease must be something that requires cortisone, a hormone from the adrenal glands. You notice that dosages are both increased and decreased.

Step 3. Use these clues to reword the question: "What is true about adjusting cortisone dosage?"

Step 4. Consider each answer choice. Does it answer THE REWORDED QUESTION?

(1) Dosage is increased when the blood glucose level increases. Is this true about cortisone? No. This sounds like insulin. Eliminate.

(2) Dosage is decreased when dietary intake is increased. Is this true about cortisone? No. Cortisone requirements are not related to diet. Eliminate.

(3) Dosage is decreased when infection stimulates endogenous steroid secretion. Endogenous means "within the client." If the client is receiving cortisone for Addison's disease, he must have adrenal insufficiency. Therefore, infection can't stimulate steroid secretion. Eliminate.

The correct answer is (4) because it is the only choice remaining. Even if you are not confident that cortisone is increased during periods of stress, you can conclude that this is the correct answer because the other choices have been eliminated.

If you're not sure about the topic of the question, read the answer choices for clues.

Let's look at another path.

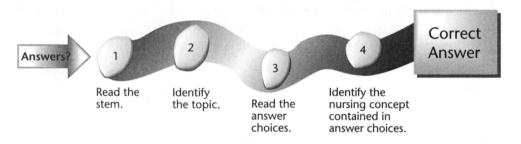

In some questions, the NCLEX-RN® exam asks you to figure out the topic of the question. In other questions you are required to use critical thinking skills to figure out what the answer choices *really* mean. The NCLEX-RN® exam can take a concept with which you are very familiar and make it difficult to recognize. The following question illustrates this point.

> A client with a history of heart failure visits the clinic. He states, "I have not been feeling like my old self for about 2 weeks." It would be MOST important for the nurse to ask which of the following questions?
>
> 1. "Do your ankles swell at the end of the day?"
> 2. "Where do you sleep at night?"
> 3. "How do you feel after you eat dinner?"
> 4. "Do you have chest pain when you inhale?"

It is not difficult to identify the topic of this question, "What is a priority for a client with heart failure?" Many students get tripped up on this question by not thinking through the answers as carefully as they should. In some questions, you have to figure out the topic of the question. In this question, you have to figure out what the answer choices mean.

Step 1. Read the stem of the question.

Step 2. Reword the question in your own words.

Step 3. Read the answer choices.

Step 4. Think: "What nursing concept should I identify in the answer choices?"

THE REWORDED QUESTION: What is a priority for a client with heart failure?

ANSWERS:

(1) "Do your ankles swell at the end of the day?" Why would you ask a client this question? Because edema is a symptom of right-sided heart failure. Is right-sided failure your priority? No, left-sided failure takes priority because it affects the lungs. Eliminate this answer.

(2) "Where do you sleep at night?" Why would you ask a client this question? If he is sleeping in his bed, his breathing is not compromised. If he has to sleep in his recliner, he is having orthopnea. Orthopnea is a symptom of left-sided failure, and this would be a priority. Keep this answer for consideration.

(3) "How do you feel after you eat dinner?" Why would you ask a client this question? Bloating after meals is a symptom of right-sided failure. This is not as important as breathing problems. Eliminate this answer.

(4) "Do you have chest pain when you inhale?" Why would you ask a client this question? It does indicate a breathing problem. The student who reacts rather than thinks may select this answer. Pain on inspiration may indicate irritation of the parietal pleura of the lung, which is not associated with heart failure. Eliminate this answer.

The correct answer is (2). In order to select this answer, you must recognize that "Where do you sleep at night?" represents orthopnea. The NCLEX-RN® exam can take important concepts such as this, and "hide" the concept in some fairly simple behaviors.

Let's try another question where you have to figure out what the answer choices really mean.

> The nurse is caring for a client immediately after a paracentesis. It is MOST important for the nurse to ask which of the following questions?
>
> 1. "Do your clothes still feel tight?"
> 2. "Do you need to void?"
> 3. "Are you feeling dizzy?"
> 4. "Do you have any pain?"

Step 1. Read the stem of the question.

Step 2. Reword the question in your own words.

Step 3. Read the answer choices.

Step 4. Think: "What nursing concept should I identify in the answer choices?"

THE REWORDED QUESTION: What is the highest priority for a client after a paracentesis?

ANSWERS:

(1) "Do your clothes still feel tight?" Why would you ask a client this question? Clothes should fit looser because the abdominal girth has decreased after fluid has been removed with a paracentesis. This is an expected outcome. Eliminate.

(2) "Do you need to void?" Why would you ask a client this question? It is imperative to empty the bladder prior to the procedure, not after the procedure. There is no compelling reason to ask the client this question. Eliminate.

(3) "Are you feeling dizzy?" What makes a client dizzy? One of the causes is a decrease in cerebral perfusion due to a fall in blood pressure. Could this client have a decreased blood pressure? Yes. Hypotension and hypovolemic shock are complications of a paracentesis due to removal of a large volume of fluid. Keep this answer for consideration.

(4) "Do you have any pain?" You ask this question to assess pain level. This client may have discomfort where the paracentesis was performed, but this is an expected outcome. Eliminate.

The correct answer is (3).

These questions illustrate why knowing nursing content is not enough to answer application/analysis-level questions. You must be able to effectively use the information you learned in nursing school to answer NCLEX-RN® exam-style test questions. Here is a brief review of some of the lessons you have learned in this chapter:

- Reword the question.
- Eliminate answer choices you know to be incorrect.
- Don't predict answers.
- Recognize expected outcomes.
- Read answer choices to obtain clues.

CHAPTER 3

NCLEX-RN® EXAM STRATEGIES

Now that you understand what kind of questions the NCLEX-RN® exam is going to ask, you need to learn more specific strategies for success on the NCLEX-RN® exam.

THE NCLEX-RN® EXAM VERSUS REAL-WORLD NURSING

Some of you are LPNs or LVNs completing your RN studies, while others are EMTs. Some of you worked during school as student techs. All of you, however, spent time in a clinical setting during your nursing education. All of this adds up to a significant amount of experience. Experience will help you get a job, but answering questions based on your experience can be dangerous on the NCLEX-RN® exam.

Look at the following question.

> On admission to the hospital, an elderly client appears disheveled and is restless and confused. During the client's second day on the unit, a nurse approaches the client to administer medication. The nurse is unable to identify the client because his armband is missing. Which of the following actions by the nurse is the *BEST?*
>
> 1. Have the client's roommate identify him.
> 2. Ask the client to state his full name.
> 3. Ask another nurse to identify the client.
> 4. Look in the chart at the picture of the client.

Let's see how someone using his or her real-world experience would approach this question:

(1) "The roommate is never involved in identification of a client."

(2) "A confused client cannot be relied on for an accurate identification."

(3) "Sounds reasonable. I have seen this done in some circumstances."

(4) "A picture? What picture? I've never seen a picture of a client in a chart!"

Possible conclusions drawn by this person would include: *"OK, I've seen one nurse ask another for information so (3) must be the answer,"* or *"Well, maybe the client isn't all that confused, so I'll select (2)."*

According to nursing textbooks, asking another health care professional is not the correct way to identify a client. Many acute-care settings now include a photo of the client in the chart for just this type of situation. The correct answer to this question is (4). Many students reject this answer because there are rarely pictures of clients in the charts. Real-world experience doesn't count, though; in this case, the client does have a picture in his chart.

The NCLEX-RN® exam is a standardized exam administered by NCSBN. Because the NCLEX-RN® exam is a national exam, students should be aware that in some parts of the country, nursing is practiced slightly differently. However, to ensure that the test is reflective of national trends, questions and answers are all carefully documented. The test makers ensure that the correct answers are documented in at least two standard nursing textbooks, or in one textbook and one nursing journal.

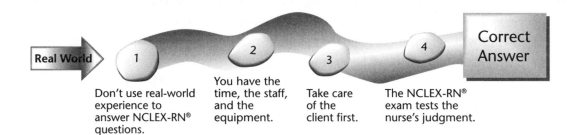

When you are unsure of an answer choice, don't ask yourself, "What do they do on my floor?" but "What does the medical/surgical textbook writer Brunner say?" or "What do Potter and Perry say to do?" This test does not necessarily reflect what happens in the real world, but is based on textbook nursing.

Remember the following when taking the NCLEX-RN® exam:

- You have all of the time and resources you need to provide appropriate care to your client. (Checking for bowel sounds for five minutes in all four quadrants, no problem!)
- You have all of the equipment you need. (Remember the bath thermometer you learned to use in the nursing lab? For the NCLEX-RN® exam, you will have one available to test the temperature of bath water.)

- There are no staffing problems on the NCLEX-RN® exam. You are caring only for the client described in the question, and that person is your only concern.
- All care given to clients is "by the book." No shortcuts are used. (You would not turn off an IV solution, flush the line, give another IV solution, flush the line, and then restart the original IV solution that was ordered to be run continuously.)

Answer the following question.

> A client is treated in the emergency room for acute alcohol intoxication. He has a five-year history of alcohol abuse. He is agitated and verbally abusive. His admission orders include chlordiazepoxide (Librium) 50 mg IM or PO every 4–6 hours for agitation. The nurse should take which of the following precautions after Librium is administered?
>
> 1. Place the client in restraints.
> 2. Leave the client in a room by himself until the tranquilizer takes effect.
> 3. Assign a practical nurse to stay with the client and assess his condition.
> 4. Ask the security guard to stay with the client.

Let's look at this using real-world logic.

(1) "Place the client in restraints." Yes, that is done in the real world.

(2) "Leave the client in a room by himself until the tranquilizer takes effect." Yes, that is done in the real world, but most students recognize that it is not the best answer.

(3) "Assign a practical nurse to stay with the client and assess his condition." Sounds good, but what if you don't have enough staffing to assign an LPN/LVN to sit with this client?

(4) "Ask the security guard to stay with the client." Yes, in the real world, security is called when clients are agitated.

According to real-world logic, the correct answer must be (1) or (4). However, textbook theoretical nursing practice states that this client should not be left alone while in an agitated state. A professional should remain with the client. Therefore, the correct answer is (3).

Use your real-world experience to help you visualize the client described in the test question, but select your answers based on what is found in nursing textbooks.

Your nursing faculty has probably been conscientious about instructing you in the most up-to-date nursing practice. According to the National Council, the primary source for documenting correct answers is in nursing textbooks, and the most up-to-date practice might not always agree with the textbooks. When in doubt, always select the textbook answer!

The next question illustrates this point.

> A woman is admitted to the hospital and delivers a healthy 7 lb., 2 oz. girl. The mother decides to bottle-feed her infant. Which of the following statements by the mother after a teaching session indicates to the nurse that the client needs further instruction?
>
> 1. "I'll pump my breasts and use warm packs to relieve breast pain."
> 2. "I'll use a tight bra and ice packs to relieve engorgement discomfort."
> 3. "I'll take the medication prescribed by the doctor for pain."
> 4. "I'll take the pills ordered by my doctor to help stop the production of milk."

Let's look at these answers more closely.

(1) Pumping the breasts will stimulate milk production. This is clearly wrong.

(2) Wearing a tight bra and using ice packs are appropriate interventions for a nonbreastfeeding mother.

(3) Taking a medication (mild analgesic) is an appropriate intervention for a nonbreastfeeding mother.

(4) Medication to prevent lactation is not frequently prescribed because of potentially dangerous side effects. However, a medication may be prescribed to prevent lactation. This would be considered an appropriate intervention.

The correct answer is (1).

First Take Care of the Client, Then the Equipment

The NCLEX-RN® exam tests your ability to use critical thinking skills to make nursing judgments. It is very important that you remember to:

- Take care of the client first.
- Take care of the equipment second.

Look at the following question.

> A client sustains a fractured left femur in a car accident. She is placed in balanced suspension skeletal traction using a Thomas splint and a Pearson attachment. The client tells the nurse that she has "terrible" pain in her left thigh. Which of the following should the nurse do *FIRST?*
>
> 1. Determine that all the weights and ropes from the traction apparatus are in line and hanging free.
> 2. Ask the client for more information about the location and characteristics of her pain.
> 3. Check the Thomas splint and Pearson attachment to make sure they are appropriately positioned.
> 4. Explain to the client that the pain she is experiencing in the affected leg is a common occurrence.

Let's review the answers:

(1) All weights should be hanging free in balanced suspension skeletal traction. This answer choice has you checking the equipment, not the client. Your first concern should be the client, not the traction.

(2) The nurse should focus on assessing the client and her problem before assessing the function of the equipment. All complaints of pain should be thoroughly investigated by the nurse.

(3) This answer choice has you checking the equipment, not the client. Your first concern should be the client, not the traction.

(4) Any complaints of pain are considered abnormal, and you should investigate them thoroughly.

The correct answer is (2).

Laboratory Values

Answering questions about lab values is another example of how the real world does not work on the NCLEX-RN® exam. In nursing school, you learned lab values for a specific test and you may not have remembered them after the test. While you were in the clinical setting, the emphasis was on interpretation of lab values. Because most lab slips contained a listing of normal values, you were able to compare the client's results to the normal levels. Questions on the NCLEX-RN® exam will not provide you with a listing of normal lab values.

To answer questions on the NCLEX-RN® exam, you must:

- Know normal lab test results.
- Correctly interpret normal or abnormal lab test results.

Compare the following two questions.

> A client is admitted to the hospital with flu-like symptoms. When taking the history, the nurse learns that the client has been taking digoxin (Lanoxin) 0.125 mg PO daily and furosemide (Lasix) 40 mg PO daily for 3 years. Last month her physician changed the prescription for digoxin to 0.25 mg qd. The nurse would expect the physician to order which of the following laboratory tests?
>
> 1. Serum electrolytes and digoxin level
> 2. White blood cell count, hemoglobin, and hematocrit
> 3. Cardiac enzymes and an arterial blood gas
> 4. Blood cultures and urinalysis

You are probably familiar with the concepts presented in this question. The physician has increased the client's dose of digoxin. Lasix is a potassium-wasting diuretic. The client will likely develop digitalis toxicity if she has a low potassium level. Serum electrolytes and digoxin level (1) is the correct answer.

Now look at this question.

> The nurse plans care for a teenager admitted with complaints of fever, vomiting, and diarrhea. The nurse writes the following nursing diagnosis on the client's care plan: "fluid volume deficit." Which of the following changes in laboratory values would demonstrate an improvement in the client's condition?
>
> 1. Urine specific gravity, 1.015; hematocrit, 37%
> 2. Urine specific gravity, 1.020; hematocrit, 45%
> 3. Urine specific gravity, 1.032; hematocrit, 52%
> 4. Urine specific gravity, 1.025; hematocrit, 35%

In order to correctly answer this question, you must know:

- The specific gravity of urine (1.010–1.030) and the normal levels of hematocrit (male 42–50%, female 40–48%)
- How the specific gravity and hematocrit levels are affected by a fluid volume deficit

Fluid volume deficit occurs when water and electrolytes are lost in the same proportion as they exist in the body. When a client is dehydrated, both the specific gravity of urine and the hematocrit become elevated. The correct answer is (2).

Answer the following question.

> A client is hospitalized with a diagnosis of atrial fibrillation. Heparin 5,000 units is ordered every 12 hours to be given subcutaneously. The physician orders daily partial thromboplastin times (PTT). The result of the client's most recent PTT is 55. Which of the following actions should be taken by the nurse?
>
> 1. Document the results and administer the heparin.
> 2. Withhold the heparin.
> 3. Notify the physician.
> 4. Have the test repeated.

In order to answer this question you need to know:

- The normal range for a PTT is 20–45 seconds.
- The therapeutic range for a client receiving heparin, an anticoagulant, is 1.5–2 times the control or normal level.
- To calculate the therapeutic range, take the lower number for the normal range for a PTT (20) and multiply it by 1.5. The result is 30. Multiply the higher number (45) by 2. The result is 90. Thus the therapeutic range goes from 30 to 90. If a PTT reading is between those endpoints, no medication is needed.

Evaluate the answer choices:

(1) "Document the results and administer the heparin." The client's most recent PTT is 55. This is within the therapeutic range of 30 to 90, so no medication should be given.

(2) "Withhold the heparin." The PTT level is within what is considered an effective therapeutic level. This client does not need the anticoagulant.

(3) "Notify the physician." There is no reason to notify the physician. The client has reached the therapeutic level of heparin.

(4) "Have the test repeated." There is no reason to have the test repeated. The client has achieved the therapeutic level.

The correct answer is (2).

Medication Administration

An important function in providing safe and effective care to clients is the administration of medications. Because this is one of the responsibilities of a beginning practitioner, questions about medications are often an important part of the NCLEX-RN® exam. The nurse who is minimally competent is knowledgeable about medications and uses the "six rights" when administering medication.

In nursing school, most questions about medication followed the same pattern. You were told the client's diagnosis and the name of the medication, and then were asked a question. Even if you didn't know the information about the medication, sometimes you were able to select the correct answer by knowing the diagnosis.

The NCLEX-RN® exam does not give you any clues from the context of the question. The questions on this exam include the name of the medication, almost always identifying it by both trade and generic names. Most of the time, you will not be given the reason the client is receiving the medication.

Let's look at some medication questions.

> The physician orders furosemide (Lasix) and spironolactone (Aldactone) for a client. Prior to administering the medication, the nurse determines that the client's potassium is 3.2 mEq/L. In addition to notifying the physician, the nurse should anticipate taking which of the following actions?
>
> 1. Do not administer the Lasix or Aldactone.
> 2. Administer the Aldactone only.
> 3. Administer the Lasix only.
> 4. Administer the Lasix and Aldactone.

This is a typical exam-style medication question. The question concerns the side effects and nursing implications of Lasix and Aldactone.

(1) The potassium level is below normal (3.5–5.0 mEq/L). Lasix is a potassium-wasting diuretic. Aldactone is a potassium-sparing diuretic. There is no reason to hold the Aldactone because the client has a low potassium level. Eliminate this answer.

(2) The Aldactone should be administered.

(3) Do not administer the Lasix because it is a potassium-wasting diuretic. The client's potassium level is already low. Eliminate.

(4) Do not administer the Lasix. Eliminate.

The correct answer is (2).

Let's try this next question.

> A client returns to the clinic 2 weeks after being started on allopurinol (Zyloprim) 200 mg PO daily. The nurse reviews information about this medication with the client. Which of the following statements by the client indicates that the teaching was effective?
>
> 1. "I should take my medication on an empty stomach."
> 2. "I should take my medication with orange juice."
> 3. "I should increase my intake of protein."
> 4. "I should drink at least 8 glasses of water every day."

To answer this question you need to know information about Zyloprim, an antigout agent that reduces uric acid.

(1) Zyloprim is best tolerated with or immediately after meals to reduce gastrointestinal (GI) irritation. Eliminate.

(2) Orange juice makes the urine acidic. Zyloprim is more soluble in alkaline urine. Eliminate.

(3) It is not necessary to increase the intake of protein when taking Zyloprim. Eliminate.

(4) Zyloprim can cause renal calculi. The client should drink 3,000 mL/day to reduce the risk of kidney stone formation.

The correct answer is (4). You must know the side effects and nursing implications of medications for the NCLEX-RN® exam.

Notify the Physician

Another behavior that commonly occurs in the real world is calling the physician. In nursing school you were encouraged to notify your instructor of changes in your client's condition. Be very careful how you handle this on the NCLEX-RN® exam. More often than not, the answer choice that states "call the physician," "contact the social worker," or "refer to the chaplain" is the WRONG answer. Usually there is something you need to do first before you make that call. The NCLEX-RN® exam does not want to know what the physician is going to do. The NCLEX-RN® exam wants to know what you, the registered professional nurse, will do in a given situation.

Answer this question.

> A client is receiving packed red blood cells. Several minutes after the infusion is started, the client complains of itching and develops hives on his chest and abdomen. Which of the following actions should the nurse take *FIRST?*
>
> 1. Slow the rate of the transfusion.
> 2. Call the physician for an order for an antihistamine.
> 3. Mix IV fluid with the blood to dilute it.
> 4. Stop the transfusion.

THE REWORDED QUESTION: What should you do *first* for this client?

It sounds like the client is having an allergic reaction to the transfusion. If this is what's going on, what should you do?

(1) If the client is having a transfusion reaction, slowing the rate of the transfusion is not the right action.

(2) Antihistamines are given for allergic reactions. The doctor needs to be notified. This answer might be a possibility, but is there something you should do first?

(3) Mixing IV fluids with blood is done to decrease the viscosity of RBCs. This doesn't have anything to do with an allergic transfusion reaction. Eliminate.

(4) If the client was having a transfusion reaction, the best action is to stop the transfusion. This is the correct action to take first, before the physician is called.

The correct answer is (4). After the transfusion is stopped, you will contact the physician and antihistamines will probably be ordered.

Before you want to choose the answer choice that involves "call the physician," look at the other answer choices very carefully. Make sure that there isn't an answer that contains an assessment or action you should do before making the phone call. The test makers want to know what you would do in a situation, not what the doctor would do!

Here is one more real-world question.

> Upon returning from lunch, the nurse is approached in the elevator by a hospital employee from another unit. The employee states that her close friend is a client on the nurse's unit. The employee asks how her friend is doing and if all of her tests were normal. The nurse should do which of the following?
>
> 1. Answer the employee's questions softly so other people on the elevator will not hear.
> 2. Refuse to discuss her friend's medical condition. Suggest that she visit her friend.
> 3. Give the employee the name of the client's physician to call for this information.
> 4. Tell the employee about the results of the client's tests because they were within normal limits.

THE REWORDED QUESTION: What should a nurse do when asked about a client by a hospital employee?

(1) Discussing client information in a public place is a breach of confidentiality. Eliminate.

(2) Refusing to discuss a client's medical condition does not violate the client's right to privacy and confidentiality. Keep in consideration.

(3) Providing any information about a client to someone not directly involved in the client's care is a breach of privacy. Eliminate.

(4) It is a breach in the client's right to privacy to share information with others without the client's permission. Eliminate.

The correct answer is (2).

Expect to see real-world situations on your NCLEX-RN® exam, but make sure that you do not choose real-world answers! These strategies should help you use your previous nursing experience without encountering any pitfalls.

STRATEGIES FOR PRIORITY QUESTIONS

You will recognize priority questions on the NCLEX-RN® exam because they will ask you what is the "best," "most important," "first," or "initial response" by the nurse.

Take a look at this sample question.

> An hour after admission to the nursery, the nurse observes a newborn baby having spontaneous jerky movements of the limbs. The infant's mother had gestational diabetes mellitus (GDM) during pregnancy. Which of the following actions should the nurse take *FIRST?*
>
> 1. Give dextrose water.
> 2. Call the physician immediately.
> 3. Determine the blood glucose level.
> 4. Observe closely for other symptoms.

As you read this question you are probably thinking, "All of these look right!" or "How can I decide what I will do first?" The panic sets in as you try to decide what the best answer is when they all seem "correct."

As a registered professional nurse, you will be caring for clients who have multiple problems and needs. You must be able to establish priorities by deciding which needs take precedence over the other needs. You probably recognized the baby's jerky movements as an indication of hypoglycemia. Don't forget that an important part of the assessment process is *validating* what you observe. You must complete an assessment before you analyze, plan, and implement nursing care. The correct answer is (3).

The following situation might sound familiar: You are called to a client's room by a family member and find the client lying on the floor. He is bleeding from a wound on the forehead, and his indwelling catheter is dislodged and hanging from the side of the bed. Where do you begin? Do you call for help? Do you return him to bed? Do you apply pressure to the cut? Do you reinsert the catheter? Do you call the doctor? What do you do *first*? This is why establishing priorities is so important.

Your nursing faculty recognized the importance of teaching you how to establish priorities. They required you to establish priorities both in clinical situations and when answering test questions. These are the type of questions that nursing students find most controversial.

Here is an example of a nursing school test question:

> Which of the following would most concern the nurse during a client's recovery from surgery?
>
> (1) Safety
> (2) Hemorrhage
> (3) Infection
> (4) Pain control

A conversation in class with your instructor may then go something like this:

Instructor: "The correct answer is (2)."

Student: "Why isn't infection the correct answer? It says right here [pointing to textbook] that infection is a major complication after surgery."

Instructor: "Yes, infection is an important concern after surgery. But if the client has a life-threatening hemorrhage, then the fact that the wound is infected is immaterial."

Student: "But you can't count this answer wrong!"

In some situations, the faculty member will give you partial credit for your answer, or will "throw the question out" because there is more than one right answer. But you won't get the opportunity to argue about questions on the NCLEX-RN® exam. You either select the answer the test makers are looking for, or you get the question wrong. In the question above, all of the answers listed are important when caring for a postoperative client, but only one answer is the *best*.

The critical thinking required for priority questions is for you to recognize patterns in the answer choices. By recognizing these patterns, you will know which path you need to choose to correctly answer the question. There are three strategies to help you establish priorities on the NCLEX-RN® exam:

- Maslow strategy
- Nursing process strategy
- Safety strategy

We will outline each strategy, describe how and when it should be used, and show you how to apply these strategies to exam-style questions. By using these strategies, you will be able to eliminate the second-best answer and correctly identify the highest priority.

Strategy One: Maslow

Maslow's hierarchy of needs (Figure 1) is crucial to establishing priorities on the NCLEX-RN® exam. Maslow identifies five levels of human needs: physiological, safety or security, love and belonging, esteem, and self-actualization.

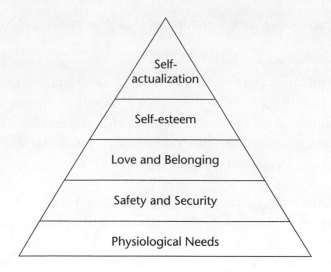

Figure 1: Maslow's Hierarchy of Needs

Because *physiological needs* are necessary for survival, they have the highest priority and must be met first. Physiological needs include oxygen, fluid, nutrition, temperature, elimination, shelter, rest, and sex. If you don't have oxygen to breathe or food to eat, you really don't care if you have stable psychosocial relationships!

Safety and security needs can be both physical and psychosocial. Physical safety includes decreasing what is threatening to the client. The threat may be an illness (myocardial infarction), accidents (a parent transporting a newborn in a car without using a car seat), or environmental threats (the client with COPD who insists on walking outside in 10° F [−12° C] temperatures).

To attain psychological safety, the client must have the knowledge and understanding about what to expect from others in his environment. For example, it is important to teach the client and his family what to expect after a cerebrovascular accident (CVA). It is also important that you allow a woman preparing for a mastectomy to verbalize her concerns about changes that might occur in her relationship with her partner.

To achieve *love and belonging,* the client needs to feel loved by family and accepted by others. When a client feels self-confident and useful, he will achieve the need of *self-esteem* as described by Maslow.

The highest level of Maslow's hierarchy of needs is *self-actualization.* To achieve this level, the client must experience fulfillment and recognize his or her potential. In order for self-actualization to occur, all of the lower-level needs must be met. Because of the stresses of life, lower-level needs are not always met, and many people never achieve this high level of functioning.

The Maslow Four-Step Process

The first strategy to use in establishing priorities is a four-step process, beginning with Maslow's hierarchy. To use the Maslow strategy, you must first recognize the pattern in the answer choices.

Step 1. Look at your answer choices.

Determine if the answer choices are both physiological and psychosocial. If they are, apply the Maslow strategy detailed in Step 2.

Step 2. Eliminate all psychosocial answer choices. If an answer choice is physiological, don't eliminate it yet. Remember, Maslow states that physiological needs must be met first. Although pain certainly has a physiological component, reactions to pain are considered "psychosocial" on this exam and will become a lower priority.

Step 3. Look at each of the answer choices that you have not yet eliminated and ask yourself if the answer choice makes sense with regard to the disease or situation described in the question. If it makes sense as an answer choice, keep it for consideration and go on to the next choice.

Step 4. Can you apply the ABCs?

Look at the remaining answer choices. Can you apply the ABCs? The ABCs stand for airway, breathing, and circulation. If there is an answer that involves maintaining a patent airway, it will be correct. If not, is there a choice that involves breathing problems? It will be correct. If not, go on with the ABCs. Is there an answer pertaining to the cardiovascular system? It will be correct. What if the ABCs don't apply? Compare the remaining answer choices and ask yourself, "What is the highest priority?" This is your answer.

 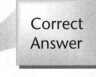

Maslow

1 — Recognize that answers are both physical and psychosocial.

2 — Eliminate psychosocial answers.

3 — "Does this make sense?"

4 — Apply ABCs.

Correct Answer

Let's apply this technique to a few sample exam-style test questions.

> A woman is admitted to the hospital with a ruptured ectopic pregnancy. A laparotomy is scheduled. Preoperatively, which of the following goals is *MOST* important for the nurse to include on the client's plan of care?
>
> 1. Fluid replacement
> 2. Pain relief
> 3. Emotional support
> 4. Respiratory therapy

Look at the stem of the question. The words *most important* mean:

- This is a priority question.
- There probably will be more than one answer choice that is a correct nursing action, but only one will be the most important or highest priority action.

Step 1. Look at the answer choices.

You see that both physical and psychosocial interventions are included. Apply Maslow.

Step 2. Eliminate all psychosocial answer choices.

Answer choice (2), which is pain relief, should be discarded. Remember, pain is considered a psychosocial problem on the NCLEX-RN® exam. Answer choice (3), emotional support, is also a psychosocial concern. Eliminate this answer. You have now eliminated two of the possible choices.

Step 3. Now look at the remaining answer choices and ask yourself if they make sense.

Answer choice (1), fluid replacement, makes sense because this client has a ruptured ectopic pregnancy. An ectopic pregnancy is implantation of the fertilized ovum in a site other than the endometrial lining, usually the fallopian tube. Initially, the pregnancy is normal; but as the embryo outgrows the fallopian tube, the tube ruptures, causing extensive bleeding into the abdominal cavity. Answer choice (4), respiratory therapy, does not make sense with a ruptured ectopic pregnancy. The obstetrical client is not likely to need respiratory care prior to surgery. Eliminate this answer choice.

You are left with the correct answer, (1). After reading this question, many students select answer choices (2) or (3) as the correct answer. They justify this by emphasizing the importance of managing this woman's pain, or addressing her grief about losing the pregnancy. Neither answer choice takes priority over the physiological demand of fluid replacement prior to surgery.

Ready for another question? Try this one.

> The nurse obtains a diet history from a pregnant 16-year-old girl. The girl tells the nurse that her typical daily diet includes cereal and milk for breakfast, pizza and soda for lunch, and a cheeseburger, milk shake, fries, and salad for dinner. Which of the following is the *MOST* accurate nursing diagnosis based on this data?
>
> 1. Altered nutrition: more than body requirements related to high-fat intake
> 2. Knowledge deficit: nutrition in pregnancy
> 3. Altered nutrition: less than body requirements related to increased nutritional demands of pregnancy
> 4. Risk for injury: fetal malnutrition related to poor maternal diet

The first thing you should notice about this question stem is the phrase *"most accurate."* This alerts you that there may be more than one answer choice that could be considered correct.

Step 1. Look at the answer choices.

You will see that both physical and psychosocial interventions are included. Apply the Maslow strategy.

Step 2. Eliminate all psychosocial answer choices. In this case, that means answer choice (2). Knowledge deficit is a psychosocial need.

Step 3. Ask yourself whether the remaining answer choices make sense.

(1) "Altered nutrition: more than body requirements related to high-fat intake" does make sense. This diet is high in fat.

(3) "Altered nutrition: less than body requirements related to increased nutritional demands of pregnancy" also makes sense. This diet has an adequate number of calories, but it is deficient in the needed vitamins and minerals.

(4) "Risk for injury: fetal malnutrition related to poor maternal diet" does not make sense. There is an adequate number of calories to support fetal growth. Eliminate this choice.

You have now eliminated two of the choices. Let's go on.

Step 4. Answer choices (1) and (3) remain. Can you apply the ABCs to these choices? No. So compare the answer choices. Which is higher priority: the fact that this pregnant 16-year-old's diet contains too much fat, or that the diet does not have enough nutrients? Insufficient nutrients is a higher priority, so the correct answer is (3).

Many students, when they first read this question, choose (2), knowledge deficit. According to Maslow, physiological needs always take priority over psychosocial needs. Using this strategy on the NCLEX-RN® exam will enable you to choose the correct answer.

Now, let's try another question.

> The nurse plans care for a 14-year-old girl admitted with an eating disorder. On admission, the girl weighs 82 lb. and is 5'4" tall. Lab tests indicate severe hypokalemia, anemia, and dehydration. The nurse should give which of the following nursing diagnoses the *HIGHEST* priority?
>
> 1. Body image disturbance related to weight loss
> 2. Self-esteem disturbance related to feelings of inadequacy
> 3. Altered nutrition: less than body requirements related to decreased intake
> 4. Decreased cardiac output related to the potential for dysrhythmias

The first thing you should notice in this question stem is the phrase *"highest priority."* This alerts you that there may be more than one answer that could be considered correct.

Step 1. Look at the answer choices.

Both physical and psychosocial interventions are included. Apply the Maslow strategy.

Step 2. Eliminate all phychosocial answer choices.

It is easy to see that answer choice (1), body image disturbance, is a psychosocial concern. The same is true of answer choice (2), self-esteem disturbance. Answer choices (3) and (4) are physiological. You have now eliminated all but two answer choices.

Step 3. Ask yourself whether the remaining answer choices make sense.

Answer choice (3), "Altered nutrition: less than body requirements related to decreased intake," does make sense. Remember, the client has anorexia, is 5'4" tall, and weighs 82 lb. Answer choice (4), "Decreased cardiac output related to the potential for dysrhythmias," also makes sense. Dysrhythmias are a concern for a client with severe hypokalemia, which often occurs with anorexia.

You still have work to do.

Step 4. Can you apply the ABCs? Yes.

Decreased cardiac output is a higher priority than altered nutrition. One answer choice remains: (4).

When you first read this question, you probably identified each of the answer choices as appropriate for a client with anorexia. Only one nursing diagnosis can be the highest priority. By using strategies involving Maslow and the ABCs, you will choose the correct answer on your NCLEX-RN® exam.

Strategy Two: Nursing Process (Assessment versus Implementation)

A second strategy that will assist you in establishing priorities involves the assessment and implementation steps of the nursing process. As a nursing student, you have been drilled so that you can recite the steps of the nursing process in your sleep—assessment, analysis, planning, implementation, and evaluation. In nursing school, you did have some test questions about the nursing process, but you probably did not use the nursing process to assist you in selecting a correct answer on an exam. On the NCLEX-RN® exam, you will be given a clinical situation and asked to establish priorities. The possible answer choices will include both the correct assessment and implementation for this clinical situation. How do you choose the correct answer when both the correct assessment and implementation are given? Think about these two steps of the nursing process.

Assessment is the process of establishing a data profile about the client and his or her health problems. The nurse obtains subjective and objective data in a number of ways: talking to clients, observing clients and/or significant others, taking a health history, performing a physical examination, evaluating lab results, and collaborating with other members of the health care team.

Once you collect the data, you compare it to the client's baseline or normal values. On the NCLEX-RN® exam, the client's baseline may not be given, but as a nursing student you have acquired a body of knowledge. On this exam, you are expected to compare the client information you are given to the "normal" values learned from your nursing textbooks.

Assessment is the first step of the nursing process and takes priority over all other steps. It is essential that you complete the assessment phase of the nursing process before you implement nursing activities. This is a common mistake made by NCLEX-RN® exam takers: don't implement before you assess. For example, when performing cardiopulmonary resuscitation (CPR), if you don't access the airway before performing mouth-to-mouth resuscitation, your actions may be harmful!

Implementation is the care you provide to your clients. Implementation includes: assisting in the performance of activities of daily living (ADLs), counseling and educating the client and the client's family, giving care to clients, and supervising and evaluating the work of other members of the health team. Nursing interventions may be independent, dependent, or interdependent. Independent interventions are within the scope of nursing practice and do not require supervision by others. Instructing the client to turn, cough, and breathe deeply after surgery is an example of an independent nursing intervention. Dependent interventions are based on the written orders of a physician. On the NCLEX-RN® exam, you should assume that you have an order for all dependent interventions that are included in the answer choices.

This may be a different way of thinking from the way you were taught in nursing school. Many students select an answer on a nursing school test (that is later counted wrong) because the intervention requires a physician's order. Everyone walks away from the test review muttering, "Trick question." It is important for you to remember that there are no trick questions on the NCLEX-RN® exam. You should base your answer on an understanding that you have a physician's order for any nursing intervention described.

Interdependent interventions are shared with other members of the health team. For instance, nutrition education may be shared with the dietitian. Chest physiotherapy may be shared with a respiratory therapist.

The following strategy, utilizing the assessment and implementation phases of the nursing process, will assist you in selecting correct answers to questions that ask you to identify priorities.

Step 1. Read the answer choices to establish a pattern.

If the answer choices are a mix of assessment/validation and implementation, use the Nursing Process (Assessment vs. Implementation) strategy.

Step 2. Refer to the question to determine whether you should be assessing or implementing.

Step 3. Eliminate answer choices, and then choose the best answer.

If after Step 2 you find that, for example, it is an assessment question, eliminate any answers that clearly focus on implementation. Then choose the best assessment answer.

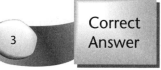

Nursing Process

1 — Recognize both assess and implement answers.

2 — Read stem to decide whether to assess or implement.

3 — Select best assessment or implementation.

Correct Answer

Try this strategy on the next question.

> The mother of a boy with type 1 diabetes calls the physician's office to discuss the child's self-monitoring blood glucose (SMBG) home reading. He is being tightly regulated with a combination of NPH and regular insulin before breakfast and supper. The past two mornings his blood sugar readings were 220 mg/dL and 210 mg/dL. Which of the following should the nurse tell the boy's mother?
>
> 1. "Continue with his medication regimen."
> 2. "Check his blood sugar during the night."
> 3. "Give his NPH insulin later in the evening."
> 4. "Serve his bedtime snack earlier in the evening."

THE REWORDED QUESTION: What advice should the nurse give the mother about her diabetic child who is hyperglycemic in the morning?

Step 1. Read the answer choices to establish a pattern.

There is one assessment answer, (2), and three implementation answers, (1), (3), and (4). You can use the Nursing Process (Assessment vs. Implementation) strategy.

Step 2. Refer to the question to determine whether you should be assessing or implementing.

The child's mother tells you that blood sugars have been elevated the last two mornings. This indicates that there is a problem. According to the nursing process, you should assess first.

Step 3. Eliminate answer choices, and then choose the best answer.

Eliminate answers (1), (3), and (4), which are implementation answers. You are left with only one answer choice, (2). This question is about the Somogyi effect, which is rebound hyperglycemia that occurs in response to a rapid decrease in blood glucose during the night. Treatment includes adjusting the evening diet, changing the insulin dose, and altering the amount of exercise to prevent nocturnal hypoglycemia. Even if you've never heard of the Somogyi effect, you are still able to correctly answer this question using the Nursing Process (Assessment vs. Implementation) strategy.

Let's look at another question.

> A boy was riding his bike to school when he hit the curb. He fell and hurt his leg. The school nurse was called and found him alert and conscious, but in severe pain with a possible fracture of the right femur. Which of the following is the *FIRST* action that the nurse should take?
>
> 1. Immobilize the affected limb with a splint and ask him not to move.
> 2. Make a thorough assessment of the circumstances surrounding the accident.
> 3. Put him in semi-Fowler's position for comfort.
> 4. Check the pedal pulse and blanching sign in both legs.

The words *"first action"* tell you that this is a priority question.

THE REWORDED QUESTION: What is the highest priority for a fractured femur?

Step 1. Read the answer choices to establish a pattern.

The answer choices are a mix of assessment/validation and implementation. Use the Nursing Process (Assessment vs. Implementation) strategy.

Step 2. Refer to the question to determine whether you should be assessing or implementing.

According to the question, the nurse has determined that the boy has a possible fracture. This implies that the nurse has completed the assessment step. It is now time to implement.

Step 3. Eliminate answer choices, and then choose the best answer.

Eliminate answers (2) and (4) because they are assessments. This leaves you with choices (1) and (3). Which takes priority: immobilizing the affected limb, or placing the boy in a semi-Fowler's position to facilitate breathing? The question does not indicate any respiratory distress. The correct answer is (1), immobilize the affected limb.

Some students will choose an answer involving the ABCs without thinking it through. Students, beware. Use the ABCs to establish priorities, but make sure that the answer is appropriate to the situation. In this question, breathing was mentioned in one of the answer choices. If you thought of the ABCs immediately without looking at the context of the question, you would have answered this question incorrectly.

Look at this question in another form.

> A boy was riding his bike to school when he hit the curb. The boy tells the school nurse, "I think my leg is broken." Which of the following actions is the *FIRST* action the nurse should take?
>
> 1. Immobilize the affected limb with a splint and ask the client not to move.
> 2. Ask the client to explain what happened.
> 3. Put the client in semi-Fowler's position to facilitate breathing.
> 4. Check the appearance of the client's leg.

In this question, the client has stated, "My leg is broken." This statement is not the nurse's assessment. This alerts the nurse that there is a problem, and the nurse should begin the steps of the nursing process. The first step is assessment, so eliminate answers (1) and (3); these are implementations. So what takes priority? Assessment of the leg takes priority over an assessment of what happened to cause the accident. The correct answer is (4).

Strategy Three: Safety

Nurses have the primary responsibility of ensuring the safety of clients. This includes clients in health care facilities, in the home, at work, and in the community. Safety includes: meeting basic needs (oxygen, food, fluids, etc.), reducing hazards that cause injury to clients (accidents, obstacles in the home), and decreasing the transmission of pathogens (immunizations, sanitation).

Remember that the NCLEX-RN® exam is a test of minimum competency to determine that you are able to practice safe and effective nursing care. Always think *safety* when selecting correct answers on the exam. When answering questions about procedures, this strategy will help you to establish priorities.

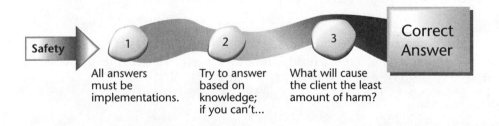

Step 1. Are all the answer choices implementations? If so, use the Safety strategy illustrated above.

Step 2. Can you answer the question based on your knowledge? If not, continue to Step 3.

Step 3. Ask yourself, "What will cause the client the least amount of harm?" and choose the best answer.

Apply this strategy to the following question.

> A child undergoes a tonsillectomy for treatment of chronic tonsillitis unresponsive to antibiotic therapy. After surgery, the child is brought to the recovery room. Which of the following actions should the nurse include in the child's plan of care?
>
> 1. Institute measures to minimize crying.
> 2. Perform postural drainage every 2 hours.
> 3. Cough and deep-breathe every hour.
> 4. Give ice cream as tolerated.

THE REWORDED QUESTION: What should you do after a tonsillectomy?

Step 1. Are all the answer choices implementations? Yes.

Step 2. Can you answer the question based on your knowledge of a tonsillectomy? If not, continue to Step 3.

Step 3. Ask yourself, "What will cause the client the least amount of harm?"

Answer choice (1), minimizing crying, will help prevent bleeding. Keep in consideration. Answer choice (2), postural drainage, may cause bleeding. Eliminate. Answer choice (3), coughing and deep-breathing, may cause bleeding. Eliminate. Answer choice (4), giving ice cream, may cause the child to clear his throat, causing bleeding. Eliminate. The correct answer is (1). The nurse must prevent postoperative hemorrhage, a complication seen after this type of surgery. Crying would irritate the child's throat and increase the chance of hemorrhage.

Let's try another question.

> A client is receiving intravenous cimetidine (Tagamet). After 20 minutes of the infusion, the client complains of a headache and dizziness. Which of the following actions should the nurse take *FIRST?*
>
> 1. Stop the infusion.
> 2. Take the client's vital signs.
> 3. Reposition the client.
> 4. Call the pharmacist.

THE REWORDED QUESTION: What should you do if a client is having side effects to a medication being administered?

Step 1. Are all answers implementations? Yes.

Step 2. Can you answer this question based on your knowledge? If not, proceed to Step 3.

Step 3. Ask yourself, "What will cause the client the least amount of harm?"

(1) Stopping the infusion would not harm the client. If the symptoms described are due to a side effect of the medication, this action would help the client. Retain this choice.

(2) Taking vital signs would not harm the client. Retain it for consideration.

(3) Repositioning the client would not harm the client, but would not help the client. Eliminate.

(4) Calling the pharmacist would not harm the client, but would not help him. Eliminate.

Choices (1) and (2) are left to consider. The infusion may be the cause of the client's reported symptoms. The client's vital signs can be taken after the infusion is stopped. Choice (1) is the correct answer.

Let's look at one more question.

> A client is admitted with a diagnosis of dementia. He attempts several times to pull out his nasogastric tube. An order for cloth wrist restraints is received by the nurse. Which of the following actions by the nurse is *MOST* appropriate?
>
> 1. Attach the ties of the restraints to the bed frame.
> 2. Perform range of motion to the restrained extremities once a shift.
> 3. Remove the restraints when the client is up in a wheelchair.
> 4. Explain the need for restraints only to the family because the client is confused.

THE REWORDED QUESTION: What is the safest way to apply restraints?

Step 1. Are all answers implementations? Yes.

Step 2. Can you answer based on your knowledge? If not, proceed to Step 3.

Step 3. Ask yourself, "What will cause the client the least amount of harm?"

(1) Attaching the restraint ties to the bed frame will not harm the client. Retain this answer.

(2) Performing range of motion once a shift will not harm the client. However, it should be performed more frequently. Retain this answer.

(3) Removing the restraints when the client is up in a wheelchair will be harmful to the client. Restraints should not be removed when the client is unattended. Eliminate.

(4) Explaining the need for restraints only to the family can cause harm to the client. Restraints can increase the confusion or combativeness of the client. Even though the client is confused, he needs to receive an explanation. Eliminate.

You are now considering answer choices (1) and (2). What will cause the least amount of harm to the client—attaching the ties of the restraint to the bed frame, or performing range of motion to the extremities once a shift? Range of motion should be performed every 2–4 hours to prevent loss of joint mobility. Eliminate (2). The correct answer is (1). Attaching the ties of the restraint to the bed frame will allow the nurse to raise and lower the side rail without injury to the client.

Priority questions are an important component of the NCLEX-RN® exam. To help you select correct answers, think:

- Maslow
- The Nursing Process
- Safety

Answer the following three questions using the appropriate priority strategy. The explanations follow the questions.

Question 1

The nurse cares for a client with a diagnosis of cerebrovascular accident (CVA). The nurse is feeding the client in a chair when he suddenly begins to choke. Which of the following actions should the nurse take *FIRST?*

1. Check for breathlessness by placing an ear over the client's mouth and observing the chest.
2. Leave the client in the chair and apply vigorous abdominal or chest thrusts from behind the client.
3. Ask the client, "Are you choking?"
4. Return the client to the bed and apply vigorous abdominal or chest thrusts while straddling the client's thighs.

Question 2

A client with a history of bipolar disorder is admitted to the psychiatric hospital. She was found by the police attempting to climb onto the wing of a plane at the airport. Her husband reports that she has not eaten or slept in 2 days, and he suspects she has stopped taking lithium. On admission, the nurse should place the *HIGHEST* priority on which of the following client care needs?

1. Teaching the client about the importance of taking lithium as prescribed
2. Providing the client with a safe environment with few distractions
3. Arranging for food and rest for the client
4. Setting limits on the client's behavior

Question 3

> The physician orders a nasogastric (NG) tube inserted and connected to low intermittent suction for a client with an intestinal obstruction. Two hours after insertion of the NG tube, the client vomits 200 mL. While irrigating the NG tube, the nurse notes resistance. Which of the following actions should the nurse take FIRST?
>
> 1. Replace the NG tube with a larger one.
> 2. Turn the client on his left side.
> 3. Change the suction from intermittent to continuous.
> 4. Continue the irrigation.

Let's see if you were able to correctly identify which strategy you should use to determine priorities.

Question 1

The answer choices include both assessments and implementations. Use the Nursing Process strategy to select the correct answer.

Step 1. Read the answer choices to establish a pattern.

Choices (1) and (3) are assessments; choices (2) and (4) are implementations.

Step 2. Refer to the question to determine whether you should be assessing or implementing. According to the situation, the client has begun to choke. This alerts the nurse that there is a problem. The first step of the nursing process is to assess.

Step 3. Eliminate answer choices, and then choose the best answer.

Eliminate answer choices (2) and (4) because they are implementations. Now choose the best answer from the remaining answer choices, (1) and (3).

What takes priority—assessing for breathlessness by placing an ear over the client's mouth, or assessing the client by asking, "Are you choking?" Inability to speak or cough indicates the airway is obstructed. Breathlessness should be checked only in an unconscious client. The correct answer is (3).

Question 2

Look at the answer choices. They include both physiological and psychosocial interventions. Apply the Maslow strategy.

Step 1. Look at the answer choices and identify which are physiological—choices (2) and (3)—and which are psychosocial—choices (1) and (4).

Step 2. Eliminate all psychosocial answer choices—(1) and (4).

Step 3. Ask yourself if the remaining answer choices make sense. Choice (2), providing the client with a safe environment, does make sense. Retain this answer. Choice (3), arranging for food and rest, also makes sense. Retain this answer.

Step 4. Can you apply the ABCs to the remaining answer choices? No; neither choice refers to airway, breathing, or circulation. Since the ABCs don't apply, ask yourself "What is the highest priority—providing for a safe environment, or providing for food and rest?" According to Maslow, food and rest take highest priority. The correct answer is (3).

Question 3

This question is about a procedure: What should the nurse do when resistance is met while irrigating an NG tube? If you are unsure about a procedure, think *safety*.

Step 1. Are all the answer choices implementations? Yes.

Step 2. Can you answer the question based on your knowledge? If not, continue to Step 3.

Step 3. Ask yourself, "What will cause the client the least amount of harm?"

(1) Replacing the nasogastric tube with a larger one could harm the client by damaging the mucosa. Eliminate.

(2) Turning the client to his left side would not hurt the client. Retain this answer.

(3) Changing the suction from intermittent to continuous is never done because it will erode the mucosa. Eliminate.

(4) Continuing the irrigation when there is resistance might be harmful. Never force an irrigation. Eliminate.

The correct answer is (2). The tip of the tube may be against the stomach wall. Repositioning the client might allow the tip to lay unobstructed in the stomach.

Using these critical thinking strategies will help you unlock the secrets of correctly answering priority questions. Now let's look at some strategies for answering another type of question, Management of Care.

STRATEGIES FOR MANAGEMENT OF CARE QUESTIONS

Every three years, the National Council conducts a job analysis study to determine the activities required of a newly licensed registered nurse. Based on this study, the National Council adjusts the content of the test to accurately reflect what is happening in the workplace. This ensures that the NCLEX-RN® exam tests what is needed to be a safe and effective nurse.

The role of the nurse has expanded in today's health care environment. In addition to providing quality client care, the nurse is also responsible for coordination and supervision of care provided by other health care workers. Many health care settings are staffed by registered nurses, licensed practical nurses/licensed vocational nurses (LPN/LVN), and nursing assistive personnel (NAPs) such as nursing assistants and support staff. It is the responsibility of the registered nurse to coordinate the efforts of these health care workers to provide affordable quality client care. Appropriate supervision of LPN/LVN and/or NAPs by the registered professional nurse is essential for safe and effective client care.

To reflect these changes, the NCLEX-RN® exam contains questions about delegation and assignment of client care. There are several reasons why you may find these questions difficult to answer correctly on the NCLEX-RN® exam:

- Many nursing schools test the content presented in the management course with essay questions rather than multiple-choice questions.
- You may have received lectures regarding management of care, but your clinical rotation in management may have been less than ideal. Regardless, do not choose answers based on decisions you may have observed during your clinical experience in the hospital or clinic setting. Remember, the NCLEX-RN® exam is ivory-tower nursing. Always ask yourself, "Is this textbook nursing care?"
- Your experience may have been restricted to caring for one or two clients without any opportunity to supervise others, or you may have spent time on a hospital unit providing client care under the supervision of a preceptor.

Even if you have no direct experience in these areas, the Rules of Management will get you through the test. They will help you choose more right answers when answering management questions on the NCLEX-RN® exam.

The Rules of Management

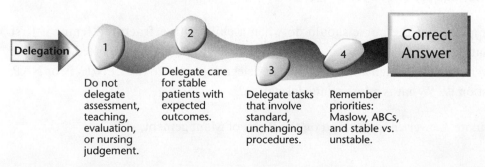

Rule #1: Do not delegate the functions of assessment, evaluation, and nursing judgment.

During your nursing education, you learned that assessment, evaluation, and nursing judgment are the responsibility of the registered professional nurse. You *cannot* give this responsibility to someone else.

Rule #2: Delegate activities for stable clients with predictable outcomes.

If the client is unstable, or the outcome of an activity not assured, it should not be delegated.

Rule #3: Delegate activities that involve standard, unchanging procedures.

Activities that frequently reoccur in daily client care can be delegated. Bathing, feeding, dressing, and transferring clients are examples. Activities that are complex or complicated should not be delegated.

Rule #4: Remember priorities!

Remember Maslow, the ABCs, and "stable versus unstable" when determining which client the RN should attend to first. Keep in the mind that you can see only one client or perform one activity when answering questions that require you to establish priorities.

Let's use the Rules of Management to eliminate answer choices in exam-like Management of Care questions.

> A child with a compound fracture of the left femur is being admitted to a pediatric unit. Which of the following actions is *BEST* for the nurse to take?
>
> 1. Ask the NAP to obtain the child's vital signs while the nurse obtains a history from the parents.
> 2. Ask the LPN/LVN to assess the peripheral pulses of the child's left leg while the nurse completes the admission forms.
> 3. Ask the LPN/LVN to stay with the child and his parents while the nurse obtains phone orders from the physician.
> 4. Ask the NAP to obtain equipment for the child's care while the nurse talks with the child and his parents.

Step 1. Reword the question in your own words.

The question asks what the nurse should do when a child with a fractured femur is first admitted. That question is very broad. To establish *exactly* what is being asked, you must read the answer choices. In each answer, the RN is delegating tasks to the LPN/LVN or NAP. The real question is, "What is appropriate delegation?"

Step 2. Eliminate answer choices based on the Rules of Management.

(1) Obtaining vital signs is an important part of assessment. According to Rule #1, the registered nurse cannot delegate assessment. Eliminate this answer choice.

(2) Checking the peripheral pulses is an important assessment for this client because of the diagnosis of a fractured left femur. The nurse needs to assess the client before delegating activities to someone else. Assessment of the client is much more important than completing paperwork. Eliminate.

(3) There is no assessment, evaluation, or nursing judgment involved in this option, so leave it in for consideration.

(4) The nurse is with the child and his parents while the NAP obtains needed equipment. There is no assessment, evaluation, or nursing judgment when gathering equipment, so leave this choice in for consideration.

Step 3. Select an answer from the remaining choices.

You are left with answer choices (3) and (4). You are halfway to the correct answer!

Answer (3) indicates that the nurse is on the phone and the LPN/LVN is with the client. Have you seen this done in the real world? Probably. Is this what nursing textbooks and journals say should be done in this situation? Probably not. Eliminate this answer. Remember, on the NCLEX-RN® exam, emphasis is placed on providing care to clients according to how nursing care is defined in textbooks and journals.

The correct answer is (4). The nurse is caring for the child and his parents while delegating tasks to nursing assistive personnel.

Let's look at another Management of Care question.

> **Which of the following tasks is appropriate for the nurse to delegate to an experienced NAP?**
>
> 1. Obtain a 24-hour diet recall from a client recently admitted with anorexia nervosa.
> 2. Obtain a clean-catch urine specimen from a client suspected of having a urinary tract infection.
> 3. Observe the amount and characteristics of the returns from a continuous bladder irrigation for a client after a transurethral resection.
> 4. Observe a client newly diagnosed with diabetes mellitus practice injection techniques using an orange.

Step 1. Reword the question.

"What task will you assign to an NAP?" The fact that the NAP is "experienced" is a distracter.

Step 2. Eliminate answer choices based on the Rules of Management.

(1) Obtain 24-hour diet recall from a client with anorexia nervosa. Some students may consider this answer choice because eating is certainly a recurring daily activity, but this answer isn't about feeding a client. Eating has special significance for a client with anorexia nervosa. An important assessment that the nurse must make is the quantity of food consumed by this client. The nurse cannot delegate assessment. Eliminate.

(2) Obtain a clean-catch urine specimen from a client with suspected UTI. Rule #4 states, "Delegate activities that involve standard, unchanging procedures." There is no indication that the client has a catheter, so this is a routine procedure. Keep for consideration.

(3) Observe bladder irrigation returns after a transurethral resection. The color of the fluid needs to be assessed to determine if hemorrhage is occurring. This is an assessment. Eliminate.

(4) Observe a newly diagnosed DM client practicing injection techniques. This answer choice involves the evaluation of client teaching. According to Rule #1, the nurse cannot delegate evaluation of client care. Eliminate.

Step 3. Select an answer from the remaining choices.

That leaves only answer choice (2), the correct answer.

Let's look at one more question.

> Which of the following clients should the nurse on a pediatric unit assign to an LPN/LVN?
>
> 1. A 3-year-old girl admitted yesterday with laryngotracheobronchitis who has a tracheostomy
> 2. A 5-year-old girl admitted after gastric lavage for Tylenol ingestion
> 3. A 6-year-old boy admitted for a fracture of the femur, in balanced suspension traction
> 4. A 10-year-old boy admitted for observation after an acute asthmatic attack

Step 1. Reword the question.

The question is asking for the appropriate assignment for an LPN/LVN.

Step 2. Eliminate answer choices based on the Rules of Management.

After reading the answer choices, you may have already seen that Rule #3 (Delegate activities for stable clients with predictable outcomes) will be particularly helpful.

(1) Ask yourself, is this a stable client with a predictable outcome? A 3 year-old with a new tracheostomy is not stable or predictable. Eliminate this answer choice.

(2) This child may be unstable and the outcome of a poisoning is unpredictable. Eliminate this answer choice.

(3) This child has a problem that has a predictable outcome. No information is provided in the choice to lead you to believe that this child is unstable at this time. Keep this answer choice in consideration.

(4) Because of the narrow airway of a child, this child may be unstable and the outcome is unpredictable. Eliminate this answer choice.

Step 3. Select an answer from the remaining choices.

Answer choice (3) is the correct answer.

STRATEGIES FOR POSITIONING QUESTIONS

Because many illnesses affect body alignment and mobility, you must be able to safely care for these clients in order to be an effective nurse. These topics are also important on the NCLEX-RN® exam. The successful test taker must correctly answer questions about impaired mobility and positioning.

Immobility occurs when a client is unable to move about freely and independently. To answer questions on positioning, you need to know the hazards of immobility, normal anatomy and physiology, and the terminology for positioning.

Many graduate nurses are not comfortable answering these questions because:

- They don't understand the "whys" of positioning.
- They don't know the terminology.
- They have difficulty imagining the various positions.

If you have difficulty answering positioning questions, the following strategy will assist you in selecting the correct answer.

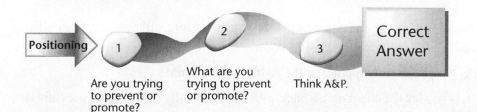

Step 1. Decide if the position for the client is designed to prevent something or promote something.

Step 2. Identify what it is you are trying to prevent or promote.

Step 3. Think about anatomy, physiology, and pathophysiology ("A & P").

Step 4. Which position best accomplishes what you are trying to prevent or promote?

Does this sound a little confusing? Hang in there. Let's walk through a question using this strategy.

> **Immediately after a percutaneous liver biopsy, the nurse should place the client in which of the following positions?**
>
> 1. Supine
> 2. Right side-lying
> 3. Left side-lying
> 4. Semi-Fowler's

Before you read the answers, let's go through the four steps outlined above.

Step 1. By positioning the client after a liver biopsy, are you trying to prevent something or promote something? Think about what you know about a liver biopsy. You position a client after this procedure to prevent something.

Step 2. What are you trying to prevent? The most serious and important complication after a percutaneous liver biopsy is hemorrhage.

Step 3. Think about the principles of anatomy, physiology, and pathophysiology. What do you do to prevent hemorrhage? You apply pressure. Where would you apply pressure? On the liver. Where is the liver? On the right side of the abdomen under the ribs.

Step 4. How should the client be positioned to prevent hemorrhage from the liver, which is on the right side of the body? Look at your answer choices.

(1) Supine. If you lay the client flat on his back, no pressure will be applied to the right side. Eliminate.

(2) Right side-lying. If you lay the client in a right side-lying position, will pressure be applied to the right side? Yes. Keep it in for consideration.

(3) Left side-lying. No pressure is applied to the right side. Eliminate.

(4) Semi-Fowler's. If you lay the client on his back with head partially elevated, no pressure is applied to the right side. Eliminate.

The correct answer is (2). Some students select (3) because they don't know normal anatomy and physiology. Some students select (4) because semi-Fowler's position is used for a lot of reasons.

Things to Remember

- Even if you didn't memorize what position to use before, during, and after a procedure, think about the question for a moment. You can figure out what position is needed.

- You cannot figure out the correct position if you do not know what the terms (such as supine or Fowler's) mean.

- You cannot figure out a correct position if you do not know anatomy and physiology. If you think the liver is on the left side of the body, you are in trouble!

- You cannot figure out a correct position if you do not know what you are trying to accomplish. If you couldn't remember that a complication after a liver biopsy is hemorrhage, you will simply be taking a random guess at the correct answer.

- If you think in images, you should form a mental image of each position. Picture yourself placing the client in each position, and then see if the position makes sense.

Let's try another question using the strategies for positioning.

> An angiogram is scheduled for a client with decreased circulation in her right leg. After the angiogram, the nurse should place the client in which of the following positions?
>
> 1. Semi-Fowler's with right leg bent at the knee
> 2. Side-lying with a pillow between the knees
> 3. Supine with right leg extended
> 4. High Fowler's with right leg elevated

Let's go through the steps.

Step 1. By positioning the client after an angiogram, are you trying to prevent something or promote something? You are trying to promote something.

Step 2. What are you trying to promote? Adequate circulation of the right leg.

Step 3. Think about the principles of anatomy, physiology, and pathophysiology. What promotes adequate circulation in the right leg? Keeping the leg at or below the level of the heart so blood flow is not constricted.

Step 4. How will the client be positioned after an angiography to prevent constriction of vessels and keep the right leg at or below the level of the heart? Look at the answer choices.

(1) "Semi-Fowler's with the right leg bent at the knee." The head of the bed is elevated 30–45 degrees in this position. The leg is lower than the heart. If the right leg is bent at the knee, this could constrict arterial blood flow. Eliminate.

(2) "Side-lying with a pillow between the knees." Use of a pillow in this position could create pressure points in the right leg. You don't want the knees bent. Eliminate.

(3) "Supine with the right leg extended." In this position, the leg is at the level of the heart. Circulation will not be constricted because the leg is straight. Keep for consideration.

(4) "High Fowler's with her right leg elevated." The head of the bed is elevated 60–90 degrees in this position. Elevating the leg promotes venous return. Eliminate.

The correct answer is (3). The client is on bed rest for 8–12 hours in a supine position after an angiogram.

If you didn't know the specific positioning needed after an angiogram, you can apply your knowledge to select the correct answer by just thinking about it.

Let's look at another question.

> The nurse cares for a client after a lumbar laminectomy. Which of the following statements *BEST* describes the method of turning a client following a lumbar laminectomy?
>
> 1. The head of the bed is elevated 30 degrees; the client locks her knees when turning.
> 2. A pillow is placed between the client's legs; her body is turned as a unit.
> 3. The client straightens her back and grasps the side rail on the opposite side of the bed.
> 4. The head of the bed is flat; the client bends her knees and rolls to the side.

This question isn't about positioning after a procedure. It asks how to turn the client after surgery.

Step 1. When turning the client after a laminectomy, are you trying to prevent or promote something? Promote.

Step 2. What are you trying to promote? A straight back. The client can't bend or twist the torso.

Step 3. Think about the principles of anatomy, physiology, and pathophysiology. A laminectomy is removal of one or more vertebral laminae. After a laminectomy, the back should be kept straight.

Step 4. How should the client be turned in order to keep the back straight?

(1) If the head of the bed is elevated 30 degrees, the back will not be straight. Eliminate.

(2) If a pillow is placed between the legs and the body is rolled as a unit, the client's back will be kept straight. Keep in for consideration.

(3) If the client grabs the opposite side rail, the client's torso will twist. The back will not be straight even though the client straightened her back before turning and twisting. Eliminate.

(4) If the head of the bed is flat, the client's back will be straight. If the client bends her knees and rolls to her side, her back will not be kept straight. Eliminate.

The correct answer is (2). That is a textbook description of log-rolling. But if you didn't recall log-rolling, you were able to select the correct answers by thoughtfully considering each answer choice.

Sometimes a positioning question will be difficult to identify, such as in the following example.

> The nurse cares for a client after an appendectomy. The client continues to complain of discomfort to the nurse shortly after receiving an analgesic. Which of the following measures by the nurse would be *MOST* appropriate?
>
> 1. Notify the physician.
> 2. Place the client in Fowler's position.
> 3. Massage his abdomen.
> 4. Provide him with reading material.

As you can see, not all of the answer choices involve positioning! How should you approach this question?

First, reword the question so you know what to focus on in the answer choices. The question really being asked is, "What should the nurse do to help this client with pain relief?" Let's look at the answer choices.

(1) Calling the doctor, as you know, is almost never the right answer. See if another answer choice is more appropriate.

(2) Fowler's position. Why change this client's position? To promote pain relief. Will Fowler's position decrease the client's pain? Yes, by relieving pressure on the client's abdomen. This answer is a possibility.

(3) Massaging his abdomen will increase the client's pain. Eliminate.

(4) Providing him with reading materials might distract him from his discomfort, but this is not an appropriate intervention for a client in pain. Eliminate.

The correct answer is (2).

Positioning is an important part of the NCLEX-RN® exam. You must be able to answer these questions correctly in order to prove your competence. If you use the strategies just discussed, you will be thinking about nursing principles and you will select correct answers!

Essential Positions to Know for the NCLEX-RN® Exam

POSITION	THERAPEUTIC FUNCTION
Flat (supine)	Avoids hip flexion, which can compress arterial flow
Dorsal recumbent	Supine with knees flexed; more comfortable
Side lateral	Allows drainage of oral secretions
Side with leg bent (Sims')	Allows drainage of oral secretions; used for rectal exam
Head elevated (Fowler's) • High Fowler's: 80–90 degrees • Fowler's: 45–60 degrees • Semi-Fowler's: 30–45 degrees • Low Fowler's: 15–30 degrees	Increases venous return; allows maximal lung expansion
Feet and leg elevated	Increases blood return to heart
Feet elevated and head lowered (Trendelenburg)	Used to insert central venous pressure (CVP) line, or for treatment of umbilical cord compression
Feet elevated 20 degrees, knees straight, trunk flat, and head slightly elevated (modified Trendelenburg)	Increases venous return; used for shock; may be used to prevent shock
Elevation of extremity	Increases venous return; decreases blood volume to extremity
Flat on back, thighs flexed, legs abducted (lithotomy)	Increases vaginal opening for examination
Prone	Promotes extension of hip joint; not well tolerated by persons with respiratory or cardiovascular difficulties
Knee-chest	Provides maximal visualization of rectal area

STRATEGIES FOR COMMUNICATION QUESTIONS

Communication is emphasized on the NCLEX-RN® exam because it is critical to your success as a beginning practitioner. Therapeutic communication means listening to and understanding the client while promoting clarification and insight. It enables the nurse to form a working relationship with both the client and the health care team, using both verbal and nonverbal communication. Remember that nonverbal communication is the most accurate reflection of attitude. Therapeutic responses include the following:

RESPONSE	GOAL/PURPOSE
Using silence	Allows the client time to think and reflect; conveys acceptance. Allows the client to take the lead in conversation.
Using general leads or broad opening	Encourages the client to talk. Indicates your interest in the client. Allows the client to choose the subject.
Clarification	Encourages recall and details of a particular experience. Encourages description of feelings. Seeks explanation; pinpoints specifics.
Reflecting	Paraphrases what client says. Reflects on what client says, especially the feelings conveyed.

There are many questions on the NCLEX-RN® exam that require you to select the correct therapeutic communication response. As with other NCLEX-RN® exam questions, one of the biggest errors that test takers commit when trying to answer this type of question is to look for the correct answer. Remember, you are selecting the *best* answer from the four possible answers that you are given.

To select the best answer, you must eliminate answer choices. Let's look at some different answer choices you can eliminate:

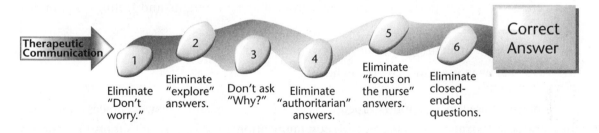

- **"Don't worry" answers:** Eliminate answer choices that offer false reassurance. These type of responses discourage communication between the nurse and the client by not allowing the client to explore his or her own ideas and feelings. False reassurance also discounts what the client is feeling. Examples include:
  - "It's going to be OK."
  - "Don't worry. Your doctors will do everything necessary for your care."

- **"Let's explore" answers:** Another incorrect answer choice that many graduate nurses select is the choice that includes the word "explore." On the NCLEX-RN® exam, avoid being a junior psychiatrist. It isn't the nurse's role to delve into the reasons why the client is feeling a particular way. The client must be allowed to verbalize the fact that he or she is sad, angry, fearful, or overwhelmed. Examples include:
  - "Let's talk about why you didn't take your medication."
  - "Tell me why you really injured yourself."

- **"Why" questions:** Eliminate answer choices that include "why" questions: ones that seek reasons or justification. "Why" questions imply disapproval of the client, who may become defensive. A "why" question can come in many forms, and need not always begin with "why." Any response that puts the client on the defensive is nontherapeutic and therefore incorrect. Examples include:
  - "What makes you think that?"
  - "Why do you feel this way?"

- **Authoritarian answers:** Eliminate answer choices in which the nurse is telling the client what to do without regard for the client's desires or feelings. Examples include:
  - Insisting that the client follow unit rules
  - Insisting that the client do what you command immediately

- **Nurse-focused answers:** Eliminate answer choices in which the focus of the comment is on the nurse. Be careful, because these answer choices may sound very empathetic. The focus of your communication should always be on the client. Examples include:
  - "That happened to me once."
  - "I know from experience this is hard for you."

- **Closed-ended questions:** Eliminate answer choices that include closed-ended questions that can be answered with the words yes, no, or another monosyllabic response. Closed-ended questions discourage the client from sharing thoughts and feelings. Examples include:
  - "Are you feeling guilty about what happened?"
  - "How many children do you have?"

Eliminating these types of nontherapeutic responses that appear as answer choices is an effective strategy when answering therapeutic communication questions. Don't simply look for the specific words that you see here; you may need to "translate" the answer choices into the above errors of therapeutic communication.

So how do you select the correct response? By choosing from the answer choices that are left! The correct response will usually contain one or both of the following elements:

- **Gives correct information:** Offering information encourages further communication from the client. Examples of giving correct information include:
  - "You are experiencing acute alcohol withdrawal; you may see and feel things that aren't real."
  - "There are many reasons for memory loss; tell me more about what you have noticed."

- **Is empathetic and reflects the client's feelings:** *Empathy* is the ability to perceive what another person experiences using that person's frame of reference. *Reflection* communicates to the client that the nurse has heard and understands what the client is trying to communicate. When reflecting feelings, the nurse focuses on the feelings and not the content of what is said. The following are examples of empathetic, reflective statements include:

  - "I can see that you are frightened about being here."

  - "You seem very upset. Tell me how you're feeling."

Let's practice therapeutic communication with a few exam-style questions.

A client is admitted to the emergency room with a diagnosis of acute myocardial infarction. The client tells the nurse, "I'm scared. I think I'm going to die." Which of the following responses by the nurse would be *MOST* appropriate?

1. "Everything is going to be fine. We'll take good care of you."
2. "I know what you mean. I thought I was having a heart attack once."
3. "I'll call your doctor so you can discuss it with him."
4. "It's normal to feel frightened. We're doing everything we can for you."

Step 1. Eliminate incorrect answer choices.

(1) This is a "don't worry" response. There is no acknowledgment of the client's fears. Eliminate.

(2) The focus of this response is on the nurse, not the client. Eliminate.

(3) It is within the scope of nursing practice for the nurse to respond to the client's feelings. Don't pass the responsibility to the physician. Eliminate.

(4) This answer choice responds to feelings and provides information. Keep it in consideration.

Step 2. Select an answer from the remaining choices.

One answer was not eliminated: (4). This is the correct answer. The nurse is empathetic, acknowledging that the client feels frightened, and provides information.

Let's look at another question.

> A mother is to undergo a breast biopsy. She tells the nurse, "If lose my breast, I know my husband will no longer find me attractive." Which of the following responses by the nurse would be *MOST* appropriate?
>
> 1. "You don't know if you are going to lose your breast. They are just doing the biopsy now."
> 2. "You should focus on your children. They are young and they need you."
> 3. "You seem to be concerned that your relationship with your husband might change."
> 4. "Why don't you wait and see what your husband's reaction is before you get upset."

Step 1. Eliminate answer choices.

(1) This response gives false reassurance and discounts the client's feelings. Eliminate it.

(2) This response is authoritarian: the nurse tells the client what to do. Eliminate it.

(3) This response reflects the fears of the client. The response is open-ended and allows the client to express what she is feeling. Keep it in for consideration.

(4) This response dismisses the feelings that the client is experiencing and gives advice. Eliminate it.

Step 2. Select an answer from the remaining choices.

You have eliminated three of the four answer choices. The correct answer is the only answer choice remaining, (3).

Let's look at one more question.

> A client in the psychiatric unit asks the nurse, "Am I in a special radioactive shelter? When was it last checked for radioactivity?" Which of the following responses by the nurse would be *MOST* appropriate?
>
> 1. "This is a hospital, and we do not have a Nuclear Medicine Department here."
> 2. "Don't worry, you're safe. There's no radioactivity here."
> 3. "I'm sure your safety is of concern to you, but this is a hospital."
> 4. "Please share with me what makes you think there is radioactivity here."

Step 1. Eliminate answer choices.

(1) This response provides information. Leave it in for consideration.

(2) This response offers false reassurances. Eliminate it.

(3) This response reflects the client's concern about safety and provides information. Keep it in for consideration.

(4) This response allows the client to verbalize, but you don't want to encourage a client with psychological problems to talk about hallucinations or delusions. Rather, you want your discussion to focus on the feelings that accompany them. Eliminate this choice.

Step 2. Select an answer from the remaining choices.

You have more than one possible answer choice: (1) and (3). Look for the answer choice that reflects feelings and gives information. The correct answer is (3).

YOUR NCLEX-RN® EXAM STUDY PLAN

Now that you've read about the various Kaplan test-taking strategies, you are probably thinking, "Wow! This is great!" Most of you have started identifying why you are having difficulty answering application/analysis-level test questions. Some of you have already formulated a plan to master your NCLEX-RN® exam questions using the strategies outlined in this book, and are confident that you will pass the exam. Others are thinking, "This sounds great, but can I really answer questions using these strategies?"

The authors of this book work for Kaplan, the oldest test prep company in the nation. We have been preparing graduate nurses and international nurses for the NCLEX-RN® exam for more than 25 years. We know what works to prepare for the exam and what doesn't work.

Ineffective Ways to Prepare

Here are a few of the biggest mistakes some NCLEX-RN® exam test takers make before Test Day.

Relying on False Hopes

Some students use what is known as the "hope" method of study. "I hope that I don't have questions about chest tubes on the test." "I hope that I don't have questions about medication on my test." "I hope that I have questions about ABGs because I did great on that test in school." The "hope" method usually doesn't work very well. The test pool contains thousands of questions. How many topics do you "hope" won't be on your test?

Lacking Respect for the Exam

Many candidates for the NCLEX-RN® exam are good students in school. Because of their school success, they expect to pass the exam with minimal preparation. After all, it's just a test of minimum competency. These students do some studying, but they really believe there is no chance they might fail this exam. You might think that you can't possibly fail, but if you do not respect this exam and prepare for it correctly, you run the risk of failure.

All students know why they take the NCLEX-RN® exam. However, after interviewing hundreds of students, we have discovered that many graduate nurses have no idea what the exam content is. How can you effectively study for a test if you don't know what content the exam tests? Learn what is on the NCLEX-RN® exam, and then you will realize that preparation with a review course or a planned method of study is essential.

Cramming

Some students completed nursing school with a minimal understanding of nursing content. These students studied long and hard on the night before a nursing school test, cramming as many facts into their heads as they could remember. Because the test questions primarily involved recognition and recall, cramming worked for tests in nursing school. But as we said earlier, the NCLEX-RN® exam is not an exam about facts. It tests your ability to apply the knowledge that you have learned and to think critically. Recognition and recall will not work!

Poor Planning

As with all standardized exams, you must work on your areas of weaknesses. This is hard to do because there's usually a reason you're weak in an area. Some graduate nurses, for example, profess a weakness in or dislike for obstetrical nursing. Some students didn't understand the theory, while other students had a poor clinical experience or didn't get to see many deliveries; still other students simply didn't like this rotation. Whatever the reason, it causes them to have a weakness in this particular area. In order to pass a standardized test, you must work on your areas of weakness.

Some students don't establish a plan of study. Other students establish a plan of study but don't follow it. You can enroll in a review course or buy review books, but if you don't apply yourself, they will do you no good.

Effective Methods of Preparation

To pass the NCLEX-RN® exam, you not only need to know nursing content, you also need to be able to apply the critical thinking skills we've just reviewed. Next, you need to be an expert on the content of the exam. What topics are usually included on the NCLEX-RN® exam? How is the content organized? And finally, you need to create a study plan, and make sure that you are able to cope with the testing experience.

So let's start by talking about some of the issues that you may be asking yourself.

Question: "I'm terrible at standardized tests. Is this really going to help me?"

Answer: Yes, these strategies will help you choose more correct responses when you take the NCLEX-RN® exam. Read this book—more than once if necessary—to review the content being tested on the exam and learn the strategies. Then practice, practice, practice. Use the strategies to answer many, many practice test questions, and you will find yourself answering more and more questions correctly. Tear out the Chart of Critical Thinking Paths in Appendix A and consult it while you are answering practice test questions. This will help you become more comfortable with putting the strategies into practice. As you answer more and more questions, put the diagram aside and rely on your memory to identify and implement a critical thinking strategy.

Question: "Am I going to have enough time when I take the NCLEX-RN® exam to figure out which strategy to use?"

Answer: Timing is a concern on the NCLEX-RN® exam. You need to maximize your efforts on each test question. Practice answering test questions using the various strategies we've outlined. As you get more proficient, you will discover that it takes you less time to identify the strategy or path that will lead you to the correct answer.

Question: "I don't have to use these strategies on every question, do I? I think I'll use them only when I can't figure out the correct answer on my own."

Answer: Wrong! You should use critical thinking to answer every question on the NCLEX-RN® exam to make sure that you pass. Go through the steps that we have outlined for every practice question that you answer as you prepare for the exam. If you practice these steps, you will not need to randomly guess the correct answer on the NCLEX-RN® exam.

Question: "So all I have to do is memorize the strategies, right?"

Answer: Just memorizing the various strategies will not ensure your success on the NCLEX-RN® exam. Remember, the exam does not test your ability to memorize either critical thinking strategies or nursing content. The NCLEX-RN® exam tests your ability to think critically and use the nursing knowledge that you have. It's relatively easy to just memorize nursing content. The hard part is to figure out how to use this knowledge to make nursing judgments. It's relatively easy to memorize the critical thinking strategies. The hard part is to figure out which strategy to use on each and every question. That takes practice.

Question: "What if I use the strategies but still can't figure out the correct answer?"

Answer: It's not unusual that students will read a question, read the answers, and think "Huh? Something is missing!" If you feel like something is missing, reread the question to determine if you have correctly identified what the question is asking. If you have identified the question correctly, then read the answer choices to make sure you haven't missed the nursing concept contained in the answer choices.

Question: "Will these strategies work on every practice question that I answer?"

Answer: The critical thinking strategies discussed in this book will enable you to answer all kinds of multiple-choice test questions. The critical thinking strategies apply to test questions written at the application/analysis level and do not work with knowledge-based test questions. If you feel that the strategies don't work with the practice questions you are answering, determine the level of difficulty of the questions you are working with. Are the practice questions knowledge-based, or are they at the application/analysis level of difficulty? Remember, the majority of questions that are of a passing level of difficulty on the NCLEX-RN® exam are at the application/analysis level of difficulty.

It's time for you to start your successful preparation for the NCLEX-RN® exam! Begin by identifying your strengths and weaknesses, as follows:

- Take as many diagnostic exams as you can.
- Identify your weaknesses in nursing content.
- Identify your weaknesses in test-taking skills.

Next, decide if you need to take a review course. If you decide that this is the best way for you to prepare, ask yourself these questions:

- Is the course mainly a review of nursing content or memory techniques? This type of review won't help you put it all together on Test Day. You can know everything about heart failure, but if you don't know how to use this information to answer a question about heart failure correctly on the NCLEX-RN® exam, you will have difficulty on the exam. Are the strategies specific for the NCLEX-RN® exam?

- Are there plenty of opportunities for practice testing? You need to prove your competence by answering NCLEX-RN® exam-style test questions, so you should practice answering these questions. If the exam were about opening a sterile pack, what would you spend your time doing to prepare for the exam? Reading about opening a sterile pack or practicing opening a sterile pack? Are there exam-style questions included in the course? Do the questions require recall and recognition of facts or application of nursing care principles? Remember, your NCLEX-RN® exam will consist mainly of application-level questions.

- What do students who have taken the course have to say about how it helped them prepare for the exam? If a review course boasts of a particularly high pass rate, ask to see their statistics. Be an informed consumer.

- Is there a guarantee? There are guarantees and there are empty promises. Make sure the course you are considering puts the guarantee in writing. Study the small print. Is your total tuition refunded? Do you have to fail the exam more than once?

- How much does it cost? This sounds easy, but "extras" can add up. Are there additional charges for books? Software? Registration fees?

- Is this course right for me?

And finally, create a realistic study schedule that works for you. Then make a vow to stick to that plan and reward yourself when you do. Spend at least 3 weeks before your exam date preparing. Don't cram! Your content focus should be in understanding the principles of nursing care, not memorizing facts.

Stay away from people who are "prophets of doom." You know the type. With the proper preparation you can and will pass the NCLEX-RN® exam. Keep a positive attitude.

You may need to consider some techniques for battling stress and managing the test day experience. Do any of these statements apply to you?

> *"I always freeze up on tests."*
>
> *"I need to pass to get my new job/promotion/commission."*
>
> *"My best friend/girlfriend/sister/brother did really well, but I won't."*
>
> *"My hospital/family/parents paid for my test prep course. They won't like it if I fail."*
>
> *"I'm afraid of losing concentration."*
>
> *"I'm afraid I'm not spending enough time preparing."*

If these sound familiar, you may want to mentally prepare yourself by understanding ways to manage test stress. Forcing yourself to identify and face fears may make you edgy at first, but will significantly alleviate test stress in the long run by adding another dimension to your preparation.

Mental Preparation*

1. Visualize

You have probably learned how to do this with clients; now it's your turn. Sit back and let your shoulders and arms relax. Close your eyes and imagine yourself in a relaxing situation—it can be fictional, but a real-life memory is best. Make it as detailed as possible. Think about the sights, the sounds, the smells, even the tastes that you associate with the relaxing situation. Keep your eyes shut; keep sinking back into your chair. Now that you're in that situation, start bringing your test in—think about the experience of taking the test while *in* that relaxing situation. Imagine how much easier it would be if you could take your test in that situation. Notice how much easier your test seems in that situation.

Here's another variation. Close your eyes and think about a situation in which you did well on a test. If you can't come up with one, pick a situation in which you did some good academic work that you were really proud of, or some other kind of genuine accomplishment. Not a fiction, mind you: it has to be from real life. Make it as detailed as possible. Think about the sights, the sounds, the smells, and even the tastes that you associate with this experience of academic success. Now think about your test in line with that experience. Don't make comparisons between them. Just imagine taking your test with that same feeling of relaxed control.

---

* Some of these methods were originally conceptualized by Dr. Émile Coué, who in the 1920s told everyone that the key to a happy life was to constantly repeat the phrase, "Every day in every way I am getting better and better." As advice to test takers, that isn't bad at all!

2. Exercise

Whether it be jogging, walking, yoga, push-ups, or a pickup basketball game, physical exercise is a great way to stimulate the mind and body and improve one's ability to think and concentrate. A surprising number of those who prepare for standardized tests don't exercise regularly because they spend so much time preparing. Sedentary people—this is a medical fact—get less oxygen in the blood, and therefore to the brain, than active people.

Do the Following on Exam Day

- *Keep moving forward.* By test day, do enough preparation with a review course or practice questions so that it becomes an instinct to keep moving forward instead of getting bogged down in a difficult question. You don't need to get everything right to pass, so don't linger on a question that is going nowhere. The best test takers don't get bothered by difficult questions because they accept that everyone encounters them on the NCLEX-RN® exam.

- *Don't listen to negative words or behavior.* Don't be distracted by the ignorant babble or the behavior of other, less-prepared, less-skilled candidates around you. Negative thoughts lead to negative feelings and may interfere with performing your best on Test Day.

- *Don't be anxious if other test takers seem to be working harder or answering questions more quickly.* Continue to spend your time patiently but persistently thinking through your answers; it's going to lead to higher-quality test taking and better results. Set your own pace and stick to it.

- *Keep breathing!* Weak standardized test takers tend to share one major trait: forgetting to breathe steadily as the test proceeds. They do not to know the value of proper breathing. They start holding their breath without realizing it, or begin breathing erratically or arrhythmically. This can hurt confidence and accuracy. Do what you can to instill an awareness of proper breathing before and during each study or testing session.

- *Do some quick isometrics during the test.* This is helpful especially if your concentration is wandering or energy is waning. For example, put your palms together and press intensely for a few seconds.

Here is a brief review of the various strategies that you have learned in this chapter:

- The NCLEX-RN® exam isn't the real world, so don't rely on your real-world experience to answer NCLEX-RN® exam questions.

- To answer priority questions correctly, think Maslow, the nursing process, and safety.

- The Rules of Management will help you answer questions about delegation and assignment of client care.

- Use the Positioning strategy when you encounter questions about positioning and mobility.

- The Therapeutic Communication strategy will help you eliminate incorrect answer choices in communication questions.

- Identify your strength and weaknesses, and choose an effective method of study that works for you.

- Use mental preparation techniques to alleviate stress and manage your test day experience.

PART 2

NCLEX-RN® Exam Content Review and Practice

CHAPTER 4

SAFE AND EFFECTIVE CARE ENVIRONMENT: MANAGEMENT OF CARE

One of the most important parts of your job in client care is keeping the care environment safe for all involved. In addition, it's also important to provide care effectively. Providing a safe and effective care environment involves both proper management of care, and safety and infection control.

Management of care refers specifically to the way nursing care is provided and directed so that the client receives proper treatment, and so that health care personnel remain safe. It also covers management, delegation, and other skills you are expected to have, as well as your ethical and legal obligations regarding client care.

On the NCLEX-RN® exam, you can expect approximately 20 percent of the questions to relate to Management of Care. Exam content related to this subcategory includes, but is not limited to, the following areas:

- Advance directives
- Advocacy
- Case management
- Client rights
- Collaboration with interdisciplinary teams
- Concepts of management
- Confidentiality/information security
- Consultation
- Continuity of care
- Delegation
- Establishing priorities
- Ethical practice
- Information technology
- Informed consent

- Legal rights and responsibilities
- Performance improvement (quality improvement)
- Referrals
- Supervision

Now let's review the most important concepts covered by the Management of Care subcategory on the NCLEX-RN® exam.

ADVANCE DIRECTIVES

An advance directive is a legal document, such as a living will, a health care proxy, or a Durable Power of Attorney for Health Care (DPAHC). Advance directives provide guidance to caregivers about the client's wishes and are followed if a client's decision-making powers become impaired. The 1990 Patient Self-Determination Act requires that upon admission to hospitals, long-term care facilities, and home health agencies, patients be informed that they have the right to accept or refuse medical care, as well as to specify in advance (through advance directives) what their wishes are.

Your role as a nurse is to integrate advance directives into the client care plan. To accomplish this, evaluate client status regarding advance directives, and help to determine whether family members and/or significant others should be involved in conversations and decision-making. If the client, a family member, significant other, or staff member is not familiar with the details of advance directives, provide the information as needed.

You must also ensure that copies of advance directives are placed in the client's medical record. This includes information on organ or tissue donation for clients over 18 years of age. The Uniform Anatomical Gift Act, for example, governs organ donations for transplantation and how to donate one's cadaver as an anatomical gift.

ADVOCACY

Client advocacy—promoting your clients' rights and interests—is an important part of nursing. Discuss treatment options with clients, including what the options are, how they work, and what the side effects may be, so the client understands all available choices. You must respect client decisions even if you do not agree with them. You may need to provide information regarding these discussions to other staff members so you can advocate for your client. When necessary, use an interpreter or translator for non-English-speaking clients. Know when it is appropriate to engage others higher in the chain of command or with different areas of expertise, such as a social worker, on your client's behalf.

CASE MANAGEMENT

It is important to assist your clients in achieving and/or maintaining their independence by identifying and utilizing the resources available to them. The individualized care plan you develop for each client should be aimed at providing safe, cost-effective care for the client. The plan is based on your assessment of client needs as well as goals, such as providing self-care. You should also incorporate evidence-based research from medical literature and other resources, where applicable, into the care plan. In addition to initiating the care plan for each client, you are expected to evaluate and revise that plan, as needed.

When a client leaves the hospital, provide the client with information on discharge procedures to home, hospice, or community living, whichever may be relevant to the client's situation. This includes information about medications the client should be taking, follow-up visits, future lab tests, and so on.

CLIENT RIGHTS

Part of your job as a health care provider is to discuss treatment options and decisions with your clients, and educate them about client rights and responsibilities. As noted previously, the Patient Self-Determination Act requires that upon admission to hospitals, long-term care facilities, and home health agencies, patients be informed that they have the right to accept or refuse medical care. At times, you may need to recognize the client's right to refuse treatment. The Health Insurance Portability and Accountability Act (HIPAA) protects personally identifying information, such as the client's name, social security number, date of birth, and information about diagnosis and treatment. HIPAA provides that such information should only be shared with individuals directly involved in the client's care, the payment of care, and/or the management of the client's care.

The Patients' Bill of Rights, adopted by the President's Advisory Commission on Consumer Protection and Quality in the Health Care Industry, is a statement about the rights to which individuals are entitled as recipients of health care, and their responsibilities. It covers the following areas:

- **Information disclosure:** The client has a right to accurate and easily understood information about health plans, health care professionals, and health care facilities.
- **Choice of providers and plans:** The client has the right to choose health care providers who can provide high-quality health care when needed.
- **Access to emergency services:** The client has the right to be screened and stabilized using emergency services whenever and wherever the client needs them, without having to wait for authorization, and without any financial penalty.

- **Participation in treatment decisions:** The client has the right to know about treatment options and take part in decisions about care. Parents, guardians, family, and significant others can represent the client if the client cannot make his or her own decisions.
- **Confidentiality of health information:** The client has the right to talk privately with health care providers and have health care information protected; it also includes the right to read and copy one's own medical records.
- **Complaints and appeals:** The client has the right to a fair, fast, and objective review of any complaint against a health plan, a physician, other health care personnel, or a hospital.
- **Consumer responsibilities:** This includes, among other things, a client's responsibility to provide information about medications and past illnesses.

Evaluate the client's understanding of his or her rights and responsibilities, including the right to informed consent and the difference between privileged communication and the duty to disclose, as well as staff understanding of client rights.

COLLABORATION WITH INTERDISCIPLINARY TEAMS

The term *interdisciplinary* or *multidisciplinary* refers to situations in which various disciplines are involved in reaching a common goal, with each contributing his or her specific expertise. The interdisciplinary interaction between different health care professions such as nursing, medicine, and social work is known as *collaboration*. Such collaboration in the management of a particular disorder enables caregivers to provide a more comprehensive and individualized approach. Collaboration with an interdisciplinary team requires cooperation, integration, and teamwork.

Because nurses are often the caregivers that clients see most often, be prepared to identify the need for interdisciplinary conferences regarding a client, and know how to initiate such conferences. This includes identification of significant information to report to other disciplines, including health care providers, pharmacists, social workers, and respiratory therapists.

You should be ready to act as the point person to review the care plan and ensure continuity across disciplines, and to collaborate with health care members in other disciplines to provide efficient and effective client care.

CONCEPTS OF MANAGEMENT

It's important to identify the roles and responsibilities of all members of the health care team. You'll often need to act as the liaison between those team members and the client to coordinate and manage care.

As issues arise regarding client treatment, apply the principles of conflict resolution, as needed, when working with health care staff. You should also be able to plan overall strategies to address client problems. Know how to supervise care provided by others (see the "Delegation" and "Supervision" sections later in this chapter), and know which staff members can perform particular procedures related to client care.

Confidentiality/Information Security

Like all health care providers, you should maintain client confidentiality and take the necessary steps to ensure that client information security is not breached. An individual not involved in the care of the client does not have a legitimate need to access the client's medical record. Know the provisions of HIPAA (summarized in the Client Rights section of this chapter) and protect the client's right to privacy. Ensure that only authorized individuals access medical records, that no medical records are viewable by the general public, and that no conversations about client information can be overheard by unauthorized persons.

You may need to intervene when confidentiality is breached by other staff members. You'll also be expected to assess staff members' and your clients' understanding of confidentiality requirements, such as those governed by HIPAA.

Consultation

Consultation involves communication with another nurse or health care professional, such as a dietician or pharmacist, about an aspect of client care. Determine when a consultation with other health care providers is appropriate, and then initiate such consultations as needed. You should also be able to identify the expected outcomes of consultations, and revise the care plan if the client's needs change.

Continuity of Care

Continuity of care is the process by which a client and health care providers are cooperatively involved in the ongoing health care management of the client, with the goal of providing high-quality and cost-effective health care. Ideally, all people involved in a client's health care, including the client, communicate with one another to coordinate care, as well as agree and understand the goals of health care for the client.

To help ensure continuity of care, know the proper procedures to admit, transfer, and discharge a client. This includes maintaining continuity of care between/among health care agencies when clients are transferred or handed off from one department to another, or from one agency to another. It also includes using documents and proper forms to enter client information into medical records or on transfer/referral forms. You may also need to follow up on unresolved issues regarding client care (e.g., laboratory results and client requests) and provide reports on assigned clients.

DELEGATION

Delegation is a crucial skill. You must be able to identify an appropriate person to carry out a specific task or set of tasks, explain the tasks clearly, and make sure you are understood. It is also your responsibility to make sure the person to whom you are delegating a task has the authority to do the job. Good delegators provide support and monitoring, provide sufficient time to complete the task, retain responsibility for knowing the outcome, and praise and acknowledge a job well done.

Do not delegate the following to nonprofessional staff:

- Nursing assessments
- Diagnosis, care goals, or progress plans
- Interventions that require professional knowledge and skill

Remember the five "rights" of delegation:

- **Right task:** Can the task be safely delegated?
- **Right circumstance:** Is the client stable, and is the outcome predictable?
- **Right person:** Does the person to whom the task will be delegated have the necessary knowledge and appropriate skills?
- **Right direction/communication:** Has the nurse communicated appropriate instructions for accomplishing the task?
- **Right supervision:** Will the delegating nurse remain responsible for the task and outcomes?

You can delegate activities for stable clients with predictable outcomes, and activities that involve standard, unchanging procedures, such as bathing, feeding, dressing, and transferring clients. Do not delegate an activity if the client is unstable, if the outcome of the activity is not assured, or if the activity is complex or complicated.

ESTABLISHING PRIORITIES

There are several other frameworks for establishing the priority of client care. They include:

- ABCs (airway, breathing, circulation/cardiovascular system)
- Maslow's hierarchy of needs (physiological needs, safety and security, love and belonging, self-esteem, and self-actualization)
- Agency policies and procedures
- Time
- Client and family preferences

- Care related to client activity
- Priorities in medication therapy

Assess/triage (French for *sort*) clients to prioritize order of care delivery, and focus on the least stable clients first. Use your knowledge of pathophysiology when establishing priorities for interventions with multiple clients. Once you have provided care to multiple clients, evaluate and adjust your care plans as needed.

The following general problems indicate priority needs:

- Postoperative clients just out of surgery
- Clients whose status has deteriorated from their normal baseline
- Clients exhibiting signs of shock
- Clients with allergic reactions
- Clients with chest pain
- Postdiagnostic-procedure clients who require temporary monitoring
- Clients who tell you they have unusual symptoms
- Clients with malfunctioning equipment or tubing

ETHICAL PRACTICE

Ethical principles help you determine whether an action is right or wrong. In addition to understanding basic ethics and morals, you should be familiar with the American Nurses Association (ANA) Code of Ethics for Nurses. These guidelines delineate values and standards for professional practice.

Make sure you understand the following ethical principles:

- **Autonomy:** The right of individuals to make decisions for themselves
- **Beneficence:** A nurse's duty to do what is in the best interests of the client
- **Justice:** A fair, equitable, and appropriate treatment
- **Nonmaleficence:** A nurse's duty to do no harm
- **Fidelity:** Keeping faithful to ethical principles and the ANA Code of Ethics for Nurses
- **Virtues:** Compassion, trustworthiness, integrity, and veracity (truthfulness)
- **Confidentiality:** Maintaining the client's privacy by not disclosing personal information about the client
- **Accountability:** Responsibility for one's actions

You should be able to identify ethical issues affecting staff or clients, provide information on ethics, and intervene appropriately to promote ethical practice. You'll also be expected to review outcomes of interventions to promote ethical practice.

INFORMATION TECHNOLOGY

Electronic medication administration records have the potential to reduce medication administration errors and improve access to client information at the point of care. You must know how to use information technology and information systems to enter computer documentation in a client's medical record and other databases in a timely and accurate manner. You may also need to access data for clients and staff through online databases and journals.

Whenever you access a client record, apply your knowledge of the facility's specific regulations. You'll also be expected to receive and/or transcribe primary health care provider orders.

You should also know how to use information technology (e.g., a computer or video) to enhance the care provided to a client. Telehealth, for example, uses transmissions via telecommunications technology to transmit health information remotely.

INFORMED CONSENT

Informed consent is the right of clients to be adequately informed of the risks and benefits of a proposed procedure or treatment before determining whether or not to consent to that procedure or treatment. The components of informed consent include an explanation of the following:

- Details of the procedure or treatment
- Risks and benefits of the procedure or treatment, including the potential for serious injury or death
- Alternative procedures or treatments
- Potential consequences of refusing the procedure or treatment

Typically, the health care provider who is performing the procedure or providing the treatment (usually the physician) is responsible for obtaining the client's informed consent. One of your roles in the process is to advocate for the client by ensuring he or she has been provided the necessary information to make an informed decision. In cases where the client does not speak English, provide written materials in the client's native language, when possible. Another one of your roles is to ensure that a client has actually given informed consent for treatment before that treatment occurs. One way to do so is to act as a witness to the informed consent. As a witness, you confirm that the client gave his or her informed consent voluntarily, the client's signature is authentic, and the client is competent to give consent. You may be called upon to evaluate clients to determine whether they are capable of providing informed consent, and identify an appropriate person to do so, such as a parent or legal guardian, if the client is a minor.

If the client waives consent, ensure it is documented in the medical record. If the client is deemed incompetent to give informed consent, a court-appointed guardian may do so on the client's behalf.

The requirement to obtain the client's informed consent can be waived in an emergency situation in which the client is incapacitated and the situation requires immediate treatment.

LEGAL RIGHTS AND RESPONSIBILITIES

Know the confines of applicable laws and understand the parameters of your nursing license. Legal limits and the scope of practice for nursing are dictated by federal and state laws, such as the Nurse Practice Acts (NPAs) and related guidelines, and are regulated by each state's Board of Nursing. Nurses are accountable and responsible for incorrect or inappropriate actions or inactions. These may include negligence, malpractice, or other legal charges. Negligence involves the unintentional failure to act as a reasonable person would in similar circumstances that results in an injury to the client. Elements include a breach of a duty of care, with a resultant injury that has been proximately caused (i.e., there is reasonably close connection between the nurse's actions and the resulting injury), and actual damages to the injured party. Malpractice involves the failure by a medical professional to carry out or perform his or her duties that result in injury to the client. The specific requirements for malpractice are typically defined by the statutes and rules/regulations of each state.

There are specific areas with which you should be familiar. They include:

- Identifying legal issues affecting clients (e.g., refusing treatment) and knowing how to respond appropriately
- Recognizing tasks and assignments you are not prepared to perform and seeking assistance
- Identifying and managing clients' valuables according to facility or agency policy
- Educating clients and staff on legal and ethical issues
- Complying with state and/or federal regulations for reporting client conditions (e.g., abuse/neglect, communicable disease, gunshot wound, or dog bite)
- Reporting unsafe practices of health care personnel to internal or external entities
- Intervening appropriately when you observe unsafe practices by staff members

PERFORMANCE IMPROVEMENT (QUALITY IMPROVEMENT)

Each institution may define it differently, but a standard definition of quality involves meeting or exceeding the expectations of customers and standards, and achieving planned outcomes. Quality management principles include total quality management (TQM), continuous quality improvement (CQI), and evidence-based decision making, among others. Quality improvement includes activities such as identifying opportunities and developing policies for improving the quality of nursing practice. Methods include establishing a comprehensive quality management plan, establishing benchmarks, completing performance appraisals, performing intradisciplinary and interdisciplinary assessments, performing nursing audits, conducting peer reviews and utilization reviews, and managing outcomes. Mock codes can improve performance by encouraging teamwork, improving communication and skill building, and enhancing confidence of caregivers.

You must report identified client care issues or problems to appropriate personnel (e.g., the nurse manager or risk manager). A nurse is also expected to participate in the performance improvement and quality assurance process, which may include data collection or participation on a team.

You may be asked to utilize research and other references when determining how best to improve performance, and you will be expected to evaluate the impact of performance improvement measures on client care and resource utilization using a variety of specific indicators.

Nurse-sensitive indicators are measurements of client care that are impacted by nursing interventions. Examples include maintenance of skin integrity, pressure ulcer prevalence and incidence, fall injury rate, medication incident rate, restraint utilization rate, client satisfaction with pain management, client satisfaction with overall nursing care, and nurse satisfaction.

REFERRALS

Nurses often have a role to play in assisting and coordinating client care that requires referrals. There are different types of referrals: authorization for care or a service, recommendation of a specific provider, referral to specialists, and referral to a different facility for care. Some of these may require specific approvals, although in some cases you can refer a client directly to a dietary or wound care specialist.

Assess the need to refer clients for assistance with actual or potential problems (physical therapy, speech therapy), and match community resources to the client's needs (respite care, social services, shelters). In all referral situations, you need to know which documents to include when referring a client, such as a medical record or referral form.

SUPERVISION

Leadership will be critical to your success. You should be able to create a common vision for staff, and promote a sense of urgency. This helps connect daily activities to a larger strategic plan, and keeps nursing activities in line with the overall goals of the institution.

A supervisor is someone who has authority to manage other employees. Supervision includes guidance and direction, evaluation, and follow-up to ensure tasks are accomplished. A good supervisor provides the following:

- Clear direction and communication
- Timely follow-up
- Active listening
- Complete technical knowledge of supervised work
- Feedback and resolution of problems and conflicts

As a supervisor, you are expected to select and implement strategies for interventions with staff members as necessary, to report staff member performance, and to evaluate the skills and abilities of staff members, particularly as they relate to time management.

Types of staff members you might be called upon to supervise include other RNs, licensed practical nurses (LPNs), licensed vocational nurses (LVNs), and nursing assistive personnel (NAPs).

CHAPTER QUIZ

1. A 58-year-old man with head and neck cancer is admitted to the hospital and tells the nurse he does not want parenteral nutritional therapy as his cancer progresses. The nurse explains he can specify his wishes by creating an advance directive. The nurse knows that the requirement to provide clients with this type of information can be found in which of the following?

   1. The Patient Self-Determination Act
   2. Nursing Scope and Standards of Practice
   3. The Patient Protection and Affordable Care Act
   4. The Patients' Bill of Rights

2. A 14-year-old girl newly diagnosed with diabetes is preparing for discharge. Which of the following activities *BEST* describes the nurse's role as a client advocate?

   1. Arranging for a visit with a home health nurse
   2. Providing written medication instructions to the client's parents
   3. Instructing the client to follow up with her provider in 4 weeks
   4. Teaching the client how to administer insulin injections

3. A client is seen for an outpatient appointment and asks the nurse if he can obtain a copy of his medical record. The nurse knows the client has the right to read and copy his medical records, and that this is guaranteed by virtue of which of the following?

   1. The Code of Ethics for Nurses
   2. The Health Insurance Portability and Accountability Act (HIPAA)
   3. The Patient Self-Determination Act
   4. The Americans with Disabilities Act

4. After receiving report at the start of the evening shift, which of the following clients should the nurse attend to *FIRST*?

   1. A 34-year-old man undergoing treatment for non-Hodgkin lymphoma with a potassium level of 7.5 mEq/L
   2. A 21-year-old woman with sickle-cell anemia with pain of 6 on a scale of 1–10
   3. A 55-year-old woman with ovarian cancer waiting to be discharged
   4. A 72-year-old man with chronic obstructive pulmonary disease (COPD) and a pulse oximetry of 96% on room air

5. A 34-year-old woman who developed Stevens-Johnson syndrome while undergoing treatment with carbamazepine (Tegretol) is being transferred in stable condition from the intensive care unit to the medical unit. There are 4 beds available. The nurse knows the *BEST* choice of roommates for this client is which of the following?

   1. A 40-year-old man with methicillin-resistant *Staphylococcus aureus* (MRSA)
   2. A 28-year-old woman diagnosed with diarrhea
   3. A 72-year-old man with fever of unknown origin
   4. A 68-year-old woman with atrial fibrillation

6. A 72-year-old man who had a stroke is being transferred from a medical unit to a rehabilitation center. The nurse case manager is assisting in the process. The nurse knows that the goals of case management include which of the following? **Select all that apply.**

   1. Improving the coordination of care
   2. Increasing referrals to local organizations
   3. Reducing the fragmentation of care
   4. Discharging clients quickly

7. An 18-year-old client with acute lymphocytic leukemia is admitted to the bone marrow transplantation unit. His family is having trouble dealing with the emotional and financial pressures of his disease. The nurse, case manager, physician, and social worker meet to discuss the plan of care. The nurse knows this type of interdisciplinary interaction is *BEST* referred to as which of the following?

   1. Case management
   2. Collaboration
   3. Cooperation
   4. Collegiality

8. A pregnant woman at 15 weeks' gestation is scheduled for an amniocentesis. As the client is being prepped for the procedure, it becomes clear to the nurse that the client doesn't fully understand the risks and benefits associated with the procedure. Which of the following describe the nurse's role in obtaining informed consent? **Select all that apply.**

   1. Explain the risks and benefits associated with the procedure.
   2. Describe alternatives to the procedure.
   3. Witness the client's signature on the consent form.
   4. Advocate for the client by ensuring she is making an informed decision.

9. The nurse noticed an increase in the prevalence of pressure ulcers among clients in an intensive care unit. She documented her findings and worked with her manager to develop and implement a new policy using a pressure ulcer risk assessment scale. Which of the following *BEST* describes the nurse's actions?

   1. Quality improvement
   2. Collaboration
   3. Advocacy
   4. Case management

10. The nurse is working on a surgical unit. Which of the following tasks would be appropriate for the nurse to delegate to nursing assistive personnel (NAP)?

    1. Assist a new postoperative client to the bathroom.
    2. Set up the clients' lunch trays.
    3. Change a central line dressing.
    4. Teach a client how to administer discharge medications.

11. The nurse has been asked to administer a drug by IV push. She is uncertain whether or not this task falls within her scope of practice. The nurse knows that which of the following are the *BEST* sources to refer to for information related to her scope of practice in this situation? **Select all that apply.**

    1. Hospital and unit policies and procedures
    2. Nurse Practice Act
    3. Ordering physician
    4. Hospital pharmacist

12. A 20-year-old client with leukemia has consented to a blood transfusion against the wishes of his family, who are all Jehovah's Witnesses. The nurse knows that which of the following ethical principles *BEST* supports this decision?

    1. Autonomy
    2. Beneficence
    3. Nonmaleficence
    4. Justice

13. The nurse wants to delegate the task of showering an elderly client in a wheelchair to the nursing assistive personnel (NAP). Before delegating a task to the NAP, the nurse should *FIRST* ensure which of the following is accomplished?

1. The UAP is supervised at all times.

2. The UAP demonstrated competency for the task during orientation.

3. The UAP has performed the task before.

4. The UAP has received the assignment during report.

14. A well-known actor has been admitted to an ambulatory surgical unit. The nurse notices a staff member who is not involved in the client's care reading his medical record. The nurse knows she should *FIRST* do which of the following?

    1. Nothing. The staff member has a hospital ID badge and is authorized to read the medical record.

    2. Inform the staff member that without a legitimate need for the information, staff should not be reading the medical record.

    3. Tell the client his medical records have been read by an unauthorized individual.

    4. Page the physician and ask if it's acceptable for the staff member to access the medical records.

15. The nurse is learning how to use the hospital's new electronic medication administration record. The nurse knows this tool has the potential to do which of the following? **Select all that apply.**

    1. Reduce medication administration errors.

    2. Improve access to information at the point of care.

    3. Eliminate the need for the nurse to document medication administration.

    4. Eliminate the need for the nurse to verify dose calculations.

16. The nurse uses the Internet to receive electrocardiogram results from a client living in a nursing home. The nurse knows this type of information technology is *BEST* described as which of the following?

    1. Encryption

    2. Telecommunications

    3. Telehealth

    4. Nursing informatics

17. The nurse is preparing to transfer a client to the operating room. She knows that adhering to the hospital policy for client handoffs *BEST* ensures which of the following?

    1. Case management

    2. Continuity of care

    3. Confidentiality protection

    4. Collaboration

18. The nurse is preparing to perform an admission assessment on a 28-year-old man being admitted for Crohn's disease. The nurse knows that according to the Patients' Bill of Rights, this client is responsible for which of the following? **Select all that apply.**

    1. Consenting to treatment

    2. Providing information about medications

    3. Providing proof of insurance

    4. Providing information about past illnesses

19. The nurse is caring for a 41-year-old man with a new colostomy. As part of the care planning for this client, the nurse knows a referral to which of the following will be the priority?

    1. A certified wound, ostomy, and continence nurse (CWOCN)

    2. Social services

3. Physical therapy

4. Occupational therapy

20. An RN is in charge of a team on a medical/surgical unit that includes an LPN. The RN understands that which of the following is an activity that falls within the scope of practice of an LPN?

1. Administer oral medications to a client.

2. Collaborate with social services to develop a discharge plan.

3. Formulate a nursing diagnosis.

4. Develop a policy.

21. The nurse in a maternity unit is caring for a client who has just delivered twins. The client voices concern about her ability to manage when she gets home. Which of the following statements *BEST* illustrates quality care delivery by the nurse? **Select all that apply.**

1. "Just focus on how lucky you are to have two healthy babies."

2. "We can arrange for follow-up visits with a home health nurse."

3. "Here is some information on support groups for parents of multiples."

4. "You will find it easier to formula-feed your babies at home."

22. After responding to a code, several staff nurses express concerns over their confidence levels and performance to the nurse in charge of the hospital's performance improvement program. The nurse in charge knows the *BEST* way to evaluate and improve performance is to implement which of the following?

1. A program that collects and analyzes performance data

2. Mock codes

3. Inservice training

4. Written competency exams

23. A client is being treated for uncontrolled hypertension. The nurse knows that the involvement of nursing, pharmacy, cardiology, and nutritional services is an example of which of the following approaches?

1. Managed care

2. Multidisciplinary

3. Case management

4. Performance improvement

24. The nurse is caring for a client newly diagnosed with diabetes, and performs the following tasks. Place the tasks the nurse would perform in the appropriate order. **All options must be used.**

1. The nurse establishes a goal with the client to be able to self-administer insulin injections.

2. The nurse assesses the client's level of knowledge about how to administer insulin injections.

3. The nurse evaluates the client while self-administering insulin injections.

4. The nurse establishes the diagnosis of knowledge deficit.

25. The nurse administers the first dose of chemotherapy to a client on an oncology unit. The nurse knows that which of the following activities is appropriate to delegate to the LPN?

1. Obtain the client's blood pressure.

2. Provide teaching about the side effects of chemotherapy.

3. Administer the second dose of chemotherapy.

4. Flush the client's central line with heparin.

CHAPTER QUIZ ANSWERS AND EXPLANATIONS

1. The Answer is 1

A 58-year-old man with head and neck cancer is admitted to the hospital and tells the nurse he does not want parenteral nutritional therapy as his cancer progresses. The nurse explains he can specify his wishes by creating an advance directive. The nurse knows that the requirement to provide clients with this type of information can be found in which of the following?

Category: Advance directives

(1) CORRECT: The 1990 Patient Self-Determination Act was passed by Congress to ensure that upon admission to hospitals, long-term care facilities, and home health agencies, patients are informed that they have the right to accept or refuse medical care, as well as to specify in advance (through advance directives) what their wishes are.

(2) Nursing Scope and Standards of Practice do not address advance directives.

(3) The Patient Protection and Affordable Care Act does not address advance directives.

(4) The Patients' Bill of Rights does not address advance directives.

2. The Answer is 4

A 14-year-old girl newly diagnosed with diabetes is preparing for discharge. Which of the following activities *BEST* describes the nurse's role as a client advocate?

Category: Advocacy

(1) Arranging for a visit with a home health nurse may be important in the overall management of this client's care, but does not directly assist in teaching the client the necessary skills to manage her diabetes.

(2) Providing written medication instructions to the client's parents may be important in the overall management of this client's care, but does not directly assist in teaching the client the necessary skills to manage her diabetes.

(3) Instructing the client to follow up with her provider in 4 weeks may be important in the overall management of this client's care, but does not directly assist in teaching the client the necessary skills to manage her diabetes.

(4) CORRECT: Teaching the client how to administer her own medication is the best example of the nurse's role as a client advocate, because this action directly helps the client develop self-advocacy skills.

3. The Answer is 2

A client is seen for an outpatient appointment and asks the nurse if he can obtain a copy of his medical record. The nurse knows the client has the right to read and copy his medical records, and that this is guaranteed by virtue of which of the following?

Category: Client rights

(1) The Code of Ethics for Nurses does not address this issue.

(2) CORRECT: HIPAA protects the patient's right to review, copy, and request amendments to his medical records.

(3) The Patient Self-Determination Act does not address whether a patient may read and copy his medical records.

(4) The Americans with Disabilities Act does not address whether a patient may read and copy his medical records.

4. The Answer is 1

After receiving report at the start of the evening shift, which of the following clients should the nurse attend to *FIRST?*

Category: Establishing priorities

(1) CORRECT: Hyperkalemia is a potentially serious condition that, in a client undergoing treatment for non-Hodgkin lymphoma, could indicate tumor lysis syndrome.

(2) A 21-year-old woman with sickle-cell anemia with pain of 6 on a scale of 1–10 should be

attended to, but her condition is not as urgent as the client's condition described in answer choice (1).

(3) A 55-year-old woman with ovarian cancer waiting to be discharged should be attended to but does not require immediate attention.

(4) A 72-year-old man with COPD and a pulse oximetry of 96% on room air does not require immediate attention.

5. The Answer is 4

A 34-year-old woman who developed Stevens-Johnson syndrome while undergoing treatment with carbamazepine (Tegretol) is being transferred in stable condition from the intensive care unit to the medical unit. There are 4 beds available. The nurse knows the *BEST* choice of roommates for this client is which of the following?

Category: Concepts of management

(1) A client with MRSA may be an infection risk for an individual with altered skin integrity.

(2) A client diagnosed with diarrhea may be an infection risk for an individual with altered skin integrity.

(3) A client with fever of unknown origin may be an infection risk for an individual with altered skin integrity.

(4) CORRECT: A client with Stevens-Johnson syndrome is likely to have severe skin integrity issues, including blistering and skin shedding, which can place the client at high risk for infection. Atrial fibrillation is not an infectious process.

6. The Answer is 1 and 3

A 72-year-old man who had a stroke is being transferred from a medical unit to a rehabilitation center. The nurse case manager is assisting in the process. The nurse knows that the goals of case management include which of the following? **Select all that apply.**

Category: Case management

(1) CORRECT: One of the primary goals of case management is to improve the coordination of care.

(2) Although case managers do make referrals to local organizations, this is not a goal of case management.

(3) CORRECT: One of the primary goals of case management is to reduce fragmentation of care.

(4) Although case managers help to make discharges more efficient, this is not a goal of case management.

7. The Answer is 2

An 18-year-old client with acute lymphocytic leukemia is admitted to the bone marrow transplantation unit. His family is having trouble dealing with the emotional and financial pressures of his disease. The nurse, case manager, physician, and social worker meet to discuss the plan of care. The nurse knows this type of interdisciplinary interaction is *BEST* referred to as which of the following?

Category: Collaboration with interdisciplinary team

(1) Case management refers to the coordination of care to reduce fragmentation and improve quality and outcomes, as well as to reduce costs.

(2) CORRECT: The interdisciplinary interaction between different health care professions, such as nursing, medicine, and social work, is known as collaboration.

(3) Although the health care team may have been cooperating, or operating as a team, the term "cooperation" does not specifically refer to the concept of interdisciplinary action.

(4) Although the health care team may have been operating in a collegial (cooperative and professional) manner, this term does not specifically refer to the concept of interdisciplinary action.

8. The Answer is 3 and 4

A pregnant woman at 15 weeks' gestation is scheduled for an amniocentesis. As the client is being prepped for the procedure, it becomes clear to the nurse that the client doesn't fully understand the risks and benefits associated with the procedure. Which of the following describe the nurse's role in obtaining informed consent? **Select all that apply.**

Category: Informed consent

(1) It is the physician's duty to provide information to the client-related to risks and benefits.

(2) It is the physician's duty to provide information to the client related to alternatives.

(3) CORRECT: One of the nurse's roles in the informed consent process is to witness the signature on the consent form.

(4) CORRECT: One of the nurse's roles in the informed consent process is to advocate for the client by ensuring she has been provided the necessary information to make an informed decision.

9. The Answer is 1

The nurse noticed an increase in the prevalence of pressure ulcers among clients in an intensive care unit. She documented her findings and worked with her manager to develop and implement a new policy using a pressure ulcer risk assessment scale. Which of the following *BEST* describes the nurse's actions?

Category: Performance improvement (quality improvement)

(1) CORRECT: Quality improvement includes activities such as identifying opportunities and developing policies for improving the quality of nursing practice. Identifying an increase in pressure ulcers and implementing a policy aimed at improving the assessment and prevention of pressure ulcers best fits the definition of quality improvement.

(2) The nurse may have collaborated (or worked together) with colleagues, but this is not the best choice.

(3) Advocacy refers to the nurse's duty to act on behalf of the client. Although reducing pressure ulcers may indirectly advocate for the client, it is not the best answer choice.

(4) Case management refers to the coordination of care to reduce fragmentation and costs, as well as to improve quality and outcomes.

10. The Answer is 2

The nurse is working on a surgical unit. Which of the following tasks would be appropriate for the nurse to delegate to nursing assistive personnel (NAP)?

Category: Delegation

(1) Assisting a new postoperative client to the bathroom is a task the registered nurse or another licensed individual, such as an LVN/LPN, should perform.

(2) CORRECT: Setting up the client's lunch trays is an appropriate task to delegate to the UAP.

(3) Changing a central line dressing is a task the registered nurse or another licensed individual, such as an LVN/LPN, should perform.

(4) Teaching a client how to administer discharge medications is a task the registered nurse or another licensed individual, such as a pharmacist, should perform.

11. The Answer is 1 and 2

The nurse has been asked to administer a drug by IV push. She is uncertain whether or not this task falls within her scope of practice. The nurse knows that which of the following are the *BEST* sources to refer to for information related to her scope of practice in this situation? **Select all that apply.**

Category: Legal rights and responsibilities

(1) CORRECT: Hospital and unit policies and procedures may outline specific information about who can administer which drugs by what route.

(2) CORRECT: Nurse Practice Acts (NPAs) are laws in each state that define the scope of practice for nursing.

(3) Although the ordering physician may be able to provide helpful information related to the drug itself, the ordering physician is not the best source of information related to nurse licensing and scope-of-practice issues.

(4) Although the hospital pharmacist may be able to provide helpful information related to the drug itself, the pharmacist is not the best source of information related to nurse licensing and scope-of-practice issues.

12. The Answer is 1

A 20-year-old client with leukemia has consented to a blood transfusion against the wishes of his family, who are all Jehovah's Witnesses. The nurse knows that which of the following ethical principles *BEST* supports this decision?

Category: Ethical practice

(1) CORRECT: Autonomy refers to the right of individuals to make decisions for themselves.

(2) Beneficence refers to the nurse's duty to do what is good for the client.

(3) Nonmaleficence refers to the nurse's duty to do no harm.

(4) Justice refers to the concept of fair and equitable treatment.

13. The Answer is 2

The nurse wants to delegate the task of showering an elderly client in a wheelchair to nursing assistive personnel (NAP). Before delegating a task to the NAP, the nurse should *FIRST* ensure which of the following is accomplished?

Category: Delegation

(1) Supervising the NAP does not ensure that the NAP's competency has been verified.

(2) CORRECT: Prior to delegating a task appropriate for the NAP, the nurse should first ensure that competency has been verified during the NAP's orientation.

(3) The fact that the NAP has performed the task before does not ensure that the NAP's competency has been verified.

(4) The fact that the NAP has received the assignment during report does not ensure that the NAP's competency has been verified.

14. The Answer is 2

A well-known actor has been admitted to an ambulatory surgical unit. The nurse notices a staff member who is not involved in the client's care reading his medical record. The nurse knows she should *FIRST* do which of the following?

Category: Confidentiality and information security

(1) A staff member who is not involved in the client's care is not authorized to access private information.

(2) CORRECT: An individual not involved in the care of the client does not have a legitimate need to access the medical record. The nurse should

protect the client's right to privacy by ensuring only authorized individuals access medical records.

(3) The nurse should do more than simply inform the client of the breach.

(4) The nurse should do more than simply ask a physician if it's acceptable for the staff member to access the client's medical records.

15. The Answer is 1 and 2

The nurse is learning how to use the hospital's new electronic medication administration record. The nurse knows this tool has the potential to do which of the following? **Select all that apply.**

Category: Information technology

(1) CORRECT: Electronic medication administration records have the potential to reduce medication administration errors.

(2) CORRECT: Electronic medication administration records have the potential to improve access to client information at the point of care.

(3) It is always the nurses' responsibility to document medication administration.

(4) It is always the nurses' responsibility to verify the doses of drugs being administered.

16. The Answer is 3

The nurse uses the Internet to receive electrocardiogram results from a client living in a nursing home. The nurse knows this type of information technology is *BEST* described as which of the following?

Category: Information technology

(1) Encryption refers to the conversion of information to code during transmission to keep the information secure.

(2) Telecommunications refers to the electronic transmission of data over phone-based lines.

(3) CORRECT: Telehealth uses transmissions via telecommunications technology to transmit health information remotely.

(4) Nursing informatics refers to a specialty of nursing that integrates nursing and computer science.

17. The Answer is 2

The nurse is preparing to transfer a client to the operating room. She knows that adhering to the hospital policy for client handoffs *BEST* ensures which of the following?

Category: Continuity of care

(1) Case management does not address the issue of handoffs between caregivers.

(2) CORRECT: Improving handoff communication allows each caregiver to communicate completely, effectively, and consistently as the client transitions to different departments in the hospital. This process improves the continuity of care.

(3) Confidentiality protection does not address the issue of handoffs between caregivers.

(4) Collaboration does not address the issue of handoffs between caregivers.

18. The Answer is 2 and 4

The nurse is preparing to perform an admission assessment on a 28-year-old man being admitted for Crohn's disease. The nurse knows that according to the Patients' Bill of Rights, this client is responsible for which of the following? **Select all that apply.**

Category: Client rights

(1) Consenting to treatment is not a patient responsibility delineated in the Patients' Bill of Rights; it is a patient right.

(2) CORRECT: According to the American Hospital Association, patients' responsibilities include (among other things) providing information about medications.

(3) Providing proof of insurance is not a patient responsibility delineated in the Patients' Bill of Rights.

(4) CORRECT: According to the American Hospital Association, patients' responsibilities include (among other things) providing information about past illnesses.

19. The Answer is 1

The nurse is caring for a 41-year-old man with a new colostomy. As part of the care planning for this client, the nurse knows a referral to which of the following will be the priority?

Category: Referral

(1) CORRECT: A referral to a certified wound, ostomy, and continence nurse (CWOCN), if available, is important to the management of a client with a colostomy during and after hospitalization.

(2) Although a referral to social services might be necessary based on other factors, it is not the priority in the situation described.

(3) Although a referral to physical therapy might be necessary based on other factors, it is not the priority in the situation described.

(4) Although a referral to occupational therapy might be necessary based on other factors, it is not the priority in the situation described.

20. The Answer is 1

An RN is in charge of a team on a medical/surgical unit that includes an LPN. The RN understands that which of the following is an activity that falls within the scope of practice of an LPN?

Category: Supervision

(1) CORRECT: Administering oral medications is an appropriate activity for the LPN.

(2) Collaborating with social services to develop a discharge plan is an activity that falls within registered nurses' scope of practice.

(3) Formulating a nursing diagnosis is an activity that falls within registered nurses' scope of practice.

(4) Developing policies are activities that fall within registered nurses' scope of practice.

21. The Answer is 2 and 3

The nurse in a maternity unit is caring for a client who has just delivered twins. The client voices concern about her ability to manage when she gets home. Which of the following statements *BEST* illustrate quality care delivery by the nurse? **Select all that apply.**

Category: Referrals

(1) This is not an appropriate answer to a new mother expressing concerns about her ability to cope.

(2) CORRECT: A referral to home health care provides the client with opportunities for support and assistance during this transition.

(3) CORRECT: A referral to support groups provides the client with opportunities for support and assistance during this transition.

(4) This is not an appropriate answer to a new mother expressing concerns about her ability to cope.

22. The Answer is 2

After responding to a code, several staff nurses express concerns over their confidence levels and performance to the nurse in charge of the hospital's performance improvement program. The nurse in charge knows the *BEST* way to evaluate and improve performance is to implement which of the following?

Category: Performance improvement (quality improvement)

(1) Although collecting and analyzing performance data can be helpful in understanding performance issues, it is not the best way to improve performance.

(2) CORRECT: Mock codes can improve performance by encouraging teamwork, improving communication and skill-building, and enhancing confidence of caregivers.

(3) Studies suggest that, although important for learning, training courses are not the best way to improve performance.

(4) A written competency exam is not the best way to evaluate and improve performance because it tests knowledge rather than performance.

23. The Answer is 2

A client is being treated for uncontrolled hypertension. The nurse knows that the involvement of nursing, pharmacy, cardiology, and nutritional services is an example of which of the following approaches?

Category: Collaboration with interdisciplinary team

(1) The concept of managed care is not related to a multidisciplinary approach.

(2) CORRECT: A multidisciplinary approach involves members from nursing, medicine, and other health care teams in the management of a particular disorder, in order to provide a more comprehensive and individualized approach.

(3) Case management is not related to a multidisciplinary approach.

(4) The concept of performance improvement is not related to a multidisciplinary approach.

24. The Answer is 2, 4, 1, 3

The nurse is caring for a client newly diagnosed with diabetes, and performs the following tasks. Place the tasks the nurse would perform in the appropriate order. **All options must be used.**

Category: Establishing priorities

(1) Establishing outcomes/planning is the third step in the nursing process.

(2) Assessment is the first step in the nursing process.

(3) Evaluation is the last step in the nursing process.

(4) Diagnosis is the second step in the nursing process.

25. The Answer is 1

The nurse administers the first dose of chemotherapy to a client on an oncology unit. The nurse knows that which of the following activities is appropriate to delegate to an LPN?

Category: Delegation

(1) CORRECT: An LPN may obtain the client's blood pressure.

(2) Providing teaching about the side effects of chemotherapy is not an activity that should be performed by an LPN.

(3) Administering a dose of chemotherapy is not an activity that should be performed by an LPN.

(4) Flushing the client's central line is not an activity that should be performed by an LPN.

CHAPTER 5

SAFE AND EFFECTIVE CARE ENVIRONMENT: SAFETY AND INFECTION CONTROL

Safety and infection control are closely linked areas that are particularly important in keeping clients healthy or helping them get well. Both home safety and safety in a hospital setting are covered in this topic area. An important part of hospital safety is the control of infections that clients might acquire while they are in the hospital (called *nosocomial infections*). These infections might not be related to their original condition or reason for admission but may have tremendous impact on their ability to heal.

On the NCLEX-RN® exam, you can expect approximately 12 percent of the questions to relate to Safety and Infection Control. This subcategory focuses on protecting clients and health care personnel from health and environmental hazards.

Exam content related to the Safety and Infection Control subcategory includes, but is not limited to, the following areas:

- Accident/injury prevention
- Emergency response plan
- Ergonomic principles
- Error prevention
- Handling hazardous and infectious materials
- Home safety
- Reporting of incident/event/irregular occurrence/variance
- Safe use of equipment
- Security plan
- Standard precautions/transmission-based precautions/surgical asepsis
- Use of restraints/safety devices

SAFETY BACKGROUND

Begin your review of safety issues by making sure you understand the various elements that are involved in client safety and accident prevention, including developmental- or age-related risks specific to infants, toddlers, school-age children, adolescents, adults, and older adults (geriatric clients), as follows:

- **Infants:** Educate parents or caretakers regarding infant safety and their responsibility to take proper precautions to prevent injury. Infants should be placed on their backs after eating and while sleeping, and transported using car seats. This age group has a high risk for falls and burns.

- **Toddlers:** Mobility and curiosity create safety issues including poisoning, choking, and drowning. Keep medications, poisons, and cleaning supplies in locked cabinets. Toddlers should be transported only in car seats.

- **School-age children:** Time spent in school and playing with friends creates new safety risks. Emphasize traffic safety, water safety, fire safety, and the dangers of strangers. Car seats and/or booster seats should be used for children until adult seat belts fit correctly, which typically does not occur until the child reaches 4′9″, weighs at least 80 lb., and is between ages 8 and 12. (Age and height/weight requirements vary by state.)

- **Adolescents:** Their sense of independence and invincibility, and access to cars, creates risk. Emphasize driver education, alcohol and substance abuse education, and sexual health information.

- **Adults:** Safety risks for this age group include home, workplace, and leisure activities. Educate adults about motor vehicle, fire, and firearm safety.

- **Older adults:** Aging issues, both physical and cognitive, impact safety, particularly regarding falls and side effects of medication. Possibilities of elder abuse and motor vehicle accidents also increase for older adults.

You also need to understand the elements that are involved in client safety and accident prevention related to the care environment. For example, in a hospital setting, fall risks are most common in infants and geriatric clients. Know the elements of a fall prevention program, including the different steps taken based on the age of the client. Safety also involves the use of restraints to limit mobility, and taking proper seizure precautions. You should be able to explain these precautions, which include the use of physical restraints, and the need for suction and oxygen equipment.

INFECTION CONTROL BACKGROUND

To correctly answer questions about infection control, begin by making sure you understand some basic information about etiologic agents and the chain of infection.

An *etiologic agent* is any pathogen that can cause an infection. Etiologic agents include bacteria, fungi, protozoa, rickettsiae, and helminthes.

There are six elements in the chain of infection:

1. **Pathogen:** An infectious agent, like a bacteria or virus.

2. **Reservoirs:** Any environment that is favorable for growth and reproduction of infectious agents. A reservoir may be animate or inanimate. Human systems that can act as reservoirs include blood, respiratory, gastrointestinal, reproductive, and urinary.

3. **Portal of exit:** A place where the infectious organisms get out of a host. Any of the above-mentioned systems may be portals of exit.

4. **Method of transmission:** The way an infectious organism is transferred from reservoir to host. This happens in one of three ways: direct contact, indirect contact via a vector, or through the air (airborne).

5. **Portal of entry:** A place where an infectious agent enters the susceptible host. A portal of entry may also be through a system that can act as a reservoir.

6. **Susceptible host:** A client, staff member, or other individual at risk for infection.

Now let's review the most important concepts covered by the Safety and Infection Control subcategory on the NCLEX-RN® exam.

ACCIDENT/INJURY PREVENTION

To help protect clients from accident and injury, you should assess risk factors upon the client's admission and identify appropriate methods to minimize risk of injury. This includes knowledge of the developmental stages mentioned previously in the Safety Background section, the client's lifestyle, and his or her knowledge of safety precautions.

You should know how to identify specific deficits, such as sight, hearing, and other sensory perceptions that may impact client safety. It's also important to be able to teach families how to properly install and use infant and child car seats.

EMERGENCY RESPONSE PLAN

The Joint Commission requires hospitals to have a disaster plan and periodically practice response to the plan. You are responsible for knowing your role in disaster response.

Know all of the steps involved in fire safety in a hospital setting. If a fire occurs, first get clients out of danger, then work to contain the fire, and finally determine the order in which to evacuate clients, including identification of clients who must be evacuated in beds or on stretchers (horizontally). You must also know how to teach clients about fire safety at home, such as knowing emergency numbers, installing and testing smoke alarms, acquiring fire extinguishers, and so on.

ERGONOMIC PRINCIPLES

You must understand ergonomic principles when caring for clients. This includes using assistive devices and proper lifting techniques. Assess a client's ability to balance and use assistive devices, such as crutches or a walker, and use that information to help develop an appropriate care plan.

For clients with repetitive stress injuries, provide instruction and information about body positions that can minimize or prevent these injuries. For clients with conditions that cause stress to specific skeletal or muscular groups, understand and educate the clients about necessary modifications. These may include changing positions frequently, and performing routine stretching exercises for the shoulders, neck, arms, hands, and fingers.

ERROR PREVENTION

Medication and allergies are primary areas for error. Error prevention, therefore, begins with proper identification of the client. You should be able to identify client allergies and intervene appropriately, know how to verify appropriateness and/or accuracy of a treatment or medication order, and be able to prevent treatment errors using critical thinking and by following policies.

HANDLING HAZARDOUS AND INFECTIOUS MATERIALS

It is important to be aware of the elements of employee safety. These include the safe use of equipment, safe handling of hazardous chemicals, and the use of Material Safety Data Sheets (MSDS), which are Occupational Safety and Health Administration (OSHA)-required handouts that describe all chemical agents in an employment setting.

Know the standard precautions to protect against blood-borne pathogen exposure. (OSHA has written standards that include recommendations from the Centers for Disease Control and Prevention [CDC], including the use of gloves and face and eye protection.) You must know what to do in case of a needlestick, the standards for environmental infection control, and necessary information related to latex allergies for both staff and clients. Be sure latex-free gloves and latex-free carts are available and used as necessary.

You also need to be able to identify biohazardous, flammable, and infectious materials; know how to control the spread of infectious agents; follow procedures for handling biohazardous materials; and be able to demonstrate safe handling techniques to staff and clients.

The Needlestick Safety and Prevention Act is significant legislation that was enacted to protect health care workers. Do not re-cap needles or bend or break them before disposal. Ensure that sharps containers are in each client room and medication area.

HOME SAFETY

Home safety includes evaluating the client's home care environment for fire risk, environmental hazards, and other elements that present a risk of accident or injury to the client. It also involves working with the client and the client's family and significant others to recommend modifications, such as lighting or handrails.

Home safety also includes teaching clients self-care, and teaching parents how to care for children. It also includes teaching preventive measures for home care, such as encouraging the client to use protective equipment when using devices that can cause injury.

REPORTING OF INCIDENT/EVENT/IRREGULAR OCCURRENCE/ VARIANCE

Incident reports are tools designed to provide information about potential areas of exposure to liability, and are also used to identify problems and develop solutions to prevent the same incident from happening again. Being able to accurately identify situations requiring completion of an incident or unusual occurrence report is an important skill. Although each hospital has its own procedures, the most important thing is to prevent further injury. In addition to reporting, you need to evaluate the response to the event to ensure it helped to correct the situation and to prevent further errors. Record the facts of the incident in the medical record, but do not include a copy of the incident report or make reference to its existence in the medical record.

SAFE USE OF EQUIPMENT

You must make sure that equipment needed to perform client care procedures and treatments is used safely and properly. This includes inspecting equipment to make sure it is safe to use. If a client needs to use equipment at home, you must teach the client how to use the equipment safely and properly.

uipment is not safe, or if it malfunctions, you should stop using it, label it as broken, ...ove it from any possible use, put it in a designated area for broken equipment (if avail-...le), and report the problem to the appropriate person.

SECURITY PLAN

You may be asked to triage injured or ill clients in an emergency, and to identify those in need of urgent care. The exam focuses on airway, breathing, circulation, and neurological deficits.

The order is:

1. Clear and open the airway.

2. Assess for respiratory distress.

3. Assess quality of breathing (rate, and color of skin, lips, and fingernails) and auscultate lungs.

4. Check pulse.

5. Assess for external bleeding.

6. Take blood pressure.

7. Assess the level of consciousness and papillary response, and the weakness or paralysis of extremities.

You should also be aware of your facility's procedures and protocols during an evacuation, newborn nursery security event, and bomb threat. Nurses often participate in developing security and emergency plans, so you should be prepared to do so. Clinical decision-making skills and critical thinking are important components of the development and successful execution of a security plan.

STANDARD PRECAUTIONS/TRANSMISSION-BASED PRECAUTIONS/SURGICAL ASEPSIS

There are a variety of different precautions that should be used to prevent the spread of infection. These include "standard" precautions that should always be used, precautions specifically aimed at the transmission of pathogenic microorganisms, and surgical asepsis (sterile techniques).

Standard Precautions

In addition to understanding the chain of infection, you should be able to apply standard precautions (such as handwashing, wearing gloves and gowns, and using face protection, such as masks, goggles, and face shields) with respect to hand hygiene, blood, bodily fluids, excretions, and secretions. These principles apply whether or not the skin and mucous membranes are intact, and should always be used in caring for clients across all diagnoses and all care settings.

Be aware of how, and in what order, to correctly put on and remove personal protective equipment (PPE). Perform hand hygiene first. Then before making contact with the client, and preferably outside the room, put on PPE: gown first, then the mask, then eye protection, and gloves last. The steps reverse for removing PPE: remove gloves first, then eye protection, then mask, then gown, with hand hygiene coming last.

Transmission-based Precautions

Transmission-based precautions limit the spread of pathogenic microorganisms. You should be able to compare and contrast airborne, droplet, and contact precautions; know when to use each; and know when multiple precautions may be needed. For example, when small (< 5 mcm) pathogen-infected droplets remain suspended in the air over time and travel distances greater than 3 feet, use airborne precautions. Pathogens may include measles (rubeola), chickenpox (varicella), and tuberculosis, among others. Use droplet precautions for larger (> 5 mcm) pathogen-infected droplets that travel 3 feet or less via coughing, sneezing, and so on. An example of this type of pathogen is *Haemophilus influenzae.* Use contact precautions with known or suspected microorganisms transmitted by direct hand-to-skin contact or indirect contact with surfaces (*Clostridium difficile*, herpes simplex, impetigo, etc.).

You should also be able to identify infectious agents that require transmission-based precautions, and specific precautions used in cases of drug-resistant infections.

Surgical Asepsis

You need to understand the principles of surgical asepsis—the practices necessary to maintain objects and areas free of microorganisms—also known as *sterile techniques.* Know how to use these techniques in implementing a variety of procedures, including IV therapy and urinary catheterization.

The basic principles of surgical asepsis are:

- Every object used in a sterile field must be sterile.
- If a sterile object touches an unsterile object, it is no longer sterile.
- If a sterile object is out of view, or below waist level, it is considered unsterile.
- A sterile object can become unsterile through exposure to airborne microorganisms.
- Fluids flow in the direction of gravity.
- Moisture passing through a sterile object can draw microorganisms from unsterile surfaces above or below through capillary action.
- The edges of a sterile field are unsterile.
- The skin cannot be sterilized.

USE OF RESTRAINTS/SAFETY DEVICES

You need to understand the difference between chemical (medication) and physical restraints (bedside rails, jacket, and extremity strap restraints). In addition, you need to know how to utilize restraints safely, effectively, and only when necessary, as well as how and with what frequency to monitor clients who are restrained. It's also important to understand the legal implications of restraining clients, as well as agency-specific policies and procedures. This includes understanding that seizures may necessitate restraint.

CHAPTER QUIZ

1. The physician orders an MRI of the brain for an adult male client. Which of the following findings in the client's history should the nurse report to the physician?

   1. Allergy to contrast dye
   2. Implanted cardiac pacemaker
   3. Chronic obstructive pulmonary disease (COPD)
   4. Hernia repair

2. The nurse is developing a care plan for a client with hepatitis C. The nurse knows that the primary route of transmission of this hepatitis virus is which of the following?

   1. Contaminated food
   2. Feces
   3. Blood
   4. Sputum

3. The nurse is preparing to discharge a client with rheumatic heart disease who is recovering from endocarditis. Which of the following statements from the client indicates that the client understands the teaching?

   1. "I'm so glad I don't need any more antibiotics now that I'm feeling better."
   2. "I can restart my exercise program in a day or two."
   3. "I will watch for signs of relapse the first few days after discharge."
   4. "I will inform my dentist should I ever need any dental work."

4. The nurse is preparing to test a client who has allergies from an unknown cause. Which of the following tests should the nurse perform?

   1. Tzanck test
   2. Patch test
   3. Rinne test
   4. Stress test

5. The nurse is preparing a client with acquired immunodeficiency syndrome (AIDS) for discharge to home. Which of the following instructions should the nurse include?

   1. "Avoid sharing articles such as razors and toothbrushes."
   2. "Do not share eating utensils with family members."
   3. "Limit the time you spend in public places."
   4. "Avoid eating food from serving dishes shared with others."

6. The nurse is preparing to administer a tuberculin (Mantoux) skin test to a client suspected of having tuberculosis (TB). The nurse knows that the test will reveal which of the following?

   1. How long the client has been infected with TB
   2. Active TB infection
   3. Latent TB infection
   4. Whether the client has been infected with TB bacteria

7. An older adult has been admitted with diagnosis of stroke and a history of dementia. Which of the following nursing diagnoses has the highest priority for this client?

   1. Bathing/hygiene self-care deficit
   2. Risk for injury
   3. Impaired physical mobility
   4. Disturbed thought processes

8. The nurse has just administered insulin to a diabetic client. In which of the following ways should the nurse dispose of the needle?

   1. Re-cap the needle and discard it in the nearest puncture-resistant container.
   2. Re-cap the needle and discard it in the nearest biohazard container.
   3. Discard the needle in a puncture-resistant container.
   4. Break the needle and discard it in the nearest puncture-resistant container.

9. The nurse is preparing to administer packed red blood cells (PRBCs) to a client. Arrange the following steps in the order the nurse should perform them. **All options must be used.**

   1. Explain the procedure to the client. _3_
   2. Obtain the client's vital signs. _4_
   3. Assess that the client has a blood bank identification armband. _2_
   4. Obtain the PRBCs from the blood bank according to hospital policy and perform a visual check of the blood. _6_
   5. Perform a bedside identification and blood product verification by two licensed individuals. _7_
   6. Verify the physician order. _1_
   7. Prime the transfusion tubing with a 0.9% sodium chloride solution. _5_

10. Two nurses are preparing to lift a client up in bed. Which of the following should the nurses do to help avoid injuring their backs?

    1. Bend from the waist.
    2. Lift with the back, not with the legs.
    3. Lower the head of the bed to about 30 degrees, if the client can tolerate it.
    4. Make certain the bed is in a reasonably high position.

11. In the emergency room, the nurse assesses a 4-year-old child suspected of having measles. Which of the following kinds of precautions should the nurse initiate?

    1. Contact precautions
    2. Droplet precautions
    3. Airborne precautions ✓
    4. Reverse isolation

12. A female client comes to the Emergency Department complaining of vaginal discharge, irritation of the vagina, and the need to urinate often. The nurse suspects a sexually transmitted disease (STD), and the physician orders diagnostic testing of the vaginal discharge. Which of the following STDs does the nurse know must be reported to the Department of Public Health?

    1. Genital herpes
    2. Human papillomavirus infection
    3. Gonorrhea
    4. Trichomoniasis

13. An elderly client, who is not oriented to time, place, or person, had a total hip replacement. The client is attempting to get out of bed and pull out the IV line that is infusing antibiotics. The client has bilateral soft wrist restraints and a vest restraint. Which of the following interventions by the nurse are appropriate? **Select all that apply.**

    1. Ask the client if he needs to use the bathroom, and provide range-of-motion exercises every 2 hours. ✓
    2. Document the type of restraint used and assess the need for continued use. ✓
    3. Tie the restraints to the side rails of the bed.
    4. Obtain a new physician order for the restraint every 12 hours.
    5. Observe for correct placement of restraints. ✓
    6. Tie the restraints in a quick-release knot. ✓

14. The nurse is preparing to administer a unit of PRBCs to an anemic client. After obtaining the blood from the blood bank, the nurse must begin administering it within which of the following time periods?

   1. 15 minutes
   2. 30 minutes
   3. 45 minutes
   4. 60 minutes

15. The nurse is assessing an elderly client for risk of falls. Which of the following should the nurse collect?

   1. The facility's restraint policy
   2. Gait, balance, and visual impairment information
   3. Psychosocial history
   4. The facility's environmental safety plan

16. The nurse is administering nightly medications, which include an anticoagulant and a stool softener. Which of the following should the nurse do *FIRST* before administering the medications?

   1. Scan the medication label and the client's wristband.
   2. Ask the client his or her name to properly identify this client as the one for whom the medications were ordered.
   3. Match the client's date of birth and name on the client's wristband with the same information on the medication order.
   4. Match the client's name and room number with the medication order.

17. The physician verbally orders a medication for a client during an emergency code. Which of the following should the nurse do?

   1. Repeat the order back to the physician for confirmation and administer it.
   2. Retrieve the medication and administer it.

3. Write the order down, retrieve the medication, and administer it.
   4. Read the order to another nurse, have that nurse retrieve the medication, and stay with the client.

18. The client has a new order for placement of a Foley catheter due to urinary retention. Which of the following should the nurse do before starting the procedure? **Select all that apply.**

   1. The nurse should confirm the client's identity, because a procedure requires proper identification.
   2. The nurse should confirm the client's medical record number via the wristband and order.
   3. Ask the client his or her name only, because this is a procedure and not a medication administration.
   4. The nurse should confirm the client's name via the wristband and order.

19. Which of the following actions by the nurse is the *MOST* effective means of preventing infection?

   1. Washing hands after client contact
   2. Washing hands after removing gloves
   3. Hand hygiene between clients
   4. Hand hygiene before entry to a client's room and upon exit of a client's room

20. The client is an obese male with decubitus ulcers. Treatment of the ulcers requires frequent turning and repositioning. The nursing unit has a special lift that allows for turning of clients and placement onto a bedpan without any lifting on the part of the staff. The client urgently requests the bedpan. Because the lift apparatus takes a few minutes to set up, which of the following should the nurse do?

   1. Quickly assist the client onto the bedpan without the lift because he needs to use it urgently.

2. Encourage the client to try to be patient, and set up the apparatus.

3. Get the assistance of an aide to help lift the client.

4. Encourage the client to wear an incontinence brief.

21. The client has experienced multiple episodes of hyperglycemia not manageable by subcutaneous insulin injections. The client has an active order for infusion of an insulin drip for glycemic management to be discontinued at bedtime, after which the client is NPO. The client's most recent blood sugar level, taken at 3 P.M., was 60. Which of the following actions by the nurse is the MOST appropriate?

1. The nurse should follow the order and allow the insulin to infuse until bedtime.

2. The nurse should recheck the client's blood sugar.

3. The nurse should bring this blood sugar level to the physician's attention and discuss stopping the infusion.

4. The nurse should seek advice from other nurses.

22. The adult children of a hospice home care client inquire about whether it is safe to hug their mother, because she has had a methicillin-resistant *Staphylococcus aureus* (MRSA) infection in the past. Which of the following statements by the children would indicate a need for further teaching by the nurse?

1. "We should wash our hands frequently."

2. "We should use hand sanitizer."

3. "Those of us with poor immune systems should be extra careful."

4. "We should wear gowns and gloves at all times when having contact with our mother."

23. The nurse witnesses another nurse, wearing a gown and gloves, enter a client room labeled "Airborne Precautions." Which of the following actions by the witnessing nurse is MOST appropriate?

1. Notify the nurse manager to discuss policies with the other nurse.

2. Ask a physician to give a presentation on which precautions require which types of personal protective equipment (PPE).

3. Remind the other nurse that she needs a mask in addition to a gown and gloves for airborne-type precautions.

4. Ask the other nurse to look up the policy about precautions.

24. The nurse discovers a client on the floor in the client's hospital room. After examining the client and assisting him safely back to bed, which of the following should the nurse do FIRST?

1. File an incident report.

2. Put the bed alarm back on.

3. Institute a client observer to sit with the client and prevent further falls.

4. Notify the nurse manager.

25. The hospitalized client is receiving an infusion and the pump has malfunctioned. Which of the following actions by the nurse is MOST appropriate once the infusion has been stopped and restarted with a functioning pump?

1. Place a "Broken" sticker on the malfunctioning pump according to hospital policy, and place the pump in the designated malfunctioning equipment area.

2. Place the malfunctioning pump in the utility room.

3. Remove the malfunctioning pump from the client's room and place with other pumps.

4. Place the malfunctioning pump to the side in the client's room.

26. The nurse completes a peripherally inserted central catheter (PICC) line dressing change for a home care client. When removing the PPE, the nurse should do which of the following?

1. Remove the mask and then the gloves.

2. Remove the gloves and then the mask.

3. Remove only the gloves; there is no need to wear a mask.

4. Remove only the mask; there is no need to wear gloves.

27. The client is found on the floor by the nursing assistive personnel (NAP). Once the client is safe, which of the following should the nurse do next?

1. Document the event in the client's medical record and file an incident report.

2. File an incident report only.

3. Document the event in the client's medical record and have the NAP file an incident report.

4. Document the event in the client's medical record only.

28. The nurse is making a home visit to an elderly client during the winter. The nurse notices upon arrival that the client has the oven turned on with the oven door open, and is using it as a form of heat. Which of the following actions by the nurse is *MOST* appropriate?

1. Take care of the client's medical needs and do not get involved in the client's private matters.

2. Shut the oven off and continue with the home visit.

3. Report the event to the local Fire Department.

4. Have a meeting with the client and family and warn them of the fire and safety risks of using the oven for heat.

29. The medical center encounters a bomb threat. The emergency response team informs the staff that the threat is legitimate and that clients should start being evacuated. Which of the following clients should the nurse begin evacuating *FIRST* to the safe designated area?

1. Ambulatory clients

2. Bedridden clients

3. ICU clients

4. Infant clients

30. The nurse discovers that the last dose of intravenous antibiotic administered to a client was the wrong dose. Which of the following should the nurse do?

1. Document the event in the client's medical record only.

2. File an incident report, and document the event in the client's medical record.

3. Document in the client's medical record that an incident report was filed.

4. File an incident report, but don't document the event in the client's medical record, because information about the incident is protected.

CHAPTER QUIZ ANSWERS AND EXPLANATIONS

1. The Answer is 2

The physician orders an MRI of the brain for an adult male client. Which of the following findings in the client's history should the nurse report to the physician?

Category: Accident/injury prevention; Safe use of equipment

(1) Allergy to contrast dye is contraindicated in CT scans with contrast, not MRI.

(2) CORRECT: Metallic items, including metallic implants such as a cardiac pacemaker, are contraindicated in MRI.

(3) COPD is not a contraindication for MRI.

(4) Hernia repair is not a contraindication for MRI.

2. The Answer is 3

The nurse is developing a care plan for a client with hepatitis C. The nurse knows that the primary route of transmission of this hepatitis virus is which of the following?

Category: Standard precautions/transmission-based precautions/surgical asepsis

(1) The hepatitis A (not hepatitis C) virus is transmitted through the fecal-oral route, primarily through ingestion of contaminated food.

(2) The hepatitis A (not hepatitis C) virus is transmitted through the fecal-oral route, primarily through ingestion of contaminated food.

(3) CORRECT: The hepatitis C virus is transmitted through blood and parenteral routes.

(4) The hepatitis C virus is not transmitted through sputum.

3. The Answer is 4

The nurse is preparing to discharge a client with rheumatic heart disease who is recovering from endocarditis. Which of the following statements from the client indicates that the client understands the teaching?

Category: Standard precautions/transmission-based precautions/surgical asepsis

(1) The client must take the full course of prescribed antibiotics even if feeling better.

(2) The client must restrict activity as directed by the physician.

(3) Relapse may occur, but not until about 2 weeks after treatment stops.

(4) CORRECT: Susceptible clients must understand the need for prophylactic antibiotics before, during, and after dental work.

4. The Answer is 2

The nurse is preparing to test a client who has allergies from an unknown cause. Which of the following tests should the nurse perform?

Category: Error prevention

(1) The Tzanck test is used to detect the herpes virus.

(2) CORRECT: The patch test identifies the cause of allergic contact sensitization and is indicated in clients with suspected allergies or allergies from an unknown cause.

(3) The Rinne test compares bone conduction to air conduction in the ears.

(4) A stress test assesses cardiovascular response to increased workload.

5. The Answer is 1

The nurse is preparing a client with acquired immunodeficiency syndrome (AIDS) for discharge to home. Which of the following instructions should the nurse include?

Category: Standard precautions/transmission-based precautions/surgical asepsis

(1) CORRECT: The human immunodeficiency virus (HIV), which causes AIDS, is concentrated mostly in blood and semen. The client should not share articles that may be contaminated with blood, such as razors and toothbrushes.

(2) HIV is not transmitted by sharing eating utensils.

(3) Someone with HIV does not need to limit time in public places.

(4) HIV is not transmitted by sharing food from serving dishes used by someone with AIDS.

6. The Answer is 4

The nurse is preparing to administer a tuberculin (Mantoux) skin test to a client suspected of having tuberculosis (TB). The nurse knows that the test will reveal which of the following?

Category: Standard precautions/transmission-based precautions/surgical asepsis

(1) The test cannot detect how long a person has been infected.

(2) The test cannot detect whether the infection is latent (inactive) or active.

(3) The test cannot detect whether the infection can be passed on to others.

(4) CORRECT: A tuberculin skin test is performed to determine if a person has ever had TB.

7. The Answer is 2

An older adult has been admitted with diagnosis of stroke and a history of dementia. Which of the following nursing diagnoses has the highest priority for this client?

Category: Accident/injury prevention

(1) A bathing/hygiene self-care deficit would not be the highest priority.

(2) CORRECT: Older adults with dementia are at risk for injury due to increased risk for falls, because they may not recognize their limitations, despite immobility related to stroke.

(3) Impaired physical mobility would not be the highest priority.

(4) Disturbed thought processes would not be the highest priority.

8. The Answer is 3

The nurse has just administered insulin to a diabetic client. In which of the following ways should the nurse dispose of the needle?

Category: Handling hazardous and infectious materials

(1) Needles should not be re-capped.

(2) Needles should not be re-capped and should be placed in puncture-resistant containers, not just any biohazard container.

(3) CORRECT: Needles and sharps should be placed in the nearest puncture-resistant container.

(4) Needles should not be broken.

9. The Answer is 6, 3, 1, 2, 7, 4, 5

The nurse is preparing to administer packed red blood cells (PRBCs) to a client. Arrange the following steps in the order the nurse should perform them. **All options must be used.**

Category: Error prevention

(1) The third step is to explain the procedure to the client.

(2) The fourth step is to obtain the client's vital signs.

(3) The second step is to assess that the client has a blood bank identification armband.

(4) The sixth step is to obtain the PRBCs from the blood bank according to hospital policy and perform a visual check of the blood.

(5) The last step is to perform a bedside identification and blood product verification by two licensed individuals.

(6) The first step is to verify the physician order.

(7) The fifth step is to prime the transfusion tubing with a 0.9% sodium chloride solution.

10. The Answer is 4

Two nurses are preparing to lift a client up in bed. Which of the following should the nurses do to help avoid injuring their backs?

Category: Accident/injury prevention; Ergonomic principles

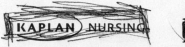

(1) When lifting or moving a client, nurses should maintain the natural curve of the spine and not bend at the waist.

(2) When lifting or moving a client, nurses should lift with the legs and not the back.

(3) When lifting or moving a client, place the bed in the Trendelenburg position if the client can tolerate it.

(4) CORRECT: The bed should be in a reasonably high position so the nurses do not have to lean.

11. The Answer is 3

In the emergency room, the nurse assesses a 4-year-old child suspected of having measles. Which of the following kinds of precautions should the nurse initiate?

Category: Standard precautions/transmission-based precautions/surgical asepsis

(1) Contact precautions are not used for measles.

(2) Droplet precautions are not used for measles.

(3) CORRECT: Airborne precautions are used to prevent the transmission of infectious agents that remain infectious over long distances when suspended in the air.

(4) Reverse isolation is not used for measles.

12. The Answer is 3

A female client comes to the Emergency Department complaining of vaginal discharge, irritation of the vagina, and the need to urinate often. The nurse suspects a sexually transmitted disease (STD), and the physician orders diagnostic testing of the vaginal discharge. Which of the following STDs does the nurse know must be reported to the Department of Public Health?

Category: Standard precautions/transmission-based precautions/surgical asepsis

(1) Genital herpes is not a reportable disease.

(2) Human papillomavirus infection is not a reportable disease.

(3) CORRECT: Gonorrhea must be reported to the Department of Public Health.

(4) Trichomoniasis is not a reportable disease.

13. The Answer is 1, 2, 5, and 6

An elderly client, who is not oriented to time, place, or person, had a total hip replacement. The client is attempting to get out of bed and pull out the IV line that is infusing antibiotics. The client has bilateral soft wrist restraints and a vest restraint. Which of the following interventions by the nurse are appropriate? **Select all that apply.**

Category: Use of restraints/safety devices

(1) CORRECT: Toileting and range-of-motion exercises should be provided every 2 hours while a client is in restraints.

(2) CORRECT: The client must be assessed frequently to ascertain when restraints can be removed, and this information must be documented.

(3) Restraints should never be tied to the side rails, because this can cause injury if the side rail is lowered without untying the restraint.

(4) A new physician's order must be obtained every 24 hours if restraints are continued.

(5) CORRECT: The nurse should observe for correct placement of restraints.

(6) CORRECT: Restraints should be tied in knots that can be released quickly and easily.

14. The Answer is 2

The nurse is preparing to administer a unit of PRBCs to an anemic client. After obtaining the blood from the blood bank, the nurse must begin administering it within which of the following time periods?

Category: Error prevention

(1) The nurse has up to 30 minutes to begin administering the blood product.

(2) CORRECT: After obtaining the blood product from the blood bank, the nurse must begin administering the product within 30 minutes.

(3) This time period is too long.

(4) This time period is too long.

15. The Answer is 2

The nurse is assessing an elderly client for risk of falls. Which of the following should the nurse collect?

Category: Accident/injury prevention

(1) The facility's restraint policy is not relevant to a fall risk assessment.

(2) CORRECT: Fall risk should include assessment of gait, balance, and visual impairment.

(3) The client's psychosocial history is important but not in relation to risk for falls.

(4) The facility's environmental safety plan is not relevant to a fall risk assessment.

16. The Answer is 3

The nurse is administering nightly medications, which include an anticoagulant and a stool softener. Which of the following should the nurse do *FIRST* before administering the medications?

Category: Error prevention

(1) Scanning the medication label and the client's wristband might be correct if the institution has a bar coding system, but it is not the first thing you would do.

(2) Asking the client his or her name might be correct, but it is not the most complete answer.

(3) CORRECT: The 2012 National Patient Safety Goals require using a minimum of two patient identifiers as a means to promote the safest care and to prevent medication errors.

(4) The room number should never be used as a client identifier.

17. The Answer is 1

The physician verbally orders a medication for a client during an emergency code. Which of the following should the nurse do?

Category: Error prevention

(1) CORRECT: In an emergency code situation, the order can be repeated back to the physician for confirmation and given, as there is another nurse recording events of the code.

(2) The medication order should be confirmed with the physician first.

(3) The order should be repeated back to the physician for verification before it is administered.

(4) The nurse should confirm the order with the physician first.

18. The Answer is 1, 2, and 4

The client has a new order for placement of a Foley catheter due to urinary retention. Which of the following should the nurse do before starting the procedure? **Select all that apply.**

Category: Error prevention

(1) CORRECT: The nurse should confirm the client's identity, because a procedure requires proper identification.

(2) CORRECT: The nurse should confirm the client's medical record number via the wristband and order.

(3) The nurse must always properly identify clients for any and all treatments, not just for medication administration.

(4) CORRECT: The nurse should confirm the client's name via the wristband and order.

19. The Answer is 4

Which of the following actions by the nurse is the *MOST* effective means of preventing infection?

Category: Standard precautions/transmission-based precautions/surgical asepsis

(1) Washing hands after client contact is appropriate but not the most effective means of preventing an infection, and alone, is not enough.

(2) Washing hands after removing gloves is appropriate but not the most effective means of preventing an infection, and alone, is not enough.

(3) Hand hygiene between clients is appropriate but not the most effective means of preventing an infection, and alone, is not enough.

(4) CORRECT: Hand hygiene should occur before entry and upon exit of all client care transactions.

20. The Answer is 2

The client is an obese male with decubitus ulcers. Treatment of the ulcers requires frequent turning and repositioning. The nursing unit has a special lift that allows for turning of clients and placement onto a bedpan without any lifting on the part of the staff. The client urgently requests the bedpan. Because the lift apparatus takes a few minutes to set up, which of the following should the nurse do?

Category: Ergonomic principles

(1) Quickly assisting the client onto the bedpan is a tempting answer and might happen frequently in real life. However, it is not the best or safest option for the client or the nurse.

(2) CORRECT: Encourage the client to wait while the apparatus is set up. It is more important to prevent potential injury to the nurse. Nurses are commonly affected by ergonomic injuries related to lifting and moving clients.

(3) This is not the best or safest option for the client or the aide.

(4) Encouraging the client to wear an incontinence brief is inappropriate.

21. The Answer is 3

The client has experienced multiple episodes of hyperglycemia not manageable by subcutaneous insulin injections. The client has an active order for infusion of an insulin drip for glycemic management to be discontinued at bedtime, after which the client is NPO. The client's most recent blood sugar level, taken at 3 p.m., was 60. Which of the following actions by the nurse is the *MOST* appropriate?

Category: Error prevention

(1) The nurse has a duty to verify the order, given the change in circumstances. The blood sugar is now low, and continuing an insulin drip has the potential to drop it to a dangerous level.

(2) The nurse would recheck the client's blood sugar level only if there was reason to believe it might be in error.

(3) CORRECT: The most appropriate action is to contact the physician and discuss stopping the infusion, based on the last blood sugar level.

(4) The nurse might ask a colleague for advice, but the most appropriate action is to discuss the situation with the physician.

22. The Answer is 4

The adult children of a hospice home care client inquire about whether it is safe to hug their mother, because she has had a methicillin-resistant *Staphylococcus aureus* (MRSA) infection in the past. Which of the following statements by the children would indicate a need for further teaching by the nurse?

Category: Standard precautions/transmission-based precautions/surgical asepsis

(1) A statement that "we should wash our hands frequently" is accurate.

(2) A statement that "we should use hand sanitizer" is accurate.

(3) A statement that "those of us with poor immune systems should be extra careful" is accurate.

(4) CORRECT: The family does not have to wear gowns and gloves when interacting with their mother. The infection occurred in the past; even if it was active, gowns and gloves would not be required. Staff wear PPE to prevent spreading these types of infections to other clients.

23. The Answer is 3

The nurse witnesses another nurse, wearing a gown and gloves, enter a client room labeled "Airborne Precautions." Which of the following actions by the witnessing nurse is *MOST* appropriate?

Category: Standard precautions/transmission-based precautions/surgical asepsis

(1) The nurse manager does not need to be notified about this event unless it was recurring behavior endangering clients and staff. The witnessing nurse may still notify the manager, but it is not the most appropriate priority action.

(2) A presentation about which precautions require which types of PPE does not need to be delivered by a physician. Precautions are within the realm of nursing practice.

(3) CORRECT: Remind the other nurse that she needs a mask in addition to a gown and gloves for airborne-type precautions.

(4) The other nurse might need to review the policy, but a gentle reminder to use a mask is the most professionally appropriate act by the witnessing nurse.

24. The Answer is 2

The nurse discovers a client on the floor in the client's hospital room. After examining the client and assisting him safely back to bed, which of the following should the nurse do *FIRST*?

Category: Accident/injury prevention

(1) The nurse would file an incident report after meeting the patient's care needs.

(2) CORRECT: Putting the bed alarm back on is the most appropriate first step to promote immediate safety of the client.

(3) Instituting a client observer might be appropriate, but not enough information about the circumstances of the client and the manner in which he got to the floor is given in the question stem.

(4) Notifying the nurse manager might be appropriate, but not enough information about the circumstances of the client and the manner in which he got to the floor is given in the question stem.

25. The Answer is 1

The hospitalized client is receiving an infusion and the pump has malfunctioned. Which of the following actions by the nurse is *MOST* appropriate once the infusion has been stopped and restarted with a functioning pump?

Category: Safe use of equipment

(1) CORRECT: The malfunctioning equipment should be labeled clearly and put in a separate area to be reviewed by the equipment department.

(2) Placing the malfunctioning pump in the utility room may inadvertently allow the pump to reenter circulation and have the potential to lead to an infusion error.

(3) Placing the pump with other pumps may inadvertently allow the pump to reenter circulation and have the potential to lead to an infusion error.

(4) Placing the pump to the side in the client's room may inadvertently allow the pump to reenter circulation and have the potential to lead to an infusion error.

26. The Answer is 2

The nurse completes a peripherally inserted central catheter (PICC) line dressing change for a home care client. When removing the PPE, the nurse should do which of the following?

Category: Standard precautions/transmission-based precautions/surgical asepsis

(1) Removing the mask with gloves on could transfer contamination from the gloves to the mask and potentially to the nurse's head.

(2) CORRECT: Gloves are removed first.

(3) Both gloves and a mask should be worn when changing a PICC line dressing.

(4) Both gloves and a mask should be worn when changing a PICC line dressing.

27. The Answer is 3

The client is found on the floor by the nursing assistive personnel (NAP). Once the client is safe, which of the following should the nurse do next?

Category: Reporting of incident/event/irregular occurrence/variance

(1) The nurse should not file the incident report—the one who discovers the event (the NAP) should document it.

(2) An incident report needs to be filed for internal purposes of learning from occurrences, but the event must also be documented for purposes of client care.

(3) CORRECT: The event should be documented in the client's medical record and the NAP should file an incident report.

(4) An incident report needs to be filed for internal purposes of learning from occurrences.

28.   The Answer is 4

The nurse is making a home visit to an elderly client during the winter. The nurse notices upon arrival that the client has the oven turned on with the oven door open, and is using it as a form of heat. Which of the following actions by the nurse is *MOST* appropriate?

Category: Home safety

(1) As the home care nurse, it is the nurse's obligation to promote client safety and to prevent hazards.

(2) Shutting the oven off and continuing with the home visit might be a tempting choice. The nurse might do this, too, but it doesn't solve the problem if no education is done with the client and family.

(3) Reporting the event to the local Fire Department is not necessary unless the nurse has a fear that this activity will be continued.

(4) CORRECT: Have a meeting with the client and family and warn them of the fire and safety risks of using the oven for heat.

29.   The Answer is 1

The medical center encounters a bomb threat. The emergency response team informs the staff that the threat is legitimate and that clients should start being evacuated. Which of the following clients should the nurse begin evacuating *FIRST* to the safe designated area?

Category: Emergency response plan

(1) CORRECT: Ambulatory clients have the potential to wander and end up in an unsafe place if not directed correctly.

(2) Bedridden clients cannot leave without assistance; therefore they would be evacuated subsequent to the ambulatory clients.

(3) ICU clients cannot leave without assistance; therefore they would be evacuated subsequent to the ambulatory clients.

(4) Infant clients cannot leave without assistance; therefore they would be evacuated subsequent to the ambulatory clients.

30.   The Answer is 2

The nurse discovers that the last dose of intravenous antibiotic administered to a client was the wrong dose. Which of the following should the nurse do?

Category: Reporting of incident/event/irregular occurrence/variance

(1) The event should be filed both in an incident report and in the client's medical record.

(2) CORRECT: The event should be filed in an incident report and in the client's medical record.

(3) Nurses should not document in the client's medical record that an incident report was filed. The incident report is for internal purposes of learning for the institution.

(4) The event should be filed in both an incident report and in the client's medical record.

CHAPTER 6

HEALTH PROMOTION AND MAINTENANCE

Health promotion and maintenance involves helping your clients achieve and continue to enjoy optimal health. You help people to identify that target state, discover their strengths and their needs, and then support their path to full health and wellness potential. Putting your enthusiasm into screening, education, and treatment efforts can make a significant difference in successful outcomes.

On the NCLEX-RN® exam, you can expect approximately 9 percent of the questions to relate to Health Promotion and Maintenance. This category focuses on the knowledge of expected growth and development principles, prevention and/or early detection of health problems, and strategies to achieve optimal health. Exam content related to Health Promotion and Maintenance includes, but is not limited to, the following areas:

- Aging process
- Ante/intra/postpartum and newborn care
- Developmental stages and transitions
- Health and wellness
- Health promotion/disease prevention
- Health screening
- High risk behaviors
- Lifestyle choices
- Principles of teaching/learning
- Self-care
- Techniques of physical assessment

Let's now review the most important concepts covered by the Health Promotion and Maintenance category on the NCLEX-RN® exam.

AGING PROCESS

The aging process unfolds gradually, starting with infancy (the first year of life). After that, school becomes the dividing marker. Thus preadolescent stages are divided into two: preschool (1–4 years) and school-age (5–12 years). Puberty marks the onset of the adolescent stage (13–18 years). Adulthood is divided into three parts: the working years (19–64 years), the retirement years (65–85 years), and the elderly years (over 85 years). As you review for the NCLEX-RN® exam, make sure you understand the special needs of each of these age groups so that you can provide the necessary care and education required.

Whichever stage your clients are in, you need to be able to assess their reactions to expected age-related changes. For example, an adolescent and an elderly person are going to react differently to a change in their residential location. A teenager will probably make that transition more easily than an elderly client who is coping with other physical and cognitive losses.

ANTE/INTRA/POSTPARTUM AND NEWBORN CARE

To ensure the health of both mother and baby, pregnancies are now closely monitored from the moment a woman knows she is expecting to several weeks after the baby is born.

Antepartum Care

Antepartum care is care given to the mother and baby before birth. It is also known as *prenatal care*. Antepartum care involves keeping track of the client's history and includes a number of important examinations.

Calculating Expected Delivery Date

Every mother wants to know her estimated date of delivery. A simple way to calculate this is to add 7 days and 9 months to the first day of the last menstrual period. Only 4 percent of women actually give birth that day.

A pregnancy is considered *full term* between weeks 37 and 42. Birth occurring prior to week 37 is considered a *premature* birth, and later than week 42 is considered to be *overdue*.

Documenting the Mother's Current Health and Previous Health History

Documenting the mother's current health and previous health history is an important part of prenatal care. You should obtain data about blood pressure, weight, lifestyle, and family and genetic history; and ask about support systems, perception of pregnancy, and previous coping mechanisms. The absence of an in-place support system can be countered by putting the client in touch with a prenatal support group, for example. A referral is also appropriate if the client sees pregnancy as an illness, or if she has previously used denial or fantasy as coping mechanisms.

You also need to know which medications the client is using—prescribed, alternative, and over-the-counter. Category X medications have such a harmful effect on the developing fetus that they are contraindicated in pregnancy. These include:

- Birth control pills
- Accutane
- Some hyperlipidemia medications
- Warfarin (Coumadin)
- Ulcer drug (Cytotec)
- Vaccines for measles, mumps, and smallpox

You also need to test for the Rh factor, unless the mother is Rh-positive (has the factor) or both parents are Rh-negative (lack the factor). If the mother is Rh-negative and the father is Rh-positive, the mother needs to have Rho (D) immune globulin (RhoGAM) in the 28th week.

Ultrasounds are used to noninvasively confirm fetal viability, gestational age, fetal anatomy, and location of the placenta.

Sometimes an *amniocentesis*—withdrawing amniotic fluid for analysis—is done after the 14th week. The test is indicated for women over age 35 and those with a family history of genetic or metabolic problems.

Documenting Fetal Health

Fetal heart rate during routine prenatal exams should be between 120–160 beats per minute.

Educating a New Mother-to-Be

Nutrition is an important part of prenatal care and education. An estimated 50 percent of pregnancies are unplanned, and the mother-to-be might not have been getting adequate nutrients. Pregnant teenagers need more protein, calcium, and phosphorus than pregnant adults, because their bones are still growing.

Weight gain should be limited to between 22 and 27 pounds—somewhat less if overweight, somewhat more if underweight. Substantial weight gain is deleterious to both mother and baby because it increases risk of preeclampsia. If the mother does not lose the extra pounds after childbirth, she increases her risk of diabetes and high blood pressure, which are linked to a greater risk of coronary artery disease, among other conditions.

You also need to be able to provide prenatal education about normal pregnancy events, such as *quickening* (the first perceptible fetal movement, typically at 17–19 weeks, but in some instances as early as 13 weeks or as late as 25 weeks). Some women might have some Braxton Hicks contractions after the 20th week.

It is equally important to educate about possible danger signals. Examples include:

- Vaginal bleeding
- Continuous headaches during the last three months
- Marked or sudden swelling of extremities during the last three months
- Dimness or blurring of vision during the last three months
- Severe, unrelenting abdominal pain
- Decreased fetal movement after 24 weeks

Recognizing Cultural Differences

Be aware of cultural differences in childbearing practices. Chinese Confucian women value modesty and self-control, so such women may remain stoic during pregnancy, asking few questions. For Mormon women, pregnancy is viewed as a time of personal and family growth, as it creates a connection with eternity. The Orthodox Jewish woman is considered ritually impure after her water breaks, so her Orthodox Jewish husband is unlikely to be in the delivery room. Instead, he prays in the waiting area.

Intrapartum Care and Education

Intrapartum care is defined as care that is given during labor and birth.

Identifying Onset of Labor

The three main factors that may cause labor to begin are the effect of hormones, the distension of the uterus, and the effect of oxytocin. Two recognizable signs of impending labor are the passage of a thick mucus plug from the cervix and rupture of the amniotic membranes. On average, the entire process from onset to birth lasts about 12–14 hours for a first baby. Subsequent labors tend to be shorter in length.

Care During Labor

Nursing care mirrors labor's four stages:

1. **From 4–10 cm:** Assess cervical effacement and dilation, and need for analgesia.
2. **From complete dilation to delivery of baby:** Assess newborn.
3. **From delivery of baby to expulsion of placenta:** Usually within 5–20 minutes after birth; assess umbilical cord for two arteries and one vein.

4. **Immediate recovery and observation:** Approximately two hours after birth; assess maternal vital signs, uterine fundal height, vaginal discharge, and bladder distention; assist breast-feeding efforts if indicated.

Postpartum Care and Education

The mother must be carefully observed after birth to identify serious complications, including the following:

- **Hemorrhage:** Report heavy clots or spurts of bleeding. Expect some blood in vaginal discharge for 3–6 weeks.
- **Infection or other illnesses:** Watch for a temperature over 100.4° F (38° C); sudden increase in perineal pain; unusually heavy or foul-smelling vaginal discharge; hot, tender, or red breast; dysuria; pain or swelling in the legs; and chest pain or cough.

Newborn Care and Education

One minute after birth, the physician rates five factors:

1. Appearance (color)
2. Pulse (heart rate)
3. Grimace (reflex irritability)
4. Activity (muscle tone)
5. Respiration (respiratory effort)

This is known as the *APGAR score.* The value of each factor is 0 (not good), 1 (OK), or 2 (good). A total score of 10 is optimum.

Inform the mother of the warning signs of complications with her newborn, and explain when to call a doctor or take the baby to an emergency room. Those complications include:

- Has sunken or swollen soft spots on the head
- Has a fever higher than 100.4° F (38° C)
- Vomits more than once in 24 hours
- Is unable to keep down food or water
- Is not breathing easily

It is also important to assist the mother in performing newborn care. This is an ideal time to answer questions about parent-infant bonding. This is also the best time to provide contraception education, if needed. The client's menstrual cycle should begin in 6–8 weeks after giving birth, unless she is breastfeeding. Make sure your client knows about normal emotional stress (the *blues*) during her second or third postpartum week. Tell her to contact her physician if she experiences significant negative mood changes.

DEVELOPMENTAL STAGES AND TRANSITIONS

The following sections provide an overview of life's milestones to review for the NCLEX-RN® exam.

Infants

Infants are 1–12 months old.

Expected Development

- **Physical:** May have swollen genitals and breasts, a misshapen head, milia (white spots) on face; exhibits sucking, grasping reflexes; able to focus; learns to grasp with thumb and finger
- **Cognitive and psychosocial:** Vocalizes sounds (coos); begins to respond selectively to words

Deviations

- Not rolling from tummy to side at 10 months
- Not transferring toys from hand to hand at 9 months

Special Needs

- Parent-infant bonding

Preschool-Age Children

Preschool-age children are 1–4 years old.

Expected Development

- **Physical:** Enjoys physical activities; has increasing bladder and bowel control; can manipulate small objects with hands; is able to dress and undress self; has refined coordination
- **Cognitive and psychosocial:** Becomes aware of limits; says "no" often; has a limited vocabulary of 500–3,000 words in very short sentences (3–4 words); believes that adults know everything; can use a pencil to draw shapes; is eager to learn; has a strong desire to please adults

Deviations

- Does not walk at 18 months
- Does not speak at least 15 words
- Does not imitate actions or words or follow simple instructions

- Talks excessively about violence or other mature topics
- Not interested in "pretend" play or other children

Special Needs

- Security and consistency of environment
- Protection from harmful situations caused by natural curiosity
- Some allowance for independence and playtime

School-Age Children

School-age children are 5–12 years old.

Expected Development

- **Physical:** Able to do a series of motions to perform activities, such as skipping or jumping rope
- **Cognitive and psychosocial:** Able to follow two-step directions; knows full name, age, and address; tends to identify with parent of the same sex

Deviations

- Bed-wetting late into childhood
- Verbal or outward expression of anxiety about school or home

Special Needs

- Developing scoliosis (sideways curvature of spine)
- Vision and hearing problems: important to discover at earliest stages

Adolescents

Adolescents are 13–18 years old.

Expected Development

- **Physical:** Shows increased interest in personal attractiveness; develops secondary sexual characteristics
- **Cognitive and psychosocial:** Struggles with sense of identity; forms strong peer allegiances; engages in risk-taking due to a sense of immortality

Deviations

- Persistent misbehavior, especially in school
- Aggression

Special Needs

- Understanding of puberty's effect on disposition and personality

Adults

Adults are 19–64 years old.

Expected Development

- **Physical:** Peak reached between 25 and 35 years old; might live for many years with a chronic condition
- **Cognitive and psychosocial:** From 19–34 years old—Erikson's stage of intimacy versus isolation; from 35–64 years old—Erikson's stage of generativity versus stagnation

Deviations

- Feeling that life is meaningless

Special Needs

- Learning lessons of workplace, long-term relationships, and parenting

Older Adults

Older adults are 65–85 years old.

Expected Development

- **Physical:** General slowing of physical functioning
- **Cognitive and psychosocial:** General slowing of cognitive functioning; Erikson's stage of ego integrity versus despair; interpersonal relationships continue despite changes and losses

Deviations

- Despair can arise from remorse for what might have been

Special Needs

- Learning lessons of successfully retiring from the workplace
- Keeping or losing long-term relationships

Very Old Adults

Very old adults are over 85 years old.

Expected Development

- **Physical:** Continued decline of physical functioning
- **Cognitive and psychosocial:** Continued decline of cognitive functioning; marked increase in changes and losses in relationships

Deviations

- Suicidal thoughts and behavior

Special Needs

- Acceptance of life's accomplishments and declines

HEALTH AND WELLNESS

Traditionally, health is the absence of disease and disability. Known as the medical model, that philosophy has changed with the recognition that people can enjoy life even while experiencing challenges. The World Health Organization defines *health* as a state of physical, mental, and social well-being. Thus the phrase "health and wellness" points to your helping each client achieve optimal functioning regardless of current health status or disability.

During the continuum of life from infancy to old age, you need to be able to educate clients about their health and help them make changes to increase their wellness. Your approach is straightforward:

1. Assess the client's perception of his or her own health status.
2. Identify the client's health-oriented behaviors.
3. At regular intervals, evaluate the client's understanding of health and wellness activities.
4. Encourage client participation in behavior modification programs, as needed.

HEALTH PROMOTION/DISEASE PREVENTION

Health promotion concerns helping people to increase control over and to improve their health. Health promotion activities seek to empower individuals and their communities to organize, prioritize, and act on health issues. Disease prevention, on the other hand, involves efforts to stop the onset of a specific illness or condition, such a cancer.

You should be able to identify the important risk factors for disease/illness. Table 1 lists the top three leading causes of death by age group, as identified by the Centers for Disease Control and Prevention.

CAUSE OF DEATH	UNDER 1	1–4	5–9	10–14	15–24	25–34	35–44	45–54	55–64	OVER 65
Birth defects	1	2	3							
Disorders related to premature birth	2									
Sudden infant death syndrome (SIDS)	3									
Unintentional injuries		1	1	1	1	1	1	3		
Cancer			2	2			2	1	1	2
Homicide		3			2	3				
Suicide				3	3	2				
Heart disease							3	2	2	1
Chronic low respiratory disease									3	3
Stroke										

*   Adapted from the Centers for Disease Control and Prevention's "10 Leading Causes of Death, United States, 2009."

Table 1

Health Promotion/Disease Prevention Programs

Health promotion/disease prevention programs include using community intervention techniques, such as holding health fairs or doing on-site education at elementary and high schools. Health promotion topics might include the following:

- **Healthy weight management:** The client's current weight should be assessed in comparison to a desirable weight. Know that a person with type 2 diabetes can improve glucose control by losing only 10–20 pounds.
- **Smoking cessation:** Factors associated with continued smoking include the strength of the nicotine addiction, continued exposure to smoking-associated stimuli (at work or in social settings), stress, depression, and habit. Continued smoking is more prevalent among those with low incomes, low levels of education, and psychosocial problems. Multiple factors often require multiple strategies.
- **Stress management:** Studies show a cause-and-effect relationship between stress and events including infectious diseases, traumatic injuries (e.g., motor vehicle crashes),

and some chronic illnesses. Teaching stress reduction prevents other additional negative consequences.

- **Exercise:** Benefits include improved circulatory and respiratory systems; decreased cholesterol; lower body weight; delayed osteoporosis; and more flexibility, strength, and endurance.

- **Special diets:** Clients with hypertension should avoid foods high in sodium, such as processed, canned foods. Clients with high cholesterol should avoid saturated fatty acids (found in fatty meats) and trans fatty acids (found in deep-fried fast foods).

- **Complementary, alternative, or homeopathic therapies:** Examples include hypnosis, acupuncture, and massage. Some clients use over-the-counter remedies, vitamins, minerals, herbal medicines, or other approaches, such as a shaman.

- **Breast self-examination (BSE):** Beginning at puberty, women should examine their breasts monthly, between day 5 and day 7 of their menstrual period. In menopause, BSE should continue monthly.

- **Testicular self-examination:** Testicular cancer is the most common cancer in men ages 15–35, and one of the most curable solid tumors. Teach clients that the best time to check is after bathing, when the scrotum is more relaxed. Any evidence of a lump or swelling should be reported to a physician.

- **Hormone replacement therapy (HRT) information updates:** HRT lowers the risk of osteoporosis-related bone fractures, but increases the risk for coronary artery disease (CAD), breast cancer, deep vein thrombosis (DVT), and stroke.

- **Immunizations:** Hepatitis B vaccine is given to newborns. Infants get most immunizations from 2–12 months. Annual flu shots can start at 6 months. Meningococcal vaccine is recommended for previously unvaccinated college freshmen living in dormitories. Seniors over age 60 need vaccinations to prevent shingles (herpes zoster) and pneumonia.

- **Oral health:** Gum disease can allow bacteria to enter the body. Clients should schedule regular visits to dentists every 6 months beginning at age 2.

- **Mental health:** Teach ways to deal with stress and encourage seeking professional help during crises.

- **Stroke and heart disease prevention:** Clients should monitor blood pressure regularly, especially if they have a positive family history of hypertension.

- **Healthy joints:** Teach clients to do weight-bearing and stretching exercises regularly.

- **Bone health:** Diets need to include vitamin D and calcium to prevent osteoporosis.

- **Skin cancer prevention:** Teach clients to counteract the negative impacts of excessive sun exposure by using sunscreen, wearing protective clothing, or limiting time outdoors.

HEALTH SCREENING

Health screening requires you to apply your knowledge of pathophysiology and risk factors linked to ethnicity and known population or community characteristics. Screening examples include:

- **Blood sugar check:** Levels more than 199 mg/dL without fasting or more than 125 mg/dL with fasting for 8 hours signal the need for a more complete workup.

- **Blood pressure check:** One-third of people whose blood pressures exceed 140/90 mm Hg do not know it. Incidence of the *silent killer* is higher in the southeastern United States, especially among African Americans. Other risk factors are age over 60 years, inactive lifestyle, and hyperlipidemia.

- **Fasting lipid profile:** Adults should have a fasting lipid profile done at least once every 5 years. The total cholesterol value should be under 200 mg/dL, triglycerides (fatty acids) should be under 150 mg/dL, the low-density lipoprotein (LDL, the "bad" cholesterol that accelerates atherosclerosis) value should be under 100 mg/dL, and the high-density lipoprotein (HDL, the "good" cholesterol that removes cholesterol) value should be greater than 40 mg/dL for men and 50 mg/dL for women.

- **Colorectal screening:** Regular screening, beginning at age 50, is the key to preventing colorectal cancer. This screening can include fecal occult blood test (FOBT), sigmoidoscopy, colonoscopy, double-contrast barium enema (DCBE), or digital rectal exam (DRE).

- **Prostate screening:** Men should get a prostate-specific antigen (PSA) test beginning at age 50.

- **Mammograms:** Women should get a baseline mammogram between ages 40 and 50, after considering risk factors.

HIGH-RISK BEHAVIORS

High-risk behaviors are those lifestyle practices that increase the likelihood of illness, disease, or death. For example, in the case of HIV/AIDS, those activities include unprotected sex (anal, vaginal, or oral), using contaminated needles or sharing syringes, and coming in contact with bodily fluids (blood, semen, vaginal fluids, and saliva). Unprotected sex can also lead to other consequences, such as sexually transmitted diseases (STDs). Most safe sexual practices take some planning, such as having condoms available. An unplanned pregnancy can be avoided by taking birth control pills regularly.

Promote accident awareness to reduce deaths due to unintentional injuries. This includes using seat belts in automobiles, wearing helmets while biking, and using crosswalks.

Lifestyle Choices

Lifestyle is a characteristic set of behaviors and practices that range from habits and conventional ways of doing things to reasoned actions. Examples of lifestyle choices include being child-free; living in urban, rural, or suburban environments; educating children in public or private schools or home-schooling; and using alternative or homeopathic health care practices. Any of these choices might have an impact on your clients' health.

Principles of Teaching/Learning

Principles of teaching and learning are techniques that allow you to share medical and health information with clients. You have been in school for some time, so it is second nature for you to absorb new information. For clients, you need to do the following:

1. Use an organized approach to assess readiness and ability to learn.

    a. Consider age and developmental stage when teaching clients. For example, teaching adolescents might best be done by pointing them to trusted Internet sites, so that they can have a sense of autonomy in discovering health advice for themselves.

    b. Take into account clients' living situations. An example is an elderly person who is socially isolated due to decreasing sight and hearing or geographically isolated due to family and friends living far away.

    c. Encourage clients to establish their own goals and evaluate their own progress.

    d. Let clients demonstrate their understanding of information and practice their skills.

    e. After teaching, evaluate the results.

2. Account for learning preference.

    a. Visual learners think in pictures, so use visual aids such as diagrams, videotapes, and handouts.

    b. Auditory learners best understand material through listening. Tell them about community lectures, discussions, and recordings.

    c. Tactile or kinesthetic learners prefer to learn via experience—moving, touching, and doing. Let the client hold a scale model of body organs to illustrate anatomy, for example.

3. Identify barriers to client learning.

    a. Physical condition, such as decreased sight or hearing

    b. Financial considerations

    c. Lack of support systems

    d. Misconceptions about disease and treatment

    e. Low literacy and comprehension skills

f.   Cultural/ethnic background and language barriers

g.   Lack of motivation

h.   Environment

i.   Negative past experiences

j.   Denial of personal responsibility

SELF-CARE

Self-care includes all activities that promote and maintain personal well-being without medical, professional, or other assistance or oversight. For developmentally delayed or elderly people, an inability to perform these tasks can curtail their ability to live independently. Your knowledge of in-home community resources might enable them to live in that environment longer. Your care plan might also need to involve clients (if able to give input), family members, friends, or paid staff inside or outside an institution.

TECHNIQUES OF PHYSICAL ASSESSMENT

You should know the four methods or techniques of performing a physical assessment:

1. **Inspection or purposeful observation:** Pay attention to outward details about the client, noting any deviations from expected age-related development. Note posture and stature, body movements, nutritional status by appearance, speech pattern, and vital signs. Individualize your approach. For example, with an obese young person, use an adult-size blood pressure cuff to get an accurate reading while assuring client comfort.

2. **Palpation:** Use fingers and palms to apply a light touch or deeper pressure to gather data about the health of superficial blood vessels, lymph nodes, the thyroid, and the organs of the abdomen and pelvis.

3. **Percussion:** Tap a part of the body and listen for the returned sound. This technique is often used on the chest and abdominal walls.

4. **Auscultation:** Use a stethoscope to listen to sounds caused by movement of air or fluid within the client's body. This provides information about breath sounds, the spoken voice, bowel sounds, cardiac murmurs, and heart sounds. The stethoscope's bell (hollow cup) part of the endpiece can assess very-low-frequency sound, such as heart murmurs. The diaphragm (disc) part of the endpiece can assess high-frequency sounds from the heart and lungs.

This chapter reviewed aspects of childbirth to features of old age, and looked at health and wellness across the life span. Whatever your clinical setting, and whatever the reason for clients seeking medical help, you can rely on your grasp of basic health promotion and maintenance concepts. That knowledge will be evident when you successfully take the NCLEX-RN® exam.

CHAPTER QUIZ

1. A 20-year-old client has just given birth. The baby looks healthy, with the exception of giving a grimace instead of a cry. Which of the following would the nurse expect the obstetrician to say?

   1. "The APGAR score is 3."
   2. "The APGAR score is 6."
   3. "The APGAR score is 9."
   4. "The APGAR score is 12."

2. The outpatient client is postmenopausal. In discussing breast self-examination, which of the following should the nurse let the client know that she can do?

   1. Switch to an annual schedule, because she does not have periods.
   2. Discontinue self-examination, because hormone changes decrease her risks.
   3. Wait until her mammogram shows some findings.
   4. Continue to palpate monthly, picking her own meaningful date.

3. A client with acne has been using isotretinoin (Accutane). She tells the nurse that she recently learned she is pregnant. She asks "Will my pregnancy interfere with the medication's effectiveness?" Which of the following is the appropriate response by the nurse?

   1. "The medication is contraindicated for pregnant women."
   2. "You will have to change the route of administration, because you are pregnant."
   3. "There is no reason you can't continue taking it."
   4. "If the medication helps you look better, that will help feel better about yourself."

4. The nurse is preparing for a women's health fair. The nurse knows that which of the following is correct when teaching about the risks and benefits of hormone replacement therapy (HRT)?

   1. HRT is related to a decreased risk of deep vein thrombosis (DVT).
   2. HRT is related to an increased risk for coronary artery disease (CAD).
   3. HRT is related to an increased risk for osteoporosis-related bone fractures.
   4. HRT is related to a decreased risk of breast cancer.

5. The nurse has been working with a 45-year-old African American who bicycles to work. Lab tests show low serum lipids. The nurse knows that the client's risk factors for primary (essential) hypertension include which of the following?

   1. Being under the age of 65
   2. Race
   3. Low serum lipids
   4. Active lifestyle

6. The nurse is designing a diet plan for a 70-year-old with poorly fitting dentures who has been recently diagnosed with type 2 diabetes. The nurse knows that which of the following is the *LEAST* likely risk to the client?

   1. Malnutrition
   2. Dehydration
   3. Hyperglycemia
   4. Low blood sugar

7. The nurse is providing education at a senior center. Which of the following measures will the nurse say is *MOST* effective in attaining normal blood sugar levels in a client with type 2 diabetes?

1. Decreasing sodium intake
2. Increasing potassium and calcium intake
3. Reaching recommended weight
4. Decreasing daily exercise

8. A local high school is having a health fair. Which of the following main courses should the nurse recommend as most healthful for a teenager whose cholesterol level is 300 mg/dL?

1. Medium-rare hamburger with only one slice of cheese
2. Vegetarian New York–style pizza
3. Grilled chicken breast
4. Salad with extra dressing

9. The nurse is talking to a client who is still grieving the loss of a parent to stomach cancer. The nurse knows that which of the following would increase the client's risk of cancer?

1. Keeping a strict high-protein diet
2. Following a low-fat, low-carbohydrate diet
3. Using considerable spices when cooking
4. Smoking cigarettes

10. A 3-month-old child accompanies her parents to a seasonal flu clinic. Assuming that the child does not have a fever, can the nurse give the child a flu shot?

1. Yes, if regular immunizations are up to date.
2. No, because the child is not old enough.
3. Yes, because then the child won't get sick later.

4. No, because it would interfere with regular immunizations.

11. The nurse gives a 35-year-old primigravida client a RhoGAM injection in her 28th week of pregnancy. Which of the following client situations requires the nurse to take this action?

1. Rh-positive mother and Rh-negative father
2. Rh-positive mother and Rh-positive father
3. Rh-negative mother and Rh-negative father
4. Rh-negative mother and Rh-positive father

12. The nurse is teaching a young male client to recognize the most common early sign of testicular cancer. The nurse emphasizes the fact that he should be aware of which of the following?

1. Lumbar pain
2. Urinary frequency
3. Urinary urgency
4. Painless testicular enlargement

13. New parents are concerned about an unexpected characteristic of their newborn baby. Which of the following would cause the nurse to initiate contact with the physician?

1. Swollen genitals and breast
2. High-pitched crying
3. Misshapen head
4. Milia

14. A public health nurse visits a client at home three days after the client gave birth. In which of the following situations should the nurse instruct the client to report to a clinician?

1. Vaginal drainage with streaks of bright red blood

2. Some discomfort at the site of her episiotomy

3. Feelings of fatigue late in the afternoon and evening

4. An elevated temperature without other symptoms

15. The pediatric nurse is providing discharge instructions to the parents of a newborn. In which of the following situations would the nurse advise the parents to call a physician? **Select all that apply.**

    1. The infant has a temperature higher than 100.4° F (38° C).

    2. The infant vomits more than once in 24 hours.

    3. The infant's respirations are even and unlabored.

    4. The infant is unable to keep down food or water.

    5. The infant has sunken or swollen soft spots on the head.

16. The client's first day of her last period was February 1. Which of the following should the nurse tell the client is her expected date of delivery?

    1. November 8

    2. October 8

    3. December 1

    4. November 20

17. The client is 7 months pregnant with her first child. She is anxious because she feels some mild contractions at times. The nurse tells her which of the following?

    1. She should increase her bed rest to prevent those contractions.

    2. The contractions are normal unless they increase in severity.

3. The contractions are a way of her body asking for more exercise.

4. She should avoid getting constipated and having gas as a result.

18. The client is 40 years old and pregnant with her first child. Her obstetrician has asked the nurse to schedule her for an amniocentesis. The client inquires why she needs that test. The nurse says which of the following as an explanation?

    1. "We routinely do an amniocentesis on all our clients to check the child's gender."

    2. "An amniocentesis is not invasive, so there is less risk than doing an ultrasound."

    3. "The standard for doing an amniocentesis is motherhood over age 35."

    4. "If we know the baby's size, you can better count on having a vaginal birth."

19. The nurse is educating a mother-to-be about possible danger signs during the last three months of pregnancy. Which of the following would *NOT* cause the nurse concern about danger signs?

    1. Rectal bleeding

    2. Continuous headaches

    3. Marked swelling of hands

    4. Blurred vision

20. A first-time parent is discussing developmental milestones with the nurse. The nurse tells the client that she can reasonably expect her child to achieve which of the following by the time the child is 1 year old? **Select all that apply.**

    1. Walking

    2. Rolling from tummy to side

    3. Transferring toys from hand to hand

    4. Beginning to respond selectively to words

    5. Vocalizing sounds (coos)

21. A parent is discussing the behavior of her 3-year-old child with the nurse. At 3 years, the nurse would expect the client's child to be doing all of the following *EXCEPT* which activity?

    1. Saying "no" often
    2. Using a limited vocabulary of 500–3,000 words
    3. Speaking in 10-word sentences
    4. Believing that adults know everything

22. The nurse is teaching a group of mothers of toddlers how to prevent accidental poisoning from medications. The nurse teaches the mothers to store medications in which of the following locations?

    1. In a secure, locked place
    2. In vials with childproof caps
    3. On the highest shelf in the room
    4. Disguised in different containers

23. The nurse is assessing an elderly couple, both 80 years old, to determine if they can safely continue to live independently. They insist they are getting along fine but need help with grocery shopping and housekeeping. The nurse determines that they have difficulty in doing which of the following?

    1. Activities of daily living (ADLs)
    2. Instrumental activities of daily living (IADLs)
    3. Daily living milestones (DLMs)
    4. Preventive health activities (PHAs)

24. The nurse is giving a lecture at the senior center about preventative health activities for people over age 60. The nurse tells the clients that the Centers for Disease Control and Prevention (CDC) now recommends which of the following vaccines for this age group?

    1. Shingles (herpes zoster)
    2. Diphtheria
    3. Pertussis (whooping cough)
    4. Meningitis

25. The nurse is teaching about the challenges of smoking cessation. Which of the following factors will the nurse identify as known challenges that clients face when attempting to quit smoking? **Select all that apply.**

    1. Stress and depression
    2. Low level of income
    3. High level of education
    4. Psychosocial problems
    5. Continued exposure to smoking-associated stimuli

26. Stress reduction techniques include biofeedback and meditation. The nurse conducting classes on these methods knows that studies have shown a cause-and-effect relationship between stress and which of the following? **Select all that apply.**

    1. Adverse medication effects
    2. Infectious diseases
    3. Traumatic injuries, such as motor vehicle accidents
    4. Some chronic illnesses

27. The nurse is performing the initial assessment of an adult from a culture the nurse is not familiar with, and asks about the client's use of alternative therapies. The client says, irritably, "Do you have to ask all these questions?" Which of the following is the *BEST* explanation for what the nurse should do in response?

    1. Ask the question, because the nurse might learn about therapies used by a different culture.

2. Ask the question, because knowledge about actual use of other therapies is imperative.

3. Don't ask the question, because it is important to not upset the irritable client any further.

4. Don't ask the question, because the client needs to choose to initiate discussion of other therapies.

28. The nurse is preparing a community educational presentation. The topic is the leading cause of death for people from ages 1–44. The nurse knows that which of the following is the leading cause?

1. Cancer
2. Heart disease
3. Unintentional injuries
4. Diabetes

29. The nurse is reviewing the client's lipid profile to determine if education is needed to reduce the risk of heart disease. The nurse knows how to match healthy target values with lab descriptions. Match the appropriate part of the profile below on the left to the values on the right. **All options must be used**.

1. Total cholesterol
2. HDL cholesterol for men
3. HDL cholesterol for women
4. LDL cholesterol
5. Triglycerides

A. More than 40 mg/dL
B. More than 50 mg/dL
C. Less than 100 mg/dL
D. Less than 150 mg/dL
E. Less than 200 mg/dL

30. The nurse is assessing the best approach to prepare three clients for surgery. Each has a different learning preference. Match the learning preference to the appropriate approach. **All options must be used**.

1. Brochures about preparation activities
2. Models of the relevant anatomy
3. Discussions about the surgery

A. Auditory
B. Visual
C. Tactile

CHAPTER QUIZ ANSWERS AND EXPLANATIONS

1. The Answer is 3

The 20-year-old client has just given birth. The baby looks healthy, with the exception of giving a grimace instead of a cry. Which of the following would the nurse expect the obstetrician to say?

Category: Ante/intra/postpartum and newborn care

(1) An APGAR score of 3 indicates a baby in poor health.

(2) An APGAR score of 6 indicates a less healthy baby.

(3) CORRECT: In 4 of the 5 categories of rating, the baby scored a 2. In the category of reflex irritability, the baby scored a 1, for a total APGAR score of 9.

(4) An APGAR score of 12 does not exist; the highest score is 10.

2. The Answer is 4

The outpatient client is postmenopausal. In discussing breast self-examination, which of the following should the nurse let the client know that she can do?

Category: Aging process

(1) Although menopause itself is not associated with increased risk of breast cancer, the rate does increase with age. The client should continue with breast self-examination.

(2) Although menopause itself is not associated with increased risk of breast cancer, the rate does increase with age. The client should continue with breast self-examination.

(3) Although menopause itself is not associated with increased risk of breast cancer, the rate does increase with age. The client should continue with breast self-examination.

(4) CORRECT: Breast self-examination is extremely important for a client in this soon-to-be high risk

group. About 70 percent of new diagnoses come after age 50.

3. The Answer is 1

A client with acne has been using isotretinoin (Accutane). She tells the nurse that she recently learned she is pregnant. She asks "Will my pregnancy interfere with the medication's effectiveness?" Which of the following is the appropriate response by the nurse?

Category: Ante/intra/postpartum and newborn care

(1) CORRECT: Severe fetal abnormalities may occur if Accutane is used during pregnancy. The nurse should stress that the priority is the high risk of fetal abnormalities that the medication can cause rather than the effectiveness of the medication.

(2) The nurse would not tell the client to continue taking this drug.

(3) The nurse would not tell the client to continue taking this drug.

(4) The nurse would not tell the client to continue taking this drug.

4. The Answer is 2

The nurse is preparing for a women's health fair. The nurse knows that which of the following is correct when teaching about the risks and benefits of hormone replacement therapy (HRT)?

Category: Health promotion/disease prevention

(1) HRT causes an increased risk of DVT.

(2) CORRECT: Current research counteracts earlier theories of a decreased risk of CAD.

(3) HRT causes a decreased risk of osteoporosis-related bone fractures.

(4) HRT causes an increased risk of breast cancer.

5. The Answer is 2

The nurse has been working with a 45-year-old African American who bicycles to work. Lab tests show low serum lipids. The nurse knows that the client's risk factors for primary (essential) hypertension include which of the following?

Category: Health promotion/disease prevention; Health screening

(1) Being under the age of 65 is associated with lower risk.

(2) CORRECT: African Americans have an increased risk for hypertension.

(3) Low serum lipids are associated with lower risk.

(4) An active lifestyle is associated with lower risk.

6. The Answer is 3

The nurse is designing a diet plan for a 70-year-old with poorly fitting dentures who has been recently diagnosed with type 2 diabetes. The nurse knows that which of the following is the *LEAST* likely risk to the client?

Category: Health promotion/disease prevention

(1) Malnutrition is a possibility due to difficulty in eating.

(2) Dehydration is a possibility.

(3) CORRECT: Hypoglycemia is more likely than hyperglycemia. Often a client with denture problems will only be able to tolerate liquid or pureed foods eaten slowly. This decreases the chances of adequate nutrition.

(4) Low blood sugar is a possibility.

7. The Answer is 3

The nurse is providing education at a senior center. Which of the following measures will the nurse say is *MOST* effective in attaining normal blood sugar levels in a client with type 2 diabetes?

Category: Health and wellness

(1) Decreasing sodium intake is not an effective way to attaining normal blood sugar levels in a client with type 2 diabetes.

(2) More potassium and calcium will not affect blood glucose.

(3) CORRECT: Losing only as much as 10–20 pounds improves blood glucose control.

(4) The client needs to increase, not decrease, daily exercise.

8. The Answer is 3

A local high school is having a health fair. Which of the following main courses should the nurse recommend as most healthful for a teenager whose cholesterol level is 300 mg/dL?

Category: Health and wellness; Health promotion/disease prevention

(1) The fat content of the main course (hamburger) needs to be lower due to the teenager's known elevated cholesterol level.

(2) The fat content of the main course (pizza) needs to be lower due to the teenager's known elevated cholesterol level.

(3) CORRECT: The fat content of a grilled chicken breast is the lowest of the choices.

(4) The fat content of the main course (salad with extra dressing) needs to be lower due to the teenager's known elevated cholesterol level.

9. The Answer is 4

The nurse is talking to a client who is still grieving the loss of a parent to stomach cancer. The nurse knows that which of the following would increase the client's risk of cancer?

Category: Health promotion/disease prevention

(1) High-protein diets have not been shown to be a risk for cancer.

(2) Low-fat, low-carbohydrate diets have not been shown to be a risk for cancer.

(3) Spicy food has not been shown to be a risk for cancer.

(4) CORRECT: Tobacco use has been shown to be a risk for cancer.

10. The Answer is 2

A 3-month-old child accompanies her parents to a seasonal flu clinic. Assuming that the child does not have a fever, can the nurse give the child a flu shot?

Category: Aging process

(1) The minimum age to receive a flu shot is 6 months; therefore the nurse cannot give the child the shot.

(2) CORRECT: The minimum age to receive a flu shot is 6 months.

(3) The minimum age to receive a flu shot is 6 months; therefore the nurse cannot give the child the shot.

(4) The minimum age to receive a flu shot is 6 months; therefore the nurse cannot give the child the shot.

11. The Answer is 4

The nurse gives a 35-year-old primigravida client a RhoGAM injection in her 28th week of pregnancy. Which of the following client situations requires the nurse to take this action?

Category: Ante/intra/postpartum and newborn care

(1) An Rh-positive mother does not need to worry about the Rh factor of the father.

(2) An Rh-positive mother does not need to worry about the Rh factor of the father.

(3) An Rh-negative mother does not need to worry about the Rh factor of the father, if it is the same as her status.

(4) CORRECT: An Rh-negative mother and Rh-positive father is the combined Rh status in which the mother could develop harmful antibodies.

12. The Answer is 4

The nurse is teaching a young male client to recognize the most common early sign of testicular cancer. The nurse emphasizes the fact that he should be aware of which of the following?

Category: Health promotion/disease prevention

(1) Among other serious causes, lumbar pain could be a sign of metastasis.

(2) Urinary frequency is not an early sign of testicular cancer.

(3) Urinary urgency is not an early sign of testicular cancer.

(4) CORRECT: Painless testicular enlargement is a common early sign of testicular cancer.

13. The Answer is 2

New parents are concerned about an unexpected characteristic of their newborn baby. Which of the following would cause the nurse to initiate contact with the physician?

Category: Ante/intra/postpartum and newborn care

(1) Swollen genitals and breast are normal due to maternal hormones.

(2) CORRECT: High-pitched crying is not normal and could be due to a neurological problem.

(3) A misshapen head is normal due to descent through the birth canal.

(4) Milia is normal due to blocked sebaceous glands.

14. The Answer is 4

A public health nurse visits a client at home three days after the client gave birth. In which of the following situations should the nurse instruct the client to report to a clinician?

Category: Ante/intra/postpartum and newborn care

(1) Vaginal drainage with streaks of bright red blood is normal for the first 3–6 weeks.

(2) The area will continue to heal and is not a cause for concern, unless the discomfort rises to the level of persistent or increasing pain.

(3) Feelings of fatigue are normal after giving birth.

(4) CORRECT: A fever above 100.4° F (38° C) is reason to call the physician.

15. The Answer is 1, 2, 4, 5

The pediatric nurse is providing discharge instructions to the parents of a newborn. In which of the following situations would the nurse advise the parents to call a physician? **Select all that apply.**

Category: Ante/intra/postpartum and newborn care

(1) CORRECT: If an infant has a fever higher than 100.4° F (38° C), the parents should call the physician.

(2) CORRECT: If an infant vomits more than once in 24 hours, the parents should call the physician.

(3) There would be no need to call the physician in this instance.

(4) CORRECT: If an infant is unable to keep down food or water, the parents should call the physician.

(5) CORRECT: A physician should evaluate the infant immediately if the infant has sunken or swollen soft spots on the head.

16. The Answer is 1

The client's first day of her last period was February 1. Which of the following should the nurse tell the client is her expected date of delivery?

Category: Ante/intra/postpartum and newborn care

(1) CORRECT: November 8 is 9 months and 7 days later.

(2) October 8 is one month too early.

(3) By December 1, the baby would be overdue.

(4) By November 20, the baby would be overdue.

17. The Answer is 2

The client is 7 months pregnant with her first child. She is anxious because she feels some mild contractions at times. The nurse tells her which of the following?

Category: Ante/intra/postpartum and newborn care

(1) Increasing bed rest is not necessary; Braxton Hicks contractions are normal at this stage in the pregnancy.

(2) CORRECT: Braxton Hicks contractions are normal at this stage in the pregnancy.

(3) More exercise is not necessary: Braxton Hicks contractions are normal at this stage in the pregnancy.

(4) Gas is not likely to be the cause of the contractions; Braxton Hicks contractions are normal at this stage in the pregnancy.

18. The Answer is 3

The client is 40 years old and pregnant with her first child. Her obstetrician has asked the nurse to schedule her for an amniocentesis. The client inquires why she needs that test. The nurse says which of the following as an explanation?

Category: Ante/intra/postpartum and newborn care

(1) The most common reason for an amniocentesis is to check chromosomal abnormalities, not to check the child's gender.

(2) The ultrasound is not invasive; the amniocentesis is invasive.

(3) CORRECT: After age 35, the risk of infant chromosomal abnormality is greater than the risk associated with the procedure.

(4) The most common reason for an amniocentesis is to check chromosomal abnormalities, not to check the baby's size.

19. The Answer is 1

The nurse is educating a mother-to-be about possible danger signs during the last three months of pregnancy. Which of the following would *NOT* cause the nurse concern about danger signs?

Category: Ante/intra/postpartum and newborn care

(1) CORRECT: Although hemorrhoids could cause rectal bleeding, it is vaginal bleeding that would concern the nurse.

(2) Continuous headaches is a symptom that would concern the nurse.

(3) Marked swelling of hands would concern the nurse.

(4) Blurred vision would concern the nurse.

20. The Answer is 2, 3, 4, and 5

A first-time parent is discussing developmental milestones with the nurse. The nurse tells the client that she can reasonably expect her child to achieve which of the following by the time the child is 1 year old? **Select all that apply.**

Category: Developmental stages and transitions

(1) The parent should not become concerned unless the child cannot walk at 18 months.

(2) CORRECT: Rolling from tummy to side is a developmental milestone that the client can expect the child to reach by age 1.

(3) CORRECT: Transferring toys from hand to hand is a developmental milestone that the client can expect the child to reach by age 1.

(4) CORRECT: Beginning to respond selectively to words is a developmental milestone that the client can expect the child to reach by age 1.

(5) CORRECT: Vocalizing sounds (coos) is a developmental milestone that the client can expect the child to reach by age 1.

21. The Answer is 3

A parent is discussing the behavior of her 3-year-old child with the nurse. At 3 years, the nurse would expect the client's child to be doing all of the following *EXCEPT* which activity?

Category: Developmental stages and transitions

(1) Saying "no" often is an appropriate behavior at this age.

(2) Using a limited vocabulary of 500–3,000 words is an appropriate behavior at this age.

(3) CORRECT: Only three- or four-word sentences can be expected at this age.

(4) Believing adults know everything is an appropriate behavior for this age.

22. The Answer is 1

The nurse is teaching a group of mothers of toddlers how to prevent accidental poisoning from medications. The nurse teaches the mothers to store medications in which of the following locations?

Category: Aging process; Developmental stages and transitions

(1) CORRECT: A secure, locked place is the only safe place.

(2) Children have been known to pull childproof caps off, especially if the cap is not fully engaged.

(3) Children have been known to climb up on counters and other surfaces, so placing medications on a high shelf is not necessarily safe.

(4) The problem is the toddler's natural curiosity, not whether the toddler recognizes the item as a medication vial. If containers are disguised, this might also cause a medication error.

23. The Answer is 2

The nurse is assessing an elderly couple, both 80 years old, to determine if they can safely continue to live independently. They insist they are getting along fine but need help with grocery shopping and housekeeping. The nurse determines that they have difficulty in doing which of the following?

Category: Aging process; Self-care

(1) ADLs are basic functions of self-care, such as feeding, dressing, and bathing.

(2) CORRECT: Grocery shopping and housekeeping are two important IADL functions.

(3) Grocery shopping and housekeeping are not milestones.

(4) Grocery shopping and housekeeping are not prevention activities.

24. The Answer is 1

The nurse is giving a lecture at the senior center about preventative health activities for people over age 60. The nurse tells the clients that the Centers for Disease Control and Prevention (CDC) now recommends which of the following vaccines for this age group?

Category: Health promotion/disease prevention

(1) CORRECT: The shingles vaccine reduces the risk of shingles by about half and the risk of postherpetic neuralgia by two-thirds.

(2) The diphtheria vaccine is given much earlier in life.

(3) The pertussis (whooping cough) vaccine is given much earlier in life.

(4) The CDC recommends that college freshmen living in dormitories get the meningitis vaccine, but this is unlikely to apply to those over age 60.

25. The Answer is 1, 2, 4, and 5

The nurse is teaching about the challenges of smoking cessation. Which of the following factors will the nurse identify as known challenges that clients face when attempting to quit smoking? **Select all that apply.**

Category: Health promotion/disease prevention; High risk behaviors

(1) CORRECT: Stress and depression are known challenges to smoking cessation.

(2) CORRECT: Continued smoking is more prevalent among those with a low level of income.

(3) A low, not high, level of education has been found to be associated with continued smoking.

(4) CORRECT: Continued smoking is more prevalent among those with psychosocial problems.

(5) CORRECT: Continued exposure to smoking-associated stimuli is a known challenge to smoking cessation.

26. The Answer is 2, 3, and 4

Stress reduction techniques include biofeedback and meditation. The nurse conducting classes on these methods knows that studies have shown a cause-and-effect relationship between stress and which of the following? **Select all that apply.**

Category: Health promotion/disease prevention

(1) No association between stress and adverse medication effects is known at present.

(2) CORRECT: Research shows a relationship between stress and infectious diseases.

(3) CORRECT: Research shows a relationship between stress and traumatic injuries, such as motor vehicle accidents.

(4) CORRECT: Research shows a relationship between stress and some chronic illnesses.

27. The Answer is 2

The nurse is performing the initial assessment of an adult from a culture the nurse is not familiar with, and asks about the client's use of alternative therapies. The client says, irritably, "Do you have to ask all these questions?" Which of the following is the *BEST* explanation for what the nurse should do in response?

Category: Health screening

(1) The client is the focus, not the nurse's education.

(2) CORRECT: The need to discuss the use of these adjunct therapies with clients in all settings is imperative. This is important because it could affect or interfere with other treatment modalities.

(3) The client might become impatient, but that does not mean that the nurse shortens her clinical review.

(4) The nurse needs to ask critical questions to get the complete clinical picture.

28. The Answer is 3

The nurse is preparing a community educational presentation. The topic is the leading cause of death for people from ages 1–44. The nurse knows that which of the following is the leading cause?

Category: Health promotion/disease prevention

(1) Cancer is not the leading cause of death for people from ages 1–44, according to the CDC.

(2) Heart disease is not the leading cause of death for people from ages 1–44, according to the CDC.

(3) CORRECT: Unintentional injuries are the leading cause of death for people ages 1–44, according to the CDC.

(4) Diabetes is not the leading cause of death for people from ages 1–44, according to the CDC.

29. The Answer is 1 (E), 2 (A), 3 (B), 4 (C), 5 (D)

The nurse is reviewing the client's lipid profile to determine if education is needed to reduce the risk of heart disease. The nurse knows how to match healthy target values with lab descriptions. Match the appropriate part of the profile below on the left to the values on the right. **All options must be used**.

Category: Health promotion/disease prevention

1. (E): Total cholesterol should be less than 200 mg/dL.

2. (A): HDL cholesterol for men should be more than 40 mg/dL.

3. (B): HDL cholesterol for women should be more than 50 mg/dL.

4. (C): LDL cholesterol should be less than 100 mg/dL.

5. (D): Triglycerides should be less than 150 mg/dL.

30. The Answer is 1 (B), 2 (C), 3 (A)

The nurse is assessing the best approach to prepare three clients for surgery. Each has a different learning preference. Match the learning preference to the appropriate approach. **All options must be used.**

Category: Principles of teaching/learning

1. (B): Brochures about preparation activities are visual: the client needs to see words and pictures.

2. (C): Models of the relevant anatomy are tactile: the client needs to touch the model.

3. (A): Discussions about the surgery are auditory: the client needs to hear the words.

CHAPTER 7

PSYCHOSOCIAL INTEGRITY

Psychosocial integrity, along with physiological integrity, is a basic health need for all clients. It is the state of dynamic psychological and sociological homeostasis, which may be affected during periods of stress, illness, or crisis. Any threats to a person's emotional, mental, and social well-being can disrupt this homeostasis. Any change in adaptive and coping responses may result in counterproductive ways of thinking, communicating, feeling, and acting. When assisting clients with psychosocial needs, you must be able to anticipate, recognize, and analyze these types of responses.

On the NCLEX-RN® exam, you can expect approximately 9 percent of the questions to relate to Psychosocial Integrity. This category focuses on promoting and supporting the emotional, mental, and social well-being of clients experiencing stressful events, as well as clients with acute or chronic mental illness.

Exam content related to Psychosocial Integrity includes, but is not limited to, the following areas:

- Abuse/neglect
- Behavioral interventions
- Chemical and other dependencies
- Coping mechanisms
- Crisis intervention
- Cultural diversity
- End of life care
- Family dynamics
- Grief and loss
- Mental health concepts
- Religious and spiritual influences on health
- Sensory/perceptual alterations
- Stress management

- Support systems
- Therapeutic communications
- Therapeutic environment

Now let's review the most important concepts covered by the Psychosocial Integrity category on the NCLEX-RN® exam.

ABUSE/NEGLECT

Abuse includes physical abuse, physical neglect, sexual abuse, and emotional abuse and neglect. You should be familiar with your state's laws for reporting suspected or known abuse. In addition, you must be able to identify risk factors and recognize signs of possible abuse and neglect and their roles in follow-up care.

All suspected cases of child abuse *must* be reported to the appropriate agency or authority. It is not sufficient just to document the suspected abuse in the medical record. Risk factors for child abuse include:

- Past or present spousal abuse
- Perception of stress
- Life changes
- Age at birth of first child
- Education
- Little or no prenatal care
- Having an unlisted phone/not having a phone
- Low income
- Current unemployment
- Evidence of harsh discipline

Elder abuse can affect either sex, but usually the victims are women who are over 75 years of age, physically or mentally impaired, and dependent on the abuser for their care. Nurses can intervene by educating caregivers about the needs of older adults and making resources available to provide support. A legally competent adult, however, cannot be forced to leave the abusive situation.

Domestic/spousal abuse affects families at all socioeconomic levels. Risk factors for domestic abuse include:

- Planning to leave or having recently left an abusive relationship
- Having been in an abusive relationship in the past
- Poverty or poor living situation
- Unemployment

- Physical or mental disability
- Separation or divorce
- Abuse as a child
- Social isolation from family and friends
- Having witnessed domestic violence as a child
- Pregnancy, especially if unplanned
- Being younger than 30 years old
- Being stalked by a partner

In any abuse situation, you should communicate openly, encourage victims to share their problems, provide counseling and information about resources and coping strategies, provide support, and educate your clients. In addition, you should know how to plan interventions for victims and suspected victims, and help direct them to a safe environment. It is also important to evaluate a client's response to interventions.

BEHAVIORAL INTERVENTIONS

Nurses can intervene, helping to restore a client's ability to evaluate reality correctly. Characteristics of altered mental processes that you should be familiar with include:

- Disorientation
- Altered behavioral patterns
- Altered mood states
- Impaired ability to perform self-maintenance activities
- Altered sleep patterns
- Altered perceptions of surroundings

The treatment plan should respond to the specific needs of the client for structure, safety, and symptom management. You should be able to evaluate the client's response to the treatment plan.

Nursing interventions that you should be familiar with include:

- Maintaining routine interactions, activities, and close observation
- Developing an open and honest relationship with respectful and clearly verbalized expectations
- Verbalizing acceptance of the client despite inappropriate behavior
- Providing role modeling through appropriate social and professional interactions with other clients and staff
- Encouraging the client to assume responsibility for his or her own behavior but verbalizing willingness to assist

- Providing positive reinforcement
- Orienting the client to reality
- Encouraging the client to attend group therapy sessions, if appropriate

You should also know how to help the client achieve and maintain behavioral self-control, including strategies that the client can use to decrease anxiety.

CHEMICAL AND OTHER DEPENDENCIES

Substance abuse is the harmful use of psychoactive substances, including alcohol and illicit drugs. A history of substance abuse may reflect several risk factors for health problems. Substance use may coexist with other psychiatric, developmental, or cognitive problems, and is closely related to certain medical complications such as pancreatitis and ulcers. Substance abuse also affects the client's relationship with the environment, family, and society. The client may deny the problem. Non-substance-related dependencies include gambling addiction, sexual addiction, and addiction to pornography, among others.

Nursing priorities when dealing with a client with chemical and other dependencies include:

- Maintaining the physiological stability of clients experiencing substance-related withdrawal or toxicity by providing symptom management. For example, benzodiazepines are often part of treating alcohol withdrawal, with its symptoms of tremors, diaphoresis, and elevated heart rate.
- Promoting client safety. This might include using restraining devices, even against a client's wishes, to ensure that the client does not get hurt.
- Educating the client about chemical and other dependency complications and dangers.
- Providing appropriate referral and follow-up.
- Encouraging and supporting involvement in an intervention process (counseling).
- Teaching friends and family members how to provide ongoing support, and encouraging their participation in support groups.
- Evaluating the client's response to the treatment plan.

COPING MECHANISMS

How a client responds to life's stressors depends on the client's coping resources—for example, social support networks and problem-solving skills. Sociocultural and religious factors can also influence how a client handles problems. Some clients may not have the resources or skills to cope with stressors. You should be able to assess these client support systems, resources, and skills, as well as a client's response to illness and the emotional reaction of a family to a client's illness.

Characteristics of the inability to cope that you should be familiar with include:

- Verbalization of the inability to cope
- Inability to make decisions or ask for help
- Destructive behavior toward self or others
- Physical symptoms
- Emotional tensions
- General irritability

Factors related to the inability to cope include, but are not limited to:

- Diagnosis of a serious illness
- Change in health status
- Unsatisfactory support system
- Inadequate psychological resources
- Situational crises

You should also be familiar with the variety of different defense mechanisms your client may employ, and be able to evaluate whether uses of these mechanisms are constructive or not, such as:

- **Denial:** Completely rejecting a thought or feeling
- **Suppression:** Vaguely aware of a thought or feeling but trying to hide it
- **Projection:** Thinking someone else has the same thought or feeling
- **Acting out:** Performing an extreme behavior in order to express thoughts or feelings the person feels incapable of otherwise expressing
- **Displacement:** Redirecting feelings to another target
- **Isolation of affect:** "Thinking" the feeling but not really feeling it
- **Intellectualization:** Avoiding the emotion of an act or feeling by substituting a rational explanation.
- **Regression:** Reverting to an old, usually immature behavior to ventilate a person's feeling
- **Reaction formation:** Turning the feeling into its opposite
- **Rationalization:** Coming up with various explanations to justify the situation (while denying personal feelings)
- **Sublimation:** Directing the feeling into a socially productive activity
- **Dissociation:** Losing track of time and/or person, and instead finding another representation of self in order to continue in the moment

Additionally, you need to provide clients with opportunities to express their thoughts and feelings, help them set realistic goals, assist them in constructive problem solving, and provide teaching on methods, support systems, and available resources to cope with stress and tension.

CRISIS INTERVENTION

A crisis is an emotionally significant event or radical change of status in a person's life. It is an unstable and/or crucial time with the possibility of an undesirable outcome—a situation that has reached a critical stage. During a crisis, you should:

- Identify the client's history of the present problem.
- Identify the client's current feelings.
- Assess the client's support systems.
- Teach crisis intervention techniques to assist the client in coping.
- Assess the client's potential for self-harm or harm to others.

Goal planning is based on nursing assessment and diagnosis, and outcomes are compared to goals and the client's response.

Goals of crisis intervention include:

- Decreasing emotional stress and protecting the client from additional stress
- Assisting the client in organizing and mobilizing resources or support systems to meet the client's needs, and reaching a solution for that situation
- Returning the client to a pre-crisis level of functioning

Assessing the risk for suicide includes asking questions (from general to specific, as well as about plans and lethality), obtaining a history, assessing mental status, and assessing the signals given by the client that may indicate that he or she is at high risk for suicide. *The highest priority for patients at risk for suicide is safety. Thus, arrangements might have to be made to provide constant observation of the high risk client.*

CULTURAL DIVERSITY

Caring varies among different racial and ethnic groups in its expressions, processes, and patterns. Cultural competence requires you to understand the client's world views as well as your own, while avoiding stereotyping. You can obtain cultural information by asking questions, and then apply the knowledge to improve the quality of client care and outcomes. This requires flexibility on your part and respect for other viewpoints. To do so, you should:

- Listen carefully to the client.
- Learn about the client's beliefs regarding health and illness.

- Show respect, understanding, and tolerance of the client's cultural background and practices.
- Provide culturally appropriate care.
- Identify language needs and use appropriate interpreters, as necessary. Avoid bias and subjectivity by arranging for nonfamily translation assistance.
- Document how the client's language needs were met.

END OF LIFE CARE

A client has the right to make informed choices about his or her end of life care that reflects personal, cultural, and religious values.

Nurses provide support, education, and impartial interpretation of medical information in a way that clients and families can understand, which may include treatment options as well as the right to refuse treatment. This requires open, honest, sensitive communication and effective teamwork. You should encourage clients and families to express their goals and wishes, and then tailor the care plan to the needs of each client and family. As a nurse, you have an ethical and legal duty to respect the client's wishes, choices, and priorities.

You also need to prepare the client and family for what to expect during the final phase of a terminal illness, which includes the physical aspects of a deteriorating condition and the act of dying. As the client's death approaches, the family may become more anxious. It is important for you to teach the family about the signs and symptoms of impending death, as well as reassure the family that the health care providers are making the client as comfortable as possible. After the death, you acknowledge the loss, express sympathy, and provide the opportunity for the family to view the body, but only after asking if they wish to do so.

FAMILY DYNAMICS

Family members ideally support each other by listening, empathizing, and reaching out to one another. When communication patterns are dysfunctional, the result can be gross misunderstanding, which may lead to hostility, anger, or silence.

You need to be able to assess a family's dynamics and ability to function constructively by closely observing how well family members communicate. You should also assess coping mechanisms that determine how families relate to stress, and evaluate resources and support systems available to the family.

Family units may be vulnerable to health problems based on various factors, such as heredity, developmental level, and lifestyle practices. You should plan interventions, such as encouraging participation in group/family therapy. That intervention can assist the family with realistic strategies that enhance family functioning, such as improving communication skills and identifying and utilizing support systems.

GRIEF AND LOSS

Grieving is a normal, subjective emotional response to loss and is essential for mental and physical health. How a client or family responds to loss, and how they express grief, varies widely. Factors that influence the process of grieving include age, stage of development, gender, culture, and personal reserves and strengths.

You should know the different stages of grieving and factors that influence how clients and families react to death to understand their responses and needs. You must also be knowledgeable about legal issues surrounding death, such as advance directives, autopsies, organ donation, and do-not-resuscitate (DNR) orders.

You also need to take the time to analyze your own feelings about death before you can effectively help others.

Additional nursing responsibilities include:

- Brainstorming ways to provide relief from loneliness, fear, and depression
- Helping clients maintain a sense of security
- Helping clients and families accept the loss
- Providing physical comfort measures
- Providing emotional support, structure, and continuity
- Allowing expression of thoughts and feelings

MENTAL HEALTH CONCEPTS

Mental health is a positive state in which one is responsible, displays self-awareness, is self-directive, is reasonably worry-free, and can cope with usual daily tensions. Such individuals function well in society, are accepted within a group, and are generally satisfied with their lives.

Influences on mental health include inherited characteristics, nurturing during childhood, and life circumstances. Influences on maintaining mental health include interpersonal communication, the use of ego defense mechanisms, and the presence of support people.

Nurses focus on different aspects of care based on the identified needs or presenting problems of patients. You should also be able to apply your knowledge of client psychopathology to mental health concepts.

RELIGIOUS AND SPIRITUAL INFLUENCES ON HEALTH

Religion and spirituality have a great influence on the health of clients and how they cope, and make a difference in physical and psychosocial outcomes. You should promote your clients' physical, emotional, and spiritual health, because this balance of well-being is essential to a client's overall health. You must strive to be an empathetic listener and attempt to identify your clients' spiritual needs. To accomplish this, the nurse should understand how spirituality influences clinical care.

Nurses should be knowledgeable about religious traditions and spiritual expressions other than their own. You should approach each client based on that client's distinct need, because people develop and nurture their own spirituality in different ways. Each client's spiritual beliefs or religious practice should influence how you care for that client. Clients have the right to receive care that respects their religious and spiritual values. At the same time, they have the right to refuse care on religious grounds.

SENSORY/PERCEPTUAL ALTERATIONS

A disruption in a client's cognitive processes can lead to faulty interpretations of their surroundings.

Alterations in sensory perception, or altered thought processes, affect a client's ability to function within his or her environment, which may place the client at risk for harm. You should assist the client to function safely in health care settings.

Some factors that influence sensory function include developmental stage, culture, stress, medications, illness, lifestyle, and personality.

You need to identify clients at risk for sensory/perceptual alterations so you can initiate preventive measures. Examples of clients at risk include those who:

- are confined in a non-stimulating environment.
- have impaired vision or hearing.
- have mobility restrictions.
- have emotional disorders.
- have limited social contact.
- are experiencing pain or discomfort.
- are acutely ill.
- are closely monitored (such as in the ICU).
- have decreased cognitive ability (as in a head injury).

When dealing with such a client, you should organize nursing care to reduce unessential stimuli; orient the client to person, place, and time during every contact; and explain all nursing care.

STRESS MANAGEMENT

Everyone experiences stress, which can result from both positive and negative experiences. A person's response to any change in homeostasis results in stress. Stress indicators can be physiologic (increased heart rate or respirations, muscle tension), psychological (anxiety, fear, anger), and/or cognitive (thinking responses). Consequences of stress may be physical, emotional, intellectual, social, spiritual, or any combination of these.

To minimize stress in a client, you should help the client to do the following:

- Determine situations that precipitate anxiety.
- Verbalize feelings, perceptions, and fears, as appropriate.
- Identify personal strengths.
- Recognize usual coping patterns.
- Identify new strategies.

You should also listen attentively, provide an atmosphere of warmth and trust, provide factual information as needed, encourage clients to participate in the plan of care, promote safety and security, and provide education. Responses to stress are called *coping mechanisms*.

SUPPORT SYSTEMS

A support system is a network of personal contacts that are available to clients for practical, emotional, or moral support when needed. Support systems are important to clients in that they enhance client learning, offer support, help the client perform required skills, and help the client maintain required lifestyle changes. Exploring the client's support system is a component of the initial assessment.

Caregivers might also need to be connected to outside resources. For example, community support groups are appropriate interventions for family members suffering from caregiver role strain.

THERAPEUTIC COMMUNICATIONS

You use therapeutic communication techniques to promote understanding and establish a constructive relationship with the client. Therapeutic communication is planned, and is client- and goal-directed. It means listening to and understanding the client while promoting clarification and insight. It enables the nurse to form a working relationship with the client and peers, using both verbal and nonverbal communication. Remember that *nonverbal communication* is the most accurate reflection of attitude.

You should be familiar with the foundations for a therapeutic relationship, which include:

- An understanding of the factors influencing communication
- Realization of the importance of nonverbal communication
- Development of effective communication skills
- Recognition of the causes of ineffective communication
- Ability to participate in a therapeutic communication process

You should also be familiar with the conditions essential for a therapeutic relationship, which include:

- Empathy
- Respect
- Genuineness
- Self-disclosure
- Concreteness and specificity
- Confrontation (limited to a well-established nurse/client relationship with an accepting, gentle manner)

It is important to understand the client's views and feelings before responding. You also need to recognize barriers to effective communication, such as:

- Failure to listen
- Improperly decoding the client's intended message
- Placing the nurse's needs above the client's needs
- Stereotyping, challenging, probing, and/or rejecting
- Being defensive
- Changing topics and subjects
- Passing judgment

Effective therapeutic responses include:

- **Using silence:** Allows the client time to think and reflect; conveys acceptance; allows the client to take the lead in the conversation
- **Using general leads or a broad opening:** Encourages the client to talk; indicates your interest in the client; allows the client to choose the subject
- **Clarification:** Encourages recall and details of a particular experience; encourages description of feelings; seeks explanation; pinpoints specifics
- **Reflecting:** Paraphrases what client says

THERAPEUTIC ENVIRONMENT

Nurses provide care for clients who constantly interact with their environment. Clients may have unmet needs, be unable to care for themselves, or be unable to adapt to the environment due to health problems. You provide therapeutic care so clients can adapt to their environment.

THE NURSING PROCESS AND PSYCHOSOCIAL INTEGRITY

You utilize the nursing process (assess, diagnose, plan, implement, and evaluate) to promote a client's psychosocial integrity by conveying understanding, sensitivity, and compassion to a client who is experiencing stress, illness, or crisis. Promoting a client's psychosocial integrity is not just for the mental health client, but for *all* clients. The nursing process respects the client's autonomy, freedom to make decisions, and involvement in nursing care.

Although you need to identify emotional disorders and behaviors that indicate mental illness, a client does not need to be mentally ill for you to include psychosocial integrity in the care plan. You must possess sound knowledge and focused clinical experiences to be prepared to recognize and effectively intervene with *any* client whose state of dynamic psychological and sociological homeostasis is being threatened—whether or not the client has a mental illness.

CHAPTER QUIZ

1. The nurse cares for an elderly client who appears fully alert and oriented. As it gets later in the day, the nurse notices the client becoming increasingly confused and agitated. It would be *MOST* appropriate for the nurse to take which of the following actions?

   1. Reorient the client, and then turn on the lights and television to distract the client from his confusion.
   2. Encourage the client's alert roommate to talk with the client.
   3. Tell the client he is at home in his own bed to get him to settle down and go to sleep.
   4. Reorient the client, pull the shades down, shut the lights and television off, and promote a quiet environment.

2. On the evening shift, the nurse is caring for a client who will be undergoing a mastectomy in the morning. A call from the front desk alerts the nurse that the client's family has arrived. It would be *MOST* appropriate for the nurse to take which of the following actions?

   1. Tell the family that they cannot come in because visiting hours are over.
   2. Tell the client you want to make sure she has some alone time to relax.
   3. Invite the family in to offer support after confirming with the client.
   4. Tell the nursing assistive personnel (NAP) to sit with the client who needs company.

3. The nurse is caring for a young man who has expressed his desire to commit suicide. He has informed the nurse of plans to pursue this. The nurse requests a sitter to stay with the client around the clock, but the client says he does not want this. Which of the following is the *MOST* appropriate response by the nurse?

   1. The nurse allows the young man to refuse, because clients do have a right to refuse care.
   2. The nurse implements the intervention, because protecting the client's safety trumps the client's right to refuse care.
   3. The nurse checks on the client every hour to be sure he is safe.
   4. The nurse asks the NAP to check on the client every 30 minutes to be sure he is safe.

4. A client is scheduled to have surgery the following day. The client tells the nurse, "I'm very scared. I have never had surgery before and am afraid that I might not make it through." Which of the following responses by the nurse is the *MOST* appropriate?

   1. "Why do you feel this way?"
   2. "Don't worry, you will be fine."
   3. "Why don't we take some time to explore why you feel this way?"
   4. "It's completely normal to be scared. You will be taken care of. Tell me how you are feeling."

5. The nurse is working on a pediatric unit. The client is a 13-month-old child diagnosed with failure to thrive. The parents report that the child cries frequently, does not like to be held, and will not eat. The nurse learns that the child's uncle lives in the house with the family. When the uncle visits in the hospital, the nurse notices the child acting differently and turning away from the uncle. Sometimes the child's heart rate increases when the uncle is present. The nurse should take which of the following actions *FIRST*?

   1. Immediately report the possible situation of abuse to the authorities.

2. Call the physician, who will probably have more long-term knowledge.

3. Discuss it with other nurses to see which approaches they have taken.

4. Encourage the team that's caring for the client to have a family meeting including the parents, but not the uncle, to gather more information.

6. The nurse learns that the client's sibling has passed away during his hospitalization, and the client is distraught by this news. Which of the following should the nurse do *FIRST*?

1. Allow the client an opportunity to verbalize feelings, and inquire if the client would like to be visited by social services, chaplaincy, or psychiatry for support.

2. Provide alone time by not going into the client's room unless absolutely necessary.

3. Call psychiatry services to arrange for them to see the client as soon as possible.

4. Find out which religion the client practices by viewing the chart and then request a chaplain from that religion to see the client.

7. The nurse is working on a busy locked psychiatric unit. The alarm gets tripped when somebody tries to go through the locked doors without permission from the front desk. Which of the following actions should the nurse take after the alarm is tripped?

1. Reset the alarm from the front desk after verifying that everybody is safe and nobody has escaped from the unit.

2. Reset the alarm from the location where the alarm was tripped after verifying that everybody is safe and nobody has escaped from the unit.

3. Reset the alarm from a client's room after doing a quick scan of the hallway.

4. Reset the alarm from the front desk once the receptionist says everybody is accounted for.

8. The client is an intoxicated male on the medical/surgical unit who attempts to get out of bed every few minutes. He is unsteady on his feet, and the nurse is concerned that he will fall if he does get out of bed. The doctor writes an order for the nurse to place wrist restraints to maintain the client's safety and prevent him from falling. The man refuses the restraints. The nurse should take which of the following actions?

1. Place the restraints in compliance with hospital policy.

2. Refrain from placing restraints to honor the client's wishes, because he has the right to refuse care.

3. Call the physician for advice on how to proceed.

4. Check on the client every hour to ensure his safety.

9. The nurse is working in an outpatient clinic. The nurse has a client who appears intoxicated and who drove to the appointment. The nurse is concerned about the client's ability to drive home. Which of the following should the nurse do *FIRST*?

1. Call the police immediately.

2. Ask the client's permission to call a family member or friend for a ride.

3. Give the client a ride home to protect his privacy.

4. Call clinic security to detain the client to protect his safety.

10. The mother of a teenage client who has permission to be involved in the plan of care is asking the nurse questions, after it has been explained to her that her child has bipolar disorder. Which of the following statements by the mother indicates that further teaching is needed?

1. "My child will be cured after being on medications for a few months."

2. "My child will require support and encouragement."

3. "My child will be on psychiatric medications probably for the rest of her life."

4. "The goal of the medication is to reduce symptoms associated with bipolar disorder and to hopefully help with the mood swings."

11. The home care nurse makes a visit to the home of an elderly client who has episodic confusion but who has remained safe at home while occasionally alone. The nurse finds the client disheveled, confused, and agitated, and the home is messy. This degree of confusion is unusual for this client. The nurse takes the client's vital signs, which are BP 115/70, HR 70, RR 16, and temperature 98.7° F (37° C). Which of the following actions should the nurse take *FIRST*?

    1. Nothing, because the client's vital signs are stable.

    2. Plan to come back the following day to reevaluate the client.

    3. Encourage the client to verbalize his or her feelings.

    4. Call the client's family to take the client to be evaluated by a physician because the client is not safe to be alone right now.

12. The nurse is on an Alzheimer's unit. A client is agitated and pulling at things. Which of the following should the nurse do?

    1. Provide the client with therapeutic sensory devices.

    2. Cohort the client with another client who is agitated, because they will calm each other.

    3. Place the client in a room with several other clients.

4. Leave the client alone for a period of time to reduce stimulation.

13. The nurse is caring for a terminally ill client who has agreed to enter hospice care. Which of the following statements by the spouse indicates a need for further teaching by the nurse?

    1. "You will help to make my spouse as comfortable as possible while in hospice care."

    2. "You will help my spouse get better so we can get back to our old life."

    3. "The goal is to make the end of my spouse's life as comfortable as possible."

    4. "You will provide me with support during this difficult time."

14. The nurse is caring for a male client. The client has exhibited some signs of anxiety and hostility. The nurse is aware that the client is a recently returned combat veteran. The nurse should assess the client for which of the following conditions?

    1. Post-traumatic stress disorder (PTSD)

    2. Bipolar disorder

    3. Schizophrenia

    4. Borderline personality disorder (BPD)

15. The nurse is caring for a client with a known past medical history for intravenous substance abuse. The client requests to go outside for a few minutes to smoke a cigarette and promises to come right back. The client has a peripheral intravenous line in. The nurse should take which of the following actions?

    1. Allow the client to go outside but set a time limit in which to return.

    2. Call security to escort the client to an approved smoking area.

3. Make a behavioral contract with the client that includes an agreement to have the NAP accompany the client outside.

4. Watch the client from the window to make sure the IV line stays open.

16. The client is a non-English-speaking elderly woman who is being admitted to the hospital for worrisome symptoms. She is accompanied by family members who speak English. The nurse admitting the client needs to ask some general admission questions. It would be *MOST* appropriate for the nurse to take which of the following actions?

1. Call the hospital's interpreter services to assist with asking the client questions in her native language.

2. Ask family members the questions and document their responses.

3. Ask family members to translate and ask the questions for the nurse.

4. Document "Unable to obtain answers, patient does not speak English."

17. The client has a medical history of alcohol abuse and had a drink yesterday. The nurse notes tremors, diaphoresis, and an elevated heart rate. The nurse should perform which of the following actions *FIRST*?

1. Call the physician to report the symptoms and administer hydromorphone (Dilaudid) per the alcohol withdrawal pathway.

2. Assess the client every hour to monitor symptoms.

3. Call the family and administer meperidine (Demerol) per the alcohol withdrawal pathway.

4. Administer lorazepam (Ativan) per the alcohol withdrawal pathway.

18. A client with post-traumatic stress disorder (PTSD) appears to be having a flashback. It would be *MOST* appropriate for the nurse to perform which of the following interventions?

1. Encourage the client to tell the nurse how the client is feeling in that moment.

2. Calmly reorient the client to the current situation.

3. Assist the client in acting out the event.

4. Tell the client loudly that what the client is experiencing is not real.

19. An elderly client asks the nurse to kill the bugs that are crawling on the floor of her room. The nurse does not see any bugs and suspects the client is hallucinating. Which of the following statements by the nurse would be *MOST* appropriate?

1. "It may seem to you that there are bugs crawling on the floor, but I do not see any bugs."

2. "I see them too. How should I kill them?"

3. "Can you tell me more about these bugs?"

4. "What do the bugs look like?"

20. The client has had a depressed mood, decreased sleep, poor concentration, and poor appetite for the past 4 months. Which of the following does the nurse expect the physician to prescribe?

1. Quetiapine (Seroquel)

2. Haloperidol (Haldol)

3. Mirtazapine (Remeron)

4. Clonazepam (Klonipin)

21. A client is experiencing a manic episode. It would be *MOST* appropriate for the nurse to perform which of the following interventions?

1. Give the client materials to make a collage.
2. Encourage the client to use an exercise bike.
3. Encourage the client to attend a group about managing feelings.
4. Ask the client to play a board game with other clients.

22. A client with bipolar disorder makes a sexually inappropriate comment to the nurse. The nurse should take which of the following actions?

   1. Ignore the comment because the client has a mental health disorder and cannot help it.
   2. Report the comment to the nurse manager.
   3. Ignore the comment, but tell the incoming nurse to be aware of the client's propensity to make inappropriate comments.
   4. Tell the client that it is inappropriate for clients to speak to any nurse that way.

23. The nurse makes a home visit to a child with a G-tube. Upon arrival, the nurse notices that the client's sibling is wearing dirty clothes that are too small. The nurse also notices that there is no food in the refrigerator or in the kitchen cabinets. Which of the following *MOST* appropriately describes how the nurse should respond to these observations?

   1. The nurse should not be concerned because the sibling is not her client and the client is being fed through a G-tube appropriately.
   2. The nurse should not be concerned because there are no signs of physical abuse.
   3. The nurse should be concerned and take action because there is no food or appropriate clothing available to the sibling.
   4. The nurse should not be concerned because her client is well cared for.

24. The nurse is caring for a hospice client who lives at home with an attentive spouse. The client's spouse quit work to care for the client. During the nurse's visit, the spouse expresses frustration and hostility toward the nurse. Which of the following are appropriate interventions by the nurse? **Select all that apply.**

   1. The nurse should encourage the spouse to verbalize feelings.
   2. The nurse should encourage the spouse to attend a caregiver support group.
   3. The nurse should encourage the spouse to go back to work part-time.
   4. The nurse should encourage the spouse not to verbalize negative feelings that may upset the client.

25. The nurse is taking a history from a client in an outpatient clinic. The client has been taking lorazepam (Ativan) for 6 months. Which of the following is the *MOST* likely side effect that the nurse would expect to see as a result of the client using Ativan for this time period?

   1. Excessive appetite
   2. Physical dependence
   3. Suicidal ideation
   4. Seizure activity

26. A client requires a lifesaving blood transfusion per hospital guidelines. The client refuses based on religious beliefs. It would be *MOST* appropriate for the nurse to take which of the following actions?

1. Confirm with the client that the client understands the potential risks of not having the blood transfusion.

2. Tell the client that, regardless of personal beliefs, the client has to have the lifesaving transfusion.

3. Call the Legal Department of the hospital immediately.

4. Try to gently encourage the client to change his or her mind.

27. The nurse monitors clients' medications in a day program for clients with disabilities. The nurse notices a teenage client who is frequently alone and often quiet. It would be *MOST* appropriate for the nurse to take which of the following actions?

    1. Allow the client alone time since the client seems to prefer this. The client has the right to make that choice.

    2. Make an effort to interact with the client periodically.

    3. Encourage the client to join a youth group.

    4. Encourage other clients in the program to interact more frequently with the client.

28. The nurse on the inpatient psychiatric ward is caring for a client with known suicidal ideation. The 24-hour observer calls the nurse to report that the client took off down the hall. The nurse is unable to immediately locate the client. Arrange the following actions by the nurse in the order that is *MOST* appropriate. **All options must be used.**

    1. Notify security that the client has eloped, and provide a description of the client. *3*

    2. Notify the nurse manager. *4*

    3. Notify other staff on the unit. *2*

    4. Ask the observer in what direction the client headed. *1*

29. The nurse discovers a hospice client has expired. The family members are regrouping in the facility's waiting room. Which of the following actions by the nurse would be the *MOST* appropriate?

    1. Tell the family it would not be in their best interests to see their loved one.

    2. Encourage the family to view the body to help accept the situation.

    3. Provide condolences to the family and offer them viewing time.

    4. Tell the family "I will give you some time to spend with your loved one. Let me know if you need anything."

30. The nurse is caring for a newly admitted client in a hospital setting. The client was recently diagnosed with cancer but is alert and oriented. The client is a Greek immigrant, but does speak English. During the admission process, the nurse inquires about advance directives with the client. The client tells the nurse: "I do not want to make any medical decisions. I want my daughter to make these decisions for me." The nurse should take which of the following actions?

    1. Make sure that the written advance directives document the client's wishes.

    2. Tell the client that, being alert and oriented, the client should make his or her own medical decisions.

    3. Tell the client that due to confidentiality, the daughter will not be informed of details of the client's care.

    4. Encourage both the daughter and the client to work together on making medical decisions.

Chapter Quiz Answers and Explanations

1. The Answer is 4

The nurse cares for an elderly client who appears fully alert and oriented. As it gets later in the day, the nurse notices the client becoming increasingly confused and agitated. It would be *MOST* appropriate for the nurse to take which of the following actions?

Category: Therapeutic environment

(1) Although the nurse would reorient the client, the nurse would not turn on the lights and television in an attempt to distract. Clients with confusion can become increasingly more agitated with stimulation, such as lights and television.

(2) Encouraging the client's roommate to talk with the client is another inappropriate attempt at distraction.

(3) Reassuring clients is usually a good practice, but it is not appropriate unless the nurse is honest with the attempt to reorient to an accurate location, time, and place.

(4) CORRECT: Promoting a quiet environment decreases stimulation to prevent agitation. It also promotes the normal sleep-wake cycle, consistent with it being "later in the day."

2. The Answer is 3

On the evening shift, the nurse is caring for a client who will be undergoing a mastectomy in the morning. A call from the front desk alerts the nurse that the client's family has arrived. It would be *MOST* appropriate for the nurse to take which of the following actions?

Category: Support systems

(1) Enforcing nursing unit rules, in this instance by telling the family they cannot come because visiting hours are over, is not considered a best answer on the NCLEX-RN® exam. On the exam, the nurse should do what is in the best interests of the client.

(2) The client may need some time alone, but the nurse would include the client in making that decision.

(3) CORRECT: During times of stress and anxiety, such as undergoing surgery, nurses should promote family support. The answer choice also states that the nurse would ask the client first. This supports including clients in their care.

(4) Telling the NAP to sit with client may be appropriate at times, but it is not the best option here.

3. The Answer is 2

The nurse is caring for a young man who has expressed his desire to commit suicide. He has informed the nurse of plans to pursue this. The nurse requests a sitter to stay with the client around the clock, but the client says he does not want this. Which of the following is the *MOST* appropriate response by the nurse?

Category: Crisis intervention

(1) Although clients do have the right to refuse care, in certain high risk-to-safety situations (for example, suicide), nurses put measures in place to prevent harm.

(2) CORRECT: Protecting the client's safety trumps the client's right to refuse care.

(3) The nurse could check in on the client every hour in combination with other interventions. However, clients at high risk for suicide cannot be left alone for any time period.

(4) This answer is incorrect for the same reasons as answer choice (3): clients at high risk for suicide cannot be left alone for any time period, even for 30 minutes.

4. The Answer is 4

A client is scheduled to have surgery the following day. The client tells the nurse, "I'm very scared. I have never had surgery before and am afraid that I might not make it through." Which of the following responses by the nurse is the *MOST* appropriate?

Category: Therapeutic communications

(1) Avoid asking "Why" questions because they imply disapproval with what the client is saying.

(2) Telling the client not to worry, and that the client will be fine, dismisses the client's feelings and provides for false reassurances.

(3) The nurse must remain within the nursing scope of practice. The nurse is not a therapist, so asking the client to explore his feelings with the nurse would not be appropriate.

(4) CORRECT: A response that tells the client that it is normal to be scared, and that he will be taken care of, and asks how he is feeling, normalizes the client's experience, provides some reassurance, and allows for him to verbalize.

5. The Answer is 4

The nurse is working on a pediatric unit. The client is a 13-month-old child diagnosed with failure to thrive. The parents report that the child cries frequently, does not like to be held, and will not eat. The nurse learns that the child's uncle lives in the house with the family. When the uncle visits in the hospital, the nurse notices the child acting differently and turning away from the uncle. Sometimes the child's heart rate increases when the uncle is present. The nurse should take which of the following actions *FIRST*?

Category: Abuse/neglect

(1) Although nurses are mandated to report child abuse in almost every state, the question stem does not present enough solid, verifiable facts to know whether abuse should be suspected. Thus the nurse should use the support of other colleagues and the interdisciplinary team to make this decision.

(2) Although the nurse might want to eventually notify the physician of abuse suspicions, this is not the first step. Most importantly, the NCLEX-RN® exam wants to see what the test taker would do rather than passing the responsibility to someone else.

(3) Although the nurse might ask for advice from peers on the client's care team, the nurse should not discuss a client's information with those who are not part of the care team.

(4) CORRECT: The nurse should utilize other disciplines in a team fashion and attempt to gather more facts before deciding appropriate further steps.

6. The Answer is 1

The nurse learns that the client's sibling has passed away during his hospitalization, and the client is distraught by this news. Which of the following should the nurse do *FIRST*?

Category: Grief and loss

(1) CORRECT: Allowing the client an opportunity to verbalize feelings, and inquiring if the client would like to be visited by social services, chaplaincy, or psychiatry are all appropriate for the nurse to do.

(2) Ignoring the client is not best practice. The client may want to be alone, but the nurse first needs to assess the situation and check with the client about his needs.

(3) The nurse would not call psychiatry services without first evaluating the client's emotional status and needs.

(4) It would be important to know if the client is practicing that religion and has current spiritual needs. But the client would dictate that and not the nurse.

7. The Answer is 2

The nurse is working on a busy locked psychiatric unit. The alarm gets tripped when somebody tries to go through the locked doors without permission from the front desk. Which of the following actions should the nurse take after the alarm is tripped?

Category: Therapeutic environment

(1) Resetting the alarm from the front desk is not proper procedure.

(2) CORRECT: An alarm is a safety mechanism meant to alert staff to somebody at risk attempting to leave. When an alarm is activated, the nurse should first make sure that all clients are accounted for and safe, and then reset the alarm by going to the place where it was tripped.

(3) The nurse must be sure, based on firsthand knowledge, that all clients are safe. Resetting the alarm without doing so would not be appropriate.

(4) The nurse must be sure, based on firsthand knowledge, that all clients are safe. Resetting the alarm without doing so would not be appropriate.

8. The Answer is 1

The client is an intoxicated male on the medical/surgical unit who attempts to get out of bed every few minutes. He is unsteady on his feet, and the nurse is concerned that he will fall if he does get out of bed. The doctor writes an order for the nurse to place wrist restraints to maintain the client's safety and prevent him from falling. The man refuses the restraints. The nurse should take which of the following actions?

Category: Chemical and other dependencies

(1) CORRECT: The nurse should place the restraints in compliance with hospital policy. This is a circumstance where the client's risk of harm and promotion of safety trumps the client's right to refuse.

(2) The client is at risk and intoxicated, so the nurse should place the restraints.

(3) The nurse, at some point, may call the physician for further assistance, but the NCLEX-RN® exam wants to know what the test taker would do rather than passing the responsibility to someone else.

(4) The nurse could check on the client every hour, but only in addition to the needed ongoing safety measure of restraints or constant observation. A client could fall within minutes; an hour is too long to leave an at-risk client alone.

9. The Answer is 2

The nurse is working in an outpatient clinic. The nurse has a client who appears intoxicated and who drove to the appointment. The nurse is concerned about the client's ability to drive home. Which of the following should the nurse do *FIRST*?

Category: Chemical and other dependencies

(1) The nurse's goal is to protect the client (and in this scenario, potentially the public as well), but calling the police immediately is not the best first option. The nurse may end up doing this but should first take the time to review other options.

(2) CORRECT: Asking the client's permission to call a family member is a better option because it includes the client in the choice. An intoxicated client may not make good choices, but the client may be amenable to good suggestions. Ideally, the nurse would find somebody (not the police) to get the client home safely. That would allow maintaining a trusting nurse-client relationship.

(3) The nurse should not overstep the boundaries and drive the client home.

(4) Calling clinic security to detain the client sounds less threatening than calling the police and might be done eventually, but the first option would be answer choice 2.

10. The Answer is 1

The mother of a teenage client who has permission to be involved in the plan of care is asking the nurse questions, after it has been explained to her that her child has bipolar disorder. Which of the following statements by the mother indicates that further teaching is needed?

Category: Mental health concepts

(1) CORRECT: Bipolar disorder is not curable. Clients can suffer from bipolar disorder throughout their entire lives. The mother's statement that the child will be cured after being on medication indicates further teaching about the disorder is needed.

(2) This is an accurate statement. Somebody suffering from this mental illness would need support and encouragement.

(3) This is an accurate statement. Psychotropic medications are used to treat bipolar disorder, usually for life.

(4) This is an accurate statement. The goal of the medication is to reduce symptoms associated with bipolar disorder and to lessen mood swings.

11. The Answer is 4

The home care nurse makes a visit to the home of an elderly client who has episodic confusion, but who has remained safe at home while occasionally alone. The nurse finds the client disheveled, confused, and agitated, and the home is messy. This degree of confusion is unusual for this client. The nurse takes the client's vital signs, which are BP 115/70, HR 70, RR 16, and temperature 98.7° F (37° C). Which of the following actions should the nurse do *FIRST*?

Category: Crisis intervention

(1) Although the vital signs are within normal limits, the onset of worsening symptoms could be an indication of something more serious, so doing nothing would not be correct.

(2) The nurse may plan to come back the following day depending on what happens to the client in the next 24 hours, but as a first choice, this is not correct.

(3) Encouraging the client to verbalize his or her feelings is not an inappropriate intervention given the presenting symptoms.

(4) CORRECT: These are new symptoms, and the client does not appear safe to be alone. By contacting the family, the nurse is performing an intervention based on the assessment of the client. In the home care setting, assessing safety is prioritized, especially with new symptoms.

12. The Answer is 1

The nurse is on an Alzheimer's unit. A client is agitated and pulling at things. Which of the following should the nurse do?

Category: Sensory/perceptual alterations

(1) CORRECT: Alzheimer's clients often pick at items, such as buttons on clothing or medical devices, which poses a danger to them. Providing them with safely designed sensory devices serves the need of stimulating the senses as well as their urge to pick.

(2) Cohorting the client with another agitated client can worsen the problem due to increased stimulation.

(3) Placing the client in a room with several other clients can worsen the problem due to increased stimulation.

(4) Leaving the client alone could lead to injuries related to the agitation and picking.

13. The Answer is 2

The nurse is caring for a terminally ill client who has agreed to enter hospice care. Which of the following statements by the spouse indicates a need for further teaching by the nurse?

Category: End of life care

(1) This is an accurate statement. The goal of hospice is to make clients as comfortable as possible during the remainder of their life.

(2) CORRECT: This is an inaccurate statement. The philosophy of hospice care is not to help a client recover, but to promote comfort and peace during the end of life. The presumption is that the client will not improve.

(3) This is an accurate statement. The goal of hospice is to make the end of life as comfortable as possible.

(4) This is an accurate statement. Hospice care involves the family as well as the client.

14. The Answer is 1

The nurse is caring for a male client. The client has exhibited some signs of anxiety and hostility. The nurse is aware that the client is a recently returned combat veteran. The nurse should assess the client for which of the following conditions?

Category: Mental health concepts

(1) CORRECT: PTSD is a known disorder from which veterans of war can suffer. Any thorough evaluation of symptoms would include one for PTSD.

(2) Although veterans can potentially suffer from bipolar disorder, PTSD is the best answer choice because of the common link.

(3) Although veterans can potentially suffer from schizophrenia, PTSD is the best answer choice because of the common link.

(4) Although veterans can potentially suffer from borderline personality disorder, PTSD is the best answer choice because of the common link.

15. The Answer is 3

The nurse is caring for a client with a known past medical history for intravenous substance abuse. The client requests to go outside for a few minutes to smoke a cigarette and promises to come right back. The client has a peripheral intravenous line in. The nurse should take which of the following actions?

Category: Chemical and other dependencies

(1) Allowing the client to go outside for a set time could potentially be a part of an agreement with the client, but review the other choices first.

(2) The client has not shown any signs of eloping and has not threatened anyone. If the client tried to elope, the nurse might then call security. At this point, the client has merely requested to go outside.

(3) CORRECT: Contracting with the client is the best choice. The nurse makes a compromise that the client can go outside but must be supervised while doing so. The client is a known abuser of intravenous substances, so sending the client outside alone could be a safety risk.

(4) Watching the client from the window is not an appropriate form of medical supervision.

16. The Answer is 1

The client is a non-English-speaking elderly woman who is being admitted to the hospital for worrisome symptoms. She is accompanied by family members who speak English. The nurse admitting the client needs to ask some general admission questions. It would be *MOST* appropriate for the nurse to take which of the following actions?

Category: Cultural diversity

(1) CORRECT: The only way to avoid bias and interjection by family members is by utilizing interpreter services at your hospital.

(2) Asking family members the questions and documenting their responses will result in obtaining answers to the questions and being able to create

some documentation, but the responses should come straight from the client.

(3) Asking family members to translate and ask the questions is not appropriate. The responses should come straight from the client.

(4) Documenting "unable to obtain answers, patient does not speak English" is a poor choice without trying another more appropriate method.

17. The Answer is 4

The client has a medical history of alcohol abuse and had a drink yesterday. The nurse notes tremors, diaphoresis, and an elevated heart rate. The nurse should perform which of the following actions *FIRST?*

Category: Chemical and other dependencies

(1) The nurse might call the physician at some point to report unmanageable symptoms, but Dilaudid is for pain and not for management of alcohol withdrawal.

(2) The nurse might assess the client every hour, but it is not the first thing the nurse would do. The nurse needs to intervene to prevent acute withdrawal.

(3) The nurse would not call the family unless the nurse had permission of the client, and would not give Demerol for withdrawal; it is for pain.

(4) CORRECT: Benzodiazepines such as Ativan are often given as part of an alcohol withdrawal pathway; this client is clearly beginning to exhibit symptoms of withdrawal by having tremors, diaphoresis, and an elevated heart rate.

18. The Answer is 2

A client with post-traumatic stress disorder (PTSD) appears to be having a flashback. It would be *MOST* appropriate for the nurse to perform which of the following interventions?

Category: Crisis intervention

(1) The patient is in crisis mode. Encouraging the client to verbalize feelings is not going to bring the client back to reality.

(2) CORRECT: The nurse wants to calmly orient the client back to the reality of the moment, to the actual safe environment.

(3) Assisting the client in acting out the event is not an appropriate intervention. The nurse wants to encourage the client back to reality and not go further into the flashback.

(4) Although the nurse wants to orient the client to reality, this would not be done loudly. This could possibly cause more hostility or violence if the client feels a sense of heightened danger.

19. The Answer is 1

An elderly client asks the nurse to kill the bugs that are crawling on the floor of her room. The nurse does not see any bugs and suspects the client is hallucinating. Which of the following statements by the nurse would be *MOST* appropriate?

Category: Crisis intervention

(1) CORRECT: This response validates what the client is seeing. To the client, a hallucination is real. However, the nurse must reorient the client to the appropriate reality and try to restore the client's feelings of safety.

(2) The nurse should not reinforce the hallucination.

(3) The nurse should not encourage verbalizing feelings during an active hallucination.

(4) It is not helpful to question or imply that the client is not seeing real bugs.

20. The Answer is 3

The client has had a depressed mood, decreased sleep, poor concentration, and poor appetite for the past 4 months. Which of the following does the nurse expect the physician to prescribe?

Category: Mental health concepts

(1) Seroquel is not typically given for depression symptoms. It is usually given for bipolar disorder.

(2) Haldol is given for symptoms of schizophrenia, not depression.

(3) CORRECT: Remeron is typically prescribed for depression.

(4) Klonipin is more typically given for panic disorders.

21. The Answer is 2

A client is experiencing a manic episode. It would be *MOST* appropriate for the nurse to perform which of the following interventions?

Category: Coping mechanisms

(1) Manic energy does not lend itself well to the patience and organization needed for a collage.

(2) CORRECT: The exercise bike would allow an outlet for the client's excessive energy.

(3) During the manic phase, clients do not have the patience to sit in a group and discuss feelings. This is not an appropriate intervention.

(4) During the manic phase, clients do not have the patience play a board game. This is not an appropriate intervention.

22. The Answer is 4

A client with bipolar disorder makes a sexually inappropriate comment to the nurse. The nurse should take which of the following actions?

Category: Mental health concepts; Behavioral interventions

(1) Clients have to be accountable for their own actions even if they have bipolar disorder. It is important to correct inappropriate behavior, and to encourage clients to interact socially in an acceptable way.

(2) The nurse's priority is to first communicate with the client; the nurse might want to report the incident to the nurse manager later.

(3) The nurse should not ignore the comment.

(4) CORRECT: The nurse should notify the client that this is inappropriate behavior and set up appropriate boundaries.

23. The Answer is 3

The nurse makes a home visit to a child with a G-tube. Upon arrival, the nurse notices that the client's sibling is wearing dirty clothes that are too small. The nurse also notices that there is no food in the refrigerator or in the kitchen cabinets. Which of the following *MOST* appropriately describes how the nurse should respond to these observations?

Category: Abuse/neglect

(1) Nurses are mandated reporters of child abuse whether or not it is their client.

(2) Although there are no signs of physical abuse, neglect is considered abuse even without violence and is reportable.

(3) CORRECT: As a mandated reporter, the nurse needs to investigate to determine if there is a reasonable explanation: for example, the sibling just came in from playing and the parents are on their way to buy food.

(4) Nurses are mandated reporters for any suspected child abuse whether or not it is their client.

24. The Answer is 1 and 2

The nurse is caring for a hospice client who lives at home with an attentive spouse. The client's spouse quit work to care for the client. During the nurse's visit, the spouse expresses frustration and hostility toward the nurse. Which of the following are appropriate interventions by the nurse? **Select all that apply.**

Category: Support systems

(1) CORRECT: Verbalizing feelings is an appropriate intervention for family members suffering from caregiver role strain.

(2) CORRECT: Attending a support group is an appropriate intervention for family members suffering from caregiver role strain.

(3) It may not be possible or practical for the spouse to go back to work part time.

(4) Encouraging the spouse not to verbalize negative feelings interferes with natural expression and personal family conversations.

25. The Answer is 2

The nursing is taking a history from a client in an outpatient clinic. The client has been taking lorazepam (Ativan) for 6 months. Which of the following is the *MOST* likely side effect that the nurse would expect to see as a result of the client using Ativan for this time period?

Category: Mental health concepts

(1) Excessive appetite is a possibility, but not the most likely.

(2) CORRECT: Clients can experience all types of side effects from benzodiazepines, but the most likely side effect from prolonged use is physical dependence.

(3) Suicidal ideation is a possibility, but not the most likely.

(4) Seizure activity is a withdrawal effect the nurse would monitor for if the client discontinued Ativan abruptly.

26. The Answer is 1

A client requires a lifesaving blood transfusion per hospital guidelines. The client refuses based on religious beliefs. It would be *MOST* appropriate for the nurse to take which of the following actions?

Category: Religious and spiritual influences on health

(1) CORRECT: The nurse must be sure the client understands the potential risks of not receiving the transfusion.

(2) Clients do have the right to refuse care on religious grounds.

(3) Although the nurse may call the Legal Department at some future time, this would not be the first course of action in this situation.

(4) The nurse must be sure that the client comprehends the choice he or she is making, including risks and benefits. However, the nurse does not want to coerce the client into changing his or her mind.

27. The Answer is 3

The nurse monitors clients' medications in a day program for clients with disabilities. The nurse notices a teenage client who is frequently alone and often quiet. It would be *MOST* appropriate for the nurse to take which of the following actions?

Category: Support systems

(1) It appears that the client has enough alone time, which could stunt the client's social growth. It could also defeat the purpose of a day program, which is to promote interaction among clients.

(2) Making an effort to interact with the client periodically does not lead to the client's personal growth. Therefore, it is not the best option.

(3) CORRECT: Participating in a youth group can help a teenage client with a disability develop social skills, use support systems, and feel more like a typical teenager.

(4) It would not be appropriate to talk about one client with other clients, for reasons of confidentiality and privacy.

28.   The Answer is 4, 3, 1, 2

The nurse on the inpatient psychiatric unit is caring for a client with known suicidal ideation. The 24-hour observer calls the nurse to report that the client took off down the hall. The nurse is unable to immediately locate the client. Arrange the following actions by the nurse in the order that is *MOST* appropriate. **All options must be used.**

Category: Crisis intervention

(1) Security is the third step because, although they are not immediately on hand, they can have multiple people search from different directions.

(2) Notifying your nurse manager is the last step, because the manager may not be readily available. Your priority is locating client and ensuring the client's safety.

(3) Notifying other staff is the second step because they know the client and are readily available to search locally.

(4) Asking the observer which direction the client headed is the first step. This enables the nurse to give accurate information to staff, and if necessary, security to help locate the client.

29.   The Answer is 3

The nurse discovers a hospice client has expired. The family members are regrouping in the facility's waiting room. Which of the following actions by the nurse would be the *MOST* appropriate?

Category: Grief and loss

(1) It is not the nurse's decision whether a family wants to view a body or not. This is a paternalistic attitude to be avoided in this setting.

(2) The nurse should react to that particular family's needs or wishes, and not encourage or discourage in either direction.

(3) CORRECT: The nurse acknowledges the loss, expresses sympathy, and offers the viewing opportunity.

(4) This statement assumes the family wants to view the body without the nurse inquiring first.

30.   The Answer is 1

The nurse is caring for a newly admitted client in a hospital setting. The client was recently diagnosed with cancer but is alert and oriented. The client is a Greek immigrant, but does speak English. During the admission process, the nurse inquires about advance directives with the client. The client tells the nurse: "I do not want to make any medical decisions. I want my daughter to make these decisions for me." The nurse should take which of the following actions?

Category: Cultural diversity

(1) CORRECT: As long as the client is not pressured into this decision and the nurse believes that it is being made of the client's free will, it is acceptable for the daughter to take over medical decision making for the ill parent.

(2) The client is entitled to have her daughter make the medical decisions for the client, if that is what the client wishes to do.

(3) The client is entitled to allow her daughter to be informed of the details of the client's care.

(4) The client is entitled to have her daughter make the medical decisions for the client, and the nurse should not encourage her to do otherwise.

CHAPTER 8

PHYSIOLOGICAL INTEGRITY: BASIC CARE AND COMFORT

Providing basic care and comfort for your clients is one of your most important roles. Ensuring that your clients have adequate nutrition and hydration, personal hygiene, and rest and sleep, and that their elimination needs are being properly attended to, are important priorities. Being able to help your clients with non-pharmacological comfort interventions, mobility issues, and assistive devices are also part of providing them with basic care and comfort.

On the NCLEX-RN® exam, approximately 9 percent of the questions will relate to Basic Care and Comfort. Exam content related to this subcategory includes, but is not limited to, the following topics:

- Assistive devices
- Elimination
- Mobility/immobility
- Non-pharmacological comfort interventions
- Nutrition and oral hydration
- Personal hygiene
- Rest and sleep

Let's now review the most important concepts covered by these subtopics on the NCLEX-RN® exam.

ASSISTIVE DEVICES

It is important to assess your clients for communication, speech, vision, and hearing issues, and help them learn how to compensate for deficits by using appropriate strengthening exercises, assistive devices, positioning, and/or other compensatory techniques. You will help clients select and learn how to use appropriate assistive devices, such as crutches, walkers, canes, hearing aids, and prosthetics, and evaluate whether the client is using them correctly.

Being able to communicate with clients who have visual and auditory deficits is also important. The following summarizes some techniques that you can employ.

Communicating with the Client with Visual Deficits

- Announce yourself and say your name when entering a client room.
- Stay in the client's field of vision, if possible.
- Use a warm, pleasant speaking voice; do not speak loudly.
- Explain procedures before starting them.
- Announce when you are leaving the room.

Communicating with the Client with Auditory Deficits

- Move where you can be seen by the client, or touch the client gently so the client knows where you are standing, before starting a conversation.
- Keep background noise to a minimum.
- Speak in a normal voice; do not shout.
- Look at the client when speaking so he or she can see your face/mouth for lip reading.
- Mime, write, or spell words, if needed.
- Pronounce words carefully.
- When changing the subject, slow down or use key words to indicate the change.

ELIMINATION

Clients' elimination needs are important to their basic care and comfort, as well to as their health. You need to provide appropriate interventions for a client who has an alteration in elimination.

Urinary Issues

One of the most common urinary problems is a urinary tract infection (UTI).

Lower Urinary Tract Issues

- Urethritis, inflammation of urethra
- Cystitis, inflammation of the bladder
- Prostatitis, inflammation of the prostate

Upper Urinary Tract Issues

- Pyelonephritis, inflammation of the pelvis and parenchyma

- Incontinence
  - Stress
  - Reflex
  - Urge
  - Functional

Other Urinary Issues

- Urgency
- Pain or difficulty (dysuria)
- Frequency
- Hesitancy
- Polyuria (large volume at one time)
- Nocturia (excessive at night, interrupting sleep)
- Hematuria (red blood cells in urine)
- Retention

Be familiar with common urinary tests, including the bladder scan at the bedside. It is also important to teach clients how to maintain a healthy urinary tract—provide information and instruction about adequate hydration (1,500–2,000 mL/day), emptying the bladder completely, the impact of caffeine and alcohol, proper personal hygiene, and Kegel exercises. In addition, teach clients to recognize the signs of a UTI.

Foley catheters are used to drain urine. Catheters can cause infection, so it is highly important to use proper sterile techniques when inserting, maintaining, and removing them. You should also know how to perform irrigations of the bladder, eyes, and ears.

Bowel Issues

Be able to recognize potential bowel issues based on the age and health of a client. Common bowel problems include constipation (hard, dry stools that are difficult to pass), impaction (an accumulated mass of stool that cannot be passed), diarrhea (frequent passage of unformed/liquid stool), incontinence (inability to retain urine or stool), flatulence, and hemorrhoids. Bowel problems are diagnosed by abdominal x-ray, upper gastrointestinal (GI) barium test, barium enema, and upper (oral) and lower (rectal) endoscopy.

Treatments include the following:

- **Constipation:** Increase fluid intake, including hot liquids and fruit juices; advise a high-fiber diet.
- **Diarrhea:** Understand and treat underlying cause (which may be a virus, reaction to certain foods or medications, GI tract infection, etc.); typically, advise bland foods and

a low-fiber diet, as well as to avoid spicy foods, alcohol, and caffeine while symptoms continue.

- **Flatulence:** Limit gum, carbonated beverages, cabbage, cauliflower, beans, and onions.

Care for ostomies (a surgically created opening in the abdominal wall through which feces can pass) is also an important part of basic care and comfort. Types and locations are as follows:

- **Ileostomy:** An opening into the distal end of the small intestine
- **Colostomy:** An opening into the colon

Ostomy care includes regularly assessing the condition of the stoma (the opening), making sure the skin around the stoma is clean and dry, and teaching the client how to care for the ostomy, including proper diet, fluid intake, and hygiene, and how to remove a food blockage.

It is also important to use proper skin care for clients who are incontinent, including the use of barrier creams and ointments. You should also be able to evaluate whether client elimination is restored to normal and whether it's maintained.

MOBILITY/IMMOBILITY

It is a nurse's responsibility to assess a client's mobility, gait, strength, motor skills, and use of assistive devices. You should be able to identify common causes of immobility, and the complications associated with each. The main causes are:

- Pain
- Motor/nervous system impairment
- Functional problems
- Generalized weakness
- Psychological problems
- Side effect of medication

Complications of immobility can be physiological and/or psychological in nature. Physical complications can include:

- Atrophy, joint contracture
- Disuse osteoporosis
- Pressure ulcers
- Orthostatic hypotension
- Deep vein thrombosis
- Pneumonia and pulmonary embolisms
- Decreased peristalsis, constipation
- Kidney stones

Psychological complications can include body image issues, lack of social interaction, sensory deprivation, and depression.

Interventions should be implemented to counteract physiological and psychological complications. Active and passive range of motion exercises, positioning, and mobilization can be used to promote circulation. Turning, repositioning, and pressure-relieving support surfaces can be used to maintain skin integrity and prevent skin breakdown. Anti-embolic stockings and sequential compression devices can be used to promote venous return.

It is also important to know when orthopedic and assistive devices, such as crutches, walkers, canes, splints, traction, braces, or casts, are needed; you should be able to teach the client how to use them properly to maintain correct body alignment.

NON-PHARMACOLOGICAL COMFORT INTERVENTIONS

It is important to be able to apply your knowledge of client pathophysiology to non-pharmacological interventions. Assess the client's need for pain management and implement comfort measures, as needed.

Therapies for comfort and treatment of inflammation/swelling can include heat, cold, or elevation of limbs. Use the pain scale and verbal reports to assess the effectiveness of the intervention.

Palliative Care

Nurses have an important role to play in palliative care, particularly in relation to pain and symptom management and the coordination of care. Assess a client's need for palliative care and provide counseling, as needed. Call in specialists from other disciplines, including doctors, psychologists, social workers, and clergy, as appropriate.

You should be able determine whether interventions are working and whether they are meeting the client's goals. The client's care may include pain management to improve comfort and quality of life, but may exclude painful treatments or heroic interventions.

You must respect a client's palliative care choices, and review those choices with the client periodically because they may change during the course of a client's disease. Assisting a client in receiving appropriate end-of-life symptom management, particularly as the client enters the active dying phase, is also important.

NUTRITION AND ORAL HYDRATION

It is important to know the principles of nutrition, such as the basic food groups, their functions, and which foods fall within those groups. These include:

- **Carbohydrates:** Are converted to glucose, which the body uses for energy. Sources of carbohydrates include grain products (bread, pasta, and rice), fruits, milk, and products with high sugar content.
- **Proteins:** Are used to build and repair body tissue, such as muscles, and also for many essential body processes, such as nutrient transport and muscle contraction. Sources of protein include meat, poultry, fish, eggs, nuts, beans, peas, and lentils.
- **Fats:** Are used to insulate the body, provide energy, and store certain vitamins such as A, D, E, and K, which are soluble in fats and insoluble in water. Sources of fat include whole milk and milk products, oils, nuts, and certain meats.

Be familiar with general dietary guidelines, key nutritional concepts across a client's life span, and types of diets appropriate for specific conditions, for example, which foods would be appropriate for a client with heart disease (foods with low fat and low cholesterol) or inappropriate (foods with high fat and high cholesterol). You should also be able to apply your knowledge of mathematics to nutrition (e.g., body mass index [BMI] calculations).

You can use the following to assess a client's ability to eat:

- Documented history
  - From patient
  - Nutritional screening initiatives (NSIs)
- Anthropomorphic measures
  - Height, weight, and body size
  - BMI
  - Basal metabolic rate (BMR)
  - Distribution of body fat (obesity)
- Lab/diagnostic measures
  - Albumin levels
  - Total lymphocyte count (TLC)
  - Hemoglobin levels
- Ability to chew and swallow

Assess clients for specific food/medication interactions, and consider client choices regarding nutritional requirements and dietary restrictions. Also monitor client hydration status. For example, be familiar with the signs and symptoms of both edema (excess fluid) and dehydration.

For clients unable to eat on their own, nutrition can be provided through continuous or intermittent tube feedings. This includes nasogastric, enterostomy (surgical), or percutaneous tubes. You should know how to maintain the tube insertion site, monitor it for infection and proper function, as well as ensure that the proper volume of formula is getting through. You should also recognize mechanical or metabolic problems and intervene, as needed. These include:

- Formula selection
- Formula adjustment
- Skin irritation
- Clogging
- Aspiration

Monitor the client's underlying condition to ensure the right dietary/feeding choices are made. Factors you must monitor include weight, protein measures, TLC, blood urea nitrogen (BUN), and creatinine levels, making adjustments as needed.

PERSONAL HYGIENE

It is important to assess your clients' personal hygiene and assist them in performance of both activities of daily living (ADLs) and instrumental activities of daily living (IADLs). Provide information on adaptations, such as shower chairs and hand rails.

Personal hygiene topics to know include care of skin, eyes, ears, nose, mouth, feet, nails, hair and scalp, perineal area, and prostheses. Care of the skin is particularly important. Know the measures to keep skin clean and moist, and how to prevent pressure points. Keeping skin clean can help prevent skin breakdowns and infections.

You should also know how to perform post-mortem care. After the patient is pronounced dead, nurses prepare the body for viewing by the family and transport to the morgue or funeral home. Family members should be given the option of seeing their loved one before or after post-mortem care is provided, or not at all, if that is their choice.

REST AND SLEEP

It is important to know the physiology of sleep, the phases, normal sleep patterns, and how sleep differs at each developmental stage. Your knowledge of each client's pathophysiology will help you to provide the appropriate interventions, which could include the following:

- Keeping the environment conducive to quiet relaxation
- Promoting bedtime routines
- Promoting comfort
- Avoiding heavy meals before bedtime
- Promoting appropriate activity
- Providing pharmaceutical aids (sedatives or hypnotics) as needed

CHAPTER QUIZ

1. The nurse is assessing an irritable 6-month-old infant during a well-baby checkup. The infant's weight is 19 lb., 6.4 oz. (8.8 kg). The infant does not have an elevated temperature, the heart rate is 102, and the respiratory rate is 32. The mother states that the infant wakes every hour or two throughout the night. The infant wants a bottle, and falls asleep while eating, but doesn't stay asleep. Which of the following instructions should the nurse give the parents?

   1. Instruct the parents to offer acetaminophen (Tylenol) 325 mg orally for comfort, and diphenhydramine (Benadryl) 25 mg orally for sleep.

   2. Instruct the parents to offer high-calorie solid foods during daytime hours so the infant does not wake up hungry during the night.

   3. Instruct the parents to offer the last feeding as late as possible, and put the infant to bed awake without a bottle.

   4. Suggest using pacifiers, taking the infant to the parent's bed, or rocking the infant to sleep.

2. The nurse caring for a child burned over 20% of her body assists the physician in performing dressing changes on day 5 after the initial injury. The child appears disoriented, has a fever of 101° F (38.3° C), and is crying in pain. Which of the following nursing interventions would be the *MOST* appropriate in caring for this client?

   1. Gather equipment for the dressing change and explain the procedure to the child.

   2. Do a complete physical assessment and notify the physician of the findings.

   3. Administer appropriate analgesics and gather equipment for the dressing change.

   4. Offer the child an enticing distraction from pain, such as a video, music, or toy.

3. The nurse is taking care of a young child a few hours after a tonsillectomy. Which of the following nursing interventions would be appropriate to promote adequate nutrition and oral hydration for this child?

   1. Offer the child warm soup, watch for signs of bleeding, and suction vigorously to remove old blood.

   2. Offer ice chips after the child awakens; advance to cool, clear liquids; and suction gently to remove oral secretions without causing the child to cough or gag.

   3. Maintain the intravenous fluids appropriate for the child's weight for the next 24 hours and keep the child NPO.

   4. Offer soft, warm foods so the child will not be hungry; orange juice to provide vitamin C; and milk shakes for calories.

4. The nurse is caring for a child who had an adenoidectomy and tonsillectomy 10 hours ago. The parents are in the room and preparing the child for bedtime. Which of the following nursing interventions would be helpful to promote rest and sleep for this client?

   1. Provide a cool water rinse, adjust the head of the bed to a 30–45-degree angle, and offer an ice collar for comfort.

   2. Encourage the parents to leave so the child can sleep.

   3. Suction vigorously before the child falls asleep to ensure the child has a patent airway.

4. Provide a water rinse, offer an ice collar for discomfort, and assist the child in finding a position of comfort while promoting a patent airway for sleep.

5. The nurse has been assigned to an adult male client who is less than 24 hours post-op. In report, the nurse learns that he rings his call light frequently, is anxious, and has had pain medication as ordered. Which of the following nondrug nursing interventions should the nurse include when caring for this client?

   1. Assure the client his anxiety is understandable, because the pain medication needs time to take effect.
   2. Assess other clients first, giving this client time to relax before evaluating his level of pain.
   3. Call the client's physician to increase the amount or frequency of pain medications ordered.
   4. Provide a quiet environment, offer repositioning, straighten the bed linens, offer fluids, and assess his pain level.

6. The nurse is taking care of an adult male with bilateral leg fractures. He has a long leg cast on his right leg as well as traction applied to the left femur. Which of the following is the *MAIN* purpose served by the cast for this client?

   1. Immobilizes the tibia and fibula and corrects deformities
   2. Keeps the client, who is in traction, more comfortable
   3. Immobilizes the pelvic bones for better healing
   4. Encircles the trunk and stabilizes the spine

7. The nurse is taking care of an elderly male client who has shortness of breath, cough, and fluid in his pleural space. The physician asks the nurse to assist in the performance of a therapeutic and diagnostic thoracentesis. Which of the following nursing interventions should the nurse perform to assist this client?

   1. Make certain the consents are signed, witnessed, and filed in the chart.
   2. Offer oral fluids, because the client will not be able to take a drink during the procedure.
   3. Help the client to lie flat with a pillow under his feet for comfort during the procedure.
   4. Help the client to sit up and place his arms over a bedside table, encouraging him to remain still during the procedure.

8. The nurse has been assigned to a 2-day-old male infant on the mother/baby unit of an acute care facility. The infant will undergo a circumcision procedure in the afternoon, before being discharged the following morning. Which of the following non-pharmacologic interventions should the nurse teach the parents to keep this infant comfortable while the circumcision heals?

   1. Fasten his diaper tightly to avoid having it move around the wound.
   2. Apply petroleum jelly to gauze and place over the end of the penis when changing the diaper, leaving the diaper slightly loose when fastening.
   3. Offer feedings more often to soothe the child who is in pain.
   4. Wash the end of the penis vigorously to prevent infection.

9. The nurse is taking care of a quadriplegic young man who suffers from a C2-C3 fracture after an auto accident 3 months prior. He has a tracheotomy, is ventilator-dependent, and has been discharged to home with skilled home nursing care. The nurse knows that this client is at risk for autonomic dysreflexia. Which of the following measures should this nurse take to keep the client comfortable, manage his elimination needs, and prevent common causes of autonomic dysreflexia?

   1. Turn the client at least every two hours and look for skin breakdown.

   2. Allow the client to sleep 8–10 hours without interruption each night to promote rest.

   3. Offer appetizing fluids at least every two hours during the day to promote hydration.

   4. Straight catheterize the client to prevent bladder distention and maintain a regular bowel program to prevent impaction.

10. The nurse is taking care of a child after an open reduction of the radius and ulna of her right arm. The child is now immobilized in a plaster cast splint reinforced with an Ace wrap. Which of the following non-pharmacological nursing interventions will promote comfort for this child?

   1. Apply a heat pack to the approximate area of the surgical incision.

   2. Position the child so the cast is flat on the mattress for firm support.

   3. Elevate the cast on a pillow, apply an ice pack to the approximate area of the surgical incision, and reposition the child every two hours.

   4. Do not move any part of the child's arm until the physician orders a specific position.

11. The nurse is taking care of an elderly client with left-sided heart failure. Which of the following are the *MOST* appropriate nursing interventions to reduce the workload of the heart and to promote comfort and rest? **Select all that apply.**

   1. Assist the client on short walks at least two times per shift to increase circulation.

   2. Provide a comfortable armchair or raise the head of the bed to increase the reserve of the heart and to decrease the work of breathing.

   3. Allow the client to lie flat to sleep.

   4. Help the client walk to the bathroom rather than using a bedside commode.

12. The nurse is instructing a male client on the proper use of crutches for an ankle injury. He will be required to be non-weight bearing for 4–6 weeks. Which of the following crutch gaits should the nurse teach this client for safe ambulation?

   1. The two-point gait

   2. The three-point gait

   3. The four-point gait

   4. None, there is no special gait for crutch training

13. The nurse is working in an extended care facility when a nursing assistive personnel (NAP) reports that an elderly client is crying in pain. The nurse finds the client in the bathroom complaining of severe constipation. What would be the appropriate order of nursing interventions to assist this client with his immediate elimination needs? **All options must be used.**

   1. Offer oral fluids to ease the constipation.

   2. Notify the physician.

   3. Offer PRN medications orally, if ordered.

4. Use a gloved hand with lubricant to manually assess for fecal impaction and to stimulate the rectal wall to loosen the fecal matter.

14. The nurse is caring for a young child who has recently had a vesicostomy. Which of the following nursing interventions should the nurse undertake to assist this child with basic comfort and elimination?

    1. Offer fluids, apply an absorbent diaper or incontinence pads, and dilate the opening once or twice a day as ordered by the physician.
    2. Double-diapering the area is the only intervention needed.
    3. Apply a urine bag and change it daily.
    4. Double-diaper the area after applying a urine bag.

15. A client who has chronic pain asks the nurse about alternative therapy in conjunction with traditional treatment. Which of the following forms of alternative therapy could the nurse provide for this client?

    1. Music therapy or guided imagery
    2. Acupuncture
    3. Kegel exercises
    4. None, nurses do not participate in providing alternative treatments

16. The nurse is taking care of an adult client with a fractured femur who must be maintained in traction for several days before surgical interventions can take place. The client has several abrasions, his hair is dirty, and he has healing wounds in his mouth. Which of the following nursing interventions should the nurse use in caring for the personal hygiene of this client?

    1. Place everything within the reach of the client so he can bathe himself.

2. Assist with a bed bath, with teeth brushing, and by washing his hair with soap and water or a non-shampoo product for bed-bound clients.
3. Allow a family member to bathe the client.
4. Offer an oral rinse for hygiene, but postpone the bath until a later time due to the traction.

17. The nurse is taking care of an adult client with a long-bone fracture. The nurse encourages the client to move fingers and toes hourly, to change positions slightly every hour, and to eat high-iron foods as part of a balanced diet. Which of the following foods or beverages should the nurse advise the client to avoid while on bed rest?

    1. Fruit juices
    2. Large amounts of milk or milk products
    3. Cranberry juice cocktail
    4. No need to avoid any foods while on bed rest

18. The nurse working in an outpatient clinic has the opportunity to teach an insulin-dependent client. Which of the following topics would be *MOST* appropriate for the nurse to include when teaching personal hygiene?

    1. Oral care is not a top priority.
    2. Hair care is the most important part of personal hygiene for the diabetic client.
    3. It is most important to keep skin clean and dry, especially the feet.
    4. Personal hygiene is not included in diabetic teaching because it is an individual choice.

19. The nurse is taking care of a child in the ambulatory care clinic. The parents relate a 24-hour period of gastrointestinal complaints, including vomiting several times and 3 watery stools. Which of the following should the nurse do to assist in maintaining nutrition for this child?

 1. Educate the parents on the signs of dehydration and the slow introduction of fluids to rehydrate the child.

 2. Offer no advice to the parents other than to suggest parents offer whatever foods the child feels like taking.

 3. Encourage the parents to offer the child milk products for the vitamins and rehydration.

 4. Encourage the parents to offer solid foods to improve the nutritional status quickly.

20. An 11-lb. (5-kg) infant is NPO after a minor surgical procedure. What would be the appropriate rate of infusion of intravenous fluids if the physician ordered fluids to run at 15 mL/kg/day? Record your answer using one decimal place.

_____ mL/hr

21. An adult diagnosed with pancreatic cancer is having a consultation with the nurse about nutrition and hydration. Which of the following suggestions might the nurse include when providing education to this client?

 1. Drink clear water, progress diet rapidly as tolerated, and weigh daily.

 2. Puree foods, choose low-protein foods for easier digestion, and weigh weekly.

 3. Take herbal therapies, avoid vitamins, and don't monitor weight.

 4. Use spices to stimulate taste buds, eat cool foods to decrease odor, and eat small but frequent high-protein and high-carbohydrate meals.

22. The nurse is caring for an elderly client who has been on long-term nutritional support. The nurse is reviewing the infusion procedure with the client's daughter. The nurse states which of the following as the rationale for removing the formula from the refrigerator and infusing it through the gastrostomy tube at room temperature?

 1. "The formula tastes better at room temperature."

 2. "This method will be the least likely to give your father gastric discomfort."

 3. "There is no need to bring the formula to room temperature."

 4. "Room-temperature prepared formula reduces aspiration."

23. The nurse is working with a middle-aged female after a knee injury. Ambulation is still difficult for the client, and the physical therapist has suggested the client use a cane. The nurse states which of the following with respect to using a cane rather than a walker for this injury?

 1. "The cane is just a reminder to use good posture."

 2. "The cane can be more dangerous than helpful, and another type of assistive device should be considered for this client."

 3. "The cane will help with fatigue while assisting the client with balance and support."

 4. "A cane does not offer any relief on weight-bearing joints."

24. The nurse is preparing for a pediatric trauma admission in which traction will be applied to immobilize a femur fracture for a child. The nurse reviews the forms of traction and the purposes for each before gathering equipment prior to the child's arrival. Match the type of traction on the left with the type of injury or indication on the right. **All options must be used.**

1. Bryant's traction E.
2. Russell's traction D,
3. 90-degree traction B.
4. Buck's traction C.
5. Cervical traction A.

A. Stabilizes a spinal fracture or muscle spasm
B. Used on the femur if skin traction isn't suitable
C. Temporarily immobilizes a fractured leg
D. May reduce fractures of the hip or femur
E. Used in children younger than age 2 to reduce femur fractures or stabilize hips

25. It is important to evaluate pain in the neonate. Look at the chart below. What would the pain score be for an infant with a high-pitched cry, O_2 saturation of 96%, a grimace, and frequent periods of wakefulness?

	Score		
	0	*1*	*2*
Crying	No	High-pitched	Inconsolable
Requires O_2	No	< 30%	> 30%
Expression	None	Grimace	Grimace/grunt
Sleepless	No	Wakes frequently	Always awake

1. Score of 0
2. Score of 2
3. Score of 3
4. Not enough information

CHAPTER QUIZ ANSWERS AND EXPLANATIONS

1. The Answer is 3

The nurse is assessing an irritable 6-month-old infant during a well-baby checkup. The infant's weight is 19 lb., 6.4 oz. (8.8 kg). The infant does not have an elevated temperature, the heart rate is 102, and the respiratory rate is 32. The mother states that the infant wakes every hour or two throughout the night. The infant wants a bottle and falls asleep while eating, but doesn't stay asleep. Which of the following instructions should the nurse give the parents?

Category: Rest and sleep

(1) Tylenol may be appropriate for teething pain, and Benadryl is an antihistamine that may cause drowsiness, but the doses as given are for adults.

(2) The infant's weight is within normal limits, so high-calorie foods may not be appropriate.

(3) CORRECT: The infant is having sleep disturbances related to nighttime feeding. Feeding late and putting the infant to bed awake help the infant learn to recognize bedtime and to self-soothe to fall asleep.

(4) The Academy of Pediatrics does not promote putting infants to bed with parents. Rocking the infant will not help learning to self-soothe.

2. The Answer is 2

The nurse caring for a child burned over 20% of her body assists the physician in performing dressing changes on day 5 after the initial injury. The child appears disoriented, has a fever of 101° F (38.3° C), and is crying in pain. Which of the following nursing interventions would be the *MOST* appropriate in caring for this client?

Category: Non-pharmacological comfort interventions

(1) The nurse would gather equipment, but not before addressing the crying child.

(2) CORRECT: The child may be suffering from an infection. The nurse recognizes that disorientation and fever are the first signs of sepsis in burn clients. It would be most appropriate to assess

for the causes of fever and pain and notify the physician before proceeding.

(3) Analgesics may be appropriate but not before assessing the pain and source of fever and disorientation.

(4) Distractions may be offered after the assessment but they do not take priority over notifying the physician regarding the findings about the source of fever and pain.

3. The Answer is 2

The nurse is taking care of a young child a few hours after a tonsillectomy. Which of the following nursing interventions would be appropriate to promote adequate nutrition and oral hydration for this child?

Category: Nutrition and oral hydration

(1) Warm liquids may increase bleeding and should be avoided the first few hours after surgery.

(2) CORRECT: The child may first take ice chips 1–2 hours after awakening, followed by cool, clear liquids without pulp or ice pops. Gentle suctioning may be necessary to remove secretions in the mouth and to keep the child from gagging. Suctioning should be kept to a minimum to avoid traumatizing the oropharynx.

(3) The physician may maintain an intravenous infusion postoperatively, but it is not necessary to keep the child NPO after the surgery. Ice chips or cool, clear liquids are soothing.

(4) Soft foods are not given in the first few hours after surgery to prevent emesis. Orange juice is acidic, and juices should be alkaline when offered to a postoperative child. Milk products are controversial because they coat the throat and may cause the child to cough.

4. The Answer is 4

The nurse is caring for a child who had an adenoidectomy and tonsillectomy 10 hours ago. The parents are in the room and preparing the child for bedtime.

Which of the following nursing interventions would be helpful to promote rest and sleep for this client?

Category: Rest and sleep

(1) Semi-Fowler's may not be a position comfortable for some children, so other positions may need to be considered.

(2) The parents should be encouraged to stay with the child and to participate in the care and comfort of the child, if possible.

(3) Suctioning should not be vigorous after an adenoidectomy or a tonsillectomy.

(4) CORRECT: Assist the child in finding a position of comfort. This may be prone, semi-prone, or semi-Fowler's. An ice collar and a cool oral rinse will also aid in comfort.

5. The Answer is 4

The nurse has been assigned to an adult male client who is less than 24 hours post-op. In report, the nurse learns that he rings his call light frequently, is anxious, and has had pain medication as ordered. Which of the following nondrug nursing interventions should the nurse include when caring for this client?

Category: Non-pharmacological comfort interventions

(1) The client will probably be more reassured if physical comfort measures are taken, rather than just verbal assurances.

(2) Prioritizing is necessary, but avoiding an already anxious client may cause the nurse to overlook a serious symptom.

(3) Call a physician, if needed, *AFTER* offering basic comfort measures and doing an assessment.

(4) CORRECT: Changing the client's position, removing wrinkles in the bed linen, helping the client to take a drink, or limiting noise can help the client to rest and may reduce pain.

6. The Answer is 1

The nurse is taking care of an adult male with bilateral leg fractures. He has a long leg cast on his right leg as well as traction applied to the left femur.

Which of the following is the *MAIN* purpose served by the cast for this client?

Category: Mobility/immobility

(1) CORRECT: A long leg cast serves to immobilize the tibia and fibula by being placed above and below the knee and ankle joints.

(2) A long leg cast is not used for comfort for a client in traction.

(3) A long leg cast does not immobilize the pelvis.

(4) A body cast, not a long leg cast, encircles the trunk.

7. The Answer is 4

The nurse is taking care of an elderly male client who has shortness of breath, cough, and fluid in his pleural space. The physician asks the nurse to assist in the performance of a therapeutic and diagnostic thoracentesis. Which of the following nursing interventions should the nurse perform to assist this client?

Category: Non-pharmacological comfort interventions

(1) The nurse should make certain that consents are signed before the start of a procedure, but that does not affect the client's comfort.

(2) Fluids should not be offered right before a procedure to avoid nausea and vomiting if pain is experienced.

(3) Lying flat with feet elevated is not the position of choice for a thoracentesis.

(4) CORRECT: Placing the client in a sitting position over a bedside table is the most comfortable and allows the best opportunity to remove fluid at the base of the chest.

8. The Answer is 2

The nurse has been assigned to a 2-day-old male infant on the mother/baby unit of an acute care facility. The infant will undergo a circumcision procedure in the afternoon, before being discharged the following morning. Which of the following non-pharmacologic interventions should the nurse teach the parents to keep this infant comfortable while the circumcision heals?

Category: Non-pharmacological comfort interventions

(1) Leaving the diaper slightly loose when fastening will be more comfortable.

(2) CORRECT: Petroleum jelly offers lubrication and helps stop the friction of the diaper over the raw area.

(3) Offering feedings more often than necessary may cause emesis and is not the best way to soothe an infant.

(4) The end of the penis has a yellow exudate that is part of the healing process and should not be vigorously washed off. It will disappear with healing.

9.   The Answer is 4

The nurse is taking care of a quadriplegic young man who suffers from a C2-C3 fracture after an auto accident 3 months prior. He has a tracheotomy, is ventilator-dependent, and has been discharged to home with skilled home nursing care. The nurse knows that this client is at risk for autonomic dysreflexia. Which of the following measures should this nurse take to keep the client comfortable, manage his elimination needs, and prevent common causes of autonomic dysreflexia?

Category: Elimination

(1) Turning is necessary to prevent decubitus ulcers and promote comfort, but it does not necessarily prevent an increase in blood pressure as seen with autonomic dysreflexia.

(2) Sleeping 8–10 hours is not related to autonomic dysreflexia.

(3) Offering fluids is a nursing measure but may not be related to autonomic dysreflexia because a client with a spinal cord injury may have a fluid restriction to help control blood pressure.

(4) CORRECT: Bladder distension and bowel impaction can result in autonomic dysreflexia, causing a critical increase in blood pressure.

10.   The Answer is 3

The nurse is taking care of a child after an open reduction of the radius and ulna of her right arm. The child is now immobilized in a plaster cast splint reinforced with an Ace wrap. Which of the following non-pharmacological nursing interventions will promote comfort for this child?

Category: Non-pharmacological comfort interventions; Mobility/immobility

(1) Heat would not be appropriate, because it could cause, rather than reduce, swelling.

(2) The cast should be elevated for the first 24–48 hours and not be left flat on the mattress.

(3) CORRECT: Elevating the extremity and applying an ice pack will help to reduce swelling and may reduce pain. Repositioning is a comfort intervention.

(4) The child should not be totally immobile because it can lead to post-op respiratory complications.

11.   The Answer is 1 and 2

The nurse is taking care of an elderly client with left-sided heart failure. Which of the following are the *MOST* appropriate nursing interventions to reduce the workload of the heart and to promote comfort and rest? **Select all that apply.**

Category: Rest and sleep

(1) CORRECT: Taking short walks may provide distraction and increase mobility, circulation, and overall well-being if tolerated.

(2) CORRECT: Allowing the client to sit in an armchair makes it easier to breathe and is a safe alternative to an armless chair. It is also helpful to have the client raise the head of the bed when sleeping or napping. These are appropriate for a client with left-sided heart failure.

(3) A client in left-sided heart failure most likely will not tolerate lying flat, so this would not promote sleep and rest in this position.

(4) A bedside commode would reduce the work of getting to the bathroom and should be used.

12.   The Answer is 2

The nurse is instructing a male client on the proper use of crutches for an ankle injury. He will be required to be non-weight bearing for 4–6 weeks. Which of the following crutch gaits should the nurse teach this client for safe ambulation?

Category: Assistive devices

(1) The two-point gait is an advanced four-point gait and allows for faster ambulation with minimal support.

(2) CORRECT: The three-point gait is the safest to use when one leg is injured. Both crutches and the injured leg move forward, followed by swinging the stronger lower extremity as the rest of the body weight is placed on the crutches.

(3) The four-point gait is used as a slow and stable gait for those who can bear weight on each leg.

(4) Gait training is part of client education when crutches or adaptive equipment is used for ambulation.

13. The Answer is 4, 3, 2, 1

The nurse is working in an extended care facility when a nursing assistive personnel (NAP) reports that an elderly client is crying in pain. The nurse finds the client in the bathroom complaining of severe constipation. What would be the appropriate order of nursing interventions to assist this client with his immediate elimination needs? **All options must be used.**

Category: Elimination

(1) This is last in the appropriate order of nursing interventions. Oral fluids should be increased but will not impact the immediate pain and constipation.

(2) Relief of the immediate pain is the priority. After an attempt to manually remove the impaction, and offering a PRN medication, the physician should be notified.

(3) PRN medications do not offer immediate relief and may not be effective if the impaction is solid. After a manual exam assessment, and an attempt to remove the stool, it would be appropriate to offer a PRN medication orally, if ordered, to prevent a repeat incident.

(4) The first nursing intervention should be manual assessment and removal of the fecal impaction. This will offer immediate relief while helping to assess what needs to be relayed to the physician.

14. The Answer is 1

The nurse is caring for a young child who has recently had a vesicostomy. Which of the following nursing interventions should the nurse undertake to assist this child with basic comfort and elimination?

Category: Elimination

(1) CORRECT: A vesicostomy is performed when chronic neurogenic bladder and frequent urinary tract infections become problematic. Hydration, cleansing and drying of the area, absorbent diapers, and daily dilation of the opening are all appropriate care to prevent infection and to provide comfort.

(2) Double diapers alone are not enough to keep the child comfortable and free from infection.

(3) It is not customary to apply a urine bag over the opening of a vesicostomy.

(4) The addition of a urine bag to double diapers will not keep the child comfortable and free from infection.

15. The Answer is 1

A client who has chronic pain asks the nurse about alternative therapy in conjunction with traditional treatment. Which of the following forms of alternative therapy could the nurse provide for this client?

Category: Alternative therapy; Non-pharmacological comfort interventions

(1) CORRECT: Music therapy and guided imagery have been proven to increase a client's ability to perform activities of daily living by helping to focus on something other than pain.

(2) Acupuncture must be performed by a skilled practitioner and is not done by a nurse.

(3) Kegel exercises are done independently by the client to tighten the muscles of the pelvic floor. They do not provide pain relief.

(4) Nurses may participate in many forms of alternative therapies as nursing interventions when trained properly.

16. The Answer is 2

The nurse is taking care of an adult client with a fractured femur who must be maintained in traction for several days before surgical interventions can take place. The client has several abrasions, his hair is dirty, and he has healing wounds in his mouth. Which of the following nursing interventions should the nurse use in caring for the personal hygiene of this client?

Category: Personal hygiene

(1) The client may be able to do some of his bath, but it would not be possible for him to cleanse his own back and other areas while maintaining traction.

(2) CORRECT: Assisting with the bath allows inspection of the skin for any pressure areas; gentle teeth brushing and hair cleansing are nursing measures and promote comfort while maintaining the traction.

(3) A family member should not be responsible for inspecting the skin and maintaining the traction. These are nursing responsibilities.

(4) Oral care is important but the bath should not be postponed and can easily be done with the client in traction. It will promote comfort and healing.

17. The Answer is 2

The nurse is taking care of an adult client with a long-bone fracture. The nurse encourages the client to move fingers and toes hourly, to change positions slightly every hour, and to eat high-iron foods as part of a balanced diet. Which of the following foods or beverages should the nurse advise the client to avoid while on bed rest?

Category: Nutrition and oral hydration; Mobility/immobility

(1) Fruit juices can be taken while on bed rest.

(2) CORRECT: Too much milk increases the demand on the kidneys to excrete calcium and can lead to kidney stones.

(3) Cranberry juice can be taken while on bed rest and also aids in prevention of urinary tract infections.

(4) Some foods should be avoided or limited while on bed rest. For instance, milk and milk products should be avoided or limited while on bed rest to avoid kidney stone formation.

18. The Answer is 3

The nurse working in an outpatient clinic has the opportunity to teach an insulin-dependent client. Which of the following topics would be *MOST* appropriate for the nurse to include when teaching personal hygiene?

Category: Personal hygiene

(1) Oral care is an important part of diabetic hygiene to prevent cavities and infections.

(2) Hair care is not the most important part of personal hygiene, although it is important for self-esteem.

(3) CORRECT: Skin care is essential to prevent infection and skin breakdown. This is especially true for the feet, where a client may not see or feel problem areas.

(4) Personal hygiene is definitely a part of self-care teaching for an insulin-dependent client.

19. The Answer is 1

The nurse is taking care of a child in the ambulatory care clinic. The parents relate a 24-hour period of gastrointestinal complaints, including vomiting several times and 3 watery stools. Which of the following should the nurse do to assist in maintaining nutrition for this child?

Category: Nutrition and oral hydration

(1) CORRECT: Signs of dehydration would be part of parental teaching, and a slow introduction of clear liquids advancing to other liquids is appropriate.

(2) It would not be appropriate for the nurse to suggest that the parents offer whatever foods the child feels like taking, without first educating the parents about the signs of dehydration.

(3) Milk products would not be the first type of fluids offered for a child who has been vomiting, due to how irritating milk can be on the digestive system.

(4) Solid foods are introduced later, after liquids are offered over several hours, once vomiting has stopped.

20. The Answer is 3.1 mL/hour

An 11-lb. (5-kg) infant is NPO after a minor surgical procedure. What would be the appropriate rate of infusion of intravenous fluids if the physician ordered fluids to run at 15 mL/kg/day? Record your answer using one decimal place.

_____ mL/hr

Category: Nutrition and oral hydration

Multiply 5 kg by 15 mL/kg. This equals 75 mL. Then divide 75 mL by 24 hours in a day to arrive at the answer: 3.1 mL/hr. The nurse would run the IV at 3.1 mL over 24 hours to get the ordered amount of fluid.

21. The Answer is 4

An adult diagnosed with pancreatic cancer is having a consultation with the nurse about nutrition and hydration. Which of the following suggestions might the nurse include when providing education to this client?

Category: Nutrition and oral hydration

(1) It is more appropriate to progress the diet slowly to avoid nausea and vomiting.

(2) Pureed foods may cause nausea and gagging, low-protein foods do not offer enough nutrients, and daily weights are the norm.

(3) Herbal therapies have not been researched enough to be certain that they would not interfere or compromise cancer treatments when ingested. Topical herbal treatments may be of use for comfort.

(4) CORRECT: Flavored foods high in both protein and carbohydrates will help to increase calorie intake. Foods that have less odor, and small, frequent meals help ward off nausea.

22. The Answer is 2

The nurse is caring for an elderly client who has been on long-term nutritional support. The nurse is reviewing the infusion procedure with the client's daughter. The nurse states which of the following as the rationale for removing the formula from the refrigerator and infusing it through the gastrostomy tube at room temperature?

Category: Nutrition and oral hydration

(1) There would not be a taste to formula given through the G-tube.

(2) CORRECT: Cold formula through the G-tube can cause discomfort and cramping.

(3) It is most appropriate for the comfort of the client to bring the formula to room temperature before administering.

(4) Temperature has nothing to do with the risk of aspiration.

23. The Answer is 3

The nurse is working with a middle-aged female after a knee injury. Ambulation is still difficult for the client, and the physical therapist has suggested the client use a cane. The nurse states which of the following as the rationale for using a cane rather than a walker for this injury?

Category: Assistive devices

(1) A cane is not used as a reminder for good posture; it is used for comfort and support.

(2) A cane is safe when used properly.

(3) CORRECT: A cane offers support and can give the client relief of joint pain and fatigue, and promote a safe way to ambulate when a lower extremity is injured.

(4) A cane does offer relief on weight-bearing joints when used properly.

24. The Answer is 1 (E), 2 (D), 3 (B), 4 (C), 5 (A)

The nurse is preparing for a pediatric trauma admission in which traction will be applied to immobilize a femur fracture for a child. The nurse reviews the forms of traction and the purposes for each before gathering equipment prior to the child's arrival. Match the type of traction on the left with the type of injury or indication on the right. **All options must be used.**

Category: Mobility/immobility

(1) (E): Bryant's traction is used in children younger than age 2 to reduce femur fractures or stabilize hips.

(2) (D): Russell's traction may reduce fractures of the hip or femur.

(3) (B): 90-degree traction is used on the femur if skin traction isn't suitable.

(4) (C): Buck's traction is used to temporarily immobilize a fractured leg.

(5) (A): Cervical traction is used to stabilize a spinal fracture or muscle spasm.

25. The Answer is 3

It is important to evaluate pain in the neonate. Look at the chart in the exhibit below. What would the pain score be for an infant with a high-pitched cry, O_2 saturation of 96%, a grimace, and frequent periods of wakefulness?

	Score		
	0	1	2
Crying	No	High pitched	Inconsolable
Requires O_2	No	< 30%	> 30%
Expression	None	Grimace	Grimace/grunt
Sleepless	No	Wakes frequently	Always awake

Category: Rest and sleep

(1) A score of 0 is incorrect, because the infant has a grimace (1), periods of wakefulness (1), and a high-pitched cry (1).

(2) A score of 2 is incorrect, because the infant has a grimace (1), periods of wakefulness (1), and a high-pitched cry (1).

(3) CORRECT: This is the closest evaluation with the information given. The infant has a high-pitched cry (1), an adequate O_2 saturation (0), a grimace (1), and periods of wakefulness (1).

(4) Enough information is provided to answer the question.

CHAPTER 9

PHYSIOLOGICAL INTEGRITY: PHARMACOLOGICAL AND PARENTERAL THERAPIES

Pharmacological and parenteral therapies involve the provision of care related to the administration of all forms of medication as well as parenteral/IV therapy. On the NCLEX-RN® exam, you can expect 15 percent of the questions to relate to the Pharmacological and Parenteral Therapies subcategory. Exam content includes, but is not limited to, the following areas:

- Adverse effects/contraindications/side effects/interactions
- Blood and blood products
- Central venous access devices
- Dosage calculation
- Expected actions/outcomes
- Medication administration
- Parenteral/intravenous therapies
- Pharmacological pain management
- Total parenteral nutrition

Now let's review some of the most important concepts related to these subtopics.

ADVERSE EFFECTS/CONTRAINDICATIONS/SIDE EFFECTS/ INTERACTIONS

It is important to assess clients for actual and potential side effects and adverse effects of medications, including prescription, over-the-counter, and herbal medications. This requires knowledge of all medications a client is taking, and information on preexisting conditions.

Provide clients with information on common side effects and how to manage them. This includes letting clients know when to call or notify their primary health care provider regarding side effects. Also know when to contact the client's primary health care provider regarding side effects of medication or parenteral therapy for clients who are hospitalized.

Be able to identify signs and symptoms of an allergic reaction, which include the following:

- **Skin:** Redness, itching, swelling, blistering, weeping, crusting, rash, eruptions, or hives (itchy bumps or welts)
- **Lungs:** Wheezing, tightness, cough, or shortness of breath
- **Head:** Swelling of the face, eyelids, lips, tongue, or throat; headache
- **Nose:** Stuffy nose, runny nose (clear, thin discharge), or sneezing
- **Eyes:** Red (bloodshot), itchy, swollen, or watery
- **Stomach:** Pain, nausea, vomiting, diarrhea, or bloody diarrhea

In addition, you must know which procedures are appropriate for counteracting adverse effects due to medication or parenteral therapy, and how to implement them. And of course, document client response to actions taken to counteract adverse effects.

BLOOD AND BLOOD PRODUCTS

One of the most important aspects of dealing with blood products is the correct identification of clients to ensure the right products are used. Identify the client according to facility/agency policy prior to administration of red blood cells/blood products. The steps involved include reviewing the prescription for administration, ensuring the blood is the correct type, ensuring the identity of the client, checking that crossmatching is complete, and ensuring client consent.

Before administering any blood products, check the client for appropriate venous access for product administration, select the correct needle gauge, and check the integrity of the access site. Understand when it is appropriate for a client to be an autologous donor (i.e., use the client's own blood), and the procedures for autologous blood donation:

- Four to six weeks prior to surgery
- Every three days if hemoglobin levels are satisfactory
- Good for rare blood types, transfusion reactions, prevention of blood-borne disease transmission
- Not good if client has an acute infection, a low hemoglobin count, or cardiovascular disease

Know the different blood types (ABO and Rh blood group systems) and compatibilities based on blood type, Rh factors, antibody screening, and crossmatching. Be familiar with the procedures employed after blood is drawn for typing, including the use of special client identification bracelets, and how to match the bracelets with the unique blood donor number on a sample or identification tag on any unit of blood the client receives.

It is also important to know the various blood components and what they are used for:

- **Whole blood:** Not normally used; mainly situations of major hemorrhage
- **Red blood cells (RBCs):** Anemia, blood loss
- **Fresh frozen plasma (FFP):** Coagulation deficiency
- **Platelets:** Thrombocytopenia
- **Albumin:** Shock, blood loss, low protein levels due to surgery or liver failure
- **Cryoprecipitate:** Blood loss or immediately prior to an invasive procedure in clients with significant hypofibrinogenemia

To administer blood products safely, and evaluate client response to administered products, follow the procedure detailed below:

1. Verify client consent.
2. Check client's baseline vital signs.
3. Check physician's order.
4. Identify a stable vein, and then choose a needle with the proper gauge.
5. Set up equipment and start IV.
6. Obtain correct component from blood bank.
7. Verify client identification and related information (use second nurse to double-check).
8. Hang blood.
9. Begin transfusion at a slow rate (2 mL per minute).
10. Monitor client vital signs after the first 15 minutes and thereafter in accordance with facility policy.
11. After 15 minutes, increase rate of infusion.
12. Monitor client vital signs and lung sounds for one hour after transfusion is complete.
13. Document all activities in the client's medical record.

It is important to know how to respond to common complications from blood transfusions, including transfusion reactions (allergic, febrile, or hemolytic), circulatory overload, blood-borne infections, electrolyte imbalance, and iron overload. If complications occur, they must be documented in the client's medical record.

CENTRAL VENOUS ACCESS DEVICES

Provide information to clients regarding reasons for and care of central venous access devices (CVADs). Types of CVADs include the following:

- **Tunneled catheter:** A tunneled catheter is placed in a central vein, tunneled under the skin, and then brought out through the skin. Examples include Hickman and Broviac.
- **Implanted port:** A port is inserted under subcutaneous tissue and attached to a catheter, which is threaded into the superior vena cava. Examples include Mediport and Port-a-Cath.
- **Peripherally inserted central catheter (PICC):** PICCs are inserted into a basilic or cephalic vein just above or below the antecubital space of the client's right arm by a doctor or specially trained IV therapy nurse. The catheter terminates in the superior vena cava. PICCs often remain in place for long periods of time.

Know how to access an implanted CVAD to provide medication and/or nutrition for a client, as well as how to care for a client with a CVAD. This includes:

- Maintaining strict sterile procedures to minimize risk of infection
- Flushing line periodically with normal saline solution
- Checking port placement
- Changing dressing

DOSAGE CALCULATION

Medications are prescribed in specific amounts or weights per volume for liquids. You should be able to perform the calculations needed for proper medication administration. The common formulas for calculating dosages include the following:

- Ratio and proportion
- "Desired over have"
- Dimensional analysis

Be aware of rounding rules when calculating dosages, as well.

Dosages are calculated using body weight in kilograms, so you convert between pounds and kilograms. Most often, you multiply the body weight by the dosage order per kilogram. You can also calculate volume using standard pharmaceutical math calculations. To calculate single dosages, divide the total daily dose by the number of doses per day. You can also use a nomogram (a type of graph) to calculate dosages based on body surface area.

In addition to dosage calculation for medications for adults, it is important to know the differences between adult and pediatric dosages and how to calculate pediatric dosages. It's also important to know how to help children swallow pills and how to give medications to infants.

Oral Medications

When tablets are scored, they may be broken and given as partial doses. Do not break or crush extended release tablets. Abbreviations to know include the following:

- **CR:** Controlled release
- **CRT:** Controlled release tablet
- **LA:** Long acting
- **SA:** Sustained action
- **SR:** Sustained release
- **TR:** Timed release
- **XL:** Extended length
- **XR:** Extended release

Enteral Medications

Enteral medications are administered through a tube. Know the correct tube placement for the following types of tubes:

- Nasogastric (through the nose and into the stomach)
- Nasointestinal (through the nose, past the stomach, and into the small intestine)
- Percutaneous (through the skin directly into the stomach)

It is important to know how to care for a client receiving enteral medication. Flush the tube with 30 mL water before administering the medication. Use a solution/elixir form of medication, when available.

Injectable Medications

The following steps comprise the procedure for injecting medications:

1. Choose a needle based on volume and type of medication, destination site, client size, and viscosity of medication.
2. Maintain sterility when assembling the syringe and needle.
3. Withdraw medication from the vial/ampule.
4. Use anatomical landmarks (intramuscular, intravenous, and/or subcutaneous).
5. Wash hands and put on gloves.
6. Cleanse area with alcohol swabs and wait for it to dry.
7. Inject medication.

8. Discard the syringe and needle into a sharps container.

9. Remove gloves.

10. Wash hands.

Topical Medications

Understand how to administer the following types of topical medications:

- Skin
- Nasal
- Optical
- Otic (ear)
- Vaginal
- Rectal

Inhaled Medications

You should be able to explain how to use a metered-dose inhaled (MDI) medication to your clients. A spacer is a device that attaches to the MDI to help deliver the medicine to the lungs instead of the mouth.

EXPECTED ACTIONS/OUTCOMES

You are expected to obtain information on prescribed medications for clients by reviewing the formulary and consulting the pharmacist, as needed. You must also understand the likely effects and outcomes for any oral, intradermal, subcutaneous, intramuscular, or topical medications prescribed for your client.

Evaluate and document a client's use of medications over time, including prescriptions, over-the-counter medications, and home remedies. This includes explaining effects and outcomes to clients and families.

MEDICATION ADMINISTRATION

It is important to understand the general principles of medication administration, including how medications are named (generic versus brand name or trade name). Use the six "rights" when administering client medications, as follows:

1. **Right client:** Identify the client in two ways, such as checking the client's armband and asking the client to state his or her name, if able. Do not use the room number as a method to identify the client.

2. **Right drug:** Know both the generic name and its brand equivalent; also double-check the medication order.

3. **Right dose:** Make sure the dose that is administered is a safe amount.

4. **Right route:** Check the medication order to verify the route of administration, such as oral, IV, or suppository.

5. **Right time:** Verify that the medication is being given at the proper time (with meal, a.m./ p.m., etc.)

6. **Right documentation:** Document details immediately after the medication is administered.

Review pertinent data prior to administration of medication. This includes vital signs, lab results, allergies, potential medication interactions, medical history, and current diagnosis.

Know the drug name, dosage, route, frequency, and special parameters for withholding doses or administering additional doses. Check each medical order for accuracy: ensure that it includes the date, time, and client's last name, and that it is signed by the prescribing physician. This is important because you are responsible if you administer a drug based on an incorrect order.

It is important to understand the basic concepts of pharmacology, including:

- **Pharmacokinetics:** How the body absorbs, distributes, and metabolizes medications
- **Absorption routes:** GI tract, respiratory tract, and skin
- **Distribution:** How a drug moves through the body from absorption site to action site
- **Metabolism:** Conversion of a drug by enzymes into a less-active, excretable substance
- **Excretion:** Elimination of drug and metabolites from the body

The basic principles of medication administration are:

- Make sure the medication order is accurate.
- Check for client allergies.
- Assess the client to be sure the medication makes sense.
- Check all other medications the client is taking.
- Calculate the proper dosage.
- Check the expiration date of the medication.
- Label all medications.

You are responsible not only for preparing and administering but also for documenting medications given by common routes (oral or topical), as well as by parenteral routes (IV, IM, or subcutaneous). This may include mixing medications from two vials when necessary, such as when administering a mixed dose of insulin.

You are expected to be able to adjust/titrate dosages of medication based on the assessment of physiologic parameters of each client. This includes giving insulin according to blood glucose levels and titrating medication to maintain a specific blood pressure.

Nurses must properly dispose of unused medications according to facility/agency policy. In addition, it is your responsibility to educate clients about medications, including their potential side effects, how to take them, and how to handle side effects and/or allergic reactions.

PARENTERAL/INTRAVENOUS THERAPIES

It is important to know the basics of intravenous therapy, including the indicators, types of fluids used (isotonic solutions, hypertonic solutions, and hypotonic solutions), and equipment (catheters and needles, infusion pumps, electronic delivery devices, regulators, controllers, mechanical infusion devices, and tubing). There are four types of infusion therapy: peripheral, central, continuous, and intermittent. Know when each should be used.

As with medication dosages, apply mathematic concepts when administering intravenous and parenteral therapy. To calculate an IV drip rate, use the following formula to calculate drops per minute:

(Total number of milliliters divided by total number of minutes) × drip factor = gtt/minute

You will be provided with the drip factor in the question stem on the NCLEX-RN® exam.

Know which veins to access for various therapies; you should be able to prepare clients for intravenous catheter insertion, insert and remove a peripheral intravenous line, and monitor the use of an infusion pump, whether it's intravenous or patient controlled analgesia (PCA). You should also be able to maintain an epidural infusion.

If a client needs intermittent parenteral fluid therapy for nutritional purposes, educate the client and evaluate the client's response. You should also be able to monitor and maintain infusion sites and track the rates of infusion to ensure they are correct.

PHARMACOLOGICAL PAIN MANAGEMENT

To determine client need for administration of a PRN pain medication, question the client about his or her level of pain using a pain rating scale from 1–10, or a visual scale using images of faces with different expressions. Be aware of nonverbal indicators, such as facial expressions or sounds.

Know how to provide pain management appropriate for client age and different diagnoses (pregnant women, children, and older adults).

Document pain mediation administration according to facility/agency policy, and comply with regulations governing controlled substances (such as counting narcotics and wasting narcotics), and evaluate and document client use and response to pain medications.

Total Parenteral Nutrition

Total parenteral nutrition (TPN) is nutrition provided intravenously for clients who are unable to tolerate oral or enteral feedings. It may be used in both home and hospital environments.

Know how to administer, maintain, and discontinue TPN. This includes knowing the ingredients of the solution: amino acids, dextrose for carbohydrates, vitamins and minerals, trace elements, electrolytes, and water, and sometimes lipids, insulin, and heparin. You should also know the components of different solutions that need to be used depending on the client's nutritional needs and disease state. Clients who may need TPN are those with GI tract issues, who are recovering from GI surgery, or who have experienced trauma. Clients with high nutritional needs may also require TPN.

Access sites for TPN include peripheral lines through veins (for supplements only, not when a client needs nutrition replacement; these should only be used for two weeks or less) and central lines, which are more typical (often a PICC line).

Be aware of the following as you manage a client receiving TPN:

- There is a risk of pneumothorax during catheter insertion for a PICC line.
- Examine the IV insertion site during each shift for signs of infection.
- Do not use the IV line for anything other than TPN.
- Inspect the bag of solution for particles prior to hanging.
- Monitor the client's blood glucose level.
- Measure daily weight to determine/adjust fluid balance.
- Monitor other lab results, such as electrolytes, protein, prealbumin/albumin, creatinine, lymphocytic count, and liver function.

Know the rates of administration of TPN, how to monitor clients for adverse effects, and how to taper down use of TPN. (Do not discontinue TPN abruptly.) Possible complications include fluid overload, air embolism, infection/sepsis, hyperglycemia, and hypoglycemia.

Finally, you should be able to evaluate outcomes of TPN, including satisfactory weight gain and fluids, and electrolytes within normal limits.

CHAPTER QUIZ

1. The nurse is conducting a home visit with a client who has a history of angina. Which of the following *BEST* demonstrates that further teaching about nitroglycerin therapy is required?

   1. "I take a tablet about 10 minutes before I walk up the stairs."
   2. "I take no more than 3 doses in a 15-minute period of time."
   3. "I keep the tablets in a glass dish on the windowsill so they are readily available."
   4. "I will call my doctor immediately if I experience blurred vision."

2. The nurse assesses the peripheral IV site of a client receiving a doxorubicin (Adriamycin) infusion and suspects extravasation. After stopping the infusion and disconnecting the IV tubing, which of the following should the nurse do next?

   1. Apply a hot compress to the IV site.
   2. Apply a cold compress to the IV site.
   3. Elevate the affected extremity.
   4. Attempt to aspirate the residual drug.

3. The nurse is preparing to discharge a 72-year-old man on warfarin (Coumadin) therapy for a pulmonary embolism. The nurse's discharge teaching should include which of the following instructions?

   1. Follow a healthy diet by increasing ingestion of green, leafy vegetables.
   2. Take herbal remedies to manage cold symptoms.
   3. Avoid alcohol due to enhanced anticoagulant effect.
   4. Take Coumadin only on an empty stomach.

4. A 75-year-old woman has been prescribed amitriptyline hydrochloride (Elavil) to manage neuropathic pain associated with diabetic neuropathy. She reports to the nurse that her pain level has decreased from a 7 to a 3 on a scale of 1–10. However, she is experiencing severe xerostomia. Which of the following strategies should the nurse choose to help relieve this symptom?

   1. Increase caffeine intake.
   2. Decrease fluid intake.
   3. Increase dietary sodium.
   4. Chew sugar-free gum.

5. Prior to administering digoxin (Lanoxin) 0.125 mg PO to a client with chronic heart failure, the nurse determines that the apical pulse is 56. Which of the following should the nurse do *FIRST*?

   1. Administer the drug and recheck the pulse in one hour.
   2. Withhold the drug and notify the physician.
   3. Obtain an EKG.
   4. Send a blood sample to the laboratory for a digoxin level.

6. A 65-year-old man with metastatic colon cancer has been prescribed hydromorphone (Dilaudid) PO/PRN to help manage his pain. The nurse knows that the rectal route of administration is contraindicated when which of the following is present?

   1. Nausea and vomiting
   2. Difficulty swallowing
   3. Neutropenia
   4. Fever

7. A client is admitted for gastrointestinal bleeding. He has a platelet count of 15,000/mm and platelets have been ordered from the blood bank. Which of the following does the nurse know are required for platelet transfusions? **Select all that apply.**

   1. ABO compatibility
   2. Rh compatibility
   3. Crossmatching
   4. A specialized platelet filter

8. A client's red blood cell transfusion was discontinued due to an acute hemolytic transfusion reaction. Which of the following strategies should the nurse use to *BEST* minimize the risk of such a reaction?

   1. The nurse ensures the client's temperature does not increase more than 1.8° F during the transfusion.
   2. The nurse verifies all client-identifying information according to hospital protocol prior to hanging the unit of blood.
   3. The nurse administers meperidine (Demerol) for severe rigors.
   4. The nurse administers acetaminophen (Tylenol) prior to the transfusion.

9. A client is receiving a blood transfusion. The nurse observes that the client is experiencing diarrhea, abdominal pain, and chills. Which of the following actions should the nurse take *FIRST*?

   1. Assist the client to the bathroom.
   2. Stop the transfusion.
   3. Administer meperidine (Demerol).
   4. Get a warming blanket.

10. The nurse aspirates a central venous catheter prior to drug administration but is not able to verify blood return. The nurse does not feel resistance when flushing or see any fluid leakage, swelling, or redness around the catheter site. Which of the following does the nurse know are appropriate steps? **Select all that apply.**

    1. Flush the catheter with saline, using a 10-mL syringe and a push-pull technique.
    2. Request that the client cough and reattempt aspiration.
    3. Administer IV medication and observe for signs and symptoms of catheter malfunction.
    4. Follow institutional protocol to initiate a declotting protocol.

11. A client is admitted for pulmonary embolism and is receiving heparin 1,500 units/hour IV. In case of a serious bleeding reaction, the nurse has which of the following drugs readily available?

    1. Vitamin K
    2. Protamine sulfate
    3. Promethazine hydrochloride
    4. Protamine

12. A client with known heparin-induced thrombocytopenia (HIT) is undergoing chemotherapy and is having a central venous access device placed. Which of the following types of central venous access device does the nurse know *BEST* minimizes the risk of HIT-related complication?

    1. Hickman
    2. Broviac
    3. Groshong
    4. Port

13. A client has been instructed by his physician to increase his warfarin sodium (Coumadin) dose from 5 mg to 7.5 mg. He only has 5-mg tablets available. How many tablets should the nurse instruct him to take?

    1. 0.5
    2. 1
    3. 1.5
    4. 2

14. The nurse is preparing to set up an intravenous infusion of normal saline 1,000 mL over a 6-hour period. The tubing drop factor is 10 gtt/mL. Which of the following rates of infusion should the nurse choose?

    1. 12 gtt/min
    2. 28 gtt/min
    3. 33 gtt/min
    4. 36 gtt/min

15. A man weighs 165 lb. and is being treated for shock. The nurse is preparing a dopamine hydrochloride (Dopamine) infusion to start at 5 mcg/kg/min. The nurse has prepared the following to infuse: dopamine 400 mg in 250 mL D_5W. Which of the following rates of infusion should the nurse choose?

    1. 14 mL/hr
    2. 16 mL/hr
    3. 22.5 mL/hr
    4. 37.5 mL/hr

16. A 45-year-old woman with breast cancer is receiving doxorubicin (Adriamycin) 60 mg/m^2 as part of her cancer therapy. She is 5 ft. 6 in. tall and weighs 145 lb. Her body surface area is 1.75 m^2. What is the correct dose that the nurse should administer? Record your answer using one decimal place.

    _____ mg

17. A client is admitted with sickle-cell anemia and voices concerns about becoming addicted to pain medicine. The nurse explains the difference between physical dependence, tolerance, and addiction. Which of the following symptoms or behaviors does the nurse know is *BEST* associated with addiction?

    1. Withdrawal symptoms when the drug is abruptly stopped
    2. Withdrawal symptoms when the drug dose is reduced
    3. Habitual and compulsive use of a drug
    4. A state of adaptation

18. A client is admitted with severe back pain and is requesting pain medication. During her assessment, the nurse notes the client has been taking acetaminophen (Tylenol) 650 mg every 4 hours at home with minimal relief. Based on this information, which of the following PRN-ordered drug(s) should the nurse consider administering?

    1. Hydrocodone and acetaminophen (Vicodin)
    2. Acetaminophen (Tylenol)
    3. Ibuprofen (Motrin)
    4. Acetaminophen and oxycodone (Percocet)

19. A 14-year-old boy has been prescribed amphetamine and dextroamphetamine (Adderall) for attention-deficit/hyperactivity disorder (ADHD). The nurse explains that the client should be alert for which of the following adverse drug effects?

    1. Weight gain
    2. Depression
    3. Somnolence
    4. Bradycardia

20. The nurse is administering a drug by Z-track and must follow the proper technique. Place the following steps in the appropriate order. **All options must be used.**

    1. Withdraw the needle.
    2. Administer the drug intramuscularly (IM) in the dorsogluteal site.
    3. Release the skin.
    4. Displace the skin lateral to the injection site.

21. A client admitted with chronic heart failure is taking furosemide (Lasix). Which of the following statements, if made by the client, *BEST* demonstrates to the nurse that the client understands the side effects associated with this drug?

    1. "My blood pressure might be abnormally high."
    2. "I should include more foods such as bananas, apricots, and legumes in my diet."
    3. "I should take the drug before bedtime."
    4. "I should not take the pill with food."

22. The nurse is administering vancomycin 1 g every 12 hours for a soft tissue infection. The nurse reminds the client to report symptoms associated with one of the serious side effects of the drug, ototoxicity. Which of the following statements by the client indicates to the nurse that the client may be experiencing this adverse reaction?

    1. "I hear ringing in my ear."
    2. "The IV is burning."
    3. "My skin is very itchy."
    4. "I have a bad taste in my mouth."

23. A client is leaving the clinic with a new prescription for lisinopril (Zestril). Which of the following suggestions can the nurse make to minimize one of the major effects of lisinopril?

    1. Eat fruits and vegetables high in iron.
    2. Rise slowly from a lying to a sitting position.
    3. Increase fluid intake.
    4. Avoid aspirin-containing drugs.

24. The nurse is administering a doxorubicin (Adriamycin) IV push to a client with breast cancer. Which of the following should the nurse explain is to be expected during therapy with this drug?

    1. Burning at the IV site during administration
    2. Red-colored urine
    3. Permanent alopecia
    4. Teeth discoloration

25. A 60-year-old woman with anorexia nervosa is having an indwelling central venous access device placed in preparation for total parenteral nutrition (TPN) administration. Which of the following factors does the nurse know accounts for the client's increased risk of thrombophlebitis with a peripheral intravenous line? **Select all that apply.**

    1. Age
    2. Hypertonicity of the TPN
    3. Hypotonicity of the TPN
    4. Poor peripheral venous access

CHAPTER QUIZ ANSWERS AND EXPLANATIONS

1. The Answer is 3

The nurse is conducting a home visit with a client who has a history of angina. Which of the following *BEST* demonstrates that further teaching about nitroglycerin therapy is required?

Category: Adverse effects/contraindications/side effects/interactions

(1) Taking a nitroglycerin tablet prior to exertion is an appropriate way to help prevent angina-related symptoms induced by activity.

(2) Taking no more than 3 doses in a 15-minute period of time is appropriate nitroglycerin dosing instructions.

(3) CORRECT: Nitroglycerin tablets may lose effectiveness if not protected from light. Therefore, they should be stored in dark containers.

(4) Blurred vision is a significant side effect of nitroglycerin therapy that should be immediately reported to the physician.

2. The Answer is 4

The nurse assesses the peripheral IV site of a client receiving a doxorubicin (Adriamycin) infusion and suspects extravasation. After stopping the infusion and disconnecting the IV tubing, which of the following should the nurse do next?

Category: Adverse effects/contraindications/side effects/interactions

(1) Hot compresses should not be applied in an Adriamycin-associated extravasation.

(2) Although a cold compress is recommended in an Adriamycin-associated extravasation, it should not be applied until residual drug removal has been attempted.

(3) Although elevating the arm for 48 hours is recommended, this should not be done until after the residual drug has been removed.

(4) CORRECT: The first step the nurse should take is to attempt to remove any residual drug using a 1–3 mL syringe.

3. The Answer is 3

The nurse is preparing to discharge a 72-year-old man on warfarin (Coumadin) therapy for a pulmonary embolism. The nurse's discharge teaching should include which of the following instructions?

Category: Adverse effects/contraindications/side effects/interactions

(1) The intake of foods containing vitamin K should not be altered from baseline.

(2) Herbal medications may interfere with the effectiveness of Coumadin.

(3) CORRECT: Alcohol can increase the anticoagulant effect of Coumadin and should be avoided.

(4) Coumadin can be taken without regard to food intake, although gastrointestinal upset may be diminished if taken with food.

4. The Answer is 4

A 75-year-old woman has been prescribed amitriptyline hydrochloride (Elavil) to manage neuropathic pain associated with diabetic neuropathy. She reports to the nurse that her pain level has decreased from a 7 to a 3 on a scale of 1–10. However, she is experiencing severe xerostomia. Which of the following strategies should the nurse choose to help relieve this symptom?

Category: Adverse effects/contraindications/side effects/interactions

(1) Increasing caffeine intake will not relieve xerostomia.

(2) Decreasing fluid intake will not relieve xerostomia.

(3) Increasing dietary sodium will not relieve xerostomia.

(4) CORRECT: Strategies to reduce xerostomia (dry mouth) include increasing fluid intake and chewing sugar-free gum.

5. The Answer is 2

Prior to administering digoxin (Lanoxin) 0.125 mg PO to a client with chronic heart failure, the nurse determines that the apical pulse is 56. Which of the following should the nurse do *FIRST*?

Category: Adverse effects/contraindications/side effects/interactions

(1) Unless the physician's order specifies otherwise, when the client's apical pulse drops below 60, the nurse should hold the dose and notify the physician.

(2) CORRECT: Unless the physician's order specifies otherwise, when the client's apical pulse drops below 60, the nurse should hold the dose and notify the physician.

(3) Although an EKG may be indicated, it is not generally the first course of action.

(4) Although obtaining a digoxin level may be indicated, it is not generally the first course of action.

6. The Answer is 3

A 65-year-old man with metastatic colon cancer has been prescribed hydromorphone (Dilaudid) PO/PRN to help manage his pain. The nurse knows that the rectal route of administration is contraindicated when which of the following is present?

Category: Adverse effects/contraindications/side effects/interactions

(1) The rectal route of administration may be preferred when a client has nausea and vomiting.

(2) The rectal route of administration may be preferred when a client has difficulty swallowing.

(3) CORRECT: The rectal route of administration should NOT be used in clients who have anal or rectal lesions, mucositis, thrombocytopenia, or neutropenia.

(4) The rectal route of administration may also be appropriate for a client who has a fever.

7. The Answer is 1, 2, and 4

A client is admitted for gastrointestinal bleeding. He has a platelet count of 15,000/mm and platelets have been ordered from the blood bank. Which of the following does the nurse know are required for platelet transfusions? **Select all that apply.**

Category: Blood and blood products

(1) CORRECT: The donor and recipient should be ABO-compatible.

(2) CORRECT: The donor and recipient should be Rh-compatible.

(3) Crossmatching is not required for platelet transfusions.

(4) CORRECT: Platelets are administered using specialized platelet filters.

8. The Answer is 2

A client's red blood cell transfusion was discontinued due to an acute hemolytic transfusion reaction. Which of the following strategies should the nurse use to *BEST* minimize the risk of such a reaction?

Category: Blood and blood products

(1) Monitoring the client's temperature may help to promptly alert the nurse to a reaction but does not prevent it from occurring.

(2) CORRECT: The most common cause of an acute hemolytic transfusion reaction is the administration of ABO-incompatible blood. By verifying client-identifying information according to hospital policy, the nurse can minimize the risk of a client being transfused with ABO-incompatible blood.

(3) Administering Demerol may alleviate symptoms associated with a reaction but does not prevent it from developing.

(4) Administering Tylenol may be indicated to prevent hypersensitivity reactions, but this action will not minimize the risk of an acute hemolytic transfusion reaction from taking place.

9. The Answer is 2

A client is receiving a blood transfusion. The nurse observes that the client is experiencing diarrhea, abdominal pain, and chills. Which of the following actions should the nurse take *FIRST*?

Category: Blood and blood products

(1) Assisting the client to the bathroom may be an appropriate comfort measure but should not be performed first.

(2) CORRECT: Signs and symptoms of a transfusion reaction may include chills, diarrhea, fever, hives, pruritus, flushing, and abdominal or back pain. The nurse's first action should be to stop the transfusion.

(3) Demerol may alleviate rigors, which the client was not experiencing.

(4) Getting a warming blanket may be an appropriate comfort measure but should not be performed first.

10. The Answer is 1, 2, and 4

The nurse aspirates a central venous catheter prior to drug administration but is not able to verify blood return. The nurse does not feel resistance when flushing or see any fluid leakage, swelling, or redness around the catheter site. Which of the following does the nurse know are appropriate steps? **Select all that apply.**

Category: Central venous access devices

(1) CORRECT: Flushing the catheter with saline using a 10-mL syringe and a push-pull technique are appropriate steps to try to verify blood return in a central venous catheter.

(2) CORRECT: Instructing the client to cough before reattempting aspiration is an appropriate step to try to verify blood return in a central venous catheter.

(3) Administering IV medication (particularly cytotoxic medications) and fluids should not be performed until other steps are taken to verify proper placement of the catheter by assessing for patency and blood return.

(4) CORRECT: Initiating a declotting protocol per policy is an appropriate step to try to verify blood return in a central venous catheter.

11. The Answer is 2

A client is admitted for pulmonary embolism and is receiving heparin 1,500 units/hour IV. In case of a serious bleeding reaction, the nurse has which of the following drugs readily available?

Category: Central venous access devices

(1) Vitamin K is not an antidote for heparin and does not reverse the effects of the drug.

(2) CORRECT: The antidote for heparin is protamine sulfate.

(3) Promethazine hydrochloride is not an antidote for heparin and does not reverse the effects of the drug.

(4) Protamine is not an antidote for heparin and does not reverse the effects of the drug.

12. The Answer is 3

A client with known heparin-induced thrombocytopenia (HIT) is undergoing chemotherapy and is having a central venous access device placed. Which of the following types of central venous access device does the nurse know *BEST* minimizes the risk of HIT-related complication?

Category: Central venous access devices

(1) A Hickman does not contain valves and is routinely flushed with heparin.

(2) A Broviac does not contain valves and is routinely flushed with heparin.

(3) CORRECT: A Groshong is a valved catheter that does not require heparin flushing.

(4) A port does not contain valves and is routinely flushed with heparin.

13. The Answer is 3

A client has been instructed by his physician to increase his warfarin sodium (Coumadin) dose from 5 mg to 7.5 mg. He only has 5-mg tablets available. How many tablets should the nurse instruct him to take?

Category: Dose calculation

(1) Taking half a tablet would only provide 2.5 mg of warfarin sodium.

(2) Taking one tablet would only provide 5 mg of warfarin sodium.

(3) CORRECT: Taking one and a half tablets containing 5 mg of warfarin sodium (Coumadin) each will achieve a total dose of 7.5 mg.

(4) Taking two tablets would provide 10 mg of warfarin sodium.

14. The Answer is 2

The nurse is preparing to set up an intravenous infusion of normal saline 1,000 mL over a 6-hour period. The tubing drop factor is 10 gtt/mL. Which of the following rates of infusion should the nurse choose?

Category: Dose calculation

(1) 12 gtt/min is not the correct rate of infusion.

(2) CORRECT: 28 gtt/min is the correct rate of infusion, arrived at as follows: 1,000 mL/6 hours × 10 gtt/mL/60 min/hour = 27.8 or 28 gtt/min.

(3) 33 gtt/min is not the correct rate of infusion.

(4) 36 gtt/min is not the correct of infusion.

15. The Answer is 1

A man weighs 165 lb. and is being treated for shock. The nurse is preparing a dopamine hydrochloride (Dopamine) infusion to start at 5 mcg/kg/min. The nurse has prepared the following to infuse: dopamine 400 mg in 250 mL D_5W. Which of the following rates of infusion should the nurse choose?

Category: Dose calculation

(1) CORRECT: The correct rate of infusion is 14 mL/hour, arrived at as follows: First convert 165 lb. to kg by dividing by 2.2 (75 kg). Then, convert 400 mg/250 mL to mcg/mL by dividing 400 mg/250 mL and multiplying the result (1.6 mg/mL) by 1,000 (1,600 mcg/m). Next, multiply the weight (75 kg) by the ordered dose (5 mcg/kg/min), and multiply the result (375 mcg/min) by 60. This equals 22,500 mcg/hr. Calculate mL/hr by dividing 22,500 mcg/hr by 1,600 mcg/mL. The appropriate rate is 14 mL/hr.

(2) A rate of infusion of 16 mL/hour is not correct.

(3) A rate of infusion of 22.5 mL/hour is not correct.

(4) A rate of infusion of 37.5 mL/hour is not correct.

16. The Answer is 105 mg

A 45-year-old woman with breast cancer is receiving doxorubicin (Adriamycin) 60 mg/m² as part of her cancer therapy. She is 5 ft. 6 in. tall and weighs 145 lb. Her body surface area is 1.75 m². What is the correct dose that the nurse should administer? Record your answer using one decimal place.

Category: Dose calculation

Answer: 60 mg/m² × 1.75 m² = 105 mg

17. The Answer is 3

A client is admitted with sickle-cell anemia and voices concerns about becoming addicted to pain medicine. The nurse explains the difference between physical dependence, tolerance, and addiction. Which of the following symptoms or behaviors does the nurse know is *BEST* associated with addiction?

Category: Pharmacological pain management

(1) Withdrawal symptoms when the drug is abruptly stopped are associated with physical dependence on a particular drug, not addiction.

(2) Withdrawal symptoms when the drug dose is reduced are associated with physical dependence on a particular drug, not addiction.

(3) CORRECT: Addiction is characterized by compulsive use of a drug for reasons other than therapeutic benefit.

(4) A state of adaptation is associated with tolerance to a particular drug, not addiction.

18. The Answer is 3

A client is admitted with severe back pain and is requesting pain medication. During her assessment, the nurse notes the client has been taking acetaminophen (Tylenol) 650 mg every 4 hours at home with minimal relief. Based on this information, which of the following PRN-ordered drug(s) should the nurse consider administering?

Category: Pharmacological pain management

(1) Vicodin contains acetaminophen. The maximum recommended dose of acetaminophen in a 24-hour period is 4 g.

(2) Tylenol contains acetaminophen. The maximum recommended dose of acetaminophen in a 24-hour period is 4 g.

(3) CORRECT: Ibuprofen is the only pain relief medication listed that does not contain acetaminophen.

(4) Percocet contains acetaminophen. The maximum recommended dose of acetaminophen in a 24-hour period is 4 g.

19. The Answer is 2

A 14-year-old boy has been prescribed amphetamine and dextroamphetamine (Adderall) for attention-deficit/hyperactivity disorder (ADHD). The nurse explains that the client should be alert for which of the following adverse drug effects?

Category: Medication administration

(1) Adderall may be associated with weight loss, not weight gain.

(2) CORRECT: Adderall may be associated with depression.

(3) Adderall may be associated with agitation or restlessness, not somnolence.

(4) Adderall may be associated with tachycardia, not bradycardia.

20. The Answer is 4, 2, 1, 3

The nurse is administering a drug by Z-track and must follow the proper technique. Place the following steps in the appropriate order. **All options must be used.**

Category: Medication administration

(1) The third step in proper Z-track technique is to withdraw the needle.

(2) The second step in proper Z-track technique is to administer the drug IM.

(3) The last step in proper Z-track technique is the release the skin.

(4) The first step in proper Z-track technique is to displace the skin lateral to the injection site.

21. The Answer is 2

A client admitted with chronic heart failure is taking furosemide (Lasix). Which of the following statements, if made by the client, *BEST* demonstrates to

the nurse that the client understands the side effects associated with this drug?

Category: Medication administration

(1) Lasix may be associated with hypotension.

(2) CORRECT: Lasix may decrease potassium. Eating foods rich in potassium is advised.

(3) Lasix may be associated with nocturia.

(4) Lasix does not have to be taken with food.

22. The Answer is 1

The nurse is administering vancomycin 1 g every 12 hours for a soft tissue infection. The nurse reminds the client to report symptoms associated with one of the serious side effects of the drug, ototoxicity. Which of the following statements by the client indicates to the nurse that the client may be experiencing this adverse reaction?

Category: Medication administration

(1) CORRECT: Tinnitus may indicate that ototoxicity is developing.

(2) A feeling that the IV is burning is not related to the development of ototoxicity.

(3) Itchiness of the skin is not related to the development of ototoxicity.

(4) The sensation of a bad taste in the mouth is not related to the development of ototoxicity.

23. The Answer is 2

A client is leaving the clinic with a new prescription for lisinopril (Zestril). Which of the following suggestions can the nurse make to minimize one of the major effects of lisinopril?

Category: Expected actions/outcomes

(1) Eating fruits and vegetables high in iron will not minimize the side effects of lisinopril.

(2) CORRECT: The hypotensive effect of lisinopril may be reduced by rising slowly from a lying to a sitting position.

(3) Increasing fluid intake will not minimize the side effects of lisinopril.

(4) Avoiding aspirin-containing drugs will not minimize the side effects of lisinopril.

24. The Answer is 2

The nurse is administering a doxorubicin (Adriamycin) IV push to a client with breast cancer. Which of the following should the nurse explain is to be expected during therapy with this drug?

Category: Expected actions/outcomes

(1) Burning at the IV site during administration is not a side effect of doxorubicin.

(2) CORRECT: A common side effect of doxorubicin is red-colored urine.

(3) Permanent alopecia is not a side effect of doxorubicin.

(4) Teeth discoloration is not a side effect of doxorubicin.

25. The Answer is 1, 2, and 4

A 60-year-old woman with anorexia nervosa is having an indwelling central venous access device placed in preparation for total parenteral nutrition (TPN) administration. Which of the following factors does the nurse know accounts for the client's increased risk of thrombophlebitis with a peripheral intravenous line? **Select all that apply.**

Category: Total parenteral nutrition

(1) CORRECT: The risk of thrombophlebitis is increased in individuals over the age of 60.

(2) CORRECT: The risk of thrombophlebitis is increased in individuals undergoing treatment with hypertonic fluids.

(3) The risk of thrombophlebitis is increased with hypertonic, not hypotonic, IV therapy.

(4) CORRECT: The risk of thrombophlebitis is increased in individuals with poor peripheral venous access.

CHAPTER 10

PHYSIOLOGICAL INTEGRITY: REDUCTION OF RISK POTENTIAL

Reduction of risk potential involves ways in which you can help to reduce the likelihood that clients will develop complications or health problems related to existing conditions, diagnostic tests, treatments, or other procedures.

On the NCLEX-RN® exam, you can expect 12 percent of the questions to relate to Reduction of Risk Potential. Exam content for this category includes, but is not limited to, the following areas:

- Changes/abnormalities in vital signs
- Diagnostic tests
- Laboratory values
- Potential for alterations in body systems
- Potential for complications of diagnostic tests/treatments/procedures
- Potential for complications from surgical procedures and health alterations
- System specific assessments
- Therapeutic procedures

Now let's review some of the most important concepts related to these subtopics.

CHANGES/ABNORMALITIES IN VITAL SIGNS

You must be able to assess client vital signs and intervene when those vital signs are abnormal. Abnormal vital signs include fever, hypertension, bradycardia, and tachypnea.

In order to properly assess vital signs and recognize abnormalities, apply your knowledge of the client's pathophysiology. Evaluate invasive monitoring data, such as pulmonary artery pressure and intracranial pressure.

DIAGNOSTIC TESTS

It is important to understand the general principles of specimen collection. Ideally, routine specimen collection should take place early morning before a client has any food or fluids. If fasting is required, it is usually for an 8–12-hour period prior to the test. Use standard precautions and aseptic techniques to protect yourself and your clients from infection.

Label specimens with the client's name, date, exact time of collection, and type of specimen. On the laboratory requisition slip, include the client's name, age, gender, room number, physician's name, possible diagnosis, tests requested, and any factors that might interfere with the test results. To avoid hemolysis, do not shake blood specimens unless instructed to do so.

All specimens should be sent to the lab promptly. Values, or test results, that fall within predetermined laboratory reference ranges are considered normal. Abnormal values are outside the reference range, and critical values are far enough outside of the reference range that they can cause immediate risk to the client. Critical values are called in to the nurse's station and should be acted on immediately. You may be responsible for informing the client's physician about these critical lab values.

You should understand the purpose of and preparation for a variety of diagnostic tests, such as the following:

- General
    - Biopsy
    - Computed tomography (CT) scan
    - Fluoroscopy
    - Magnetic resonance imaging (MRI)
    - Nuclear scan (radionuclide imaging or radioisotope scan)
    - Positron emission tomography (PET) scan
    - Ultrasonography
    - X-rays
- Respiratory
    - Bronchoscopy
    - Pulmonary function tests
    - Ventilation scan (pulmonary ventilation scan)
- Cardiovascular
    - Angiography (angiogram)
    - Cardiac catheterization
    - Echocardiography (echocardiogram)
    - Electrocardiography (electrocardiogram or ECG, EKG)
    - Holter monitoring

- Stress/exercise tests
- Venography (venogram), also called phlebography
- Renal/Urinary
  - Cystoscopy and cystography (cystogram)
  - Intravenous pyelography (IVP)
  - Retrograde pyelography (retrograde pyelogram)
- Neurological
  - Electroencephalography (electroencephalogram or EEG)
  - Myelography (myelogram)
- Musculoskeletal
  - Arthroscopy
  - Bone densitometry
- Gastrointestinal
  - Barium enema
  - Cholangiography
  - Cholecystography (oral)
  - Colonoscopy
  - Endoscopic retrograde cholangiopancreatography (ERCP)
  - Esophagogastroduodenoscopy
  - Gastric analysis
  - Gastrointestinal (GI) series
- Reproductive
  - Fetal nonstress test
  - Amniocentesis
  - Hysteroscopy
  - Mammography
  - Papanicolaou smear (Pap smear)
- Integumentary
  - Tuberculin skin test
  - Other skin tests (allergy)

Know how to compare client diagnostic findings with pretest results, and how to perform a variety of diagnostic tests, including:

- Oxygen saturation
- Glucose monitoring
- Testing for occult blood
- Gastric pH
- Urine specific gravity

- Arterial blood gases
- Serum electrolytes

You should also know how to perform an electrocardiogram. This test measures electrical activity of the heart and detects cardiac dysrhythmias and electrolyte imbalances. Electrodes are placed on the client's extremities and chest, and the electrical activity of the heart is recorded with each heartbeat. Cardiac waveforms are recorded in 12 leads. There are no food and fluid restrictions on clients getting an electrocardiogram, and no preconsent is needed for the test. The client should be asked to lie down and to expose arms and legs for lead placement. Men should be bare-chested, women given gowns. It is your responsibility to make note of any medications the client is taking that might impact the test results. The client should be told to relax his or her muscles and to breathe normally during the procedure, which is painless.

In addition to performing an electrocardiogram on an adult, you should know how to perform fetal heart monitoring using computer-assisted auditory assessment. This involves inserting a fetal scalp electrode through the client's cervix and attaching it to the epidermis of the fetus. You should also be able to monitor the results of additional maternal and fetal diagnostic tests, including nonstress tests, an amniocentesis, and an ultrasound.

LABORATORY VALUES

You must be familiar with a wide range of laboratory values, which include the following:

- Arterial blood gases, including pH, pO_2, pCO_2, SaO_2, and HCO_3
- Serum electrolytes
- Glucose studies, such as fasting blood glucose, random blood glucose, two-hour postprandial blood glucose, glucose tolerance test (GTT), and glycosylated hemoglobin (HgbA1C)
- Coagulation studies, such as prothrombin time (PT), international normalized ratio (INR), and activated partial thromboplastin time (APTT)
- Complete blood count (CBC), which includes hematocrit (Hct), hemoglobin (Hgb), RBC count and index, platelet count and mean volume, and white blood cell (WBC) count and differential
- Cardiovascular function studies, which include serum lipids, creatine kinase (CK) or creatine phosphokinase (CPK), lactic dehydrogenase (LDH), and troponins
- Thyroid function studies, such as thyroxine (T4), triiodothyronine (T3), and thyroid-stimulating hormone (TSH)
- Renal function studies, such as blood, urea, nitrogen (BUN) and serum creatinine
- Urinalysis, which includes the detection of nitrites and leukocyte esterase

- Liver function studies, such as alanine aminotransferase (ALT) or serum glutamic-pyruvic transaminase (SGPT), aspartate aminotransferase (AST) or serum glutamic-oxaloacetic transaminase (SGOT), bilirubin, and ammonia
- Pancreatic enzymes, such as amylase and lipase
- GI function studies, such as albumin, alkaline phosphatase, total protein, and uric acid
- Immune function studies, such as human immunodeficiency virus (HIV) test, CD4 T cell counts, CD4 to CD8 ratios, and viral load testing

You should know how to measure the amount of drug circulating in the client's bloodstream, usually before the scheduled daily dose of the drug. Trough levels are drawn when the dose is at its lowest, right before the next scheduled drug administration. Peak levels are drawn when the dose is at its highest (30 minutes after infusion). You must make sure drug levels remain within the proper therapeutic range. If you find an abnormal level, alert the prescribing physician immediately.

In addition to knowing laboratory values, and how to measure drug levels, you should be able to recognize deviations from normal values of the following:

- Albumin (blood)
- ALT (SGPT) (liver enzyme test)
- Ammonia
- AST (SGOT) (liver enzyme test)
- Bilirubin
- Bleeding time
- Calcium (total)
- Cholesterol (HDL and LDL)
- Creatinine
- Digoxin
- Erythrocyte sedimentation rate (ESR), to diagnose conditions associated with inflammation
- Lithium
- Magnesium
- Partial thromboplastin time (PTT) and APTT
- INR
- Phosphorous/phosphate
- Protein (total)
- PT (clotting)
- Urine (albumin, pH, WBC count, differential)

Know how to obtain blood specimens peripherally or through a central line. Also know how to obtain specimens other than blood for diagnostic testing. This includes procedures for getting specimens from wound cultures and stool and urine samples.

Monitor client laboratory values and provide clients with information about the purpose and procedures for prescribed laboratory tests.

POTENTIAL FOR ALTERATIONS IN BODY SYSTEMS

It is important to be able to compare current client data to baseline client data, particularly to evaluate symptoms of illness/disease. Identify client potential for aspiration (e.g., feeding tube, sedation, and swallowing difficulties), skin breakdown potential due to immobility, nutritional status or incontinence, and clients with an increased risk for insufficient vascular perfusion (such as clients with immobilized limbs, who are postsurgery, or who have diabetes). You should also be able to provide treatments and/or care in response.

Monitor client output for changes from baseline (nasogastric tube, emesis, stools, and urine) and educate clients about methods to prevent complications associated with activity level or diagnosed illness/disease (such as contractures, and foot care for client with diabetes mellitus).

POTENTIAL FOR COMPLICATIONS OF DIAGNOSTIC TESTS/ TREATMENTS/PROCEDURES

You must assess a client for complications or abnormal responses following a diagnostic test or procedure, such as monitoring the client for signs of bleeding. Know how to position clients to prevent complications following tests, treatments, and procedures, by, for example, elevating the head of the bed or immobilizing an extremity. When you see a complication, it is important to recommend a change in tests, procedures, and/or treatment prescriptions based on the client's response to the initial testing and treatment.

You should be able to insert an oral/nasogastric tube, and maintain tube patency. Be able to recognize potential circulatory complications (such as hemorrhage, embolus, and shock) and know how to intervene to manage them. Examples of measures you can take to manage, prevent, or lessen possible complications include restricting fluids or sodium, raising side rails of the client's bed, or implementing suicide precautions.

You also need to know how to provide care for clients undergoing electroconvulsive therapy. This includes monitoring the airway, assessing for side effects, and teaching the client about the procedure. You should be able to intervene to prevent aspiration, and to prevent potential neurological complications. Signs of neurological complications include foot drop, numbness, and tingling. Make sure to evaluate and document responses for all procedures and treatments.

POTENTIAL FOR COMPLICATIONS FROM SURGICAL PROCEDURES AND HEALTH ALTERATIONS

Apply your knowledge of pathophysiology to monitor for complications from surgical procedures and health alterations. For example, you should recognize signs of thrombocytopenia. You should also evaluate the client's response to postoperative interventions aimed at preventing complications, such as reducing the risk of aspiration and promoting venous return and mobility.

SYSTEM-SPECIFIC ASSESSMENTS

Assess clients for abnormal peripheral pulses and neurological status after a procedure or treatment. Neurological status can be assessed by checking level of consciousness and evaluating muscle strength and mobility. You should also be able to assess clients for peripheral edema, hypoglycemia, and hyperglycemia.

It is also important to identify factors that could result in delayed wound healing and to implement appropriate treatment in response, and/or to notify the primary care provider.

Perform a risk assessment for sensory impairment, falls, level of mobility, and skin integrity. Once initial assessments are complete, perform focused assessments and reassessments based on initial findings.

THERAPEUTIC PROCEDURES

When caring for clients undergoing therapeutic procedures, assess client response to recovery from local, regional, or general anesthesia.

Educate clients about treatments and procedures, and home management and care. The education may include preoperative and/or postoperative instructions to clients and families.

Monitor a client before, during, and after a procedure or surgery, and provide preoperative and intraoperative care (positioning, maintaining sterile field, and operative assessment). To prevent further injury while moving a client with a musculoskeletal condition, for example, use the log-rolling technique or an abduction pillow.

CHAPTER QUIZ

Refer to page in notebook

1. The nurse is reviewing the chart of an older adult male client after surgery for removal of the parathyroid glands. The client complains of difficulty swallowing and a feeling of "pins and needles." The nurse expects which of the following laboratory values to be abnormal?

    1. Calcium
    2. Lipase
    3. Potassium
    4. Sodium

2. The nurse is assessing a young-adult pregnant client with no allergies who has tested positive for gonorrhea. Which of the following medications should the nurse expect to be part of the treatment plan?

    1. Tetracycline (Declomycin)
    2. Ciprofloxacin (Cipro)
    3. Azithromycin (Zithromax)
    4. Ceftriaxone (Rocephin)

3. A client is one day post-op for abdominal surgery. The nurse is teaching the client techniques to reduce pain when he moves, coughs, or breathes deeply. Which of the following statements from the client indicates that the client understands the teaching?

    1. "I can start exercising my limbs as soon as you medicate me."
    2. "I will just lie here for a few days until the pain goes away."
    3. "I will use the side rail for support when I move or turn."
    4. "I will ask for pain medication only when absolutely necessary."

4. A 36-year-old primigravid client with a history of diabetes is admitted with preeclampsia. Which of the following actions should the nurse take *FIRST*?

    1. Administer low-dose aspirin as ordered.
    2. Ask the physician for an order for calcium supplements.
    3. Monitor the client's blood pressure.
    4. Prepare the client for delivery.

5. The nurse has just answered a call light for a client who is two days post-op for abdominal surgery. The client states, "I coughed and heard this pop." The nurse assesses the surgical site and observes dehiscence of the wound. Which of the following should the nurse do *FIRST*?

    1. Stay with the client and have a colleague notify the physician.
    2. Help the client to lie with his head slightly elevated and with knees bent.
    3. Apply warm, sterile normal saline soaks.
    4. Help the client to sit up, which will reduce the harmful effects of further coughing.

6. An elderly man is admitted to the hospital from the Emergency Department during the night shift. The nurse is assessing the client's cerebellar function. Which of the following questions should the nurse ask the client?

    1. "Who is the current president of the United States?"
    2. "Do you have trouble swallowing fluids or foods?"
    3. "Do you have any muscle pain?"
    4. "Do you have problems with balance?"

7. An older adult male client with a history of myasthenia gravis is admitted to the medical/surgical unit. Which of the following tests should the nurse expect to see ordered? **Select all that apply.**

   1. Tensilon test
   2. Nerve conduction studies
   3. Lumbar puncture
   4. EEG
   5. Electromyography

8. A middle-aged female client with a history of atherosclerosis is admitted with complaints of abdominal tenderness during deep palpation. The nurse notices a pulsating mass in the periumbilical area. Which of the following does the nurse suspect?

   1. Appendicitis
   2. Abdominal aortic aneurysm
   3. Acute cholecystitis
   4. Paralytic ileus

9. An older adult client with a history of blood clots is in the emergency room with suspected deep vein thrombosis (DVT) of the left leg. The nurse starts IV heparin as ordered. Which of the following is *LEAST* likely to be included in the care plan?

   1. Ambulation as tolerated
   2. Warm, moist soaks applied to the affected area
   3. Analgesics as ordered
   4. Anti-embolism stockings

10. The nurse is caring for a client with a history of chronic liver disease and cirrhosis of the liver. Lab values reveal rising ammonia levels. Which of the following treatments should the nurse question?

    1. Calorie intake 1,800–2,400 cal/day in the form of glucose or carbohydrates
    2. Protein 100 g/day
    3. An order to administer neomycin
    4. Potassium supplements

11. The laboratory values of an adult male client reveal the presence of hepatitis B surface antigens and hepatitis B antibodies. Which of the following laboratory results should the nurse also expect to see? **Select all that apply.**

    1. Elevated serum albumin
    2. Low serum globulin
    3. Elevated serum transaminate (ALT and AST)
    4. Prolonged prothrombin time (PT)
    5. Low urine bilirubin

12. The nurse is assessing a client with Addison's disease. The nurse expects to note which of the following?

    1. Anorexia
    2. Weight gain
    3. Yellow skin coloration
    4. A craving for sweets

13. A client is having a tonic-clonic seizure. Which of the following should the nurse do *FIRST?*

    1. Check the client's breathing.
    2. Remove objects from the client's surroundings.
    3. Place a tongue blade in the client's mouth.
    4. Restrain the client.

14. A client is recovering from a bout with chronic glomerulonephritis. The nurse prepares the client for discharge and home management. Which of the following statements indicates the client understands his condition and how to control it?

   1. "I should stop taking my blood pressure medication if I feel better or have side effects."
   2. "I will take my furosemide medications as ordered every morning."
   3. "I will keep my negative feelings to myself, so I don't get stressed."
   4. "I don't need a follow-up examination unless I'm feeling poorly."

15. A nursing home client is admitted to the hospital with a pressure ulcer involving full-thickness loss extending to the bone. The nurse documents the pressure ulcer as being at which of the following stages?

   1. Stage I
   2. Stage II
   3. Stage III
   4. Stage IV

16. A client with Raynaud's disease is experiencing an acute attack. The nurse should anticipate which of the following assessment findings?

   1. Involuntary muscle contractions and twitching
   2. Unilateral facial weakness and drooping mouth
   3. Numbness and tingling of fingers and blanching of the skin at the fingertips
   4. Photophobia

17. The physician orders a CT scan of the client's chest with IV contrast. Which of the following findings in the client's history should the nurse report to the physician?

   1. Hypertension
   2. Allergy to shellfish
   3. Urinary tract infection (UTI)
   4. Allergy to penicillin

18. The oncologist examines a client in the clinic and subsequently admits the client to the hospital with severe bone marrow depression. The client's therapy included radiation and chemotherapy. Which of the following nursing diagnoses takes priority in the client's care plan?

   1. Imbalanced nutrition: less than body requirements
   2. Risk for infection
   3. Pain
   4. Risk for injury

19. The nurse is preparing to discharge a client who is stable after a sickle-cell anemia crisis. Which of the following instructions should the nurse provide to the client to avoid future crises? **Select all that apply.**

   1. Limit your fluid intake.
   2. Avoid strenuous exercise.
   3. Apply cold compresses to painful areas.
   4. Take pain medications as ordered.
   5. Avoid tight clothing.

20. The clinic nurse is updating the medications being taken by an anxious middle-aged client, and sees that the physician prescribed an antidiuretic hormone. The nurse knows the medication has which of the following effects on the kidneys?

   1. Increases water reabsorption and urine concentration
   2. Decreases water reabsorption and dilutes the urine
   3. Regulates sodium retention
   4. Controls potassium secretion

21. The nurse is performing an assessment on a client who has developed cirrhosis. Which of the following signs and symptoms should the nurse expect to see? **Select all that apply.**

    1. Dull abdominal ache
    2. Cyanosis
    3. Poor tissue turgor
    4. Bruises
    5. Fruity breath

22. The physician orders 0.5 mg of digoxin (Lanoxin) for a client with atrial fibrillation. The pharmacy has 250-mcg tablets available. How many tablets will the nurse give?

    $$0.5 \, mg \times \frac{1000 \, mcg}{1 mg} \times \frac{1 \, tab}{250 \, mcg} = 2 \, tabs$$

23. The nurse is preparing to administer a red blood cell transfusion to a client with a low hemoglobin level and low hematocrit. The nurse knows which of the following statements about blood transfusion practice is true?

    1. The client should be monitored for at least one hour after the start of the transfusion.
    2. The transfusion should be completed within 2 hours.
    3. The transfusion should be started within 30 minutes of removing the blood or blood components from the blood bank.
    4. The only solution that should be added to blood or blood components is 0.45% sodium chloride (half normal saline solution).

24. The nurse is providing discharge teaching to a client stabilized after an acute attack of primary gout. Which of the following foods should the nurse instruct the client to avoid to prevent future attacks?

Patients c gout should not eat foods that are high purine — such as an.ml products

    1. Cauliflower, asparagus, and mushrooms
    2. Anchovies, liver, and lentils
    3. Cherries, strawberries, and blueberries
    4. Cereal, pasta, and rice

25. In the emergency room, the nurse is caring for a client with complaints of substernal pain radiating to the arm and jaw, shortness of breath, and a feeling of impending doom. The client had a stroke one month ago. The client's vital signs are blood pressure 146/72, pulse 128, and respirations 36. The 12-lead ECG reveals evolving acute myocardial infarction (MI). Which of the following physician orders should the nurse question?

    1. Beta-adrenergic blocker — *metoprolol, propranolol → Beta block to help block the stress hormone to heart muscle*
    2. Morphine for pain
    3. IV nitroglycerin
    4. Thrombolytic therapy

26. An older adult female, newly diagnosed with type 2 diabetes, is ready for discharge. When providing discharge instructions, the nurse teaches the client that the key to preventing diabetic foot complications is which of the following?

    1. Taking the medication as ordered
    2. Following the recommended diet — *this key to prevention*
    3. Surgical intervention
    4. Regular evaluation of the look and feel of her feet

27. The nurse knows that the physician is most likely to order which of the following laboratory tests to evaluate a client for hypoxia?

    1. Hematocrit
    2. Sputum analysis
    3. Arterial blood gas (ABG) analysis
    4. Total hemoglobin

28. The nurse is performing a 12-lead ECG on a client who has come to the emergency room complaining of chest pain. Where should the nurse place lead V1?

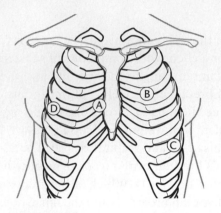

1. A
2. B
3. C
4. D

29. The nurse is assessing a client admitted with a cerebrovascular accident (CVA). The physician has ordered a swallow study. The nurse knows which of the following lobes of the cerebral hemisphere is involved in the control of voluntary muscle movement, including those necessary for the production of speech and swallowing?

1. Frontal
2. Parietal
3. Temporal
4. Occipital

30. The nurse is preparing to do the Heimlich maneuver on a choking middle-aged adult male client. Arrange the following steps in the order the nurse should perform them. **All options must be used.**

1. Make a fist with one hand.
2. Stand behind the client.
3. Wrap your other arm around the client and place that hand on top of your fist.
4. Place your thumb toward the client, below the rib cage and above the waist, and wrap one arm around the client.
5. Ask the client if he is choking.
6. Thrust upward 6–10 times.

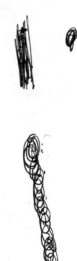

CHAPTER QUIZ ANSWERS AND EXPLANATIONS

1. The Answer is 1

The nurse is reviewing the chart of an older adult male client after surgery for removal of the parathyroid glands. The client complains of difficulty swallowing and a feeling of "pins and needles." The nurse expects which of the following laboratory values to be abnormal?

Category: Laboratory values

(1) CORRECT: Hypocalcemia is an indication of hypoparathyroidism; symptoms include dysphagia and paresthesia.

(2) Lipase levels are not indicators of hypoparathyroidism.

(3) Potassium levels are not indicators of hypoparathyroidism.

(4) Sodium levels are not indicators of hypoparathyroidism.

2. The Answer is 4

The nurse is assessing a young-adult pregnant client with no allergies who has tested positive for gonorrhea. Which of the following medications should the nurse expect to be part of the treatment plan?

Category: Potential for complications of diagnostic tests/treatments/procedures

(1) Tetracyclines are contraindicated in pregnancy.

(2) Fluoroquinolones are contraindicated in pregnancy.

(3) Azithromycin is the treatment for chlamydia.

(4) CORRECT: Ceftriaxone, a third-generation cephalosporin, is the recommended treatment for gonorrhea in pregnancy.

3. The Answer is 3

A client is one day post-op for abdominal surgery. The nurse is teaching the client techniques to reduce pain when he moves, coughs, or breathes deeply. Which of the following statements from the client indicates that the client understands the teaching?

Category: Therapeutic procedures

(1) The client should wait until the medication has taken effect.

(2) The client should frequently move the parts of his body not affected by surgery to prevent stiffness and soreness.

(3) CORRECT: The client should use the side rail for support and move slowly and smoothly without sudden movement.

(4) The client should ask for pain medication as needed so that he can move comfortably.

4. The Answer is 4

A 36-year-old primigravid client with a history of diabetes is admitted with preeclampsia. Which of the following actions should the nurse take *FIRST*?

Category: Potential for complications of diagnostic tests/treatments/procedures

(1) Using low-dose aspirin has not been successful and is not recommended for routine use in pregnancy.

(2) Using calcium supplements has not been successful and is not recommended for routine use in pregnancy.

(3) Although frequent monitoring of blood pressure is a part of the management of preeclampsia, this is not the first thing the nurse should do.

(4) CORRECT: The nurse should prepare the client for delivery, which is the most effective treatment for preeclampsia.

5. The Answer is 1

The nurse has just answered a call light for a client who is two days post-op for abdominal surgery. The client states, "I coughed and heard this pop." The nurse assesses the surgical site and observes dehiscence of the wound. Which of the following should the nurse do *FIRST*?

Category: Therapeutic procedures; Potential for complications of diagnostic tests/treatments/procedures; Potential for complications from surgical procedures and health alterations

(1) CORRECT: The nurse should stay with the client and have a colleague notify the physician first.

(2) The second thing the nurse should do is help the client lie with his head slightly elevated (low Fowler's position) with knees bent in to decrease abdominal tension and monitor the client's vital signs.

(3) The nurse should not place anything on the wound unless it has eviscerated, and then cover the extruding wound contents with warm, sterile normal saline soaks.

(4) The nurse would not help the client to sit up. Instead, the nurse would help the client to a low Fowler's position with knees bent in to decrease abdominal tension and monitor the client's vital signs.

6. The Answer is 4

An elderly man is admitted to the hospital from the Emergency Department during the night shift. The nurse is assessing the client's cerebellar function. Which of the following questions should the nurse ask the client?

Category: System specific assessments

(1) This question will not help the nurse assess the client's cerebellar function, which is related to balance and coordination.

(2) Trouble swallowing fluids or foods is not related to cerebellar function.

(3) Muscle pain is not related to cerebellar function.

(4) CORRECT: The nurse evaluates cerebellar function by testing the client's balance and coordination.

7. The Answer is 1, 2, and 5

An older adult male client with a history of myasthenia gravis is admitted to the medical/surgical unit. Which of the following tests should the nurse expect to see ordered? **Select all that apply.**

Category: Diagnostic tests; Potential for complications of diagnostic tests/treatments/procedures

(1) CORRECT: Myasthenia gravis produces sporadic but progressive weakness and abnormal

fatigue in skeletal muscles. The Tensilon test confirms the diagnosis by temporarily improving muscle function after an IV injection of edrophonium or neostigmine.

(2) CORRECT: Nerve conduction studies test for receptor antibodies.

(3) Lumbar puncture is a test used to diagnose multiple sclerosis, a result of progressive demyelination of the white matter of the brain and spinal cord.

(4) An EEG is a test used to diagnose multiple sclerosis, a result of progressive demyelination of the white matter of the brain and spinal cord.

(5) CORRECT: Electromyography helps differentiate nerve disorders from muscle disorders.

8. The Answer is 2

A middle-aged female client with a history of atherosclerosis is admitted with complaints of abdominal tenderness during deep palpation. The nurse notices a pulsating mass in the periumbilical area. Which of the following does the nurse suspect?

Category: System specific assessments; Potential for complications of diagnostic tests/treatments/procedures; Potential for complications from surgical procedures and health alterations

(1) Signs of appendicitis include loss of appetite, nausea, vomiting, fever, board-like abdominal rigidity, and increasingly severe abdominal spasm.

(2) CORRECT: Signs of abdominal aortic aneurysm include asymptomatic pulsating mass in the periumbilical area, possible systolic bruit over the aorta on auscultation, possible abdominal tenderness on deep palpation, and lumbar pain that radiates to the flank and groin (imminent rupture).

(3) Signs of acute cholecystitis include midepigastric or right upper quadrant pain radiating to the back or referred to the right scapula.

(4) Signs of paralytic ileus include severe abdominal distention, vomiting, and severe constipation.

9. The Answer is 1

An older adult client with a history of blood clots is in the emergency room with suspected deep vein thrombosis (DVT) of the left leg. The nurse starts IV heparin as ordered. Which of the following is *LEAST* likely to be included in the care plan?

Category: Potential for complications of diagnostic tests/treatments/procedures

(1) CORRECT: Treatment aims to prevent complications, relieve pain, and prevent recurrence. Ambulation is not allowed until the physician approves walking.

(2) Warm, moist soaks is an appropriate action to take.

(3) Analgesics are an appropriate action to take.

(4) When the acute episode of DVT subsides, the client may begin to walk while wearing anti-embolism stockings.

10. The Answer is 2

The nurse is caring for a client with a history of chronic liver disease and cirrhosis of the liver. Lab values reveal rising ammonia levels. Which of the following treatments should the nurse question?

Category: Potential for complications of diagnostic tests/treatments/procedures

(1) Adequate calorie intake in the form of glucose or carbohydrates helps prevent protein catabolism.

(2) CORRECT: Rising blood ammonia levels can result from cirrhosis, and hepatic encephalopathy follows. Protein is restricted to 40 g/day and increased up to 100 g/day as symptoms improve.

(3) Neomycin is administered to remove ammonia-producing substances from the GI tract and suppress bacterial ammonia production.

(4) Potassium supplements are administered to help correct alkalosis from increased ammonia levels.

11. The Answer is 3 and 4

The laboratory values of an adult male client reveal the presence of hepatitis B surface antigens and hepatitis B antibodies. Which of the following laboratory results should the nurse also expect to see? **Select all that apply.**

Category: Laboratory values

(1) In viral hepatitis, serum albumin levels are low.

(2) In viral hepatitis, serum globulin levels are high.

(3) CORRECT: In viral hepatitis, serum transaminate levels are elevated.

(4) CORRECT: In viral hepatitis, prothrombin time is prolonged.

(5) In viral hepatitis, urine bilirubin levels are elevated.

12. The Answer is 1

The nurse is assessing a client with Addison's disease. The nurse expects to note which of the following?

Category: System specific assessments; Potential for alterations in body systems

(1) CORRECT: Anorexia is associated with Addison's disease.

(2) Weight loss, not weight gain, is a sign of Addison's disease.

(3) Bronze skin coloration (not yellow skin coloration) is a sign of Addison's disease.

(4) A craving for salty foods (not sweets) is a sign of Addison's disease.

13. The Answer is 2

A client is having a tonic-clonic seizure. Which of the following should the nurse do *FIRST*?

Category: Potential for complications of diagnostic tests/treatments/procedures; Therapeutic procedures

(1) This is not the first thing the nurse should do. When the seizure stops, the nurse should check for breathing and, if necessary, initiate rescue breathing.

(2) CORRECT: The nurse's first priority during a seizure is to protect the client from injury. To do this, the nurse must first remove objects from the surroundings and pad objects that cannot be removed.

(3) Placing an object in the client's mouth can cause injury.

(4) Restraining the client can cause injury.

14. The Answer is 2

A client is recovering from a bout with chronic glomerulonephritis. The nurse prepares the client for discharge and home management. Which of the following statements indicates the client understands his condition and how to control it?

Category: Therapeutic procedures

(1) The nurse should teach the client to take his prescribed antihypertensive medication as scheduled, even if he's feeling better.

(2) CORRECT: The nurse should teach the client to take diuretics, such as furosemide (Lasix), in the morning so that sleep won't be disrupted by the need to void.

(3) The nurse should teach the client to report any adverse side effects and encourage the client to express his feelings to help him adjust to this illness.

(4) The nurse should urge the client to schedule follow-up examinations to assess renal function.

15. The Answer is 4

A nursing home client is admitted to the hospital with a pressure ulcer involving full-thickness loss extending to the bone. The nurse documents the pressure ulcer as being at which of the following stages?

Category: System specific assessments; Potential for complications of diagnostic tests/treatments/procedures

(1) In Stage I, the skin is intact with non-blanchable redness over a localized area.

(2) Stage II involves partial-thickness loss of the dermis.

(3) Stage III involves full-thickness loss, but bone, tendon, and muscle are not exposed.

(4) CORRECT: Stage IV involves full-thickness loss with exposed bone, tendon, and muscle.

16. The Answer is 3

A client with Raynaud's disease is experiencing an acute attack. The nurse should anticipate which of the following assessment findings?

Category: System specific assessments

(1) Involuntary muscle contractions and twitching may be signs of amyotrophic lateral sclerosis (ALS).

(2) Unilateral facial weakness and drooping mouth are signs of Bell's palsy.

(3) CORRECT: The cause of Raynaud's disease is unknown; however, after exposure to cold or stress, the client typically experiences blanching of the skin at the fingertips and numbness and tingling of the fingers.

(4) Photophobia is not a symptom of Raynaud's disease.

17. The Answer is 2

The physician orders a CT scan of the client's chest with IV contrast. Which of the following findings in the client's history should the nurse report to the physician?

Category: Potential for complications of diagnostic tests/treatments/procedures

(1) Hypertension is not a contraindication for a CT scan with IV contrast.

(2) CORRECT: A client with an allergy to iodine or shellfish may have an adverse reaction to the contrast medium.

(3) A UTI is not a contraindication for a CT scan with IV contrast.

(4) An allergy to penicillin is not a contraindication for a CT scan with IV contrast.

18. The Answer is 2

The oncologist examines a client in the clinic and subsequently admits the client to the hospital with severe bone marrow depression. The client's therapy included radiation and chemotherapy. Which of the following nursing diagnoses takes priority in the client's care plan?

Category: Potential for complications of diagnostic tests/treatments/procedures

(1) Imbalanced nutrition is a health-threatening but not life-threatening problem.

(2) CORRECT: Because clients with bone marrow depression have a decrease in white blood cells—those cells that fight infection—risk for infection takes priority. Nursing diagnoses should be categorized in order of priority, with life-threatening problems addressed first, followed by health-threatening concerns.

(3) Pain may be a health-threatening problem, but typically is not life-threatening.

(4) Risk for injury is a health-threatening but not life-threatening problem.

19. The Answer is 2, 4, and 5

The nurse is preparing to discharge a client who is stable after a sickle-cell anemia crisis. Which of the following instructions should the nurse provide to the client to avoid future crises? **Select all that apply.**

Category: Therapeutic procedures

(1) Clients should maintain a high fluid intake to prevent dehydration.

(2) CORRECT: Sickle-cell anemia clients should avoid strenuous exercise, which could provoke hypoxia.

(3) Clients should apply warm compresses to painful areas.

(4) CORRECT: Sickle-cell anemia clients should take pain medications as ordered to provide effective pain management.

(5) CORRECT: Sickle-cell anemia clients should avoid tight clothing that restricts circulation.

20. The Answer is 1

The clinic nurse is updating the medications being taken by an anxious middle-aged client, and sees that the physician prescribed an antidiuretic hormone. The nurse knows the medication has which of the following effects on the kidneys?

Category: Laboratory values

(1) CORRECT: Antidiuretic hormone (ADH) is produced by the pituitary gland, and acts in the distal tubule and collecting ducts to increase water reabsorption and urine concentration.

(2) ADH deficiency decreases water reabsorption, causing dilute urine.

(3) Aldosterone, produced by the adrenal gland, regulates sodium retention.

(4) Aldosterone also controls potassium secretion.

21. The Answer is 1, 3, and 4

The nurse is performing an assessment on a client who has developed cirrhosis. Which of the following signs and symptoms should the nurse expect to see? **Select all that apply.**

Category: System specific assessments; Potential for alterations in body systems

(1) CORRECT: Signs and symptoms of cirrhosis include dull abdominal ache.

(2) Jaundice, not cyanosis, is a sign of cirrhosis.

(3) CORRECT: Signs and symptoms of cirrhosis include poor tissue turgor.

(4) CORRECT: Signs and symptoms of cirrhosis include bruises due to bleeding tendencies.

(5) Musty breath, not fruity breath, is a sign of cirrhosis.

22. The Answer is 2

The physician orders 0.5 mg of digoxin (Lanoxin) for a client with atrial fibrillation. The pharmacy has 250-mcg tablets available. How many tablets will the nurse give?

Category: Potential for complications of diagnostic tests/treatments/procedures

Answer: The nurse will give 2 tablets, arrived at as follows: 500 mcg (=0.5 mg) divided by 250 = 2

23. The Answer is 3

The nurse is preparing to administer a red blood cell transfusion to a client with a low hemoglobin level and low hematocrit. The nurse knows which of the following statements about blood transfusion practice is true?

Category: Diagnostic tests; Potential for complications of diagnostic tests/treatments/procedures

(1) The client should be monitored for at least 15 minutes after the start of the transfusion.

(2) The transfusion needs to be completed within 4 hours, not 2 hours.

(3) CORRECT: The transfusion should be started within 30 minutes of removing the blood or blood components from the blood bank.

(4) The only solution that should be added to blood or blood components is 0.9% sodium chloride (normal saline solution).

24. The Answer is 2

The nurse is providing discharge teaching to a client stabilized after an acute attack of primary gout. Which of the following foods should the nurse instruct the client to avoid to prevent future attacks?

Category: Therapeutic procedures

(1) Cauliflower, asparagus, and mushrooms can be consumed unless contraindicated for a comorbid condition.

(2) CORRECT: A client with gout should avoid high-purine foods, such as anchovies, liver, sardines, and lentils.

(3) Cherries, strawberries, and blueberries can be consumed unless contraindicated for a comorbid condition.

(4) Cereal, pasta, and rice can be consumed unless contraindicated for a comorbid condition, such as diabetes.

25. The Answer is 4

In the emergency room, the nurse is caring for a client with complaints of substernal pain radiating to the arm and jaw, shortness of breath, and a feeling of impending doom. The client had a stroke one month ago. The client's vital signs are blood pressure 146/72, pulse 128, and respirations 36. The 12-lead ECG reveals evolving acute myocardial infarction (MI). Which of the following physician orders should the nurse question?

Category: Changes/abnormalities in vital signs; Potential for complications of diagnostic tests/treatments/procedures

(1) Beta-adrenergic blockers are an accepted treatment for evolving acute MI.

(2) Morphine for pain is an accepted treatment for evolving acute MI.

(3) IV nitroglycerin (in clients without hypotension or bradycardia) is an accepted treatment for evolving acute MI.

(4) CORRECT: Thrombolytic therapy is contraindicated in clients with a history of recent stroke (within the past 2 months). *could cause a hemorrhagic stroke.*

26. The Answer is 2

An older adult female, newly diagnosed with type 2 diabetes, is ready for discharge. When providing discharge instructions, the nurse teaches the client that the key to preventing diabetic foot complications is which of the following?

Category: Therapeutic procedures

(1) Although taking medication as ordered is important, following the recommended diet is key to preventing diabetic foot complications.

(2) CORRECT: Following the recommended diet is key to preventing diabetic foot complications.

(3) Surgical intervention may be a choice in preventing further complications.

(4) Although any foot problems should be evaluated, following the recommended diet is key to preventing diabetic foot complications.

27. The Answer is 3

The nurse knows that the physician is most likely to order which of the following laboratory tests to evaluate a client for hypoxia?

Category: Laboratory values

(1) Hematocrit does not assess gas exchange.

(2) Sputum analysis helps diagnose respiratory infection.

(3) CORRECT: Hypoxia deprives the body of adequate oxygen supply. ABGs assess respiratory status by helping to evaluate gas exchange in the lungs.

(4) Total hemoglobin does not assess gas exchange.

28. The Answer is 1

The nurse is performing a 12-lead ECG on a client who has come to the emergency room complaining of chest pain. Where should the nurse place lead V1?

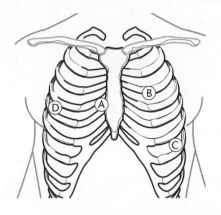

Category: Diagnostic tests

(1) CORRECT: Location A is correct. The V1 lead is placed at the fourth intercostal space to the right of the sternum. A 12-lead ECG measures electrical potential and helps make a definitive diagnosis of acute myocardial infarction. The six precordial leads—V1-V6—in combination with other leads, record potential in the horizontal plane.

(2) Location B is incorrect for the V1 lead.

(3) Location C is incorrect for the V1 lead.

(4) Location D is incorrect for the V1 lead.

29. The Answer is 1

The nurse is assessing a client admitted with a cerebrovascular accident (CVA). The physician has ordered a swallow study. The nurse knows which of the following lobes of the cerebral hemisphere is involved in the control of voluntary muscle movement, including those necessary for the production of speech and swallowing?

Category: System specific assessments

(1) CORRECT: The frontal lobe deals with higher levels of cognitive functions, such as reasoning and judgment. It also contains several cortical areas involved in the control of voluntary muscle movement, including those necessary for the production of speech and swallowing.

(2) The parietal lobe is associated with sensation, and is involved in writing and some aspects of reading.

(3) The temporal lobe is associated with auditory processing, olfaction, and word meaning.

(4) The occipital lobe is involved in vision.

30. The Answer is 5, 2, 1, 4, 3, 6

The nurse is preparing to do the Heimlich maneuver on a choking middle-aged adult male client. Arrange the following steps in the order the nurse should perform them. All options must be used.

Category: Potential for complications of diagnostic tests/treatments/procedures

(1) The third step is to make a fist with one hand.

(2) The second step is to stand behind the client.

(3) The fifth step is to wrap your other arm around the client and place that hand on top of your fist.

(4) The fourth step is to place your thumb toward the client, below the rib cage and above the waist, and wrap one arm around the client.

(5) The first step is to ask the client if he is choking.

(6) The last step is to thrust upward 6–10 times.

CHAPTER 11

PHYSIOLOGICAL INTEGRITY: PHYSIOLOGICAL ADAPTATION

Physiological adaptation involves managing and providing care for clients who may have a variety of acute, chronic, or life-threatening health conditions. To provide the proper care, you need to understand the client's stable/normal state (homeostasis), understand the internal and external factors that can influence or change it, and know how to help the client return to a stable state.

Understanding "normal" involves knowing the basics about all bodily systems, and knowing about the fluids and chemicals that keep the body functioning properly. In addition to knowing what a normal state looks like—in general and for each client—you also must know proper fluid and electrolyte balances and pH balance (water, sodium, potassium, calcium, magnesium, chloride, etc.). This is also a good time to remember the six elements of infection:

1. Susceptible host
2. Portal of entry
3. Cause
4. Reservoir
5. Portal of exit
6. Modes of transmission

It's important to know how to protect yourself and your client from infection and understand how to intervene to break the chain of infection. When a client is ill or injured, his or her body cannot respond quickly enough to internal or external events. Between your powers of observation and your understanding of pathophysiology, you should know how to determine whether there is a problem, identify the problem, and respond appropriately. This includes recognizing which body systems can be affected by the client's condition, being aware of each client's usual baselines and preexisting conditions, and incorporating that information to determine which care measures to try and whether they are effective.

On the NCLEX-RN® exam, you can expect approximately 13 percent of the questions to relate to Physiological Adaptation. Exam content for this subcategory includes, but is not limited to, the following areas:

- Alterations in body systems
- Fluid and electrolyte imbalances
- Hemodynamics
- Illness management
- Medical emergencies
- Pathophysiology
- Unexpected response to therapies

Now let's review some of the most important concepts related to these subtopics.

ALTERATIONS IN BODY SYSTEMS

Clients can experience a variety of alterations in body systems when they are ill. You should be able to monitor and assess these changes, and implement and explain appropriate interventions to clients.

You should understand the most common therapeutic activities, which include:

- Assessing tube drainage when a client has an alteration in a body system (e.g., whether the amount of fluid increased or decreased, whether the color of the fluid changed)
- Monitoring and maintaining a client on a ventilator
- Maintaining desired temperature using external devices
- Implementing and monitoring phototherapy
- Providing ostomy care
- Providing care to clients who have experienced a seizure
- Assisting with invasive procedures (central line placement, biopsy, debridement)
- Performing peritoneal dialysis
- Providing pulmonary hygiene (chest physiotherapy, spirometry)
- Performing oral nasopharyngeal suctioning
- Suctioning via an endotracheal or a tracheostomy tube
- Performing tracheostomy care
- Providing care for clients experiencing increased intracranial pressure

Providing wound care includes assisting in or performing dressing changes and removal of sutures or staples, monitoring wounds for signs and symptoms of infection, and promoting client wound healing through turning, hydration, nutrition, and skin care. In surgical cases, wound care may also include monitoring and maintaining devices and equipment used for drainage, such as chest tube suction.

It is important to identify signs of potential prenatal complications, and to provide care for clients experiencing complications from pregnancy, labor, and delivery (such as eclampsia, precipitous labor, or hemorrhage). You should also be able to assess a client's response to surgery and provide postoperative care.

In a more general sense, you should be able to educate clients about managing their health problem, whether it's a chronic illness such as diabetes or appropriate post-stroke care. Your efforts should promote progress toward recovery, and you should be able to evaluate whether the client has successfully achieved treatment goals.

FLUID AND ELECTROLYTE IMBALANCES

It is important to understand the concepts of fluid transport, capillary fluid movement, and the chemical regulation of fluid and electrolyte balances (hormones and peptides).

One of the most important elements is being able to identify the signs and symptoms of fluid or electrolyte imbalance in a client. In terms of fluids, this means identifying both dehydration and edema, knowing how to treat each one, and being able to teach the client how to prevent recurrence.

For example, a dehydrated client needs fluids, with no sugar, salt, or caffeine. If the client can take fluids orally, they should be delivered that way, but you should know when parenteral (IV) therapy is the right choice. Clients may also retain excess fluid; risk factors include age, surgery, cardiac or renal failure, and medications. A client with excess fluid should have fluid intake limited, protein intake increased, and excretion promoted, and should be carefully monitored for overcorrection.

Implement interventions to restore client fluid and/or electrolyte balance. Common electrolyte imbalances include the following:

- Hyponatremia and hypernatremia (sodium)
- Hypokalemia and hyperkalemia (potassium)
- Hypocalcemia and hypercalcemia (calcium)
- Hypomagnesemia and hypermagnesemia (magnesium)
- Hypochloremia and hyperchloremia (chlorine)
- Hypophosphatemia and hyperphosphatemia (phosphates)

HEMODYNAMICS

Your responsibility in hemodynamic monitoring is to position the transducer at the level of the right atrium, level central venous pressure (CVP) of the pulmonary artery catheter transducer into this point during each shift and before each measurement, and maintain patency of the catheter with a constant small amount of fluid delivered under pressure.

Assess clients for decreased cardiac output, and identify cardiac rhythm strip abnormalities, such as sinus bradycardia, premature ventricular contractions, ventricular tachycardia, and fibrillation.

Monitor and maintain arterial lines, and connect and maintain pacing devices, including pacemakers, biventricular pacemakers, and implantable cardioverter defibrillators. You should also be able to initiate, maintain, and evaluate telemetry monitoring.

In addition to monitoring pacemakers and defibrillators, you should be able to intervene to improve client cardiovascular status through modifying an activity schedule and initiating a protocol to manage cardiac arrhythmias.

You should be able to provide care for clients with vascular access for hemodialysis, such as via an arteriovenous shunt, a fistula, or a graft.

Finally, apply your knowledge of pathophysiology to interventions in response to client abnormal hemodynamics, and provide clients with strategies to manage decreased cardiac output, such as frequent rest periods and limiting activities.

ILLNESS MANAGEMENT

In addition to recognizing symptoms and helping to identify client health issues, it is important to implement interventions that help a client manage recovery from an illness. This includes applying your knowledge of each client's pathophysiology when determining which interventions are best.

When examining a client who is ill, examine and interpret data and know what information should be reported to the physician immediately. This means knowing a particular client's baseline values, identifying abnormal values or test results, and identifying critical values.

You play an important role in teaching clients how to manage their illnesses, so communicate appropriate and helpful information to clients with infectious illnesses such as AIDS, as well as chronic conditions such as asthma and diabetes. Evaluate and document client response to interventions, and promote continuity of care in illness management activities.

In terms of specific care, you should be able to perform gastric lavage and to administer oxygen therapy and evaluate client response.

Medical Emergencies

When a client appears to be experiencing a medical emergency, you should know how best to intervene. Although things are likely to happen very quickly, you should also be able to explain emergency interventions to the client, despite being in a pressure situation.

You should be able to perform a variety of emergency care procedures, including CPR, the Heimlich maneuver (abdominal thrusts), respiratory support, and use of an automated external defibrillator. You should also know how to provide emergency care for a wound disruption (evisceration or dehiscence). You should also be able to monitor and maintain a client on a ventilator. Once emergency procedures are implemented, evaluate and document client responses, such as restoration of breathing and return to normal pulse rate.

Nurses are typically expected to notify the clinician about unexpected responses and/or emergency situations.

Pathophysiology

It is important to understand the general principles of pathophysiology, including injury and repair, immunity, and cellular structure. You should also be able to identify and determine a client's health status based on pathophysiology.

Unexpected Response to Therapies

Most clients will respond to therapies in a predictable manner, but some will not. Assess clients for unexpected adverse responses to therapy (e.g., increased intracranial pressure or hemorrhage) and know how to intervene to counteract such complications.

CHAPTER QUIZ

1. The nurse has just completed setting up an external warming device (Bear Hugger) for a 48-year-old client and is ready to initiate therapy. The core temperature taken with a rectal probe is currently 91.4° F (33° C). Which of the following actions should the nurse perform?

   1. Active rewarming to increase the core temperature no more than 0.9° F (0.5° C) per hour
   2. Active rewarming to increase the core temperature as quickly as possible
   3. Active rewarming to increase the core temperature to 96.8° F (36° C)
   4. Active rewarming to increase the core temperature to 100.4° F (38° C)

2. The nurse is cleansing a simple surgical wound. The client is two days postoperative, and the incision has well-approximated edges with no sign of infection. A Jackson-Pratt drain is adjacent to the incision site. Which of the following should the nurse do?

   1. Cleanse the incision and drain sites while wearing standard clean gloves.
   2. Cleanse in a back-and-forth motion across the incision line and in a circular motion around the drain site.
   3. Cleanse the incision site and drain site together.
   4. Cleanse the incision and drain sites using a sterile saline solution.

3. The nurse is emptying an evacuator of a Jackson-Pratt drain. The nurse has drained the fluid into a calibrated container and has placed the container on a level flat surface. The nurse measures 20 mL of bloody fluid. Arrange the following actions the nurse should take in sequential order. **All options must be used.**

   1. Dispose of the bloody drainage.
   2. Compress the evacuator completely.
   3. Replace the plug in the evacuator.
   4. Cleanse the plug with an alcohol wipe.
   5. Document the amount, odor, and consistency of the drainage.

4. The nurse in an outpatient clinic has received an order from the physician to remove the client's sutures. The nurse should do which of the following?

   1. Use gloves when removing sutures.
   2. Apply hydrogen peroxide gauze pads to cleanse the area first, then remove the sutures.
   3. Use sterile technique when removing sutures.
   4. Nothing, suture removal is outside of the nurse's scope of practice.

5. The medical floor nurse receives report from the Emergency Department on a 42-year-old client who is admitted to the hospital for hyperphosphatemia related to end-stage renal disease. The client receives continuous ambulatory peritoneal dialysis (CAPD), and the physician has ordered continuation of treatment during hospitalization. The nurse should do which of the following?

1. Maintain a permanent peritoneal catheter with flushes of 0.9% normal saline (0.9% NS) every 4–6 hours.

2. Obtain a pump in preparation for dialysate infusion.

3. Ensure the dialysate is refrigerated until ready to infuse, and obtain a warming pad or a warming machine to warm the dialysate to body temperature prior to exchange.

4. Weigh the client at the same time every day, and use sterile technique while working with a permanent peritoneal catheter.

cleansing of track is every 8hr ... ties every 24hrs

6. An 8-year-old girl is discharged from the hospital with a new tracheostomy. The parents have received initial teaching in the hospital, and the home health nurse will reinforce this teaching. Per report, the parents are willing to learn and are grasping the concepts well. The home health nurse would expect the parents to verbalize and demonstrate which of the following?

   1. "The cleansing and dressing of the stoma will be done at least every 24 hours."

   2. "It is not always necessary to suction before tracheostomy care."

   3. "The inner cannula should be changed by the physician or home health nurse."

   4. "Hydrogen peroxide is used to cleanse the stoma area."

7. The nurse is preparing to suction a client with an endotracheal tube. After ventilating, which is the correct sequence of actions for the nurse to follow during suctioning?

   1. Apply suction, insert a sterile catheter, and withdraw while rotating the catheter.

   2. Insert a sterile catheter, begin to withdraw, apply suction, and continue to withdraw while rotating the catheter.

   3. Apply suction, insert a sterile catheter, and withdraw without rotating the catheter.

   4. Insert a sterile catheter, begin to withdraw, apply suction, and continue to withdraw without rotating the catheter.

8. The nurse assesses a client with a diagnosis of parathyroid disease. The client is having abdominal cramping, positive Chovstek's and Trousseau's signs, and tingling in the extremities. The nurse knows that these findings could be signs and symptoms of which of the following?

   1. Hypermagnesemia

   2. Hypomagnesemia

   3. Hypercalcemia

   4. Hypocalcemia

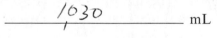

9. The physician has ordered a 2-L daily fluid restriction for a client diagnosed with congestive heart failure. The nurse is totaling the client's fluid intake for the 8-hour shift. The client drank 5 oz. of juice at breakfast, 2 oz. of water with medications, 8 oz. of soup at lunch, and 6 oz. of milk with lunch. Intravenous fluids, flushes, and intravenous antibiotics for the shift were 400 mL. Urinary output was 300 mL, 100 mL, and 250 mL. What should the nurse document, in milliliters, as the total fluid intake for the shift?

   _____ 1030 _____ mL

10. A 70-year-old male presented to the Emergency Department with shortness of breath, crackles in the bases and middle of the lung fields bilaterally, +2 pitting edema bilaterally of the lower extremities, and a weight increase of 6 lb. in one week. His heart rate is 82 and his blood pressure is 162/90. Per physician's order, the nurse administers 40 mg of furosemide (Lasix) intravenously. The nurse knows that which of the following indicates effectiveness of the medication?

1. A heart rate of 58
2. A blood pressure of 100/52
3. Urine output increase of 200 mL over the next hour
4. Diminished lung sounds bilaterally with crackles in the bases

11. The nurse takes report on a client returning from left-sided cardiac catheterization. The client also underwent a percutaneous transluminal coronary angioplasty (PTCA), with drug-eluding stents placed in the right coronary artery and left coronary artery, and the site was closed with a collagen plug. The nurse would expect to assess the entry site on the client at which of the following locations?

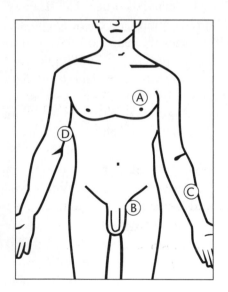

1. A
2. B
3. C
4. D

12. The progressive care unit nurse is assessing the following cardiac rhythm. Using the following exhibit, the nurse should identify this rhythm as which of the following?

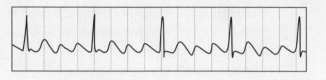

1. Atrial fibrillation
2. Atrial flutter
3. Ventricular fibrillation
4. Third-degree atrioventricular block

13. The critical care nurse is caring for a client with an arterial line (A-line). The nurse can utilize this line for which of the following?

1. Monitoring blood pressure and heart rate, and infusing medications
2. Monitoring blood pressure and heart rate, and obtaining blood gases and other laboratory samples
3. Monitoring heart rate, obtaining blood gases and other laboratory samples, and infusing medications
4. Obtaining blood gases and other laboratory samples, and infusing medications

14. An 82-year-old woman is admitted with a diagnosis of rapid atrial fibrillation. The nurse has initiated telemetry monitoring per the physician's order. Two hours after initiation of monitoring, an alarm sounds at the central monitoring station: the client is in what appears to be ventricular tachycardia. Which of the following actions should the nurse take FIRST?

1. Call a code blue.
2. Silence the alarm and change the alarm parameters.
3. Notify the physician of a change in rhythm.
4. Assess the client and check lead placement.

15. A 39-year-old client has been diagnosed with end-stage renal disease and is on the transplant waiting list. The client has been receiving dialysis through a subclavian central vein catheter while an arteriovenous fistula is maturing. Besides dialysis access, the surgical floor nurse can utilize this subclavian central vein catheter for which of the following?

1. Nothing

2. Blood draws only

3. Infusion of normal saline (0.9% NS) and obtaining blood draws

4. Infusion of medications, all intravenous fluids, and obtaining blood draws

16. A 76-year-old man is brought into the Emergency Department by his spouse. The client's spouse tells the nurse he is confused, disoriented, and weak, and has not been eating well. The nurse obtains blood work as ordered by the physician, including a complete blood count (CBC) and a comprehensive metabolic panel (CMP). For which result should the nurse immediately notify the physician?

1. Potassium (K^+) 3.8 mEq/L

2. Sodium (Na) 122 mEq/L

3. Magnesium (Mag^+) 1.9 mg/dL

4. Hemoglobin (Hgb) 12 g/dL

17. The nurse is providing discharge instructions to a client going home on enoxaparin (Lovenox). Which of the following responses by the client indicates to the nurse that the teaching was effective?

1. "Prior to injection, I will rub the site with an alcohol wipe."

2. "I will use the same site for each injection."

3. "I will not pull back the plunger after inserting the needle into the site."

4. "After injection, I will massage the site to increase absorption."

18. The nursing home nurse finds a 92-year-old client on the floor during rounds. The client is not responsive. Vital signs have been taken by the certified nursing assistant: blood pressure 98/52, heart rate 120, respirations 28, and oxygen saturation 94%. The client has a history of falls, hypertension, and an extensive cardiac history. The client's chart indicates a signed physician order that states "Do not resuscitate" and "Do not intubate" (DNR/DNI). Which of the following should the nurse do?

1. Stay with the client and have another staff member call 911.

2. Begin CPR and have another staff member call 911.

3. Move the client into the bed and call the physician.

4. Call the family and ask what they would like to have done for the client.

19. The surgical floor nurse is working with a client on coughing and deep breathing. The mildly obese client is six days postoperative, and has a large midline abdominal incision that is not well approximated. The client stops the exercise and states she felt a popping sensation in her abdominal area. Upon assessment, the nurse finds a small portion of the viscera to be protruding through the incision. Which of the following actions should the nurse take *FIRST*?

1. Do nothing; this is a normal finding for a large midline abdominal incision.

2. Call the surgeon who operated on the client and inform the physician of the finding.

3. Place sterile dressings moistened with sterile normal saline (0.9% NS) over the viscera and hold in place with a sterile gloved hand.

4. Place an abdominal binder on the area, elevate the head of the bed no more than 20 degrees, and have the client recline with her knees bent.

20. The intensive care nurse is caring for a client requiring mechanical ventilation. Which of the following are interventions the nurse should take to help prevent ventilator-associated pneumonia (VAP)? **Select all that apply.**

    1. Reposition the client at least every 2 hours and maintain the head of the bed upright at 30–45 degrees.

    2. Promote nutrition with the use of a nasogastric tube and high-calorie feedings.

    3. Suction oral and pharynx secretions, and provide thorough oral care at least every 2 hours.

    4. Assess the client for sedation reduction and weaning/extubation readiness.

    5. Perform hand hygiene before and after care of the client, and implement prophylactic intravenous antibiotic therapy.

21. The night nurse on a medical floor has just received report. On which of the following clients should the nurse make rounds *FIRST?*

    1. The 52-year-old female with pancreatitis who is experiencing abdominal pain rated 4 on a 1–10 scale

    2. The 70-year-old male who underwent a transurethral resection of the prostate (TURP) yesterday and is having a burning sensation during urination

    3. The 78-year-old male with diagnosis of left-sided heart failure who has developed a new nonproductive cough and is restless

    4. The 37-year-old female diagnosed with cellulitis of the left leg yesterday who is experiencing redness and warmth of the left leg

22. The nurse knows which of the following body systems is responsible for the production of erythropoietin?

    1. Urinary system

    2. Cardiovascular system

    3. Lymphatic system

    4. Endocrine system

23. The nurse is initiating cefazolin (Ancef) therapy following a physician's order. The nurse notes that the client has an allergy to penicillin. The client states he becomes a little short of breath and itches after receiving penicillin. The nurse should do which of the following?

    1. Call the pharmacy to therapeutically change the medication and notify the physician of this change.

    2. Hold the medication and call the physician to double-check the order.

    3. Give the medication as ordered—cefazolin is not a penicillin.

    4. After asking another nurse, give the medication as ordered.

24. A 52-year-old woman is admitted with a new diagnosis of gastrointestinal (GI) bleed. The physician has ordered the client to receive 2 units of packed red blood cells (PRBCs) for a hemoglobin (Hgb) of 6.8 g/dL. The nurse begins the infusion of the first unit at 100 mL/hr. Fifteen minutes after the start of the infusion, the client complains that she is feeling chilled, is short of breath, and is experiencing lumbar pain rated 8 on a 1–10 scale. Which of the following should be the nurse's *FIRST* action?

    1. Obtain vital signs and notify the physician of potential reaction.

    2. Slow the infusion to 75 mL/hr and reassess in 15 minutes.

    3. Stop the infusion and run normal saline (NS) to keep the vein open (KVO).

    4. Administer PRN pain medication as ordered, apply oxygen at 2 L/min, and provide an additional blanket.

25. The nurse receives report on a client with a right total knee arthroplasty who developed methicillin-resistant *Staphylococcus aureus* (MRSA) in the surgical incision. The incision was cultured and showed sensitivity to vancomycin. The client's blood urea nitrogen (BUN) is 14 mg/dL and serum creatinine (Cr) is 0.9 mg/dL. Intake and output are balanced. A peak and trough have been ordered. The third dose of vancomycin is to be given on the nurse's shift. The nurse should do which of the following?

    1. Draw a trough 30 minutes prior to dose and draw a peak 60 minutes after infusion.

    2. Draw a peak 30 minutes prior to dose and draw a trough 60 minutes after infusion.

    3. Hold the dose of vancomycin and notify the physician of the BUN and Cr levels.

    4. Give the dose of vancomycin as ordered and draw the peak and trough with other evening labs.

CHAPTER QUIZ ANSWERS AND EXPLANATIONS

1. The Answer is 1

The nurse has just completed setting up an external warming device (Bear Hugger) for a 48-year-old client and is ready to initiate therapy. The core temperature taken with a rectal probe is currently 91.4° F (33° C). Which of the following actions should the nurse perform?

Category: Alterations in body systems

(1) CORRECT: The client is in moderate hypothermia with a core temperature of 91.4° F (33° C). This would indicate the need for an external warming device and other measures to increase core temperature.

(2) The core temperature should be brought up by no more than 0.9° F (0.5° C) per hour for treatment of moderate hypothermia.

(3) Active rewarming would be discontinued when the core temperature is greater than 95° F (35° C) to prevent hyperthermia.

(4) Active rewarming would be discontinued when the core temperature is greater than 95° F (35° C) to prevent hyperthermia.

2. The Answer is 4

The nurse is cleansing a simple surgical wound. The client is two days postoperative, and the incision has well-approximated edges with no sign of infection. A Jackson-Pratt drain is adjacent to the incision site. Which of the following should the nurse do?

Category: Alterations in body systems

(1) The nurse should use a sterile/aseptic technique; standard clean gloves are not sufficient.

(2) The nurse will use a small circular motion along the wound edges, but cleanse from one end of the incision to the other. This is to prevent contamination and trauma to the wound.

(3) The drain site should be cleansed last, separately from the primary incision site, to prevent the risk of cross-contamination.

(4) CORRECT: The nurse will use a sterile/aseptic technique while cleansing and dressing the wound, including using sterile gloves, cotton-tipped applicators, sterile saline, and sterile dressings.

3. The Answer is 4, 2, 3, 1, 5

The nurse is emptying an evacuator of a Jackson-Pratt drain. The nurse has drained the fluid into a calibrated container and has placed the container on a level flat surface. The nurse measures 20 mL of bloody fluid. Arrange the following actions the nurse should take in sequential order. **All options must be used.**

Category: Alterations in body systems

(1) The fourth thing the nurse would do is dispose of the bloody drainage, typically into a toilet. This would be done after closing the Jackson-Pratt drain to potentially infective agents and after resuming negative pressure (suction).

(2) The second thing the nurse would do is compress the evacuator completely.

(3) The third thing the nurse would do is replace the plug while the evacuator is compressed. This creates a negative pressure as the evacuator expands.

(4) The first thing the nurse would do is cleanse the plug with an alcohol wipe. This is to reduce the risk of infection.

(5) The last thing the nurse would do is document the process and drainage, including amount, consistency, color, odor, date, time, and client's tolerance of the procedure.

4. The Answer is 3

The nurse in an outpatient clinic has received an order from the physician to remove the client's sutures. The nurse should do which of the following?

Category: Alterations in body systems

(1) To prevent incision contamination, this is should be a sterile procedure. Wearing regular gloves is not sufficient.

(2) To prevent incision contamination, this should be a sterile procedure. This answer choice does not provide enough information to determine if proper sterile procedures are being followed.

(3) CORRECT: A sterile field is maintained, a sterile suture removal tray is used, and sterile gloves are applied.

(4) In many facilities, nurses do remove sutures and staples following a physician's order.

5.　The Answer is 4

The medical floor nurse receives report from the Emergency Department on a 42-year-old client who is admitted to the hospital for hyperphosphatemia related to end-stage renal disease. The client receives continuous ambulatory peritoneal dialysis (CAPD), and the physician has ordered continuation of treatment during hospitalization. The nurse should do which of the following?

Category: Alterations in body systems

(1) The nurse would not flush a CAPD permanent peritoneal catheter with normal saline solution.

(2) The dialysate bag is raised to shoulder level and is infused by gravity into the peritoneal cavity after the dwell dialysate solution is drained.

(3) Dialysate for CAPD is not refrigerated but should be warmed to body temperature prior to infusion, if a warmer is available. Never use a microwave to warm the dialysate; this method creates an unpredictable temperature.

(4) CORRECT: The nurse would weigh the client at the same time daily. The nurse would use sterile technique and equipment when working with the peritoneal catheter to infuse and drain the dialysate, including having the client and nurse wear a surgical mask while the peritoneal catheter and hub are exposed.

6.　The Answer is 4

An 8-year-old girl is discharged from the hospital with a new tracheostomy. The parents have received initial teaching in the hospital, and the home health nurse will reinforce this teaching. Per report, the parents are willing to learn and are grasping the concepts well. The home health nurse would expect the parents to verbalize and demonstrate which of the following?

Category: Alterations in body systems

(1) The stoma should be cleaned and dressed at least every 8 hours and the ties every 24 hours; cleaning and dressing changes may be done more frequently to keep the dressing and ties dry to prevent infection.

(2) Suctioning the trachea and pharynx thoroughly before tracheostomy care keeps the area clean longer.

(3) The inner cannula can be cleaned and changed by the parents, and should be removed and cleaned at least every 8 hours.

(4) CORRECT: Hydrogen peroxide-soaked gauze pads or cotton-tipped applicators are used to clean the stoma area, followed by the use of sterile water-soaked gauze pads and cotton-tipped applicators to remove the hydrogen peroxide. The stoma area would then be dried using sterile gauze pads to reduce the risk of infection and irritation.

7.　The Answer is 2

The nurse is preparing to suction a client with an endotracheal tube. After ventilating, which is the correct sequence of actions for the nurse to follow during suctioning?

Category: Alterations in body systems

(1) Suctioning on insertion unnecessarily decreases oxygen in the airway. Most clients will cough when the suction catheter touches the carina.

(2) CORRECT: The nurse would ventilate the client and insert the sterile catheter without applying suction. The nurse would then withdraw the catheter about 1 inch and apply suction while rotating the catheter.

(3) Suctioning on insertion unnecessarily decreases oxygen in the airway. Most clients will cough when the suction catheter touches the carina.

(4) Failure to withdraw and rotate the catheter may result in damage to the tracheal mucosa.

8. The Answer is 4

The nurse assesses a client with a diagnosis of parathyroid disease. The client is having abdominal cramping, positive Chovstek's and Trousseau's signs, and tingling in the extremities. The nurse knows that these findings could be signs and symptoms of which of the following?

Category: Fluid and electrolyte imbalances

(1) A person with hypermagnesemia would not exhibit all of these symptoms.

(2) A person with hypomagnesemia might exhibit a positive Chovstek's sign but not the rest of the symptoms listed.

(3) A person with hypercalcemia would not exhibit all of these symptoms.

(4) CORRECT: Hypocalcemia can be demonstrated by abdominal cramping, tingling of the extremities, and tetany. Chovstek's sign refers to an abnormal reaction to the stimulation of the facial nerve such that, when tapped at the masseter muscle, the facial muscles on the same side of the face contract, causing a brief twitching of the nose or lips. Chovstek's sign can be seen in hypomagnesemia and hypocalcemia. Trousseau's sign of latent tetany is more sensitive than Chovstek's sign in hypocalcemia, and may be positive before gross manifestations of hypocalcemia, specifically tetany and hyperreflexia. A blood pressure cuff is inflated to a pressure greater than the systolic pressure and held in place for 3 minutes. This causes the occlusion of the brachial artery, and the hypocalcemia and subsequent neuromuscular irritability will induce a muscle spasm of the client's hand and forearm.

9. The Answer is 1,030 mL

The physician has ordered a 2-L daily fluid restriction for a client diagnosed with congestive heart failure. The nurse is totaling the client's fluid intake for the 8-hour shift. The client drank 5 oz. of juice at breakfast, 2 oz. of water with medications, 8 oz. of soup at lunch, and 6 oz. of milk with lunch. Intravenous fluids, flushes, and intravenous antibiotics for the shift were 400 mL. Urinary output was 300 mL, 100 mL, and 250 mL. What should the nurse document, in milliliters, as the total fluid intake for the shift?

Category: Fluid and electrolyte imbalances

Answer: The answer can be calculated as follows: 1 ounce is equal to 30 milliliters. Oral intake is 150 mL (because 5 oz. × 30 mL = 150 mL) + 60 mL (because 2 oz. × 30 mL = 60 mL) + 240 mL (because 8 oz. × 30 mL = 240 mL) + 180 mL (because 6 oz. × 30 mL = 180 mL) to equal 630 mL of oral intake. Add that to the intravenous fluids and antibiotics for a total intake of 1,030 mL (630 mL + 400 mL). Intake consists of oral intake, intravenous intake, intake through any feeding tube, intravenous blood products, liquid medications, and flushes of any tubes or IV accesses. The nurse would not include urinary output in intake totals, because that is totaled separately under output. Output includes urine, diarrhea, emesis, wound drainage, and any gastric suction.

10. The Answer is 3

A 70-year-old male presented to the Emergency Department with shortness of breath, crackles in the bases and middle of the lung fields bilaterally, +2 pitting edema bilaterally of the lower extremities, and a weight increase of 6 lb. in one week. His heart rate is 82 and his blood pressure is 162/90. Per physician's order, the nurse administers 40 mg of furosemide (Lasix) intravenously. The nurse knows that which of the following indicates effectiveness of the medication?

Category: Fluid and electrolyte imbalances

(1) A heart rate of 58 could indicate a side effect of the medication rather than effectiveness. This significant drop in heart rate would be cause for alarm, especially after the administration of furosemide.

(2) A blood pressure of 100/52 could indicate a side effect of the medication rather than effectiveness. This significant drop in blood pressure would be cause for alarm, especially after the administration of furosemide.

(3) CORRECT: The nurse would expect an increase in urine output after the administration of furosemide (Lasix). The client presented with signs and symptoms of hypervolemia or fluid overload, including shortness of breath, crackles in lung

bases, and edema. Weight gain and hypertension can also be indicative of hypervolemia. The goal of treatment using furosemide is diuresis, with care not to send the client into hypovolemia.

(4) The nurse would expect to auscultate a reduction, if not elimination, of crackles in the lung bases. The nurse would also not expect diminished lung sounds, because this could indicate atelectasis and/or decreased air flow through the lungs. The goal would be baseline or clear lung sounds bilaterally, with minimal to no crackles in the lung bases upon auscultation.

11.   The Answer is 2

The nurse takes report on a client returning from left-sided cardiac catheterization. The client also underwent a percutaneous transluminal coronary angioplasty (PTCA), with drug-eluding stents placed in the right coronary artery and left coronary artery, and the site was closed with a collagen plug. The nurse would expect to assess the entry site on the client at which of the following locations?

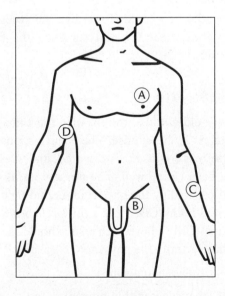

Category: Hemodynamics

(1) A: This is not the correct location.

(2) CORRECT: B is the correct answer. The nurse would expect to assess the entry site in the left femoral artery. This is the preferred site for left-sided cardiac catheterization and PTCA.

(3) C: This is not the correct location.

(4) D: This is not the correct location.

12.   The Answer is 2

The progressive care unit nurse is assessing the following cardiac rhythm. Using the following exhibit, the nurse should identify this rhythm as which of the following?

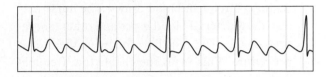

Category: Hemodynamics

(1) The atrial rhythm would be irregular in atrial fibrillation. Coarse, chaotic, asynchronous waves would be present, and the atrial and ventricular rhythms would be grossly irregular and barely discernible with rates that vary.

(2) CORRECT: This is an atrial flutter rhythm—there are no identifiable P waves, and characteristic sawtooth flutter waves are present. The PR interval is not measurable, and the atrial rate is regular and greater than the ventricular rate. This is expressed in a ratio; the example is 3:1, because there are 3 atrial beats for every 1 ventricular beat. The flutter waves should be able to be mapped across the rhythm strip. Flutter waves would mostly be visible with few occurring within the QRS and T waves. The subsequent flutter waves would occur on time.

(3) Ventricular fibrillation (VF) is characterized by atrial and ventricular rates and rhythms that cannot be determined, coarse and chaotic waves in coarse VF, and fine and chaotic waves in fine VF.

(4) Third-degree atrioventricular (AV) block, also known as complete heart block, is characterized by a regular rhythm, an independent atrial rate that is faster than the ventricular rate, an identifiable P wave that is normal and occurring without a QRS complex, and no PR interval.

13.   The Answer is 2

The critical care nurse is caring for a client with an arterial line (A-line). The nurse can utilize this line for which of the following?

Category: Hemodynamics

(1) Medications should never be infused through an arterial line.

(2) CORRECT: Arterial lines are used for monitoring blood pressure and heart rate, especially in clients requiring the use of vasopressor medications intravenously. They are also used for clients requiring frequent blood draws. The nurse may also draw arterial blood gases and other laboratory samples from the line, following the proper procedure. This saves the client from frequent arterial and venous draws.

(3) Medications should never be infused through an arterial line.

(4) Medications should never be infused through an arterial line.

14. The Answer is 4

An 82-year-old woman is admitted with a diagnosis of rapid atrial fibrillation. The nurse has initiated telemetry monitoring per the physician's order. Two hours after initiation of monitoring, an alarm sounds at the central monitoring station: the client is in what appears to be ventricular tachycardia. Which of the following actions should the nurse take *FIRST*?

Category: Hemodynamics

(1) This would be premature on the part of the nurse—assessment of the client may yield different information than what is reported by the monitor.

(2) Verify alarm limits with the physician, and only change parameters following an order from the physician.

(3) The nurse would first check the lead wires and assess the client to ensure that information given to the physician is accurate.

(4) CORRECT: Assess the client first, then the equipment for disconnections or malfunctions. Check lead placement to determine if the monitoring results are indeed accurate, and not due to interference or an artifact. If assessment of the client reveals true ventricular tachycardia, follow advance directives as established by the client, including, but not limited to, calling a code.

15. The Answer is 1

A 39-year-old client has been diagnosed with end-stage renal disease and is on the transplant wait list. The client has been receiving dialysis through a subclavian central vein catheter while an arteriovenous fistula is maturing. Besides dialysis access, the surgical floor nurse can utilize this subclavian central vein catheter for which of the following?

Category: Hemodynamics

(1) CORRECT: The nurse is not to access the subclavian central vein catheter that is being used for dialysis for blood draws, for infusions, or for any reason other than dialysis. Only in the event of a life-threatening emergency may the access be used for anything other than dialysis, and that is only under the physician's direct order.

(2) Any other use could jeopardize the access that must be patent for dialysis until the fistula matures.

(3) Any other use could jeopardize the access that must be patent for dialysis until the fistula matures.

(4) Any other use could jeopardize the access that must be patent for dialysis until the fistula matures.

16. The Answer is 2

A 76-year-old man is brought into the Emergency Department by his spouse. The client's spouse tells the nurse he is confused, disoriented, and weak, and has not been eating well. The nurse obtains blood work as ordered by the physician, including a complete blood count (CBC) and a comprehensive metabolic panel (CMP). For which result should the nurse immediately notify the physician?

Category: Illness management

(1) This lab value is within normal range.

(2) CORRECT: Symptoms of hyponatremia include confusion, disorientation, weakness, and poor appetite. The physician should be notified immediately for this critical level of sodium.

(3) This lab value is within normal range.

(4) This lab value is within normal range.

17. The Answer is 3

The nurse is providing discharge instructions to a client going home on enoxaparin (Lovenox). Which of the following responses by the client indicates to the nurse that the teaching was effective?

Category: Illness management

(1) The area would be cleansed with an alcohol wipe, with care not to rub. Rubbing may cause damage to the skin and could contribute to formation of a hematoma.

(2) Sites for injection should be rotated, focusing on areas that have an easily accessible, fatty, subcutaneous layer. This is also minimizes tissue damage from repeated injections, which may affect absorption.

(3) CORRECT: Aspiration, or pulling back the plunger after needle insertion, can cause damage to small capillaries and blood vessels and can lead to hematoma formation and bleeding.

(4) Massaging the area postinjection may cause damage to the skin and could contribute to hematoma formation.

18. The Answer is 1

The nursing home nurse finds a 92-year-old client on the floor during rounds. The client is not responsive. Vital signs have been taken by the certified nursing assistant: blood pressure 98/52, heart rate 120, respirations 28, and oxygen saturation 94%. The client has a history of falls, hypertension, and an extensive cardiac history. The client's chart indicates a signed physician order that states "Do not resuscitate" and "Do not intubate" (DNR/DNI). Which of the following should the nurse do?

Category: Medical emergencies

(1) CORRECT: The nurse should have another staff member call 911, gather paperwork, and contact the primary physician to notify of the transfer while the nurse stays with the client to continue to assess for any change in condition.

(2) The client has a pulse and is breathing spontaneously at this point, so initiation of CPR would be contraindicated. If the client would no longer have a pulse and/or stop breathing, CPR would not be initiated due to the DNR/DNI status of the client. Unless the client has advance directives that indicate no emergency treatment or no hospitalization, the nurse should continue reasonable and necessary treatment and nursing care up to the point of resuscitation and intubation. This includes calling 911 for emergency assistance.

(3) The nurse would not move the client from the floor because the client may have experienced a fracture or head trauma during the unwitnessed fall.

(4) Family notification would take place after emergency services are requested (or ordered).

19. The Answer is 3

The surgical floor nurse is working with a client on coughing and deep breathing. The mildly obese client is six days postoperative, and has a large midline abdominal incision that is not well approximated. The client stops the exercise and states she felt a popping sensation in her abdominal area. Upon assessment, the nurse finds a small portion of the viscera to be protruding through the incision. Which of the following actions should the nurse take *FIRST*?

Category: Medical emergencies

(1) This is not a normal finding for a large midline abdominal incision.

(2) It is very important for someone to stay with the client due to the anxiety that the client will be feeling. The surgeon must be notified, and possible surgery could ensue, but this is not the first thing the nurse would do.

(3) CORRECT: This medical emergency is known as wound dehiscence with evisceration. The nurse would saturate sterile dressings with normal saline and hold the dressings over the viscera, which is most likely part of the bowel loop.

(4) The nurse should attempt to minimize any additional stress on the incision by having the client lie in a low Fowler's position with knees bent. An abdominal binder is used in the prevention of dehiscence and not in the treatment of evisceration.

20. The Answer is 1, 3 and 4

The intensive care nurse is caring for a client requiring mechanical ventilation. Which of the following are interventions the nurse should take to help prevent ventilator-associated pneumonia (VAP)? **Select all that apply.**

Category: Medical emergencies

(1) CORRECT: The standard of care is to reposition the client at least every 2 hours using lateral and horizontal positioning techniques. The head of the bed should be raised 30–45 degrees unless contraindicated. This helps reduce aspiration of both secretions and gastric contents.

(2) A nasogastric tube can lead to sinusitis, which increases the likelihood of the client developing VAP. The use of an orogastric tube to aid in feeding and/or gastric decompression is recommended over the use of a nasogastric tube.

(3) CORRECT: Oral care should be done at least every 2 hours. The removal of excess secretions is also an important element in the reduction of VAP. These secretions can cause aspiration, and can also be a perfect moist breeding ground for infection.

(4) CORRECT: A reduction in the duration of mechanical ventilation and/or a reduction in sedation to assess readiness of weaning have been shown to decrease the development and incidence of VAP. No alteration in medication or weaning/extubation should be attempted without an order from the physician. The nurse can be proactive and encourage the progression of weaning through assessment and subsequent discussions with the physician.

(5) Although proper hand hygiene and the use of gloves have been shown to reduce the risk of VAP, prophylactic intravenous antibiotic therapy is not recommended. A broad-spectrum antibacterial oral rinse (chlorhexidine) has been used in conjunction with thorough oral care with good results.

21. The Answer is 3

The night nurse on a medical floor has just received report. On which of the following clients should the nurse make rounds *FIRST?*

Category: Pathophysiology

(1) The client with mild to moderate pain related to pancreatitis is not as critical as the client with potential acute pulmonary edema.

(2) The client with the burning sensation post-TURP is not as critical. In fact, this is a common finding with this procedure/diagnosis.

(3) CORRECT: This new nonproductive cough and restlessness could indicate acute pulmonary edema. The nurse would assess this client first, focusing on lung sounds and heart sounds. Acute pulmonary edema is seen in clients that have heart disease, circulatory overload (from transfusions and infusions), or lung injuries; that are postanesthesia; and other etiologies that could bring about fluid in the alveoli that impedes gas exchange. This situation can quickly escalate into a medical emergency, so the nurse should assure oxygenation and implement measures to decrease pulmonary congestion. Quick assessment and response are critical in preventing a medical emergency.

(4) The client with the redness related to cellulitis is not as critical. In fact, this is a common finding with this procedure/diagnosis.

22. The Answer is 1

The nurse knows which of the following body systems is responsible for the production of erythropoietin?

Category: Pathophysiology

(1) CORRECT: The urinary system is responsible for the production of erythropoietin, which is the primary hormone regulator that promotes the development and differentiation of red blood cells in the bone marrow and initiates the production of hemoglobin. Ninety percent of erythropoietin is produced by renal peritubular cells, with the other 10% produced in the liver. The cells that produce erythropoietin are sensitive to levels of oxygen within the blood. If the level of oxygen is low, the kidney cells release erythropoietin to stimulate the bone marrow to produce more red blood cells to increase the oxygen-carrying capability of the blood.

(2) The cardiovascular system is not responsible for the production of erythropoietin.

(3) The lymphatic system is not responsible for the production of erythropoietin.

(4) The endocrine system is not responsible for the production of erythropoietin.

23. The Answer is 2

The nurse is initiating cefazolin (Ancef) therapy following a physician's order. The nurse notes that the client has an allergy to penicillin. The client states he becomes a little short of breath and itches after receiving penicillin. The nurse should do which of the following?

Category: Unexpected response to therapies

(1) The physician should be made aware of this allergy prior to the client receiving the medication. In some instances, the physician will confirm the order and not change the medication, depending on the severity of the past or prior reaction to penicillin or cephalosporins. More often, though, the physician will change the antibiotic to a different family, but that is for the physician to decide and not the pharmacist or the nurse.

(2) CORRECT: The nurse would call the physician and double-check this order.

(3) Ancef is not a penicillin; it's a first-generation cephalosporin, which can cause a reaction in clients with penicillin allergies.

(4) It is for the physician to decide to change the medication, not the nurse.

24. The Answer is 3

A 52-year-old woman is admitted with a new diagnosis of gastrointestinal (GI) bleed. The physician has ordered the client to receive 2 units of packed red blood cells (PRBCs) for a hemoglobin (Hgb) of 6.8 g/dL. The nurse begins the infusion of the first unit at 100 mL/hr. Fifteen minutes after the start of the infusion, the client complains that she is feeling chilled, short of breath, and is experiencing lumbar pain rated 8 on a 1–10 scale. Which of the following should be the nurse's *FIRST* action?

Category: Unexpected response to therapies

(1) Vital signs should be obtained, and the physician notified after treatment is discontinued. The unit in question should not be restarted, and any other units that were issued should not be implemented.

(2) Just slowing the infusion will not resolve the issue of an allergic reaction to the treatment.

(3) CORRECT: The symptoms of feeling chilled, being short of breath, and having back pain could indicate an acute hemolytic reaction. This medical emergency requires swift action on the part of the nurse, including immediately discontinuing the infusion, flushing the IV site, and saving the unit of blood in question for testing.

(4) Treating the symptoms of the reaction will not resolve the issue of an allergic reaction to the treatment.

25. The Answer is 1

The nurse receives report on a client with a right total knee arthroplasty who developed methicillin-resistant *Staphylococcus aureus* (MRSA) in the surgical incision. The incision was cultured and showed sensitivity to vancomycin. The client's blood urea nitrogen (BUN) is 14 mg/dL and serum creatinine (Cr) is 0.9 mg/dL. Intake and output are balanced. A peak and trough have been ordered. The third dose of vancomycin is to be given on the nurse's shift. The nurse should do which of the following?

Category: Unexpected response to therapies

(1) CORRECT: The nurse would expect to draw a trough 30 minutes prior to the third dose of vancomycin, and draw a peak 60 minutes after infusion is complete. The physician orders this set of labs to be drawn, or the order is part of a hospital protocol for clients receiving vancomycin intravenously.

(2) Drawing a peak 30 minutes prior to dose and drawing a trough 60 minutes after infusion would yield an inaccurate result.

(3) The BUN and Cr levels that are given in this scenario are within normal limits.

(4) Giving the dose of vancomycin as ordered and drawing the peak and trough with other evening labs would yield an inaccurate result.

PART 3

THE PRACTICE TEST

PRACTICE TEST

Directions: Each question or incomplete statement below is followed by four suggested answers or completions. In each case, HIGHLIGHT the statement that best answers the question or completes the statement.

1. The nurse is interviewing a client who is being treated for obsessive-compulsive disorder. Which of the following is the *MOST* important question the nurse should ask this client?

   1. "Do you find yourself forgetting simple things?"
   2. "Do you find it hard to stay on a task?"
   3. "Do you have trouble controlling upsetting thoughts?"
   4. "Do you experience feelings of panic in a closed area?"

2. Which of the following actions by the nurse would be considered negligence?

   1. Obtaining a Guthrie blood test on a 4-day-old infant
   2. Massaging lotion on the abdomen of a 3-year-old diagnosed with Wilms' tumor
   3. Instructing a 5-year-old asthmatic to blow on a pinwheel
   4. Playing kickball with a 10-year-old with juvenile arthritis (JA)

3. The nurse on a postpartum unit is preparing 4 clients for discharge. It would be *MOST* important for the nurse to refer which of the following clients for home care?

   1. A 15-year-old primipara who delivered a 7-lb. male 2 days ago
   2. An 18-year-old multipara who delivered a 9-lb. female by cesarean section 2 days ago
   3. A 20-year-old multipara who delivered 1 day ago and is complaining of cramping
   4. A 22-year-old who delivered by cesarean section and is complaining of burning on urination

4. A client is telling the nurse about his perception of his thought patterns. Which of the following statements by the client would validate the diagnosis of schizophrenia?

   1. "I can't get the same thoughts out of my head."
   2. "I know I sometimes feel on top of the world, then suddenly down."
   3. "Sometimes I look up and wonder where I am."
   4. "It's clear that this is an alien laboratory and I am in charge."

5. A nursing team consists of an RN, an LPN/LVN, and an NAP. The nurse should assign which of the following clients to the LPN/LVN?

1. A 72-year-old client with diabetes who requires a dressing change for a stasis ulcer

2. A 42-year-old client with cancer of the bone complaining of pain

3. A 55-year-old client with terminal cancer being transferred to hospice home care

4. A 23-year-old client with a fracture of the right leg who asks to use the urinal

6. To determine the structural relationship of one hospital department with another, the nurse should consult which of the following?

   1. Organizational chart
   2. Job descriptions
   3. Personnel policies
   4. Policies and Procedures Manual

7. A client complains of pain in his right lower extremity. The physician orders codeine 60 mg and aspirin grains X PO every 4 hours, as needed for pain. Each codeine tablet contains 15 mg of codeine. Each aspirin tablet contains 325 mg of aspirin. Which of the following should the nurse administer?

   1. 2 codeine tablets and 4 aspirin tablets
   2. 4 codeine tablets and 3 aspirin tablets
   3. 4 codeine tablets and 2 aspirin tablets
   4. 3 codeine tablets and 3 aspirin tablets

8. The nurse is leading an inservice about management issues. The nurse would intervene if another nurse made which of the following statements?

   1. "It is my responsibility to ensure that the consent form has been signed and attached to the client's chart prior to surgery."
   2. "It is my responsibility to witness the signature of the client before surgery is performed."

3. "It is my responsibility to provide a detailed description of the surgery."

4. "It is my responsibility to answer questions that the client may have prior to surgery."

9. A nurse in the outpatient clinic evaluates the Mantoux test of a client whose history indicates that she has been treated during the past year for an AIDS-related infection. The nurse should document that there was a positive reaction if there is an area of induration measuring which of the following?

   1. 3 mm
   2. 7 mm
   3. 11 mm
   4. 15 mm

10. The nurse in the newborn nursery has just received report. Which of the following infants should the nurse see FIRST?

   1. A 2-day-old infant who is lying quietly alert with a heart rate of 185
   2. A 1-day-old infant who is crying and has a bulging anterior fontanel
   3. A 12-hour-old infant who is being held, with respirations that are 45 breaths per minute and irregular
   4. A 5-hour-old infant who is sleeping and whose hands and feet are blue bilaterally

11. While inserting a nasogastric tube, the nurse should use which of the following protective measures?

   1. Gloves, gown, goggles, and surgical cap
   2. Sterile gloves, mask, plastic bags, and gown
   3. Gloves, gown, mask, and goggles
   4. Double gloves, goggles, mask, and surgical cap

12. The nurse is caring for clients in the outpatient clinic. Which of the following phone calls should the nurse return *FIRST*?

    1. A client with hepatitis A who states, "My arms and legs are itching."
    2. A client with a cast on the right leg who states, "I have a funny feeling in my right leg."
    3. A client with osteomyelitis of the spine who states, "I am so nauseous that I can't eat."
    4. A client with rheumatoid arthritis who states, "I am having trouble sleeping."

13. The nursing team consists of 1 RN, 2 LPNs/LVNs, and 3 NAPs. The RN should care for which of the following clients?

    1. A client with a chest tube who is ambulating in the hall
    2. A client with a colostomy who requires assistance with a colostomy irrigation
    3. A client with a right-sided cerebrovascular accident (CVA) who requires assistance with bathing
    4. A client who is refusing medication to treat cancer of the colon

14. The home care nurse is visiting a client during the icteric phase of hepatitis of unknown etiology. The nurse would be *MOST* concerned if the client made which of the following statements?

    1. "I must not share eating utensils with my family."
    2. "I must use my own bath towel."
    3. "I'm glad that my husband and I can continue to have intimate relations."
    4. "I must eat small, frequent feedings."

15. A nurse plans for care of a client with anemia who is complaining of weakness. Which of the following tasks should the nurse assign to nursing assistive personnel?

    1. Listening to the client's breath sounds
    2. Setting up the client's lunch tray
    3. Obtaining a diet history
    4. Instructing the client on how to balance rest and activity

16. The nurse is caring for clients on the surgical floor and has just received report from the previous shift. Which of the following clients should the nurse see *FIRST*?

    1. A 35-year-old admitted 3 hours ago with a gunshot wound; 1.5 cm area of dark drainage noted on the dressing
    2. A 43-year-old who had a mastectomy 2 days ago; 23 mL of serosanguinous fluid noted in the Jackson-Pratt drain
    3. A 59-year-old with a collapsed lung due to an accident; no drainage noted in the previous 8 hours
    4. A 62-year-old who had an abdominal-perineal resection 3 days ago; client complains of chills

17. Which of the following actions by the nurse would certainly be considered negligence?

    1. Inserting a 16 Fr nasogastric tube and aspirating 15 mL of gastric contents
    2. Administering meperidine (Demerol) IM to a client prior to using the incentive spirometer
    3. Turning and repositioning a client once every 8 hours post-abdominal surgery
    4. Initially administering blood at 5 mL per minute for 15 minutes

18. A 1-day-old newborn diagnosed with intrauterine growth retardation is observed by the nurse to be restless, irritable, and fist-sucking, and having a high-pitched, shrill cry. Based on this data, which of the following actions should the nurse take *FIRST*?

    1. Massage the infant's back.
    2. Tightly swaddle the infant in a flexed position.
    3. Schedule feeding times every 3 to 4 hours.
    4. Encourage eye contact with the infant during feedings.

19. The nurse visits a neighbor who is at 20 weeks' gestation. The neighbor complains of nausea, headache, and blurred vision. The nurse notes that the neighbor appears nervous, is diaphoretic, and is experiencing tremors. It would be *MOST* important for the nurse to ask which of the following questions?

    1. "Are you having menstrual-like cramps?"
    2. "When did you last eat or drink?"
    3. "Have you been diagnosed with diabetes?"
    4. "Have you been lying on the couch?"

20. The school nurse notes that a first-grade child is scratching her head almost constantly. It would be *MOST* important for the nurse to take which of the following actions?

    1. Discuss basic hygiene with the parents.
    2. Instruct the child not to sleep with her dog.
    3. Inform the parents that they must contact an exterminator.
    4. Observe the scalp for small white specks.

21. A suicidal client who was admitted to the psychiatric unit for treatment and observation a week ago suddenly appears cheerful and motivated. The nurse should be aware of which of the following?

    1. The client is likely sleeping well because of the medication.
    2. The client has made new friends and has a support group.
    3. The client may have finalized a suicide plan.
    4. The client is responding to treatment and is no longer depressed.

22. The nurse is caring for clients in the GYN clinic. A client complains of an off-white vaginal discharge with a curdlike appearance. The nurse notes the discharge and vulvular erythema. It would be *MOST* important for the nurse to ask which of the following questions?

    1. "Do you douche?"
    2. "Are you sexually active?"
    3. "What kind of birth control do you use?"
    4. "Have you taken any cough medicine?"

23. The nurse is caring for a client in the prenatal clinic. The nurse notes that the client's chart contains the following information: blood type AB, Rh-negative; serology—negative; indirect Coombs test—negative; fetal paternity—unknown. The nurse should anticipate taking which of the following actions?

    1. Administer Rho (D) immune globulin (RhoGAM).
    2. Schedule an amniocentesis.
    3. Obtain a direct Coombs test.
    4. Assess maternal serum for alpha fetoprotein level.

24. The nurse is caring for a woman at 37 weeks' gestation. The client was diagnosed with insulin-dependent diabetes mellitus (IDDM) at age 7. The client states, "I am so thrilled that I will be breastfeeding my baby." Which of the following responses by the nurse is *BEST*?

    1. "You will probably need less insulin while you are breastfeeding."

    2. "You will need to initially increase your insulin after the baby is born."

    3. "You will be able to take an oral hypoglycemic instead of insulin after the baby is born."

    4. "You will probably require the same dose of insulin that you are now taking."

25. The nurse is caring for clients in a pediatric clinic. The mother of a 14-year-old male privately tells the nurse that she is worried about her son because she unexpectedly walked into his room and discovered him masturbating. Which of the following responses by the nurse would be *MOST* appropriate?

    1. "Tell your son he could go blind doing that."

    2. "Masturbation is a normal part of sexual development."

    3. "He's really too young to be masturbating."

    4. "Why don't you give him more privacy?"

26. The nurse performs a home visit on a client who delivered 2 days ago. The client states that she is bottle-feeding her infant. The nurse notes white, curdlike patches on the newborn's oral mucous membranes. The nurse should take which of the following actions?

    1. Determine the newborn's blood glucose level.

    2. Suggest that the newborn's formula be changed.

    3. Remind the caregiver not to let the infant sleep with the bottle.

    4. Explain that the newborn will need to receive some medication.

27. The nurse at the birthing facility is caring for a primipara woman in labor, who is 4 cm dilated and 25% effaced, and whose fetal vertex is at +1. The physician informs the client that an amniotomy is to be performed. The client states, "My friend's baby died when the umbilical cord came out when her water broke. I don't want you to do that to me!" Which of the following responses by the nurse is *BEST*?

    1. "If you are that concerned, you should refuse the procedure."

    2. "The procedure will help your labor go faster."

    3. "That shouldn't happen to you because the baby's head is engaged."

    4. "We will monitor you carefully to prevent cord prolapse."

28. A primigravid woman comes to the clinic for her initial prenatal visit. She is at 32 weeks' gestation and says that she has just moved from out of state. The client says that she has had periodic headaches during her pregnancy, and that she is continually bumping into things. The nurse notes numerous bruises in various stages of healing around the client's breasts and abdomen. Vital signs are: BP 120/80, pulse 72, resp 18, and FHT 142. Which of the following responses by the nurse is *BEST*?

    1. "Are you battered by your partner?"

    2. "How do you feel about being pregnant?"

    3. "Tell me about your headaches."

    4. "You may be more clumsy due to your size."

29. The nurse is teaching a class on natural family planning. Which of the following statements by a client indicates that teaching has been successful?

   1. "When I ovulate, my basal body temperature will be elevated for 2 days and then will decrease."

   2. "My cervical mucus will be thick, cloudy, and sticky when I ovulate."

   3. "Because I am regular, I will be fertile about 14 days after the beginning of my period."

   4. "When I ovulate, my cervix will feel firm."

30. The home care nurse plans care for a child in a leg cast for treatment of a fractured right ankle. The nurse enters the following nursing diagnosis on the care plan: skin integrity, risk for impaired. Which of the following actions by the nurse is BEST?

   1. Teaching the child how to perform isometric exercises of the right leg

   2. Teaching the mother to gently massage the child's right foot with emollient cream

   3. Instructing the mother to keep the leg cast clean and dry

   4. Teaching the mother how to turn and position the child

31. The nurse is caring for a client who had a thyroidectomy 12 hours ago for treatment of Graves' disease. The nurse would be MOST concerned if which of the following was observed?

   1. The client's blood pressure is 138/82, pulse 84, respirations 16, oral temp 99° F (37.2° C).

   2. The client supports his head and neck when turning his head to the right.

   3. The client spontaneously flexes his wrist when the blood pressure is obtained.

4. The client is drowsy and complains of a sore throat.

32. A client is admitted with complaints of severe pain in the right lower quadrant of the abdomen. To assist with pain relief, the nurse should take which of the following actions?

   1. Encourage the client to change positions frequently in bed.

   2. Massage the right lower quadrant of the abdomen.

   3. Apply warmth to the abdomen with a heating pad.

   4. Use comfort measures and pillows to position the client.

33. The nurse prepares a client for peritoneal dialysis. Which of the following actions should the nurse take FIRST?

   1. Assess for a bruit and a thrill.

   2. Warm the dialysate solution.

   3. Position the client on the left side.

   4. Insert a Foley catheter.

34. The nurse teaches an elderly client with right-sided weakness how to use a cane. Which of the following behaviors by the client indicates that the teaching was effective?

   1. The client holds the cane with his right hand, moves the cane forward followed by the right leg, and then moves the left leg.

   2. The client holds the cane with his right hand, moves the cane forward followed by his left leg, and then moves the right leg.

   3. The client holds the cane with his left hand, moves the cane forward followed by the right leg, and then moves the left leg.

   4. The client holds the cane with his left hand, moves the cane forward followed by his left leg, and then moves the right leg.

35. While caring for a client receiving total parenteral nutrition (TPN) through a central line, the nurse notices a small trickle of opaque fluid leaking from around the central line dressing. It is *MOST* important for the nurse to take which of the following actions?

   1. Prepare to change the central line dressing.
   2. Verify that the client is on antibiotics.
   3. Place the client's head lower than his feet.
   4. Secure the Y-port where the lipids are infusing.

36. A 46-year-old man is admitted to the hospital with a fractured right femur. He is placed in balanced suspension traction with a Thomas splint and Pearson attachment. During the first 48 hours, the nurse should assess the client for which of the following complications?

   1. Pulmonary embolism
   2. Fat embolism
   3. Avascular necrosis
   4. Malunion

37. The nurse is helping an NAP provide a bed bath to a comatose client who is incontinent. The nurse should intervene if which of the following actions is noted?

   1. The NAP answers the phone while wearing gloves.
   2. The NAP log-rolls the client to provide back care.
   3. The NAP places an incontinence diaper under the client.
   4. The NAP positions the client on the left side, head elevated.

38. A 70-year-old woman is brought to the emergency room for treatment after being found on the floor by her daughter. X-rays reveal a displaced subcapital fracture of the left hip and osteoarthritis. When comparing the legs, the nurse would most likely make which of the following observations?

   1. The client's left leg is longer than the right leg and externally rotated.
   2. The client's left leg is shorter than the right leg and internally rotated.
   3. The client's left leg is shorter than the right leg and adducted. ✓
   4. The client's left leg is longer than the right leg and is abducted.

39. The nurse is caring for a client with a cast on the left leg. The nurse would be *MOST* concerned if which of the following is observed?

   1. Capillary refill time is less than 3 seconds
   2. Client complains of discomfort and itching
   3. Client complains of tightness and pain
   4. Client's foot is elevated on a pillow

40. The nurse is discharging a client from an inpatient alcohol treatment unit. Which of the following statements by the client's wife indicates to the nurse that the family is coping adaptively?

   1. "My husband will do well as long as I keep him engaged in activities that he likes."
   2. "My focus is learning how to live my life."
   3. "I am so glad that our problems are behind us."
   4. "I'll make sure that the children don't give my husband any problems."

41. A nurse is caring for clients in the mental health clinic. A woman comes to the clinic complaining of insomnia and anorexia. The client tearfully tells the nurse that she was laid off from a job that she had held for 15 years. Which of the following responses by the nurse would be *MOST* appropriate?

   1. "Did your company give you a severance package?"
   2. "Focus on the fact that you have a healthy, happy family."
   3. "Tell me what happened."
   4. "Losing a job is common nowadays."

42. A client with a history of alcoholism is brought to the emergency room in an agitated state. He is vomiting and diaphoretic. He says he had his last drink 5 hours ago. The nurse would expect to administer which of the following medications?

   1. Chlordiazepoxide hydrochloride (Librium)
   2. Disulfiram (Antabuse)
   3. Methadone hydrochloride (Dolophine)
   4. Naloxone hydrochloride (Narcan)

43. An elderly client is admitted to the nursing home setting. The client is occasionally confused and her gait is often unsteady. Which of the following actions by the nurse would be *MOST* appropriate?

   1. Ask the woman's family to provide personal items such as photos or mementos.
   2. Select a room with a bed by the door so the woman can look down the hall.
   3. Suggest the woman eat her meals in the room with her roommate.
   4. Encourage the woman to ambulate in the halls twice a day.

44. The nurse teaches an elderly client how to use a standard aluminum walker. Which of the following behaviors by the client indicates that the nurse's teaching was effective?

   1. The client slowly pushes the walker forward 12 inches, then takes small steps forward while leaning on the walker.
   2. The client lifts the walker, moves it forward 10 inches, and then takes several small steps forward.
   3. The client supports his weight on the walker while advancing it forward, then takes small steps while balancing on the walker.
   4. The client slides the walker 18 inches forward, then takes small steps while holding onto the walker for balance.

45. A nurse is supervising a group of elderly clients in a residential home setting. The nurse knows that the elderly are at greater risk of developing sensory deprivation for which of the following reasons?

   1. Increased sensitivity to the side effects of medications
   2. Decreased visual, auditory, and gustatory abilities
   3. Isolation from their families and familiar surroundings
   4. Decreased musculoskeletal function and mobility

46. After receiving report, the nurse should see which of the following clients *FIRST?*

   1. A 14-year-old client in sickle-cell crisis with an infiltrated IV
   2. A 59-year-old client with leukemia who has received half of a packed red blood cell transfusion
   3. A 68-year-old client scheduled for a bronchoscopy

4. A 74-year-old client complaining of a leaky colostomy bag

47. The home care nurse is visiting a client with a diagnosis of hepatitis of unknown etiology. The nurse knows that teaching has been successful if the client makes which of the following statements?

1. "I am so sad that I am not able to hold my baby."

2. "I will eat after my family eats."

3. "I will make sure that my children don't use my eating utensils or drinking glasses."

4. "I'm glad that I don't have to get help taking care of my children."

48. The nurse calculates the IV flow rate for a postoperative client. The client is to receive 3,000 mL of Ringer's lactate solution IV to run over 24 hours. The IV infusion set has a drop factor of 10 drops per milliliter. The nurse should regulate the client's IV to deliver how many drops per minute?

1. 18
2. 21
3. 35
4. 40

$$\frac{3000\,mL}{24\,hr} \times \frac{10\,drops}{mL} \times \frac{1\,hr}{60\,min}$$

$$21\,drops/min$$

49. A client with emphysema becomes restless and confused. Which of the following steps should the nurse take next?

1. Encourage the client to perform pursed-lip breathing.

2. Check the client's temperature.

3. Assess the client's potassium level.

4. Increase the client's oxygen flow rate to 5 L/min.

50. The nurse is caring for a client 1 day after an abdominal-perineal resection for cancer of the rectum. The nurse should question which of the following orders?

1. Discontinue the nasogastric tube when bowel sounds are heard. Yes!

2. Irrigate the colostomy.

3. Place petrolatum gauze over the stoma.

4. Administer meperidine (Demerol) 50 mg IM for pain.

51. The nurse is caring for a client 4 hours after intracranial surgery. Which of the following actions should the nurse take immediately?

1. Turn, cough, and deep-breathe the client.

2. Place the client with the neck flexed and head turned to the side.

3. Perform passive range-of-motion exercises.

4. Move the client to the head of the bed using a turning sheet.

52. A 6-year-old child with a congenital heart disorder is admitted with congestive heart failure. Digoxin (Lanoxin) 0.12 mg is ordered for the child. The bottle of Lanoxin contains 0.05 mg of Lanoxin in 1 mL of solution. Which of the following amounts should the nurse administer to the child?

1. 1.2 mL
2. 2.4 mL
3. 3.5 mL
4. 4.2 mL

$$0.12\,mg \times \frac{1\,mL}{0.05\,mg}$$

53. The nurse is caring for a client with chest pain in the Emergency Department. Which of the following laboratory findings would MOST concern the nurse?

1. Erythrocyte sedimentation rate (ESR): 10 mm/hr

[handwritten: pernicious anemia — faulty absorption of vit. B12]

2. Hematocrit (Hct): 42%

3. Creatine phosphokinase-MB (CK-MB): 4 ng/mL

4. Serum glucose: 100 mg/dL

54. The nurse is caring for a client with cervical cancer. The nurse notes that the radium implant has become dislodged. Which of the following actions should the nurse take *FIRST*?

   1. Grasp the implant with a sterile hemostat and carefully reinsert it into the client.

   2. Wrap the implant in a blanket and place it behind a lead shield.

   3. Ensure the implant is picked up with long-handled forceps and placed in a lead container.

   4. Obtain a dosimeter reading on the client and report it to the physician.

55. The nurse in a primary care clinic is caring for a 68-year-old man. History reveals that the client has smoked 1 pack of cigarettes per day for 45 years and drinks 2 beers per day. He is complaining of a nonproductive cough, chest discomfort, and dyspnea. The nurse hears isolated wheezing in the right middle lobe. It would be *MOST* important for the nurse to complete which of the following orders?

   1. Pulmonary function tests

   2. Echocardiogram

   3. Chest x-ray

   4. Sputum culture

56. The nurse is caring for a client with pernicious anemia. The nurse knows that her teaching has been successful if the client makes which of the following statements?

   1. "In order to get better, I will take iron pills."

   2. "I am going to attend smoking cessation classes."

   3. "I will learn how to perform IM injections."

   4. "I will increase my intake of carbohydrates."

57. The nurse is caring for clients in the Emergency Department of an acute care facility. Four clients have been admitted in the last 20 minutes. Which of the following admissions should the nurse see *FIRST*?

   1. A client complaining of chest pain that is unrelieved by nitroglycerin

   2. A client with third-degree burns to the face *[handwritten: airway precaution due to swelling]*

   3. A client with a fractured left hip

   4. A client complaining of epigastric pain

58. The nurse is caring for a client with a diagnosis of COPD, bronchitis-type, in the long-term care facility. The client is wheezing, and his oxygen saturation is 85%. Four hours ago, the oxygen saturation was 88%. It is *MOST* important for the nurse to take which of the following actions?

   1. Administer beclomethasone (Vanceril), 2 puffs per metered-dose inhaler.

   2. Listen to breath sounds.

   3. Increase oxygen to 4 L per mask.

   4. Administer albuterol (Proventil), 2 puffs per metered-dose inhaler.

59. The nurse is caring for a client hospitalized for observation after a fall. The client states, "My friend fell last year, and no one thought anything was wrong. She died 2 days later!" Which of the following responses by the nurse is *BEST*?

   1. "This happens to quite a few people."

   2. "We are monitoring you, so you'll be okay."

   3. "Don't you think I'm taking good care of you?"

4. "You're concerned that it might happen to you?"

60. The nurse is caring for clients on the pediatric unit. An 8-year-old client with second- and third-degree burns on the right thigh is being admitted. The nurse should assign the new client to which of the following roommates?

    1. A 2-year-old with chickenpox
    2. A 4-year-old with asthma
    3. A 9-year-old with acute diarrhea
    4. A 10-year-old with methicillin-resistant *Staphylococcus aureus* (MRSA)

61. The nurse teaches a client about elastic stockings. Which of the following statements by the client indicates to the nurse that teaching was successful?

    1. "I will wear the stockings until the physician tells me to remove them."
    2. "I should wear the stockings even when I am asleep."
    3. "Every 4 hours I should remove the stockings for a half hour."
    4. "I should put on the stockings before getting out of bed in the morning."

62. The nurse is teaching a client who is scheduled for a paracentesis. Which of the following statements by the client to the nurse indicates that teaching has been successful?

    1. "I will be in surgery for less than an hour."
    2. "I must not void prior to the procedure."
    3. "The physician will remove 2 to 3 liters of fluid."
    4. "I will lie on my back and breathe slowly."

63. The home care nurse is performing chest physiotherapy on an elderly client with chronic airflow limitations (CAL). Which of the following actions should the nurse take FIRST?

    1. Perform chest physiotherapy prior to meals.
    2. Auscultate the chest prior to beginning the procedure.
    3. Administer bronchiodilators after the procedure.
    4. Percuss each lobe prior to asking the client to cough.

64. A client is admitted to the hospital with a diagnosis of chronic bronchitis. He has a 10-year history of emphysema. The nurse should place him in which of the following positions?

    1. Side-lying
    2. Supine
    3. High Fowler's
    4. Semi-Fowler's

65. A client is to receive 1,000 mL of 5% dextrose in 0.45 NaCl intravenous solution in an 8-hour period. The intravenous set delivers 15 drops per milliliter. The nurse should regulate the flow rate so it delivers how many drops of fluid per minute?

    1. 15
    2. 31
    3. 45
    4. 60

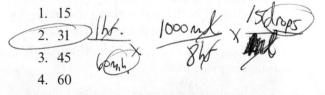

66. The nurse knows that the plan of care for a client with severe liver disease should include which of the following actions?

    1. Administer Kayexelate enemas.
    2. Offer a low-protein, high-carbohydrate diet.
    3. Insert a Sengsteken-Blakemore tube.

4. Administer salt-poor albumin IV.

67. A client with a diagnosis of delirium is admitted to the hospital. To evaluate the cause of a client's delirium, blood is sent to the laboratory for analysis. The results are as follows: Na^+ 156, Cl^- 100, K^+ 4.0, HCO_3 21, BUN 86, glucose 100. Based on these laboratory results, the nurse should record which of the following nursing diagnoses on the client's care plan?

1. Alteration in patterns of urinary elimination
2. Fluid volume deficit
3. Nutritional deficit: less than body requirements
4. Self-care deficit: feeding

68. A client is to receive 3,000 mL of 0.9% NaCl IV in 24 hours. The intravenous set delivers 15 drops per milliliter. The nurse should regulate the flow rate so that the client receives how many drops of fluid per minute?

$$\frac{3000\,mL}{24\,hr} \times \frac{1\,hr}{60\,min} \times \frac{15\,drops}{mL}$$

1. 21
2. 28
3. 31
4. 42

69. The nurse is supervising the care of a client receiving TPN through a single-lumen percutaneous central catheter. The nurse would be MOST concerned if which of the following was observed?

1. The client receives insulin through the single-lumen catheter.
2. A mask is placed on the client when changing the client's dressing.
3. The client's dressing is changed daily using sterile technique.
4. The client is weighed 2 to 3 times per week.

Don't change a central line dressing daily — only 1 to 2 times per week + PRN

70. *Guillaume - Barré syndrome* The nurse is caring for clients in the outpatient clinic. A client tells the nurse that he developed weakness and numbness in the legs the previous day and now his body feels the same way. The client's vital signs are: BP 120/60, pulse 86, and resp 20. The client denies any pain but appears anxious to the nurse. It would be MOST important for the nurse to ask which of the following questions?

1. "Have you recently fallen or had some other type of physical injury?"
2. "Have you recently had a viral infection, such as a cold?"
3. "Have you recently taken any over-the-counter medication?"
4. "Have you recently experienced headaches?"

71. The nurse is admitting a client who is jaundiced due to pancreatic cancer. The nurse should give the HIGHEST priority to which of the following needs?

1. Nutrition *— Due to profound weight loss + anorexia*
2. Self-image
3. Skin integrity
4. Urinary elimination

72. Which of the following statements by a client during a group therapy session would the nurse identify as reflecting a client's narcissistic personality disorder?

1. "I'm sick of hearing about all your life tragedies." *(lack of empathy)*
2. "I know I'm interrupting others. So what?"
3. "I just can't stop wanting to slash myself."
4. "I just have no hope for the future."

73. A teenage client is admitted to the hospital with anorexia nervosa. Which of the following statements by the client requires immediate follow-up by the nurse?

    1. "My gums were bleeding this morning."
    2. "I'm getting fatter every day."
    3. "Nobody likes me because I'm so ugly."
    4. "I'm feeling dizzy and weak today."

74. A client is admitted to the hospital for treatment of *Pneumocystis jiroveci* pneumonia and Kaposi's sarcoma. The client tells the nurse that he has been considering organ donation when he dies. Which of the following responses by the nurse is *BEST*?

    1. "What does your family think about your decision?"
    2. "You will help many people by donating your organs."
    3. "Would you like to speak to the organ donor representative?"
    4. "That is not possible based on your illness."

75. The nurse is caring for a client 5 hours after a pancreatectomy for cancer of the pancreas. On assessment, the nurse notes that there is minimal drainage from the nasogastric (NG) tube. It is *MOST* important for the nurse to take which of the following actions?

    1. Notify the physician.
    2. Monitor vital signs q 15 minutes.
    3. Check the tubing for kinks.
    4. Replace the NG tube.

76. When collecting a 24-hour urine specimen for creatinine clearance, it is *MOST* important for the nurse to do which of the following?

    1. Obtain an order from the physician for insertion of a Foley catheter.
    2. Obtain the client's weight prior to beginning the urine collection.
    3. Discard the last voided specimen prior to ending the collection.
    4. Ask if a preservative is present in the container.

77. The nurse is planning discharge teaching for a client with Parkinson's disease. To maintain safety, the nurse should make which of the following suggestions to the family?

    1. Install a raised toilet seat.
    2. Obtain a hospital bed.
    3. Instruct the client to hold his arms in a dependent position when ambulating.
    4. Perform an exercise program during the late afternoon.

78. The nurse is performing discharge teaching for a client with chronic pancreatitis. Which of the following statements by the client to the nurse indicates that further teaching is necessary?

    1. "I do not have to restrict my physical activity."
    2. "I should take pancrelipase (Viokase) before meals."
    3. "I will eat 3 meals per day." Small frequent meals preferred
    4. "I am not allowed to drink any alcoholic beverages."

79. After a laparoscopic cholecystectomy, the client complains of abdominal pain and bloating. Which of the following responses by the nurse is *BEST*?

    1. "Increase your intake of fresh fruits and vegetables."
    2. "I'll give you the prescribed pain medication."

3. "Why don't you take a walk in the hallway."

4. "You may need an indwelling catheter."

80. The nurse in an outpatient clinic is supervising student nurses administering influenza vaccinations. The nurse should question the administration of the vaccine to which of the following clients?

1. A 45-year-old male who is allergic to shellfish

2. A 60-year-old female who says she has a sore throat

3. A 66-year-old female who lives in a group home

4. A 70-year-old female with congestive heart failure

81. An arterial blood gas is ordered for a man after a myocardial infarction. After obtaining the specimen, it would be *MOST* appropriate for the nurse to take which of the following actions?

1. Obtain ice for the specimen.

2. Apply direct pressure to the site.

3. Apply a sterile dressing to the site.

4. Observe the site for hematoma formation.

82. The nurse is caring for a man who was involved in an auto accident the previous day. The client has a double-lumen tracheostomy tube with a cuff. Which of the following actions should the nurse perform?

1. Change the tracheostomy dressing every 8 hours and PRN.

2. Change the tracheostomy ties every 48 hours.

3. Keep the inner cannula of the tracheostomy in place at all times.

4. Push the outer cannula back in if it accidentally "blows out."

83. The nurse performs discharge teaching with a client with emphysema. Which statement by the client indicates that teaching was successful?

1. "Cold weather will help my breathing problems."

2. "I should eat 3 balanced meals but limit my fluid intake."

3. "My outside activity should be limited when pollution levels are high."

4. "An intensive exercise program is important in regaining my strength."

84. The nurse assists the physician with the removal of a chest tube. Before the physician removes the chest tube, which instruction should the nurse give to the client?

1. "Exhale and bear down."

2. "Hold your breath for 5 seconds."

3. "Inhale and exhale rapidly."

4. "Cough as hard as you can."

85. A client comes into the emergency room with complaints of sudden onset of severe right flank pain. While tests are being performed, it is *MOST* important for the nurse to take which of the following actions?

1. Make sure that he does not eat or drink anything.

2. Strain all his urine through several layers of gauze.

3. Check his grip strength and pupil reactivity.

4. Send blood and urine specimens to the lab for analysis.

86. The nurse is preparing discharge teaching for a client with a new colostomy. The nurse knows teaching was successful when the client chooses which of the following menu options?

1. Sausage, sauerkraut, baked potato, and fresh fruit
2. Cheese omelet with bran muffin and fresh pineapple
3. Pork chop, mashed potatoes, turnips, and salad
4. Baked chicken, boiled potato, cooked carrots, and yogurt

87. A client is seen in the outpatient clinic to rule out acute renal failure. The nurse would be *MOST* concerned if the client made which of the following statements?

1. "My urine is often pink-tinged."
2. "It is hard for me to start the flow of urine."
3. "It is quite painful for me to urinate."
4. "I urinate in the morning and again before dinner."

88. The nurse is teaching a new mother how to breastfeed her newborn. The nurse knows that teaching has been successful if the client makes which of the following statements?

1. "My baby's weight should equal her birthweight in 5 to 7 days."
2. "My baby should have at least 6 to 8 wet diapers per day."
3. "My baby will sleep at least 6 hours between feedings."
4. "My baby will feed for about 10 minutes per feeding."

89. A man is admitted to the telemetry unit for evaluation of complaints of chest pain. Eight hours after admission, the client goes into ventricular fibrillation. The physician defibrillates the client. The nurse understands that the purpose of defibrillation is to do which of the following?

1. Increase cardiac contractility and cardiac output.
2. Cause asystole so the normal pacemaker can recapture.
3. Reduce cardiac ischemia and acidosis.
4. Provide energy for depleted myocardial cells.

90. A man is brought to the emergency room complaining of chest pain. The nurse performs an assessment of the client. Which of the following symptoms would be *MOST* characteristic of an acute myocardial infarction?

1. Colic-like epigastric pain
2. Sharp, well-localized, unilateral chest pain
3. Severe substernal pain radiating down the left arm
4. Sharp, burning chest pain moving from place to place

91. The nurse is caring for clients on the medical unit. A client is admitted with a diagnosis of deep vein thrombosis (DVT). Admission orders include heparin 2,000 units per hour in 5% dextrose in water. The nurse should have which of the following available?

1. Propranolol (Inderal)
2. Protamine zinc
3. Protamine sulfate
4. Vitamin K

92. A client returns to the clinic 2 weeks after discharge from the hospital. He is taking warfarin sodium (Coumadin) 2 mg PO daily. Which of the following statements by the client to the nurse indicates that further teaching is necessary?

1. "I have been taking an antihistamine before bed."

2. "I take aspirin when I have a headache."

3. "I use sunscreen when I go outside."

4. "I take Mylanta if my stomach gets upset."

93. To enhance the percutaneous absorption of nitroglycerin ointment, it would be *MOST* important for the nurse to select a site that is which of the following?

1. Muscular

2. Near the heart

3. Non-hairy

4. Over a bony prominence

94. A client with chronic alcohol abuse has been admitted to a rehabilitation unit. The nurse knows that the client is denying alcoholism when he makes which of the following statements?

1. "My brother did this to me."

2. "Drinking always calms my nerves."

3. "I can stop drinking anytime I feel like it."

4. "Let's all plan to play cards tonight."

95. During the acute phase of a cerebrovascular accident (CVA), the nurse should maintain the client in which of the following positions?

1. Semi-prone with the head of the bed elevated 60–90 degrees

2. Lateral, with the head of the bed flat

3. Prone, with the head of the bed flat

4. Supine, with the head of the bed elevated 30–45 degrees

96. Which of the following statements by a client during a group therapy session requires immediate follow-up by the nurse?

1. "I know I'm a chronically compulsive liar, but I can't help it."

2. "I don't ever want to go home; I feel safer here."

3. "I don't really care if I ever see my girlfriend again."

4. "I'll make sure that doctor is sorry for what he said."

97. A client newly diagnosed with Alzheimer's disease is admitted to the unit. Which of the following actions by the nurse is *BEST?*

1. Place the client in a private room away from the nurses' station.

2. Ask the family to wait in the waiting room while the nurse admits the client.

3. Assign a different nurse daily to care for the client.

4. Ask the client to state today's date.

98. A female client visits the clinic with complaints of right calf tenderness and pain. It would be *MOST* important for the nurse to ask which of the following questions?

1. "Do you exercise excessively?"

2. "Have you had any fractures in the last year?"

3. "What type of birth control do you use?"

4. "Are you under a lot of stress?"

99. A mother calls the well-baby clinic to report that her 4-month-old son has an upper respiratory infection (URI) with a temperature of 104° F (40° C). The infant is scheduled to receive his DPT and TOPV immunizations later that day. The mother asks the nurse if she should bring him in for his scheduled immunizations. Which of the following responses by the nurse would be *MOST* appropriate?

1. "Keep him at home. We'll give him a double dose next time."

2. "Bring him in. His illness will not interfere with his immunizations."

3. "Keep him at home until his temperature and infection resolve."

4. "Bring him in. We'll give some antibiotics with the immunizations."

100. The nurse in the postpartum unit cares for a client who delivered her first child the previous day. During her assessment of the client, the nurse notes multiple varicosities on the client's lower extremities. Which of the following actions should the nurse perform?

1. Teach the client to rest in bed when the baby sleeps.

2. Encourage early and frequent ambulation.

3. Apply warm soaks for 20 minutes every 4 hours.

4. Perform passive range-of-motion exercises 3 times daily.

101. A man fractures his left femur in a bicycle accident. A cast is applied. The nurse knows that which of the following exercises would be MOST beneficial for this client?

1. Passive exercise of the affected limb

2. Quadriceps setting of the affected limb

3. Active range-of-motion exercises of the unaffected limb

4. Passive exercise of the upper extremities

102. The nurse plans care for a client receiving electroconvulsive treatments (ECT). Immediately after a treatment, the nurse should take which of the following actions?

1. Orient the client to time and place.

2. Talk about events prior to the client's hospitalization.

3. Restrict fluid intake and encourage the client to ambulate.

4. Initiate comfort measures to relieve vertigo.

103. A client is to receive 35 mg/hr of intravenous aminophylline. The nurse mixes 350 mg of aminophylline in 500 mL D₅W. At which of the following rates should the nurse infuse this solution?

1. 20 mL/hr

2. 35 mL/hr

3. 50 mL/hr

4. 70 mL/hr

104. The nurse prepares an adult client for instillation of eardrops. The nurse should use which of the following methods to administer the eardrops?

1. Cool the solution for better adsorption. Drop the medication directly into the auditory canal.

2. Warm the solution. Flush the medication rapidly into the ear.

3. Warm the solution. Drop the medication along the side of the ear canal.

4. Warm the solution to 104° F (40° C). Drop the medication slowly into the ear canal.

105. The nurse is inserting an IV catheter into a client's left arm. Suddenly the client exclaims, "It feels like an electric shock is going all the way down my arm and into my hand!" What is the FIRST action the nurse should take?

1. Instruct the client to take slow, deep breaths.

2. Remove the needle from the client's arm.

3. Tell the client this is a common response to IV insertion.

4. Withdraw the needle slightly and then push it forward.

106. A client comes to the emergency room with complaints of nausea, vomiting, and abdominal pain. He is a type 1 diabetic (IDDM). Four days earlier, he reduced his insulin dose when flu symptoms prevented him from eating. The nurse performs an assessment of the client that reveals poor skin turgor, dry mucous membranes, and fruity breath odor. The nurse should be alert for which of the following problems?

1. Hypoglycemia
2. Viral illness
3. Ketoacidosis
4. Hyperglycemic hyperosmolar nonketotic coma

107. The nurse knows that it is *MOST* important for which of the following clients to receive their scheduled medication on time?

1. A client diagnosed with myasthenia gravis receiving pyridostigmine bromide (Mestinon)
2. A client diagnosed with bipolar disorder receiving lithium carbonate (Lithobid)
3. A client diagnosed with tuberculosis receiving isonicotinic acid hydrazide (INH)
4. A client diagnosed with Parkinson's disease receiving levodopa (L-dopa)

108. An 11-year-old boy is admitted to the hospital for evaluation for a kidney transplant. During the initial assessment, the nurse learns that the client received hemodialysis for 3 years due to renal failure. The nurse knows that his illness can interfere with this client's achievement of which of the following?

1. Intimacy
2. Trust
3. Industry
4. Identity

109. The nurse assesses a client with a history of Addison's disease who has received steroid therapy for several years. The nurse could expect the client to exhibit which of the following changes in appearance?

1. Buffalo hump, girdle-obesity, gaunt facial appearance
2. Tanning of the skin, discoloration of the mucous membranes, alopecia, weight loss
3. Emaciation, nervousness, breast engorgement, hirsutism
4. Truncal obesity, purple striations on the skin, moon face

110. Haloperidol (Haldol) 5 mg tid is ordered for a client with schizophrenia. Two days later, the client complains of "tight jaws and a stiff neck." The nurse should recognize that these complaints are which of the following?

1. Common side effects of antipsychotic medications that will diminish over time
2. Early symptoms of extrapyramidal reactions to the medication
3. Psychosomatic complaints resulting from a delusional system
4. Permanent side effects of Haldol

111. The nurse is caring for a woman who states she was beaten and sexually assaulted by a male friend. Which of the following should the nurse do *FIRST*?

1. Encourage the client to call her family lawyer.
2. Ask for a psychiatry consult.

3. Stay with the client during the physical exam.

4. Wash and dress the client's wounds before the physical exam.

112. The nurse cares for a client after surgery for removal of a cataract in her right eye. The client complains of severe eye pain in her right eye. The nurse knows this symptom is which of the following?

1. Expected; the nurse should administer analgesic to the client.

2. Expected; the nurse should maintain the client on bed rest.

3. Unexpected and may signify a detached retina.

4. Unexpected and may signify hemorrhage.

113. A client returns to his room after a lower GI series. When he is assessed by the nurse, he complains of weakness. Which of the following nursing diagnoses should receive priority in planning his care?

1. Alteration in sensation-perception, gustatory

2. Constipation, colonic

3. High risk for fluid-volume deficit

4. Nutrition: less than body requirements

114. A client hospitalized with a gastric ulcer is scheduled for discharge. The nurse teaches the client about an anti-ulcer diet. Which of the following statements by the client indicates to the nurse that dietary teaching was successful?

1. "I must eat bland foods to help my stomach heal."

2. "I can eat most foods, as long as they don't bother my stomach."

3. "I cannot eat fruits and vegetables because they cause too much gas."

4. "I should eat a low-fiber diet to delay gastric emptying."

115. A 6-year-old boy is returned to his room after a tonsillectomy. He remains sleepy from the anesthesia but is easily awakened. The nurse should place the child in which of the following positions?

1. Sims' — for rectal or vaginal exam/action.

2. Side-lying

3. Supine

4. Prone

116. A client is preparing to take her 1-day-old infant home from the hospital. The nurse discusses the test for phenylketonuria (PKU) with the mother. The nurse's teaching should be based on an understanding that the test is MOST reliable after which of the following?

1. A source of protein has been ingested.

2. The meconium has been excreted.

3. The danger of hyperbilirubinemia has passed.

4. The effects of delivery have subsided.

117. The nurse is completing a client's preoperative checklist prior to an early morning surgery. The nurse obtains the client's vital signs: temperature 97.4° F (36° C), radial pulse 84 strong and regular, respirations 16 and unlabored, and blood pressure 132/74. Which of the following actions should the nurse take FIRST?

1. Notify the physician of the client's vital signs.

2. Obtain orthostatic blood pressures lying and standing.

3. Lower the side rails and place the bed in its lowest position.

4. Record the data on the client's preoperative checklist.

118. A woman is hospitalized with a diagnosis of bipolar disorder. While she is in the client activities room on the psychiatric unit, she flirts with male clients and disrupts unit activities. Which of the following approaches would be *MOST* appropriate for the nurse to take at this time?

    1. Set limits on the client's behavior and remind her of the rules.

    2. Distract the client and escort her back to her room.

    3. Instruct the other clients to ignore this client's behavior.

    4. Tell the client that she is behaving inappropriately and send her to her room.

119. A client is brought to the emergency room bleeding profusely from a stab wound in the left chest area. The nurse's assessment reveals a blood pressure of 80/50, pulse of 110, and respirations of 28. The nurse should expect which of the following potential problems?

    1. Hypovolemic shock
    2. Cardiogenic shock
    3. Neurogenic shock
    4. Septic shock

120. A client is admitted to the hospital for surgical repair of a detached retina in the right eye. In planning care for this client postoperatively, the nurse should encourage the client to do which of the following?

    1. Perform self-care activities.
    2. Maintain patches over both eyes.
    3. Limit movement of both eyes.
    4. Refrain from excessive talking.

121. The nurse cares for a client receiving a balanced complete food by tube feeding. The nurse knows that the *MOST* common complication of a tube feeding is which of the following?

    1. Edema
    2. Diarrhea
    3. Hypokalemia
    4. Vomiting

122. A 6-week-old infant is brought to the hospital for treatment of pyloric stenosis. The nurse enters the following nursing diagnosis on the infant's care plan: "fluid volume deficit related to vomiting." Which of the following assessments supports this diagnosis?

    1. The infant eagerly accepts feedings.

    2. The infant vomited once since admission.

    3. The infant's skin is warm and moist.

    4. The infant's anterior fontanel is depressed.

123. A client is diagnosed with thrombocytopenia due to acute lymphocytic leukemia. She is admitted to the hospital for treatment. To which of the following should the nurse assign the client?

    1. To a private room so she will not infect other clients and health care workers

    2. To a private room so she will not be infected by other clients and health care workers

    3. To a semiprivate room so she will have stimulation during her hospitalization

    4. To a semiprivate room so she will have the opportunity to express her feelings about her illness

124. A woman comes to the clinic because she thinks she is pregnant. Tests are performed and the pregnancy is confirmed. The client's last menstrual period began on September 8 and lasted for 6 days. The nurse calculates that her expected date of confinement (EDC) is which of the following?

    1. May 15
    2. June 15
    3. June 21
    4. July 8

125. A 2-month-old infant is brought to the pediatrician's office for a well-baby visit. During the examination, congenital subluxation of the left hip is suspected. The nurse would expect to see which of the following symptoms?

    1. Lengthening of the limb on the affected side
    2. Deformities of the foot and ankle
    3. Asymmetry of the gluteal and thigh folds
    4. Plantar flexion of the foot

126. After 2 weeks of receiving lithium therapy, a client in the psychiatric unit becomes depressed. Which of the following evaluations of the client's behavior by the nurse would be *MOST* accurate?

    1. The treatment plan is not effective; the client requires a larger dose of lithium.
    2. This is a normal response to lithium therapy; the client should continue with the current treatment plan.
    3. This is a normal response to lithium therapy; the client should be monitored for suicidal behavior.
    4. The treatment plan is not effective; the client requires an antidepressant.

127. A client is admitted for treatment of pulmonary edema. During the admission interview, she states she has a 6-year history of congestive heart failure (CHF). The nurse performs an initial assessment. When the nurse auscultates the breath sounds, the nurse should expect to hear which of the following?

    1. Crackling
    2. Wheezing
    3. Whistling
    4. Absent breath sounds

128. A man is diagnosed with cancer of the larynx and comes to the hospital for a total laryngectomy. When admitting this client, the nurse should assess laryngeal nerve function by doing which of the following?

    1. Assess the extent of neck edema.
    2. Check his ability to swallow.
    3. Observe for excessive drooling.
    4. Tap the side of his neck gently and observe for facial twitching.

129. The nurse supervises care at an adult day-care center. Four meal choices are available to the residents. The nurse should ensure that a resident on a low-cholesterol diet receives which of the following meals?

    1. Egg custard and boiled liver
    2. Fried chicken and potatoes
    3. Hamburger and french fries
    4. Grilled flounder and green beans

130. The nurse cares for a client with a possible bowel obstruction. A nasogastric (NG) tube is to be inserted. Before inserting the tube, the nurse explains its purpose to the client. Which of the following explanations by the nurse is *MOST* accurate?

1. "It empties the stomach of fluids and gas."

2. "It prevents spasms of the sphincter of Oddi."

3. "It prevents air from forming in the small and large intestine."

4. "It removes bile from the gallbladder."

131. The nurse cares for a client diagnosed with cholecystitis. The client says to the nurse, "I don't understand why my right shoulder hurts, when the gallbladder is not near my shoulder!" Which of the following responses by the nurse is *BEST*?

1. "Sometimes small pieces of the gallstones break off and travel to other parts of the body."

2. "There is an invisible connection between the gallbladder and the right shoulder."

3. "The gallbladder is on the right side of the body and so is that shoulder."

4. "Your shoulder became tense because you were guarding against the gallbladder pain."

132. The nurse teaches a primigravid woman how to measure the frequency of uterine contractions. The nurse should explain to the client that the frequency of uterine contractions is determined by which of the following?

1. By timing from the beginning of one contraction to the end of the next contraction

2. By timing from the beginning of one contraction to the end of the same contraction

3. By the number of contractions that occur within a given period of time

4. By the strength of the contraction at its peak

133. The nurse is teaching a woman who is receiving estrogen replacement therapy. Which of the following statements by the nurse indicates that the nurse is aware of the possible complications of estrogen therapy?

1. "Take an analgesic before you take estrogen, because estrogen may cause discomfort."

2. "Make sure you keep your clinic appointments, especially your gynecologic checkup."

3. "Limit your fluid intake, because estrogen promotes the retention of fluids."

4. "Increase roughage in your diet to avoid constipation."

134. Several days after being admitted for depression, a man is observed sitting alone in the clients' dining room. The nurse notes that the client has not finished his meal. Which of the following nursing measures would be *MOST* appropriate?

1. Allow the client to eat in his room until he becomes more comfortable eating with other clients.

2. Ask the client's family to bring foods that he likes to eat.

3. Order small, frequent meals and sit with the client while he eats in the dining room.

4. Do not focus on eating behaviors because his appetite will improve over time.

135. A client is being treated for injuries sustained in an automobile accident. The client has a central venous pressure (CVP) line in place. The nurse recognizes that CVP measurement reflects which of the following?

1. Cardiac output

2. Pressure in the left ventricle

3. Pressure in the right atrium

4. Pressure in the pulmonary artery

136. A mother brings her 4-year-old daughter to the pediatrician for treatment of chronic otitis media. The mother asks the nurse how she can prevent her child from getting ear infections so often. The nurse's response should be based on an understanding that the recurrence of otitis media can be decreased by which of the following?

   1. Covering the child's ears while bathing

   2. Treating upper respiratory infections quickly

   3. Administering nose drops at bedtime

   4. Isolating her child from other children

137. A client receives 10 units of NPH insulin every morning at 8 A.M. At 4 P.M., the nurse observes that the client is diaphoretic and slightly confused. The nurse should take which of the following actions FIRST?

   1. Check vital signs.

   2. Check urine for glucose and ketones.

   3. Give 6 oz. of skim milk.

   4. Call the physician.

138. Prior to the client undergoing a scheduled intravenous pyelogram (IVP), the nurse reviews the client's health history. It would be MOST important for the nurse to obtain the answer to which of the following questions?

   1. Does the client have difficulty voiding?

   2. Does the client have any allergies to shellfish or iodine?

   3. Does the client have a history of constipation?

   4. Does the client have frequent headaches?

139. A child with chickenpox (varicella) is brought by her parents to the physician for evaluation. The nurse knows the rash characteristic of chickenpox can be described as which of the following?

   1. Maculopapular

   2. Small, irregular red spots with minute bluish-white centers

   3. Round or oval erythematous scaling patches

   4. Petechiae

140. A primigravid woman at 28 weeks' gestation takes a 3-hour glucose tolerance test. The results indicate a fasting blood sugar of 100 mg/dL and a 2-hour post-load blood sugar of 300 mg/dL. Which of the following nursing diagnoses should be considered the HIGHEST priority at this time?

   1. Potential impaired family coping related to diagnosis of gestational diabetes mellitus (GDM)

   2. Potential noncompliance related to lack of knowledge or lack of adequate support system

   3. Potential for altered parenting related to disappointment

   4. Ineffective family coping related to anticipatory grieving

141. The nurse cares for a client admitted for a possible herniated intervertebral disk. Ibuprofen (Motrin), propoxyphene hydrochloride (Darvon), and cyclobenzaprine hydrochloride (Flexeril) are ordered PRN. Several hours after admission, the client complains of pain. Which of the following actions should the nurse do FIRST?

   1. Administer Motrin.

   2. Call the physician to determine which medication should be given.

3. Gather more information from the client about the complaint.

4. Allow the client some time to rest and see if the pain subsides.

142. When planning care for a client hospitalized with depression, the nurse includes measures to increase his self-esteem. Which of the following actions should the nurse take to meet this goal?

1. Encourage him to accept leadership responsibilities in milieu activities.

2. Set simple, realistic goals with him to help him experience success.

3. Help him to accept his illness and the adjustments that are required.

4. Assure him that when he is discharged, he will be able to resume his previous activities.

143. The nurse finds a visitor unconscious on the floor of a client's room during visiting hours at the hospital. Which of the following nursing assessments is consistent with cardiopulmonary arrest?

1. Absent pulse, fixed and dilated pupils

2. Absent respirations, fixed and dilated pupils

3. Absent pulse and respirations

4. Thready pulse and pupillary changes

144. A client is transferred to an extended care facility after a cerebrovascular accident (CVA). The client has right-sided paralysis and has been experiencing dysphagia. The nurse observes an aide preparing the client to eat lunch. Which of the following situations would require an intervention by the nurse?

1. The client is in bed in high Fowler's position.

2. The client's head and neck are positioned slightly forward.

3. The aide puts the food in the back of the client's mouth on the unaffected side.

4. The aide waters down the pudding to help the client swallow.

145. The home care nurse plans care for a client with pernicious anemia. A monthly intramuscular injection is ordered for the client. The nurse knows that in an adult, the best muscle to administer an intramuscular injection is which of the following?

1. Gluteus maximus

2. Deltoid

3. Vastus lateralis

4. Dorsogluteal

146. A man comes to the emergency room complaining of nausea, vomiting, and severe right upper quadrant pain. His temperature is 101.3° F (38.5° C) and an abdominal x-ray reveals an enlarged gallbladder. He is given a diagnosis of acute cholecystitis and is scheduled for surgery. After administering an analgesic to the client, the nurse recognizes that which of the following actions is the *HIGHEST* priority?

1. Assessing the client's need for dietary teaching

2. Assessing the client's fluid and electrolyte status

3. Examining the client's health history for allergies to antibiotics

4. Determining whether the client has signed consent for surgery

147. A mother with 4 children calls the clinic for advice on how to care for her oldest child, who has developed chickenpox. Which of the following statements by the mother indicates a need for further teaching?

1. "I should keep my child home from school until the vesicles are crusted."

2. "I can use calamine lotion if needed."

3. "I should remove the crusts so the skin can heal."

4. "I can use mittens if scratching becomes a problem."

148. The nurse is teaching a woman who comes to the clinic at 32 weeks' gestation with a diagnosis of pregnancy-induced hypertension (PIH). Which of the following statements by the client indicates to the nurse that further teaching is required?

   1. "Lying in bed on my left side is likely to increase my urinary output."

   2. "If the bed rest works, I may lose a pound or two in the next few days."

   3. "I should be sure to maintain a diet that has a good amount of protein."

   4. "I will have to keep my room darkened and not watch much television."

149. The nurse evaluates the care provided to a client hospitalized for treatment of adrenal crisis. Which of the following changes would indicate to the nurse that the client is responding favorably to medical and nursing treatment?

   1. The client's urinary output has increased.

   2. The client's blood pressure has increased.

   3. The client has lost weight.

   4. The client's peripheral edema has decreased.

150. After completing an assessment, the nurse determines that a client is exhibiting early symptoms of a dystonic reaction related to the use of an antipsychotic medication. Which of the following actions by the nurse would be MOST appropriate?

1. Reality-test with the cl[...] her that her physical sy[...] real.

2. Teach the client about common side effects of antipsychotic medications.

3. Explain to the client that there is no treatment that will relieve these symptoms.

4. Notify the physician and obtain an order for IM Benadryl.

151. The physician orders heparin for a client. In order to evaluate the effectiveness of the client's heparin therapy, the nurse should monitor which of the following laboratory values?

   1. Platelet count

   2. Clotting time

   3. Bleeding time

   4. Prothrombin time

152. A client comes to the clinic for evaluation of acute onset of seizures. A thorough history and physical examination is performed. The nurse would expect which of the following diagnostic tests to be performed FIRST?

   1. Magnetic resonance imaging (MRI)

   2. Cerebral angiography

   3. Electroencephalogram (EEG)

   4. Electromyogram (EMG)

153. The nurse performs dietary teaching with a client on a low-protein diet. The nurse knows that teaching has been successful if the client identifies which of the following meals as LOWEST in protein?

   1. Cranberries and broiled chicken

   2. Tomatoes and flounder

   3. Broccoli and veal

   4. Spinach and tofu

154. A client has a vagotomy with antrectomy to treat a duodenal ulcer. Postoperatively, the client develops dumping syndrome. Which of the following statements by the client indicates to the nurse that further dietary teaching is necessary?

1. "I should eat bread with each meal."

2. "I should eat smaller meals more frequently."

3. "I should lie down after eating."

4. "I should avoid drinking fluids with my meals."

155. A man is admitted to the hospital with a diagnosis of acquired immunodeficiency syndrome (AIDS). He is being treated for *Pneumocystis jiroveci* pneumonia. The nurse evaluates the care provided to this client by other members of the health care team. The nurse should intervene in which of the following situations?

1. A housekeeper cleans up spilled blood with a bleach solution.

2. A nursing student takes his blood pressure wearing a mask and gloves.

3. A technician wears gloves to perform a veinipuncture.

4. A nurse attendant allows visitors to enter his room without masks.

156. A woman comes to the physician's office for a routine prenatal checkup at 34 weeks' gestation. Abdominal palpation reveals the fetal position as right occipital anterior (ROA). At which of the following sites would the nurse expect to find the fetal heart tone?

1. Below the umbilicus, on the mother's left side

2. Below the umbilicus, on the mother's right side

3. Above the umbilicus, on the mother's left side

4. Above the umbilicus, on the mother's right side

157. A client is admitted to the hospital with complaints of seizures and a high fever. A brain scan is ordered. Before the scan, the client asks the nurse what position he will be in while the procedure is being done. Which of the following statements by the nurse is *MOST* accurate?

1. "You will be in a side-lying position with the foot of the bed elevated."

2. "You will be in a semi-upright sitting position, with your knees flexed."

3. "You will be lying supine with a small pillow under your head."

4. "You will be flat on your back, with your feet higher than your head."

158. A man is admitted to the psychiatric hospital with a diagnosis of obsessive-compulsive disorder. He is unable to stay employed because his ritualistic behavior causes him to be late for work. Which of the following interpretations by the nurse of the client's behavior is *MOST* accurate?

1. He is responding to auditory hallucinations and trying to gain control over his behavior.

2. He is fulfilling an unconscious desire to punish himself.

3. He is attempting to reduce anxiety by taking control of the environment.

4. He is malingering in order to avoid responsibilities at work.

159. A client diagnosed with chronic lymphocytic leukemia is admitted to the hospital for treatment of hemolytic anemia. Which of the following measures incorporated into the nursing care plan *BEST* addresses the client's needs?

1. Encourage activities with other clients in the dayroom.
2. Isolate the client from visitors and clients to avoid infection.
3. Provide a diet high in vitamin C.
4. Provide a quiet environment to promote adequate rest.

160. The nurse plans morning care for a client hospitalized after a cerebrovascular accident (CVA) resulting in left-sided paralysis and homonymous hemianopia. During morning care, the nurse should do which of the following?

1. Provide care from the client's right side.
2. Speak loudly and distinctly when talking with the client.
3. Reduce the level of lighting in the client's room to prevent glare.
4. Provide all of the client's care to reduce his energy expenditure.

161. The nurse prepares for the admission of a client with a perforated duodenal ulcer. Which of the following should the nurse expect to observe as the primary initial symptom?

1. Fever
2. Pain
3. Dizziness
4. Vomiting

162. A 3-week-old boy is admitted with a diagnosis of pyloric stenosis. The mother tells the nurse that this is her first child and asks if there is anything she can do to prevent this from happening to her next child. Which of the following statements by the nurse BEST addresses her concern?

1. "This type of thing generally happens to first children."
2. "When you have your second child, at least you'll know what signs to look for."
3. "This is a structural problem; it is not a reflection of your parenting skills."
4. "This is an inherited condition; it is not your fault."

163. The nurse cares for a client diagnosed with bipolar disorder. The client paces endlessly in the halls and makes hostile comments to other clients. The client resists the nurse's attempts to move him to a room in the unit. Which of the following actions by the nurse is MOST important?

1. Offer the client fluids every hour.
2. Inform the client about the unit rules.
3. Administer haloperidol (Haldol) IM.
4. Encourage the client to rest.

164. The nurse is caring for an Rh-negative mother who has delivered an Rh-positive child. The mother states, "The doctor told me about RhoGAM, but I'm still a little confused." Which of the following responses by the nurse is MOST appropriate?

1. "RhoGAM is given to your child to prevent the development of antibodies."
2. "RhoGAM is given to your child to supply the necessary antibodies."
3. "RhoGAM is given to you to prevent the formation of antibodies."
4. "RhoGAM is given to you to encourage the production of antibodies."

165. The nurse performs client teaching for a woman with osteoarthritis. The client asks what she can do to effectively decrease pain and stiffness in her joints before beginning her daily routine. The nurse should instruct the client to do which of the following?

1. "Perform isometric exercises for 10 minutes."

2. "Do range-of-motion exercises, then apply ointment to your joints."

3. "Take a warm bath and rest for a few minutes."

4. "Stretch all muscle groups."

166. The nurse cares for a client receiving paroxetine (Paxil). It is *MOST* important for the nurse to report which of the following to the physician?

    1. The client states there is no change in her appetite.

    2. The client states she has started taking digoxin (Lanoxin).

    3. The client states she applies sunscreen before going outside.

    4. The client states she drives her car to work.

167. A client returns to his room after a cardiac catheterization. Which of the following assessments by the nurse would justify calling the physician?

    1. Pain at the site of the catheter insertion

    2. Absence of a pulse distal to the catheter insertion site

    3. Drainage on the dressing covering the catheter insertion site

    4. Redness at the catheter insertion site

168. An 8-year-old boy is seen in a clinic for treatment of attention-deficit/hyperactivity disorder (ADHD). Medication has been prescribed for the child along with family counseling. The nurse teaches the parents about the medication and discusses parenting strategies. Which of the following statements by the parents indicates that further teaching is necessary?

1. "We will give the medication at night so it doesn't decrease his appetite."

2. "We will provide a regular routine for sleeping, eating, working, and playing."

3. "We will establish firm but reasonable limits on his behavior."

4. "We will reduce distractions and external stimuli to help him concentrate."

169. A client has been taking aluminum hydroxide (Amphojel) daily for 3 weeks. The nurse should be alert for which of the following side effects?

    1. Nausea

    2. Hypercalcemia

    3. Constipation

    4. Anorexia

170. A client recovering from a laparoscopic laser cholecystectomy says to the nurse, "I hate the thought of eating a low-fat diet for the rest of my life." Which of the following responses by the nurse is *MOST* appropriate?

    1. "I will ask the dietician to come talk to you."

    2. "What do you think is so bad about following a low-fat diet?"

    3. "It may not be necessary for you to follow a low-fat diet for that long."

    4. "At least you will be alive and not suffering that pain."

171. A client returns to his room after a transurethral resection of the prostate (TURP) for benign prostatic hypertrophy (BPH). Which of the following would cause the nurse to suspect postoperative hemorrhage?

1. Decreased blood pressure, increased pulse, increased respirations

2. Fluctuating blood pressure, decreased pulse, rapid respirations

3. Increased blood pressure, bounding pulse, irregular respirations

4. Increased blood pressure, irregular pulse, shallow respirations

172. The home care nurse screens a group of residents in a dependent living facility for risk factors to pneumonia. The nurse determines that which of the following clients is *MOST* at risk to develop pneumonia?

    1. A 72-year-old female who has left-sided hemiparesis after a cerebrovascular accident

    2. A 76-year-old male who has a history of hypertension and type 2 diabetes

    3. An 80-year-old female who walks 1 mile every day and has a history of depression

    4. An 87-year-old male who smokes and has a history of lung cancer

173. The nurse performs teaching with a client undergoing a paracentesis for treatment of cirrhosis. The client asks what position he will be in for the procedure. The nurse's reply should be based on an understanding that the *MOST* appropriate position for the client is which of the following?

    1. Sitting with his lower extremities well supported

    2. Side-lying with a pillow between his knees

    3. Prone with his head turned to the left side

    4. Dorsal-recumbent with a pillow at the back of his head

174. A man calls the Suicide Prevention Hotline and states that he is going to kill himself. Which of the following questions should the nurse ask *FIRST*?

    1. "What has happened to cause you to want to end your life?"

    2. "How have you planned to kill yourself?"

    3. "When did you start to feel as though you wanted to die?"

    4. "Do you want me to prevent you from killing yourself?"

175. A man is admitted for treatment of heart failure. The physician orders an IV of 125 mL of normal saline per hour and central venous pressure (CVP) readings every 4 hours. Sixteen hours after admission, the client's CVP reading is 3 cm/H_2O. Which of the following evaluations of the client's fluid status by the nurse would be *MOST* accurate?

    1. The client has received enough fluid.

    2. The client's fluid status remains unaltered.

    3. The client has received too much fluid.

    4. The client needs more fluid.

176. An agitated client throws a chair across the dayroom on the psychiatry floor and threatens the other clients with physical harm. Which of the following should the nurse do *FIRST*?

    1. Tell the client that his wife will be called to the hospital.

    2. Ask the client why he is so angry.

    3. Remove the other clients from the dayroom.

    4. Assemble staff and put the client in preventive seclusion.

177. The nurse is caring for a depressed client who spends most of the day sitting at a window, and is about to implement a physical activity plan for him. The nurse knows that the purpose of this plan is to do which of the following?

1. Help the client understand the problems creating the depression.
2. Reduce the client's risk for obesity and diabetes.
3. Transform self-destructive impulses into positive behaviors.
4. Encourage socialization and improve self-esteem.

178. The nurse is caring for a client with bipolar disorder. Which of the following behaviors by the client indicates to the nurse that a manic episode is subsiding?

1. The client tells several jokes at a group meeting.
2. The client sits and talks with other clients at mealtimes.
3. The client begins to write a book about his life.
4. The client initiates an effort to start a radio station on the unit.

179. A client hospitalized for treatment of delusions tells the nurse that he is really the head of the hospital system and that his "cover" is being a client to get information on client abuse. Which of the following statements by the nurse to the client is *BEST* initially?

1. "Tell me what you mean about being head of the hospital system and getting client abuse information."
2. "I think you should share this story with the other clients at dinnertime and see what they say."

3. "You are not the head of the hospital system, you are an accountant under treatment for a mental disorder."
4. "It worries me when you say these things; it means you are not responding to the medication."

180. The nurse is caring for a client in labor. The nurse palpates a firm, round form in the uterine fundus, small parts on the woman's right side, and a long, smooth, curved section on the left side. Based on these findings, the nurse should anticipate auscultating the fetal heart in which of the following locations?

1. A
2. B
3. C
4. D

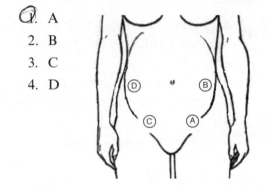

181. A 69-year-old female client admitted with pneumonia is receiving gentamicin (Garamycin). For this client, which of the following laboratory values would be *MOST* important for the nurse to monitor?

1. BUN and creatinine
2. Hemoglobin and hematocrit
3. Sodium and potassium
4. Platelet count and clotting time

182. The nurse is preparing a client newly diagnosed with Addison's disease for discharge. Which of the following statements by the client indicates a need for further instruction from the nurse?

1. "I understand that I will need lifelong cortisone replacement therapy."

2. "During times of stress, I will need to decrease my medication."

3. "I must be careful not to injure myself."

4. "I should always carry a medical identification card."

183. The nurse suspects a client has meningitis. The nurse places the client in a dorsal recumbent position, puts her hands behind the client's neck, and bends it forward. The nurse knows that pain and resistance may indicate neck injury or arthritis, but if the client also flexes the hips and knees, this positive response is which of the following?

1. Trousseau's sign

2. Brudzinki's sign

3. Homans' sign

4. Chvostek's sign

184. The nurse is assessing a client newly diagnosed with initial-stage chronic glomerulonephritis. Which of the following findings should the nurse expect to see? **Select all that apply.**

1. Hypotension

2. Proteinuria

3. Severe anemia

4. Hematuria

5. Azotemia

6. Nausea

185. A 56-year-old male client with a history of myocardial infarction is admitted for evaluation of chest pain. Several hours later, the client goes into ventricular fibrillation and a code blue is called. The Emergency Department physician defibrillates the client. The nurse knows that the purpose of defibrillation is to do which of the following?

1. Energize myocardial cells.

2. Improve left ventricular function.

3. Increase cardiac output.

4. Produce momentary asystole to allow the natural pacemaker to resume activity.

186. The physician orders 0.25 mg digoxin (Lanoxin) for a client diagnosed with heart failure. The client's pulse is 86 prior to administration of the prescribed dose. The nurse should do which of the following?

1. Give half of the prescribed dose (0.125 mg).

2. Delay the dose until the pulse is below 60.

3. Omit the dose, and record the pulse rate as the reason.

4. Give the full dose as ordered.

187. The nurse knows that atorvastatin (Lipitor) administered to a client is effective when there is a reduction in which of the following?

1. Triglycerides

2. Chest pain

3. Blood pressure

4. PTT

188. A 37-year-old female has been prescribed sumatriptan (Imitrex) for severe migraines. The nurse explains that the client should watch for which of the following adverse drug effects?

1. Constipation

2. Bradycardia

3. Somnolence

4. Sudden numbness or weakness

189. The client is resuming a diet after undergoing a Billroth II procedure. To minimize complications from eating, the nurse instructs the client to do which of the following?

1. Drink fluids with meals.
2. Increase intake of carbohydrates and salt.
3. Increase fat and protein.
4. Eat 3 large meals a day.

190. The nurse is caring for a client who is having difficulty eating due to mouth sores from chemotherapy treatments. Which of the following interventions is *MOST* appropriate to promote basic comfort and nutrition?

1. Obtain an order for TPN.
2. Keep the client NPO.
3. Administer a stool softener as ordered.
4. Provide frequent oral hygiene.

191. The nurse is caring for an adult male client who has just undergone spinal fusion for a herniated intervertebral disk. To promote comfort and minimize complications, the nurse tells the client to avoid which of the following?

1. Bending the knees when lying on one side
2. Sitting for longer than 20 minutes at a time
3. Using an extra-firm mattress
4. Sitting in a hardback chair

192. The nurse is preparing a client for surgery. When obtaining informed consent, the nurse should *INITIALLY* do which of the following?

1. Explain the risks, benefits, and alternatives of the procedure.

2. Tell the client that obtaining the signature is routine for all surgeries.
3. Witness the client's signature.
4. Assess whether the client's understanding of the procedure is sufficient to give consent.

193. The nurse is preparing to administer heparin sodium to a client diagnosed with thrombophlebitis. The nurse should ensure that which of the following is available if the client develops a significant bleeding problem?

1. Phytonadione (vitamin K)
2. Fresh frozen plasma (FFP)
3. Protamine sulfate
4. Reteplase (Retavase)

194. A client is being admitted to the hospital for elective surgery. During the admission assessment, the nurse asks the client if he has an advance directive. The nurse knows that clients have the right to play an active role in their care and treatment, and this is guaranteed by which of the following?

1. The Health Insurance Portability and Accountability Act (HIPAA)
2. The Client Self-Determination Act
3. The Civil Rights Act
4. The Americans with Disabilities Act

195. The nurse enters a client's hospital room to find the client sitting on the bathroom floor. The nurse assesses the client, obtains assistance, and assists the client back to bed. The nurse notifies the physician and completes an incident report. Which of the following is the *MOST* appropriate nursing action?

1. Document in the client's chart that an incident report has been completed.
2. Make a copy of the incident report for the nurse manager.

3. Document the incident in the client's chart.

4. Place the incident report in the client's chart.

196. The nurse is performing an initial post-operative assessment on a client who has just returned from surgery with a chest tube and water seal drainage system. The nurse should immediately intervene if she makes which of the following observations?

1. There are no dependent loops in the chest tube.

2. The chest tube is not clamped.

3. The chest tube and drainage system is above the client's chest.

4. The fluid level in the water seal is at 2 cm.

197. The nurse is present during an informed consent discussion between the client and the physician regarding recommended surgery. The physician discusses the risks, benefits, and alternatives of the procedure with the client. The nurse knows that the client's decision whether or not to have the surgery is based on which of the following ethical principles?

1. Nonmaleficence

2. Beneficence

3. Autonomy

4. Capacity

198. The nurse is caring for a terminal cancer client at home. The nurse knows that which of the following ethical principles BEST supports keeping client and family care consistent with the nurse's professional code of ethics?

1. Virtues

2. Fidelity

3. Beneficence

4. Justice

199. The nurse is caring for a client receiving intravenous therapy through a peripherally inserted central catheter (PICC). Which of the following actions implemented by the nurse will decrease the risk of infection?

1. Assess vital signs every 4 hours.

2. Ask the physician for an order for antibiotics.

3. Maintain sterile technique during all phases of PICC care.

4. Administer acetaminophen (Tylenol) before dressing changes.

200. The nurse is caring for a client with chronic obstructive pulmonary disease (COPD) and is planning to obtain an arterial blood gas (ABG). Which of the following should the nurse plan to do to prevent bleeding following the procedure?

1. Apply 2 × 2 gauze to the puncture site and hold pressure for 5 minutes.

2. Have the client hold the puncture site in a dependent position for 5 minutes.

3. Apply a warm compress to the puncture site for 15 minutes.

4. Encourage the client to open and close the hand rapidly for several minutes.

201. The nurse is caring for a client diagnosed with acute myocardial infarction (MI) and a history of severe uncontrolled hypertension. The nurse should question which of the following physician orders?

1. Limit physical activity for the first 12 hours

2. IV nitroglycerin

3. Thrombolytic therapy

4. Oxygen therapy

202. The nurse is preparing to administer warfarin (Coumadin) to a client diagnosed with atrial fibrillation. The nurse knows that which of the following nursing diagnoses takes priority?

1. Risk for imbalanced fluid volume
2. Risk for injury
3. Constipation
4. Risk for unstable blood glucose

203. Prior to administering a tuberculin (Mantoux) skin test, the nurse in an outpatient clinic is educating a client suspected of having tuberculosis (TB). The nurse determines that the client understands the teaching when the client states which of the following?

1. "I know the test will tell me how long I've been infected with TB."
2. "This test will tell me if I am contagious."
3. "I will need to come back and have a nurse look at the site in a week."
4. "The test will tell us if I've ever been infected with TB bacteria."

204. The nurse is preparing to enter the private, well-ventilated isolation room of a client with active tuberculosis (TB). Which of the following actions should the nurse take before entering the room?

1. Wash her hands and wear a gown and gloves.
2. Wash her hands.
3. Wash her hands and place a particulate filter respirator over her nose and mouth.
4. Ask the client to don a mask.

205. The nurse is preparing a female client for a cardiac catheterization with the femoral approach. The nurse should do which of the following when the client returns to her room after the procedure?

1. Elevate the head of the bed 45 degrees.
2. Keep the client's arm immobilized for the first 24 hours.
3. Keep the client's leg immobilized for the first 12 hours.
4. Tell the client to lie on the procedural side for 2 hours.

206. A 65-year-old woman with metastatic breast cancer has been admitted to the hospital with neutropenic fever. She informs the nurse that she does not want CPR or artificial ventilation to be performed under any circumstances. The nurse explains that this information can be outlined in an advance directive. The nurse understands that which of the following addresses the client's right to identify treatment desires in advance?

1. The Patient's Bill of Rights
2. The Patient Self-Determination Act
3. The Health Insurance Portability and Accountability Act (HIPAA)
4. The Americans with Disabilities Act

207. After receiving morning report on a medical/surgical unit, which of the following clients should the nurse address FIRST?

1. A 36-year-old man who underwent surgery to repair multiple fractures in his left leg after an automobile accident reports coughing up blood.
2. A 56-year-old woman newly diagnosed with diabetes has a fasting blood sugar of 83 mg/dL.
3. A 68-year-old man with head and neck cancer receiving a continuous 5-fluorouracil infusion reports feeling nauseated.
4. A 28-year-old woman with sickle cell anemia reports a pain level of 6 on a scale of 1–10.

208. A 58-year-old Spanish-speaking woman is being discharged after having a central venous access device placed. Which of the following *BEST* describes the nurse's role in advocating for her client?

    1. The nurse uses a translator when she provides the client with discharge instructions.

    2. The nurse provides both written and verbal discharge instructions.

    3. The nurse ensures the client has transportation home upon discharge.

    4. The nurse provides discharge instructions in a private room.

209. A 26-year-old man being admitted for an emergency appendectomy asks the nurse why she is asking about his medications and history of previous illnesses. In addition to explaining why it is relevant to the care of the client, the nurse knows this client responsibility has been outlined in which of the following?

    1. The Americans with Disabilities Act

    2. The Patient's Bill of Rights

    3. Nursing Scope and Standards of Practice

    4. The Health Insurance Portability and Accountability Act (HIPAA)

210. A nurse is working on the medical/surgical unit. The nurse knows that which of the following tasks should *NOT* be delegated to nursing assistive personnel (NAP)?

    1. Setting up a meal tray for a 75-year-old client with Alzheimer's disease

    2. Assessing a newly postoperative client's pain level

    3. Setting up a water basin for a 45-year-old client who wishes to shave at the bedside

    4. Transferring a 70-year-old client awaiting discharge from the bed to a wheelchair

211. A nurse receives a phone call from a family member asking for health-related information on a client being treated for suspected myocardial infarction in the Emergency Department. The nurse explains she cannot disclose personal information about the client without the client's consent. The nurse knows this represents which of the following ethical principles?

    1. Accountability

    2. Autonomy

    3. Beneficence

    4. Confidentiality

212. A nurse is caring for a 48-year-old man with a new colostomy. Which of the following activities *BEST* describes the nurse's role as an advocate for the client?

    1. Ensuring the skin is dry before re-adhering the pouch

    2. Teaching the client how to change and care for the ostomy pouch

    3. Providing the client's wife with a list of foods to avoid

    4. Explaining to the client that psychological adjustment to an ostomy can take time

213. A client who has scabies has been admitted to the medical/surgical unit. The nurse knows he should use which of the following precautions when caring for this client?

    1. Droplet precautions

    2. Airborne precautions

    3. Contact precautions

    4. Precautions are not necessary with this client

214. A client who has a localized herpes simplex virus (HSV) infection is admitted to the maternity unit. The nurse knows the client should *IDEALLY* be placed in which of the following?

1. Any available room
2. A single, unoccupied room
3. A double room with a client who underwent a cesarean section 3 days prior
4. A double room with a curtain divider

215. A 38-year-old client with breast cancer will be self-administering filgrastim (Neupogen) subcutaneously. The nurse knows that teaching should include which of the following?

1. Dispose of needles in a puncture-resistant container.
2. Wear chemotherapy-resistant gloves.
3. Recap the needles for reuse.
4. Neupogen has been prescribed to boost platelets.

216. A 76-year-old woman has been admitted to a rehabilitation center after a hip replacement. During an episode of confusion in which she became a danger to herself, the client was placed in a vest restraint. The nurse knows that which of the following are also considered types of restraints? **Select all that apply.**

1. Administering a haloperidol (Haldol) injection
2. Raising 4 bed side rails
3. Assigning a nurse's aide to sit and observe the client
4. Applying wrist cuffs and tying them to the bed.
5. Clipping a tray across the front of the client's wheelchair

217. A physician has written an order for escitalopram oxalate (Lexapro) 10 mg PO daily for a 15-year-old client with depression. After performing an initial assessment, the nurse calls the physician to verify the order. Which of the following *BEST* explains the nurse's concern about the safety of the order?

1. The client reported a history of facial swelling and difficulty breathing while on citalopram (Celexa).
2. The drug has not been approved for use in the client's age group.
3. The ordered dose is higher than the suggested range.
4. The ordered dose is lower than the suggested range.

218. A 75-year-old client has an unsteady gait and requires assistance with ambulation. The nurse decides to use a gait belt. The nurse knows she should do which of the following when using a gait belt? **Select all that apply.**

1. Secure the gait belt loosely around the client's waist.
2. Twist her upper body to position the client.
3. Remove the gait belt after use.
4. Place the gait belt over the client's clothes with the clip in front.
5. Use the gait belt to help lift the client from a sitting into a standing position

219. After receiving report at the start of a night shift, the nurse finds an elderly client lying on the floor with the bedrails down. When documenting findings, which of the following *BEST* describes what the nurse should do?

1. Complete an incident report at the end of his shift, when he is less busy.

2. Complete an incident report using clear, concise, and factual language.

3. Complete an incident report and place a copy of it in the client's medical record.

4. Ask the evening shift nurse to complete an incident report because the fall occurred on her shift.

220. A nurse is caring for an 8-year-old girl with urinary retention. The nurse is preparing to insert a Foley catheter. Which of the following catheter sizes is *MOST* appropriate for this client?

1. Number 8 French
2. Number 16 French
3. Number 20 French
4. Number 22 French

221. A 42-year-old male client weighs 196 lbs. (89.1 kg) and is 65 inches (1.65 meters) tall. Based on the client's body mass index (BMI), the nurse knows this client would fall into which of the following categories?

1. Underweight
2. Normal weight
3. Overweight
4. Obese

222. A 10-year-old girl is being seen in the Pediatric Emergency Department following a motor vehicle accident. She has been stabilized but reports a pain level of 8 on a scale of 1 to 10. The nurse is preparing to transfer the client to x-ray. The nurse knows that which nonpharmacologic intervention should *NOT* be used to help reduce pain in this client?

1. Offer choices when possible.
2. Reassure the client that the procedure will not hurt.

3. Provide complete explanations about what is going to happen.

4. Use distraction, relaxation, and imagery.

223. In preparation for doxorubicin (Adriamycin) administration, the nurse is assessing a client's arm to determine where to attempt venipuncture. The nurse knows which of the following veins is the *BEST* choice to start the IV?

1. The non-dominant antecubital fossa
2. The distal forearm
3. The wrist
4. A vein used for venipuncture within the previous 24 hours

224. A 24-year-old client with anorexia has had a nasogastric (NG) tube placed in preparation for intermittent enteral feedings. The nurse knows to do which of the following when administering medications via an NG tube?

1. Crush the enteric coated aspirin.
2. Mix the medications with the client's feeding formula.
3. Flush the tube using a 15-mL syringe.
4. Administer each medication separately.

225. A 3-year-old client with acute otitis media has been prescribed ofloxacin (Floxin) ear drops. The nurse knows that which of the following statements by the father demonstrates that he understands how to properly administer the ear drops?

1. "I can stop giving the ear drops as soon as my daughter's fever is gone."

2. "I should give the drops directly on the eardrum to help get rid of the infection quickly."

3. "I should warm the ear drops before giving them by wrapping the bottle in my hand."

4. "My daughter should lie flat while I give the drops."

226. A 68-year-old woman recently diagnosed with hypertension has started taking furosemide (Lasix) 40 mg PO twice daily. During a clinic appointment, she reports new onset muscle weakness and abdominal cramping. Lab tests are performed. The nurse knows which of the following results is the best explanation for the symptoms experienced by the client?

   1. Potassium 3.0 mEq/L
   2. Creatinine 1.5 mg/dL
   3. Fasting glucose 145 mg/dL
   4. Total calcium 10.0 mg/dL

227. A 64-year-old man with heart failure has recently been told by his physician to increase his digoxin (Lanoxin) dose to 0.25 mg. He has 125 mcg tablets on hand. Which of the following statements by the client to the home health nurse indicates the client has understood the teaching provided about the medication?

   1. "I should take one tablet."
   2. "I should notify my doctor if I experience diarrhea."
   3. "I don't need to follow up with my doctor unless I'm having a problem."
   4. "I can take over-the-counter medications without the approval of my physician."

228. The nurse is preparing to administer a tuberculin skin test to a pregnant 26-year-old client. The nurse knows which of the following statements about tuberculin skin testing is *TRUE*?

   1. The test should not be administered during pregnancy.
   2. The test should be read between 24 and 48 hours after administration.
   3. The reaction is measured in millimeters of the induration.
   4. The test should be administered into the outer surface of the forearm.

229. The nurse takes report on a client who underwent a thyroidectomy 24 hours ago. The nurse understands that the client is at risk for hypocalcemia. Which of the following assessment findings indicate the client may be hypocalcemic? **Select all that apply.**

   1. Positive Trousseau's sign
   2. Negative Chvostek's sign
   3. Numbness around the mouth.
   4. Positive Moro reflex test
   5. "Pins and needles" sensation in client's feet

230. A 58-year-old client is receiving the monoclonal antibody rituximab (Rituxan) and develops an infusion reaction manifested by chest pain and dyspnea. The nurse should do which of the following *FIRST*?

   1. Assess the client's airway.
   2. Stop the infusion.
   3. Slow down the rate of infusion.
   4. Administer epinephrine.

231. The nurse is assigned as the team leader on a busy medical/surgical unit. Which of the following *BEST* describes the "rights" of delegation the nurse must consider when assigning tasks to other members of the health care team?

   1. Right task, right timing, right client, right person, and right date

2. Right task, right client, right direction, right supervision, and right date

3. Right client, right direction, right day, right medication, and right unit

4. Right task, right circumstance, right person, right direction, and right supervision

232. Which of the following pediatric clients should the nurse provide assessment and intervention for *FIRST*?

1. A 15-month-old who has developed hives

2. A 2-year-old who is ventilated but stable

3. A 12-year-old recovering from surgical repair of a fractured femur who complains of some difficulty breathing

4. A 2-month-old whose apnea alarm is sounding with an oxygen saturation reading of 82%

233. The nurse knows that she would *NOT* be required to use airborne precautions for which of the following clients?

1. A young adult with possible tuberculosis who is also HIV positive

2. A middle-aged adult with herpes simplex

3. A teenager with chicken pox and a sore throat

4. A college student with possible rubella

234. The nurse is caring for an elderly female with dementia. The nurse knows that which of the following should be the priority for care for this client?

1. Nutrition

2. Hygiene

3. Fall risk

4. Cardiac care

235. The nurse is planning the care of an elderly male client with very poor oral hygiene and gum disease. The nurse knows that the teeth and gums can be which of the following in the chain of infection?

1. The method of transmission for bacteria

2. A portal of entry for bacteria

3. The pathogen

4. A portal of exit

236. In the event of a fire, the nurse should do which of the following *FIRST*?

1. Leave the building.

2. Attempt to get clients out of immediate danger.

3. Work to contain the fire.

4. Determine the order in which to evacuate clients.

237. The nurse knows that which of the following *BEST* describes the role of a nursing supervisor?

1. Chooses and implements interventions

2. Attends meetings to keep staff up to date

3. Does not require special skills to oversee other professionals

4. Is friendly and can make contributions to an employee evaluation

238. The nurse is conversing with a young adult client regarding an ordered blood transfusion. It is clear to the nurse that the client does not understand the risks involved with the procedure. Which of the following statements *BEST* describes the nurse's role regarding informed consent for this procedure?

1. The nurse tells the client not to worry because blood transfusions are very common.

2. The nurse informs the ordering physician that the client does not understand the risks and will need further explanation.

3. The nurse has someone else witness the signature on the consent.

4. The nurse describes alternative treatments.

239. The nurse is caring for a famous basketball player who may have sustained a career-changing injury. When asked by coworkers about the status of the client, she responds that she is not able to discuss her client. Which of the following ethical principles *BEST* supports her statement?

1. Justice
2. Beneficence
3. Confidentiality
4. Accountability

240. The nurse is on duty on a busy cardiac telemetry unit. Which of the following situations requires the nurse's immediate attention?

1. The wife of a cardiac client states that his IV pump is alarming and he is not receiving the pain medication dose due to the pump malfunctioning.

2. The daughter of an elderly client states that her mother is uncomfortable and that her electrodes have come off.

3. The new CNA reports that she cannot wake her elderly client to take his blood pressure because he is sleeping soundly and snoring, but she obtained his pulse and it is 30. She wants you to come to see if you can wake him.

4. The new admission from earlier today is complaining that he has not been assessed in over an hour and he would like to order dinner.

241. The nurse knows that which of the following terms *BEST* defines the multidisciplinary care planning for a young adult with breast cancer?

1. Team work
2. Team building
3. Case management
4. Collaboration

242. The charge RN is preparing assignments on a busy medical unit. For this shift, there are several LPNs, several RNs, and one CNA. Which of the following assignments by the charge RN is appropriate? **Select all that apply.**

1. The CNA is assigned to give morning baths.

2. An LPN is assigned to perform an initial assessment on a newly admitted client.

3. An LPN is assigned to clients who are prescribed oral medications, and will do vital signs on those clients.

4. The clients with IV medications are divided among the RNs.

5. AN LPN is assigned to insert a urinary cathether.

243. The nurse is educating new nursing staff members about safety on the pediatric unit. Which of the following comments by one of the new staff members *BEST* demonstrates that teaching has been successful?

1. "A toddler may be taken to the car in a wheelchair when discharged and, after that, the hospital is not responsible for how the child is transported in the family car."

2. "School-aged children do not require booster seats if they are less than 80 pounds, and they do not require bicycle helmets when they are more than 80 pounds."

3. "Medications can be left at the bedside for pediatric clients, and the parent will dispense when needed."

4. "All medications and cleaning supplies must be locked in a child-proof cabinet on the pediatric unit at all times."

244. The nurse knows that which of the following is the *MOST* appropriate infection control method when caring for clients on a surgical unit?

    1. Hand hygiene before charting or using the keyboard

    2. Handwashing before and after contact with each client

    3. Use of gloves

    4. Use of gowns with each client

245. The nurse on the adult medical unit assesses an elderly client with vertigo. Which of the following interventions demonstrates that the nurse understands the symptoms of vertigo?

    1. The nurse recognizes this client as at risk for falls and relays this to the other team members.

    2. The nurse allows the client to ambulate alone.

    3. The nurse encourages the client to sit up quickly before standing.

    4. The nurse makes no change in routine precautions because vertigo is an expected symptom for this age group.

246. The nurse is preparing to change a sterile surgical dressing. While repositioning herself, the client touches a sterile sponge. Which of the following is the *BEST* nursing intervention to promote and maintain surgical asepsis?

    1. Reassure the client and continue with the dressing change.

    2. Reassure the client but instruct her to keep her hands free from the sterile field. Clear the contaminated area, rewash hands, and assemble another sterile field to start over.

    3. Have the client sterilize her hands so the episode is not repeated.

    4. Continue with the dressing change, avoiding the items that came in contact with the client's hands.

247. The nurse is caring for a client who has just undergone an open laparotomy with ileostomy. The nurse knows that client education should include which of the following topics?

    1. Constipation management

    2. Limited activity

    3. Stoma care and skin care

    4. Urinary incontinence

248. The nurse is assessing a client who has multiple sclerosis and can no longer live alone due to immobility. Which of the following statements by the nurse demonstrates her understanding of this client's impaired physical mobility?

    1. "Do you have any areas of pain, pressure, or open ulcers on your legs, ankles, or hips?"

    2. "They do make motor wheelchairs. Maybe we can look into that."

    3. "How often do you have episodes of diarrhea?"

4. "What kinds of meals would you like prepared while in the hospital?"

249. The nurse is educating a client who is scheduled for surgery in the near future about autologous blood donation. Which of the following statements by the client indicates the teaching has been successful?

    1. "I cannot donate blood for myself because of my age."
    2. "I will not need a transfusion after major surgery."
    3. "I can be an autologous blood donor 6 weeks before my surgery in the event that I may need a transfusion."
    4. "I cannot get a transfusion reaction with my own blood."

250. The RN is providing education to the LPN about administrating oral medications. Which of the following statements demonstrates to the RN that the LPN understands the teaching?

    1. "Giving oral medications is simple and requires little training."
    2. "If the client can't swallow a time-released tablet, I will crush it."
    3. "It is okay to crush the client's extended-release tablet to put it in applesauce."
    4. "I can break this scored tablet for the partial dose ordered for the client."

251. The nurse is reviewing the lab work of a pediatric client admitted for chemotherapy treatment. For which of the following laboratory values should the nurse call the physician?

    1. BUN 5, creatinine 0.7
    2. WBC 0, hemoglobin 2
    3. Hemoglobin 9.5, WBC 14
    4. Magnesium 2

252. The nurse is doing a follow-up telephone call with a new mother regarding her newborn. The mother states the baby's eyes look yellow. Which of the following is the *MOST* appropriate response by the nurse?

    1. "How often are you nursing your baby?"
    2. "Are you breastfeeding or bottle feeding?"
    3. "Do you know what your baby's bilirubin level was before discharge?"
    4. "Has your baby been seen by the pediatrician?"

253. The nurse is assessing a young adult client who begins to have a grand mal seizure for the first time. Which of the following actions should the nurse do *FIRST*?

    1. Protect the client's airway.
    2. Restrain the client.
    3. Record the length of the seizure.
    4. Report this to the physician.

254. The nurse is educating a client with a history of hyponatremia on diet choices. Which of the following statements by the client *BEST* indicates the teaching was successful?

    1. "I should maintain a low-sodium diet."
    2. "I can drink as much beer as I want to."
    3. "I should avoid caffeine."
    4. "I should drink a lot of water."

255. The nurse is caring for an alert and oriented teen with a head injury who complains of a slight headache. Which of the following symptoms exhibited by the client would require immediate intervention by the nurse?

1. The client complains of a continued headache and becomes drowsy.

2. The headache becomes worse and the client shows a decrease in the level of consciousness.

3. The client vomits one time and continues to have a slight headache.

4. The client has no headache but has little memory of the incident.

256. The nurse is admitting a client to the neurology unit at the medical center. The nurse has arrived at the advance directive section of the initial nursing assessment flowsheet. The nurse assisting with the admission would intervene if the primary admitting nurse made which of the following statements to the client?

   1. "Do you have someone who would be a surrogate decision maker for you if you were unable to make decisions for yourself?"

   2. "Are you familiar with what an advance directive is?"

   3. "I should find out if you want an advance directive, but you seem tired and confused so I will ask you later."

   4. "Let me tell you a little bit about what an advance directive is so that you can decide if you want one set up."

257. The nurse is caring for a client on the medical/surgical unit who is receiving an intravenous insulin drip due to severe uncontrollable episodic hyperglycemia. After several hours of administering the insulin and monitoring blood glucose levels regularly, the glucose levels are normalizing. The physician orders the nurse to maintain the IV insulin drip despite the nurse's concerns. Which of the following actions by the nurse is the *MOST* appropriate?

1. The nurse should explain the procedure of administering the insulin intravenously to the client.

2. The nurse should maintain the intravenous medication according to the physician's orders.

3. The nurse should wait until the next blood glucose level check is due and make a decision then about next steps.

4. The nurse should contact the nursing supervisor and possibly the supervisor of the physician who ordered the medication.

258. The home care nurse is caring for an elderly client who lives alone. The nurse notices that the client is beginning to show signs of failure to thrive at home and has no family to assist him. The nurse is unsure how long this client will be able to remain in his home alone. Which of the following is the next step the nurse should take based on this assessment?

   1. The nurse should consult with the case manager employed by the home care agency.

   2. The nurse should call 911 for an emergency response due to concerns for safety.

   3. The nurse should call the client's community center for advice.

   4. The nurse should call the client's neighbors to ask them to look in on the client.

259. The new staff nurse working on the intensive care unit is concerned about her client's status. The client has continued to decline throughout the shift. The client's blood pressure, heart rate, and oxygen saturation have progressively dropped in a relatively short period of time. The nurse inquires with the charge nurse assigned to

that shift. The charge nurse says "Don't worry, the client will be fine, he always does that." Which of the following actions should the nurse take?

1. The nurse should call the nursing supervisor on duty to assist.
2. The nurse should wait and see how the client does.
3. The nurse should agree with the charge nurse because that nurse has more experience.
4. The nurse should discuss this with other nurses on the unit.

260. The nurse on a busy surgical unit has just received report from the previous shift on the clients assigned to that shift. Which of the following clients should the nurse see FIRST?

1. A young adult client who fractured his arm while playing football, had surgical repair of the fracture, and is awaiting discharge
2. A middle-aged client recovering from a knee replacement who is currently on the continuous passive motion machine with the physical therapist
3. A middle-aged client recovering from abdominal surgery who is complaining of wheezing and has a new oxygen requirement
4. An elderly client 1-day post-op for a hip replacement whose blood pressure is elevated

261. On a medical/surgical unit, each nurse is paired with nursing assistive personnel (NAP) for the night shift. The nurse should assign which of the following clients to the NAP?

1. A middle-aged client receiving chemotherapy and complaining of nausea and vomiting

2. A middle-aged client who is an unstable diabetic requiring a blood glucose level check
3. An elderly client complaining of pain from restless leg syndrome
4. A young adult client recovering from a drug overdose requesting to leave the unit against medical advice

262. The nurse is working on a state-of-the-art nursing unit with completely electronic medical records. The rooms are semi-private, with two clients to a room, and equipped with a computer for each client. Which of the following actions by the nurse is the MOST appropriate?

1. After each use of the computer and upon leaving the client room, log off from the computer.
2. After each use of the computer and upon leaving the client room, face the computer away from where visitors would be able to see the screen.
3. The nurse should not be concerned about the security of the information because there is a single computer for each client and therefore no risk of the information being seen.
4. The nurse should pull the curtain to cover the computer screen so that visitors cannot view it.

263. The nurse is working on a unit that is equipped with electronic medication administration processes. This includes a computer at the bedside that allows for scanning a bar code on the medication order, the medication label, and the client's identification band. Which of the following is the BEST method for the nurse to practice regularly?

1. The nurse should rely solely on the bar-coding scanner because it promotes safer medication administration practices.

2. The nurse should rely on a combination of nursing judgment and decision-making along with the computerized system.

3. The nurse should never give a medication that a bar-coding system scans as "incorrect medication."

4. The nurse should override any medication that the machine scans as "incorrect medication" and administer it.

264. The nurse is administering medications to a client on an inpatient psychiatric unit. The client states "I don't usually take a pink pill" when the nurse gives a cup holding 4 different pills to the client. Which of the following is the *MOST* appropriate response by the nurse?

1. The nurse checks the medication administration record, determines it is correct, and tells the client to take the medication.

2. The nurse discounts the client's concern because he is a psychiatric client and doesn't know any better.

3. The nurse asks the client for a list of medications he routinely takes, and tells the client that she will review and confirm the order with the physician.

4. The nurse tells the client that sometimes drugs come in different colors depending on what pharmacy they come from.

265. The nurse is working at a skilled nursing facility. The nurse enters the client's room and sees the client attempting to pull himself up from a sitting position on the floor. The nurse inquires with the client as to what happened. The client responds "I fell." Which of the following should the nurse document in the incident report?

1. The nurse should file an incident report stating "Client fell, no injury noted."

2. The nurse should file an incident report stating "Client fell on floor."

3. The nurse should document the event only in the client's medical record and not in an incident report.

4. The nurse should file an incident report stating "Client found on floor. Client stated "I fell." Assessment completed, no injury noted, physician notified."

YOUR PRACTICE TEST SCORES

The test included in this book is designed to provide practice answering exam-style questions along with a review of nursing content. Your results on this test indicate where you are *now*. It is *not* designed to predict your ability to pass the NCLEX-RN® exam.

- If you scored 70 percent or better, you have a good understanding of essential nursing content, and you are able to utilize the critical thinking skills required to answer exam-style questions.
- If you scored 60 to 69 percent, you have areas of essential nursing content that need further review, or you may need continued work to master the critical thinking skills needed to correctly answer exam-style questions.
- If you scored 59 percent or less, you need concentrated study of nursing content and continued practice utilizing the critical thinking skills required to be successful on the NCLEX-RN® exam.

If you are looking for additional preparation materials for the NCLEX-RN® exam, Kaplan has classroom-based and online courses to prepare you for the NCLEX-RN® exam. These courses are designed to develop both your knowledge of the nursing content as well as your critical thinking skills. And Kaplan has courses specifically designed to fit *your* lifestyle and budget. Learn more at: *kaplannursing.com* or call 1-800-533-8850 (outside the United States and Canada call 1-212-997-5883).

ANSWER KEY

1.	**3**	37.	**1**	73.	**4**	109.	**4**
2.	**2**	38.	**3**	74.	**4**	110.	**2**
3.	**4**	39.	**3**	75.	**3**	111.	**3**
4.	**4**	40.	**2**	76.	**4**	112.	**4**
5.	**1**	41.	**3**	77.	**1**	113.	**3**
6.	**1**	42.	**1**	78.	**3**	114.	**2**
7.	**3**	43.	**1**	79.	**3**	115.	**2**
8.	**3**	44.	**2**	80.	**2**	116.	**1**
9.	**2**	45.	**2**	81.	**2**	117.	**4**
10.	**1**	46.	**1**	82.	**1**	118.	**2**
11.	**3**	47.	**3**	83.	**3**	119.	**1**
12.	**2**	48.	**2**	84.	**1**	120.	**3**
13.	**4**	49.	**1**	85.	**2**	121.	**2**
14.	**3**	50.	**2**	86.	**4**	122.	**4**
15.	**2**	51.	**4**	87.	**4**	123.	**2**
16.	**4**	52.	**2**	88.	**2**	124.	**2**
17.	**3**	53.	**3**	89.	**2**	125.	**3**
18.	**2**	54.	**3**	90.	**3**	126.	**3**
19.	**2**	55.	**3**	91.	**3**	127.	**1**
20.	**4**	56.	**3**	92.	**2**	128.	**2**
21.	**3**	57.	**2**	93.	**3**	129.	**4**
22.	**3**	58.	**4**	94.	**3**	130.	**1**
23.	**1**	59.	**4**	95.	**4**	131.	**2**
24.	**1**	60.	**2**	96.	**4**	132.	**3**
25.	**2**	61.	**4**	97.	**4**	133.	**2**
26.	**4**	62.	**3**	98.	**3**	134.	**3**
27.	**3**	63.	**2**	99.	**3**	135.	**3**
28.	**1**	64.	**3**	100.	**2**	136.	**2**
29.	**3**	65.	**2**	101.	**2**	137.	**3**
30.	**1**	66.	**2**	102.	**1**	138.	**2**
31.	**3**	67.	**2**	103.	**3**	139.	**1**
32.	**4**	68.	**3**	104.	**3**	140.	**2**
33.	**2**	69.	**3**	105.	**2**	141.	**3**
34.	**3**	70.	**2**	106.	**3**	142.	**2**
35.	**3**	71.	**1**	107.	**1**	143.	**3**
36.	**2**	72.	**1**	108.	**3**	144.	**4**

145. **3**	176. **4**	206. **2**	236. **2**
146. **2**	177. **4**	207. **1**	237. **1**
147. **3**	178. **2**	208. **1**	238. **2**
148. **4**	179. **1**	209. **2**	239. **3**
149. **2**	180. **1**	210. **2**	240. **3**
150. **4**	181. **1**	211. **4**	241. **4**
151. **2**	182. **2**	212. **2**	242. **1, 3, 4, and 5**
152. **3**	183. **2**	213. **3**	243. **4**
153. **1**	184. **2 and 4**	214. **2**	244. **2**
154. **1**	185. **4**	215. **1**	245. **1**
155. **2**	186. **4**	216. **1, 2, 4, and 5**	246. **2**
156. **2**	187. **1**	217. **1**	247. **3**
157. **3**	188. **4**	218. **3 and 4**	248. **1**
158. **3**	189. **3**	219. **2**	249. **3**
159. **4**	190. **4**	220. **1**	250. **4**
160. **1**	191. **2**	221. **4**	251. **2**
161. **2**	192. **4**	222. **2**	252. **2**
162. **3**	193. **3**	223. **2**	253. **1**
163. **3**	194. **2**	224. **4**	254. **3**
164. **3**	195. **3**	225. **3**	255. **2**
165. **3**	196. **3**	226. **1**	256. **3**
166. **2**	197. **3**	227. **2**	257. **4**
167. **2**	198. **2**	228. **3**	258. **1**
168. **1**	199. **3**	229. **1, 3, and 5**	259. **1**
169. **3**	200. **1**	230. **2**	260. **3**
170. **3**	201. **3**	231. **4**	261. **2**
171. **1**	202. **2**	232. **4**	262. **1**
172. **4**	203. **4**	233. **3**	263. **2**
173. **1**	204. **3**	234. **3**	264. **3**
174. **2**	205. **3**	235. **2**	265. **4**
175. **4**			

PRACTICE TEST ANSWERS AND EXPLANATIONS

1. The Answer is 3

The nurse is interviewing a client who is being treated for obsessive-compulsive disorder. Which of the following is the *MOST* important question the nurse should ask this client?

Reworded Question: What are the signs and symptoms of obsessive-compulsive disorder?

Strategy: "*MOST* important" indicates there may be more than one correct response.

Needed Info: Obsessive-compulsive disorder is characterized by a history of obsessions and compulsions. Obsessions are recurrent and persistent thoughts, ideas, impulses, or images that are experienced as intrusive and senseless. The client knows that the thoughts are ridiculous or morbid but cannot stop, forget, or control them. Compulsions are repetitive behaviors performed in a certain way to prevent discomfort and neutralize anxiety.

Category: Assessment/Psychosocial Integrity

(1) "Do you find yourself forgetting simple things?"—should be used to assess client with suspected cognitive disorder

(2) "Do you find it hard to stay on a task?"—assesses for disorders that disrupt the ability to concentrate, such as depression

(3) "Do you have trouble controlling upsetting thoughts?"—CORRECT: one feature of obsessive-compulsive disorder is the client's inability to control intrusive thoughts that repeat over and over

(4) "Do you experience feelings of panic in a closed area?"—appropriate for client with suspected panic disorder related to closed spaces or claustrophobia

2. The Answer is 2

Which of the following actions by the nurse would be considered negligence?

Reworded Question: What is an incorrect behavior?

Strategy: Think about the consequence of each action.

Needed Info: Negligence is the unintentional failure of the nurse to perform an act that a reasonable person would or would not perform in similar circumstances; can be an act of commission or omission. Standards of care: the actions that other nurses would do in the same or similar circumstances that provide for quality client care. Nurse practice acts: state laws that determine the scope of the practice of nursing.

Category: Analysis/Safe and Effective Care Environment/Management of Care

(1) Obtaining a Guthrie blood test on a 4-day-old infant—obtain after ingestion of protein, no later than 7 days after delivery

(2) Massaging lotion on the abdomen of a 3-year-old diagnosed with Wilms' tumor—CORRECT: manipulation of mass may cause dissemination of cancer cells

(3) Instructing a 5-year-old asthmatic to blow on a pinwheel—exercise that will extend expiratory time and increase expiratory pressure

(4) Playing kickball with a 10-year-old with juvenile arthritis (JA)—excellent moving and stretching exercise

3. The Answer is 4

The nurse on a postpartum unit is preparing 4 clients for discharge. It would be *MOST* important for the nurse to refer which of the following clients for home care?

Reworded Question: Who is the most unstable client?

Strategy: Think ABCs.

Needed Info: Need to meet the client's needs. Physical stability is the nurse's first concern. Most unstable client should be seen first.

Category: Implementation/Safe and Effective Care Environment/Management of Care

(1) A 15-year-old primipara who delivered a 7-lb. male 2 days ago—stable situation, no indication of problems with mother or baby

(2) An 18-year-old multipara who delivered a 9-lb. female by cesarean section 2 days ago—stable situation, no indication of problems with mother or baby

(3) A 20-year-old multipara who delivered 1 day ago and is complaining of cramping—stable client, cramping due to uterine contraction

(4) A 22-year-old who delivered by cesarean section and is complaining of burning on urination—CORRECT: unstable client, indicates urinary tract infection, requires follow-up

4. The Answer is 4

A client is telling the nurse about his perception of his thought patterns. Which of the following statements by the client would validate the diagnosis of schizophrenia?

Reworded Question: What behaviors or thought patterns characterize schizophrenia?

Strategy: Consider each answer in turn. Which is relevant to schizophrenia?

Needed Info: Schizophrenia is generally characterized by delusions (grandiose, religious, paranoid, nihilistic, or delusions of reference or influence), confusion, hallucinations, and illusions (misinterpretations of real external stimuli).

Category: Assessment/Psychosocial Integrity

(1) "I can't get the same thoughts out of my head."—recurrent, intrusive thoughts are characteristic of obsessive-compulsive disorder

(2) "I know I sometimes feel on top of the world, then suddenly down."—rapid, changing moods are characteristic of the manic phase of bipolar disorder

(3) "Sometimes I look up and wonder where I am."—confused, disoriented thoughts are characteristic of cognitive disorders

(4) "It's clear that this is an alien laboratory and I am in charge."—CORRECT: illogical, disorganized thoughts are typical of schizophrenia

5. The Answer is 1

A nursing team consists of an RN, an LPN/LVN, and an NAP. The nurse should assign which of the following clients to the LPN/LVN?

Reworded Question: Which client is an appropriate assignment for the LPN/LVN?

Strategy: Think about the skill level involved in each client's care.

Needed Info: LPN/LVN: assists with implementation of care; performs procedures; differentiates normal from abnormal; cares for stable clients with predictable conditions; has knowledge of asepsis and dressing changes; administers medications (varies with educational background and state nurse practice act).

Category: Planning/Safe and Effective Care Environment/Management of Care

(1) A 72-year-old client with diabetes who requires a dressing change for a stasis ulcer—CORRECT: stable client with an expected outcome

(2) A 42-year-old client with cancer of the bone complaining of pain—requires assessment; RN is the appropriate caregiver

(3) A 55-year-old client with terminal cancer being transferred to hospice home care—requires nursing judgment; RN is the appropriate caregiver

(4) A 23-year-old client with a fracture of the right leg who asks to use the urinal—standard, unchanging procedure; assign to the NAP

6. The Answer is 1

To determine the structural relationship of one hospital department with another, the nurse should consult which of the following?

Reworded Question: How does the nurse determine the relationship of one hospital department to another?

Strategy: Think about each answer.

Needed Info: The lateral lines on an organizational chart define the division and specializations of labor; the vertical lines explain the lines of authority and responsibility.

Category: Implementation/Safe and Effective Care Environment/Management of Care

(1) Organizational chart—CORRECT: delineates the overall organization structure, showing which departments exist and their relationships with one another both laterally and vertically

(2) Job descriptions—focus is not on departmental relationships

(3) Personnel policies—define policies for the organization's employees

(4) Policies and Procedures Manual—defines standards of care for an institution

7. The Answer is 3

A client complains of pain in his right lower extremity. The physician orders codeine 60 mg and aspirin grains X PO every 4 hours, as needed for pain. Each codeine tablet contains 15 mg of codeine. Each aspirin tablet contains 325 mg of aspirin. Which of the following should the nurse administer?

Reworded Question: What amount of medication should you give?

Strategy: Remember how to calculate dosages.

Needed Info: 60 mg = 1 grain.

Category: Implementation/Physiological Integrity/Pharmacological and Parenteral Therapies

(1) 2 codeine tablets and 4 aspirin tablets—inaccurate

(2) 4 codeine tablets and 3 aspirin tablets—inaccurate

(3) 4 codeine tablets and 2 aspirin tablets—CORRECT: $60/x = 15/1$, $x = 4$; 10 grains = 600 mg; $325/1 = 600/x$, $x = 1.8$ (round to 2)

(4) 3 codeine tablets and 3 aspirin tablets—inaccurate

8. The Answer is 3

The nurse is leading an inservice about management issues. The nurse would intervene if another nurse made which of the following statements?

Reworded Question: What are the nurse's responsibilities regarding obtaining consent?

Strategy: Think about each answer. Does it describe the nurse's responsibility for consent?

Needed Info: Requirements: capacity-age (adult), competent, voluntary; info must be given in understandable form. Legal responsibility: physician's responsibility to get consent form signed; when nurse witnesses a signature it means there's reason to believe client is informed about upcoming treatment.

Category: Evaluation/Safe and Effective Care Environment/Management of Care

(1) "It is my responsibility to ensure that the consent form has been signed and attached to the client's chart prior to surgery."—describes the nurse's responsibility

(2) "It is my responsibility to witness the signature of the client before surgery is performed."—signature indicates that the nurse saw the client sign the form

(3) "It is my responsibility to provide a detailed description of the surgery."—CORRECT: physician should provide explanation

(4) "It is my responsibility to answer questions that the client may have prior to surgery."—describes the nurse's responsibility

9. The Answer is 2

A nurse in the outpatient clinic evaluates the Mantoux test of a client whose history indicates that she has been treated during the past year for an AIDS-related infection. The nurse should document that there was a positive reaction if there is an area of induration measuring which of the following?

Reworded Question: What is a positive reaction for a client who is immunocompromised?

Strategy: Think about each answer choice.

Needed Info: Given intradermally in the forearm; read in 48–72 hours. 10 mm induration (hard area under skin) = significant (positive) reaction. Greater than 5 mm for clients with AIDS = positive reaction. Does not mean active disease is present but indicates exposure to TB or the presence of inactive (dormant) disease. Multiple puncture test done for routine screening.

Category: Analysis/Safe and Effective Care Environment/Safety and Infection Control

(1) 3 mm—nonsignificant reaction

(2) 7 mm—CORRECT: greater than 5-mm area positive for client with HIV-infection history

(3) 11 mm—area of 10 mm or more indicates positive reaction for client without an HIV infection

(4) 15 mm—area of 10 mm or more indicates positive reaction for client without an HIV infection

10. The Answer is 1

The nurse in the newborn nursery has just received report. Which of the following infants should the nurse see *FIRST*?

Reworded Question: Which infant is most unstable?

Strategy: Remember ABCs (airway, breathing, circulation).

Needed Info: Need to meet client's needs. Physical stability of client is nurse's first concern. Most unstable client should be seen first.

Category: Evaluation/Safe and Effective Care Environment/Management of Care

(1) A 2-day-old infant lying quietly alert with a heart rate of 185—CORRECT: infant has tachycardia; normal resting rate is 120–160; requires further investigation

(2) A 1-day-old infant crying, with a bulging anterior fontanel—crying causes increased intracranial pressure, which causes fontanel to bulge

(3) A 12-hour-old infant being held; the respirations are 45 breaths per minute and irregular—normal respiratory rate is 30–60 breaths per minute with apneic episodes

(4) A 5-hour-old infant sleeping with the hands and feet blue bilaterally—acrocyanosis is normal for 2–6 hours postdelivery due to poor peripheral circulation

11. The Answer is 3

While inserting a nasogastric tube, the nurse should use which of the following protective measures?

Reworded Question: What is the correct universal precaution?

Strategy: Think about each answer choice. How is each measure protecting the nurse?

Needed Info: Mask, eye protection, face shield protect mucous membrane exposure; used if activities are likely to generate splash or sprays. Gowns used if activities are likely to generate splashes or sprays.

Category: Planning/Safe and Effective Care Environment/Safety and Infection Control

(1) Gloves, gown, goggles, and surgical cap—surgical caps offer protection to hair but aren't required

(2) Sterile gloves, mask, plastic bags, and gown—plastic bags provide no direct protection and aren't part of universal precautions

(3) Gloves, gown, mask, and goggles—CORRECT: must use universal precautions on *all* clients; prevent skin and mucous membrane exposure when contact with blood or other body fluids is anticipated

(4) Double gloves, goggles, mask, and surgical cap—surgical cap not required; unnecessary to double-glove

12. The Answer is 2

The nurse is caring for clients in the outpatient clinic. Which of the following phone calls should the nurse return *FIRST*?

Reworded Question: Which client should the nurse call back first?

Strategy: Think ABCs.

Needed Info: Need to meet client's needs. Physical stability is nurse's first concern. Most unstable client should be contacted first.

Category: Analysis/Safe and Effective Care Environment/Management of Care

(1) A client with hepatitis A who states, "My arms and legs are itching."—caused by accumulation

of bile salts under the skin; treat with calamine lotion and antihistamines

(2) A client with a cast on the right leg who states, "I have a funny feeling in my right leg."—CORRECT: may indicate neurovascular compromise; requires immediate assessment

(3) A client with osteomyelitis of the spine who states, "I am so nauseous that I can't eat."—requires follow-up, but not highest priority

(4) A client with rheumatoid arthritis who states, "I am having trouble sleeping."—requires assessment, but not a priority

13. The Answer is 4

The nursing team consists of 1 RN, 2 LPNs/LVNs, and 3 NAPs. The RN should care for which of the following clients?

Reworded Question: Which client is an appropriate assignment for the RN?

Strategy: Think about the skill level involved in each client's care.

Needed Info: Determine nursing care required to meet clients' needs; take into account time required, complexity of activities, acuity of client, infection control issues. Consider knowledge and abilities of staff members and decide which staff person is best able to provide care. Give assignments to staff members (assign responsibility for total client care; avoid assigning only procedures). Provide additional help as needed.

Category: Planning/Safe and Effective Care Environment/Management of Care

(1) A client with a chest tube who is ambulating in the hall—LPN/LVN can care for client

(2) A client with a colostomy who requires assistance with a colostomy irrigation—assign to the LPN/LVN

(3) A client with a right-sided cerebral vascular accident (CVA) who requires assistance with bathing—assign to an NAP

(4) A client who is refusing medication to treat cancer of the colon—CORRECT: requires the assessment skills of the RN

14. The Answer is 3

The home care nurse is visiting a client during the icteric phase of hepatitis of unknown etiology. The nurse would be *MOST* concerned if the client made which of the following statements?

Reworded Question: What is an incorrect statement about caring for a client with hepatitis?

Strategy: "*MOST* concerned" indicates you are looking for an incorrect statement.

Needed Info: Hepatitis A (HAV): high risk groups include young children, institutions for custodial care, international travelers; transmission by fecal/oral, poor sanitation; nursing considerations include prevention, improved sanitation, treat with gamma globulin early post-exposure, no preparation of food. Hepatitis B (HBV): high risk groups include drug addicts, fetuses from infected mothers, homosexually active men, transfusions, health care workers; transmission by parenteral, sexual contact, blood/body fluids; nursing considerations include vaccine (Heptavax-B, Recombivax HB), immune globulin (HBIG) post-exposure, chronic carriers (potential for chronicity 5–10%). Hepatitis C (HVC): high risk groups include transfusions, international travelers; transmission by blood/body fluids; nursing considerations include great potential for chronicity. Delta hepatitis: high risk groups same as for HBV; transmission coinfects with HBV, close personal contact.

Category: Evaluation/Safe and Effective Care Environment/Safety and Infection Control

(1) "I must not share eating utensils with my family."—prevents transmission; handwashing before eating and after toileting very important

(2) "I must use my own bath towel."—prevents transmission; don't share bed linens

(3) "I'm glad that my husband and I can continue to have intimate relations."—CORRECT: avoid sexual contact until serologic indicators return to normal

(4) "I must eat small, frequent feedings."—easier to tolerate than 3 standard meals; diet should be high in carbohydrates and calories

15. The Answer is 2

A nurse plans for care of a client with anemia who is complaining of weakness. Which of the following tasks should the nurse assign to nursing assistive personnel (NAP)?

Reworded Question: What is an appropriate assignment for an NAP?

Strategy: Think about the skill level involved in each task.

Needed Info: Nursing assistive personnel (NAPs): assist with direct client care activities (bathing, transferring, ambulating, feeding, toileting, obtaining vital signs/height/weight/intake/output, housekeeping, transporting, stocking supplies); includes nurse aides, assistants, technicians, orderlies, nurse extenders; scope of nursing practice is limited.

Category: Planning/Safe and Effective Care Environment/Management of Care

(1) Listen to the client's breath sounds—requires assessment; should be performed by RN

(2) Set up the client's lunch tray—CORRECT: standard, unchanging procedure; decreases cardiac workload

(3) Obtain a diet history—involves assessment; should be performed by RN

(4) Instruct the client on how to balance rest and activity—assessment and teaching required; should be performed by RN

16. The Answer is 4

The nurse is caring for clients on the surgical floor and has just received report from the previous shift. Which of the following clients should the nurse see *FIRST?*

Reworded Question: Which client is the least stable?

Strategy: Think ABCs.

Needed Info: Need to meet the client's needs. Physical stability is the nurse's first concern. Most unstable client should be seen first.

Category: Analysis/Safe and Effective Care Environment/Management of Care

(1) A 35-year-old admitted 3 hours ago with a gunshot wound; 1.5-cm area of dark drainage noted on the dressing—does not indicate acute bleeding; small amount of blood

(2) A 43-year-old who had a mastectomy 2 days ago; 23 mL of serosanguinous fluid noted in the Jackson-Pratt drain—expected outcome

(3) A 59-year-old with a collapsed lung due to an accident; no drainage noted in the previous 8 hours—indicates resolution

(4) A 62-year-old who had an abdominal-perineal resection 3 days ago; client complains of chills—CORRECT: at risk for peritonitis; should be assessed for further symptoms of infection

17. The Answer is 3

Which of the following actions by the nurse would certainly be considered negligence?

Reworded Question: What is negligent behavior?

Strategy: Think about the consequences of each action.

Needed Info: Negligence: unintentional failure of nurse to perform an act that a reasonable person would or would not perform in similar circumstances; can be an act of commission or omission. Standards of care: the actions that other nurses would do in same or similar circumstances that provide for quality client care. Nurse practice acts: state laws that determine the scope of the practice of nursing.

Category: Evaluation/Safe and Effective Care Environment/Management of Care

(1) Inserting a 16 Fr nasogastric tube and aspirating 15 mL of gastric contents—correct procedure; verify placement by checking the pH

(2) Administering meperidine (Demerol) IM to a client prior to using the incentive spirometer—reducing the client's pain enables the client to take a deep breath

(3) Turning and repositioning a client every shift after post-abdominal surgery—CORRECT: Postoperative clients should be turned and repositioned every 2 hours after surgery to promote circulation and reduce the risk of skin breakdown (except if contraindicated, such as in neurologic or musculoskeletal surgery demanding immobilization)

(4) Initially administering blood at 5 mL per minute for 15 minutes—correct procedure; start blood with normal saline and 19-gauge needle

18. The Answer is 2

A 1-day-old newborn diagnosed with intrauterine growth retardation is observed by the nurse to be restless, irritable, and fist-sucking, and having a high-pitched, shrill cry. Based on this data, which of the following actions should the nurse take *FIRST*?

Reworded Question: What do you do for a newborn experiencing withdrawal?

Strategy: Determine the outcome of each answer.

Needed Info: Drug withdrawal may manifest from as early as 12 hrs after birth up to 10 days after delivery. Symptoms: high-pitched cry, hyperreflexia, decreased sleep, diaphoresis, tachypnea, excessive mucus, vomiting, uncoordinated sucking. Nursing care: assess muscle tone, irritability, vital signs; administer phenobarbital as ordered; report symptoms of respiratory distress; reduce stimulation; provide adequate nutrition/fluids; monitor mother/child interactions.

Category: Implementation/Health Promotion and Maintenance

(1) Massage the infant's back—may result in overstimulation of the infant

(2) Tightly swaddle the infant in a flexed position—CORRECT: promotes infant's comfort and security

(3) Schedule feeding times every 3–4 hours—small, frequent feedings are preferable

(4) Encourage eye contact with the infant during feedings—may result in overstimulation of infant

19. The Answer is 2

The nurse visits a neighbor who is at 20 weeks' gestation. The neighbor complains of nausea, headache, and blurred vision. The nurse notes that the neighbor appears nervous, is diaphoretic, and is experiencing tremors. It would be *MOST* important for the nurse to ask which of the following questions?

Reworded Question: What is the priority assessment question?

Strategy: "*MOST* important" indicates there may be more than one correct response.

Needed Info: Assessment: irritability, confusion, tremors, blurring of vision, coma, seizures, hypotension, tachycardia, skin cool and clammy, diaphoresis. Plan/Implementation: liquids containing sugar if conscious, skim milk is ideal if tolerated; dextrose 50% IV if unconscious, glucagon; follow with additional carbohydrate in 15 minutes; determine and treat cause; client education; exercise regimen.

Category: Assessment/Health Promotion and Maintenance

(1) "Are you having menstrual-like cramps?"—symptoms of preterm labor

(2) "When did you last eat or drink?"—CORRECT: classic symptoms of hypoglycemia; offer carbohydrate

(3) "Have you been diagnosed with diabetes?"—need to determine if she is hypoglycemic

(4) "Have you been lying on the couch?"—not relevant to hypoglycemia

20. The Answer is 4

The school nurse notes that a first-grade child is scratching her head almost constantly. It would be *MOST* important for the nurse to take which of the following actions?

Reworded Question: What is the best assessment?

Strategy: Determine if assessment or implementation is appropriate.

Needed Info: Pediculosis (lice). Assessment: scalp—white eggs (nits) on hair shafts, itchy; body—macules and papules; pubis—red macules. Nursing consideration: OTC pyrethrin (RID, A-200), permethrin 1% (Nix); kills both lice and nits with 1 application; may suggest repeating in 7 days if necessary.

Category: Assessment/Health Promotion and Maintenance

(1) Discuss basic hygiene with parents—makes an assumption; must assess first

(2) Instruct the child not to sleep with her dog—must first assess to determine the problem

(3) Inform the parents that they must contact an exterminator—not enough information to make this determination

(4) Observe the scalp for small white specks—CORRECT: nits (eggs) appear as small, white, oval flakes attached to hair shaft

21. The Answer is 3

A suicidal client who was admitted to the psychiatric unit for treatment and observation a week ago suddenly appears cheerful and motivated. The nurse should be aware of which of the following?

Reworded Question: What is the significance of sudden mood changes in a depressed client?

Strategy: Know the signs of impending suicide.

Needed Info: Assessment for suicidal ideation, suicidal gestures, suicidal threats, and actual suicidal attempt. Clients who have developed a suicide plan are more serious about following through, and are at grave risk. Clients emerging from severe depression have more energy with which to formulate and carry out a suicide plan (for which they had no energy before treatment). The nurse should determine risk for suicide; suspect suicidal ideation in depressed client; ask the client if he is thinking about suicide; ask the client about the advantages and disadvantages of suicide to determine how the client sees his situation; evaluate client's access to a method of suicide; develop a formal "no suicide" contract with client; and support the client's reason to live.

Category: Analysis/Psychosocial Integrity

(1) The client is likely sleeping well because of the medication—improved sleep patterns would not explain the client's sudden mood change

(2) The client has made new friends and has a support group—support on the nursing unit would not explain the mood change

(3) The client may have finalized a suicide plan—CORRECT: as depressed clients improve, their risk for suicide is greater because they are able to mobilize more energy to plan and execute suicide

(4) The client is responding to treatment and is no longer depressed—sudden cheerful and energetic mood does not indicate resolution of depression

22. The Answer is 3

The nurse is caring for clients in the GYN clinic. A client complains of an off-white vaginal discharge with a curdlike appearance. The nurse notes the discharge and vulvular erythema. It would be *MOST* important for the nurse to ask which of the following questions?

Reworded Question: What is a predisposing factor to developing candidiasis?

Strategy: "*MOST* important" indicates there may be more than one correct response.

Needed Info: *Candida albicans.* Symptoms: odorless, cheesy white discharge; itching, inflames vagina and perineum. Treatment: topical clotrimazole (Gyne-Lotrimin), nystatin (Mycostatin).

Category: Assessment/Health Promotion and Maintenance

(1) "Do you douche?"—not a factor in the development of candidiasis

(2) "Are you sexually active?"—candidiasis not usually sexually transmitted; predisposing factors include glycosuria, pregnancy, and oral contraceptives

(3) "What kind of birth control do you use?"—CORRECT: oral contraceptives predispose individuals to candidiasis

(4) "Have you taken any cough medicine?"—no relationship between cough medicine and candidiasis

23. The Answer is 1

The nurse is caring for a client in the prenatal clinic. The nurse notes that the client's chart contains the following information: blood type AB, Rh-negative; serology—negative; indirect Coombs test—negative; fetal paternity—unknown. The nurse should anticipate taking which of the following actions?

Reworded Question: What should the nurse do in this situation?

Strategy: Determine if it is appropriate to assess or implement.

Needed Info: RhoGAM: given to unsensitized Rh-negative mother after delivery or abortion of an

Rh-positive infant or fetus to prevent development of sensitization. Direct Coombs test done on cord blood after delivery; if both are negative and neonate is Rh-positive, mother is given RhoGAM. RhoGAM is usually given to unsensitized mothers within 72 hours of delivery, but may be effective up to 3–4 weeks after delivery. Administration of RhoGAM at 26–28 weeks' gestation also recommended. RhoGAM is ineffective against Rh-positive antibodies already present in the maternal circulation.

Category: Implementation/Health Promotion and Maintenance

(1) Administer Rho (D) immune globulin (RhoGAM)—CORRECT: no indication of sensitization; RhoGAM will prevent possibility that she'll become sensitized; given at 28 weeks' gestation if Coombs test is negative

(2) Schedule an amniocentesis—amniotic fluid aspirated by needle through abdominal and uterine walls to detect a genetic disorder

(3) Obtain a direct Coombs test—obtained from newborns, not from pregnant woman

(4) Assess maternal serum for alpha fetoprotein level—predicts neural tubal defects, done between 16 and 18 weeks

24. The Answer is 1

The nurse is caring for a woman at 37 weeks' gestation. The client was diagnosed with insulin-dependent diabetes mellitus (IDDM) at age 7. The client states, "I am so thrilled that I will be breastfeeding my baby." Which of the following responses by the nurse is *BEST*?

Reworded Question: What are the insulin requirements of the breastfeeding diabetic?

Strategy: Determine the outcome of each answer choice.

Needed Info: Nursing care of diabetic during pregnancy: reinforce need for careful monitoring throughout pregnancy; evaluate understanding of modifications in diet/insulin coverage. Teach client and significant other: diet (eat prescribed amount of food daily at same times); home glucose monitoring; insulin (purpose, dosage, administration, action,

side effects, potential change in amount needed during pregnancy as fetus grows and immediately after delivery); no oral hypoglycemics (teratogenic). Assist with stress reduction; fetal surveillance.

Category: Planning/Health Promotion and Maintenance

(1) "You will probably need less insulin while you are breastfeeding."—CORRECT: breastfeeding has an antidiabetogenic effect; less insulin is needed

(2) "You will need to initially increase your insulin after the baby is born."—insulin needs will decrease due to antidiabetogenic effect of breastfeeding and physiological changes during immediate postpartum period

(3) "You will be able to take an oral hypoglycemic instead of insulin after the baby is born."—client has IDDM: insulin required

(4) "You will probably require the same dose of insulin that you are now taking."—during third trimester, insulin requirements increase due to increased insulin resistance

25. The Answer is 2

The nurse is caring for clients in a pediatric clinic. The mother of a 14-year-old male privately tells the nurse that she is worried about her son because she unexpectedly walked into his room and discovered him masturbating. Which of the following responses by the nurse would be *MOST* appropriate?

Reworded Question: What is the most therapeutic response?

Strategy: Remember therapeutic communication.

Needed Info: Male changes in puberty: increase in genital size; breast swelling; pubic, facial, axillary, and chest hair; deepening voice; production of functional sperm; nocturnal emissions. Psychosexual development: masturbation as expression of sexual tension; sexual fantasies; experimental sexual intercourse.

Category: Implementation/Health Promotion and Maintenance

(1) "Tell your son he could go blind doing that."—false information

(2) "Masturbation is a normal part of sexual development."—CORRECT: true statement provides opportunity for sexual self-exploration

(3) "He's really too young to be masturbating."—boys typically begin masturbating in early adolescence

(4) "Why don't you give him more privacy?"—judgmental; doesn't take advantage of opportunity to teach

26. The Answer is 4

The nurse performs a home visit on a client who delivered 2 days ago. The client states that she is bottle-feeding her infant. The nurse notes white, curdlike patches on the newborn's oral mucous membranes. The nurse should take which of the following actions?

Reworded Question: What is the treatment for thrush?

Strategy: Determine the outcome of each answer choice.

Needed Info: Thrush (oral candidiasis): white plaque on oral mucous membranes, gums, or tongue; treatment includes good handwashing, nystatin (Mycostatin).

Category: Implementation/Health Promotion and Maintenance

(1) Determine the newborn's blood glucose level—thrush in newborns is caused by poor handwashing or exposure to an infected vagina during birth

(2) Suggest that the newborn's formula be changed—not related to thrush

(3) Remind the caregiver not to let the infant sleep with the bottle—not related to thrush

(4) Explain that the newborn will need to receive some medication—CORRECT: thrush most often treated with nystatin (Mycostatin)

27. The Answer is 3

The nurse at the birthing facility is caring for a primipara woman in labor, who is 4 cm dilated and 25% effaced, and whose fetal vertex is at +1. The physician informs the client that an amniotomy is to be performed. The client states, "My friend's baby died when the umbilical cord came out when her water broke. I don't want you to do that to me!" Which of the following responses by the nurse is *BEST*?

Reworded Question: What is the most therapeutic response?

Strategy: "*BEST*" indicates that there may be more than one correct response.

Needed Info: Amniotomy: artificial rupture of membranes. Presenting part should be engaged to prevent cord prolapse. Obtain FHR before and after procedure. Assess color, odor, consistency of amniotic fluid. Check maternal temperature q 2 hrs; notify head care provider if temp is 100.4° F (38° C) or higher.

Category: Implementation/Health Promotion and Maintenance

(1) "If you are that concerned, you should refuse the procedure."—giving advice, nontherapeutic

(2) "The procedure will help your labor go faster."—doesn't respond to client's concerns

(3) "That shouldn't happen to you because the baby's head is engaged."—CORRECT: umbilical prolapse usually occurs when the presenting part isn't engaged

(4) "We will monitor you carefully to prevent cord prolapse."—monitoring will not prevent prolapsed cord

28. The Answer is 1

A primigravid woman comes to the clinic for her initial prenatal visit. She is at 32 weeks' gestation and says that she has just moved from out of state. The client says that she has had periodic headaches during her pregnancy, and that she is continually bumping into things. The nurse notes numerous bruises in various stages of healing around the client's breasts and abdomen. Vital signs are: BP 120/80, pulse 72, resp 18, and FHT 142. Which of the following responses by the nurse is *BEST*?

Reworded Question: What is the best assessment?

Strategy: Determine if it is appropriate to assess or implement.

Needed Info: Symptoms of domestic abuse: frequent visits to physician's office or emergency room for unexplained trauma; client being cued, silenced, or threatened by an accompanying family member; evidence of multiple old injuries, scars, healed fractures seen on x-ray; fearful, evasive, or inconsistent replies, or nonverbal behaviors such as flinching when approached or touched. Nursing care: provide privacy during initial interview to ensure perpetrator of violence does not remain with client; carefully document all injuries (with consent); determine safety of client by asking specific questions about weapons, substance abuse, extreme jealousy; develop with client a safety or escape plan; refer client to community resources.

Category: Assessment/Health Promotion and Maintenance

(1) "Are you battered by your partner?"—CORRECT: evidence of injury should be investigated; assess head, neck, chest, abdomen, breasts, upper extremities

(2) "How do you feel about being pregnant?"—injuries take priority

(3) "Tell me about your headaches."—injuries take priority

(4) "You may be more clumsy due to your size."—assumption; need to assess

29. The Answer is 3

The nurse is teaching a class on natural family planning. Which of the following statements by a client indicates that teaching has been successful?

Reworded Question: What is a true statement about natural family planning?

Strategy: Think about each statement. Is it true about natural family planning?

Needed Info: Natural family planning—Action: periodic abstinence from intercourse during fertile period; based on regularity of ovulation; variable effectiveness. Teaching: fertile period may be determined by a drop in basal body temp before and a slight rise after ovulation, and/or a change in cervical mucus from thick, cloudy, and sticky during nonfertile period to more abundant, clear, thin, stretchy, and slippery during ovulation.

Category: Evaluation/Health Promotion and Maintenance

(1) "When I ovulate, my basal body temperature will be elevated for 2 days and then will decrease."—basal body temp decreases prior to ovulation; after ovulation, temp increases

(2) "My cervical mucus will be thick, cloudy, and sticky when I ovulate."—fertile mucus appears clear, thin, watery, and stretchy

(3) "Because I am regular, I will be fertile about 14 days after the beginning of my period."—CORRECT: ovulation occurs approx. 14 days after start of menstrual period

(4) "When I ovulate, my cervix will feel firm."—cervix softens slightly during ovulation

30. The Answer is 1

The home care nurse plans care for a child in a leg cast for treatment of a fractured right ankle. The nurse enters the following nursing diagnosis on the care plan: skin integrity, risk for impaired. Which of the following actions by the nurse is *BEST*?

Reworded Question: What is the priority action to prevent skin breakdown?

Strategy: Determine the outcome of each answer choice.

Needed Info: Immediate nursing care for plaster cast: don't cover cast until dry (48 hours), handle with palms not fingertips; don't rest on hard surfaces; elevate affected limb above heart on soft surface until dry; don't use head lamp; check for blueness or paleness, pain, numbness, tingling (if present, elevate area; if it persists, contact physician); child should remain inactive while cast is drying. Intermediate nursing care: mobilize client, isometric exercises; check for break in cast or foul odor; tell client not to scratch skin under cast and not to put anything underneath cast; if fiberglass cast gets wet, dry with hair dryer on cool setting. After-cast nursing care: wash skin gently, apply baby powder/cornstarch/baby oil; have client gradually adjust to movement without support of cast; swelling is common, elevate limb and apply elastic bandage.

Category: Implementation/Physiological Integrity/Reduction of Risk Potential

(1) Teaching the child how to perform isometric exercises of the right leg—CORRECT: contraction of

muscle without moving joint; promotes venous return and circulation, prevents thrombi; quadriceps setting (push back knees into bed) and gluteal setting (push heels into bed)

(2) Teaching the mother to gently massage the child's right foot with emollient cream—will help prevent dryness of foot but does not address skin under cast

(3) Instructing the mother to keep the leg cast clean and dry—because client is a young child, should be included in teaching of cast care; improving circulation is best way to prevent impaired skin integrity under cast

(4) Teaching the mother how to turn and position the child—no info provided about mobility of child; will prevent hazards of immobility

31. The Answer is 3

The nurse is caring for a client who had a thyroidectomy 12 hours ago for treatment of Graves' disease. The nurse would be *MOST* concerned if which of the following was observed?

Reworded Question: What is a complication after a thyroidectomy?

Strategy: "*MOST* concerned" indicates a complication.

Needed Info: Nursing care for Graves' disease/hyperthyroidism: limit activities and provide frequent rest periods; advise light, cool clothing; avoid stimulants; use calm, unhurried approach; administer antithyroid medication, irradiation with I131 PO. Post-thyroidectomy care: low or semi-Fowler's position; support head, neck, shoulders to prevent flexion or hyperextension of suture line; tracheostomy set at bedside; observe for complications—laryngeal nerve injury, thyroid storm, hemorrhage, respiratory obstruction, tetany (decreased calcium from parathyroid involvement), check Chvostek's and Trousseau's signs.

Category: Assessment/Physiological Integrity/Reduction of Risk Potential

(1) The client's blood pressure is 138/82, pulse 84, respirations 16, oral temp 99° F (37.2° C)—vital signs within normal limits

(2) The client supports his head and neck when turning his head to the right—prevents stress on the incision

(3) The client spontaneously flexes his wrist when the blood pressure is obtained—CORRECT: carpal spasms indicate hypocalcemia

(4) The client is drowsy and complains of a sore throat—expected outcome after surgery

32. The Answer is 4

A client is admitted with complaints of severe pain in the lower right quadrant of the abdomen. To assist with pain relief, the nurse should take which of the following actions?

Reworded Question: What is an appropriate non-pharmacological method for pain relief?

Strategy: Determine the outcome of each answer choice.

Needed Info: Establish a 24-hour pain profile. Teach client about pain and its relief: explain quality and location of impending pain; slow, rhythmic breathing to promote relaxation; effects of analgesics and benefits of preventative approach; splinting techniques to reduce pain. Reduce anxiety and fears. Provide comfort measures: proper positioning; cool, well ventilated, quiet room; back rub; allow for rest.

Category: Implementation/Physiological Integrity/Basic Care and Comfort

(1) Encourage the client to change positions frequently in bed—unnecessary movement will increase pain, should be avoided

(2) Massage the lower right quadrant of the abdomen—if appendicitis is suspected, massage or palpation should never be performed as these actions may cause the appendix to rupture

(3) Apply warmth to the abdomen with a heating pad—if pain is caused by appendicitis, increased circulation from heat may cause appendix to rupture

(4) Use comfort measures and pillows to position the client—CORRECT: non-pharmacological methods of pain relief

33. The Answer is 2

The nurse prepares a client for peritoneal dialysis. Which of the following actions should the nurse take *FIRST*?

Reworded Question: What is the priority action for a client undergoing peritoneal dialysis?

Strategy: Determine if it is appropriate to assess or implement.

Needed Info: Peritoneal dialysis: takes place within peritoneal cavity to remove excess fluids and waste products usually removed by the kidneys. Procedure: rubber catheter surgically inserted into abdominal cavity; 1–2 liters of fluid infused into peritoneal space by gravity; fluid stays in cavity for approx. 20 minutes; fluid drained by gravity. Complications: peritonitis, abdominal pain, insufficient return of fluid. Nursing care before procedure: obtain baseline vitals, breath sounds, weight, glucose, and electrolyte levels. During procedure: take vital signs, ongoing assessment for respiratory distress, pain, discomfort; use aseptic technique; check abdominal dressing around catheter for wetness.

Category: Implementation/Physiological Integrity/ Reduction of Risk Potential

(1) Assess for a bruit and a thrill—used with hemodialysis through an AV fistula, graft, or shunt

(2) Warm the dialysate solution—CORRECT: solution should be warmed to body temp in warmer or with heating pad; don't use microwave oven; cold dialysate increases discomfort

(3) Position the client on the left side—client should be in supine or low Fowler's position wearing a mask

(4) Insert a Foley catheter—unnecessary, client can void without a catheter

34. The Answer is 3

The nurse teaches an elderly client with right-sided weakness how to use a cane. Which of the following behaviors by the client indicates that the teaching was effective?

Reworded Question: What is the appropriate technique used to ambulate with a cane?

Strategy: Determine the outcome of each answer choice.

Needed Info: Cane tip should have concentric rings (shock absorber for stability). Flex elbow 30 degrees and hold handle up; tip of cane should be 15 cm lateral to base of the 5th toe. Hold cane in hand opposite affected extremity; advance cane and affected leg; lean on cane when moving good leg. To manage stairs, step up on good leg, place the cane and affected leg on step; reverse when going down ("up with the good, down with the bad"); same sequence used with crutches.

Category: Evaluation/Physiological Integrity/Basic Care and Comfort

(1) The client holds the cane with his right hand, moves the cane forward followed by the right leg, and then moves the left leg—should hold cane with the stronger (left) hand

(2) The client holds the cane with his right hand, moves the cane forward followed by his left leg, and then moves the right leg—should hold cane with the stronger (left) hand

(3) The client holds the cane with his left hand, moves the cane forward followed by the right leg, and then moves the left leg—CORRECT: the cane acts as a support and aids in weight-bearing for the weaker right leg

(4) The client holds the cane with his left hand, moves the cane forward followed by his left leg, and then moves the right leg—cane needs to be a support and aid in weight-bearing for the weaker right leg

35. The Answer is 3

While caring for a client receiving total parenteral nutrition (TPN) through a central line, the nurse notices a small trickle of opaque fluid leaking from around the central line dressing. It is *MOST* important for the nurse to take which of the following actions?

Reworded Question: What is the best action if the nurse suspects a break in the central line?

Strategy: "*MOST* important" indicates there may be more than one correct response.

Needed Info: TPN: method of supplying nutrients to the body by the IV route. Nursing care: site of catheter changed every 4 weeks, change IV tubing and filters every 24 hours, dressing changed 2–3 times a week and PRN; initial rate of infusion 50 mL/hr and gradually increased (100–125 mL/hr) as client's fluid and electrolyte tolerance permits; increased rate of infusion causes hyperosmolar state (headache, nausea, fever, chills, malaise); slowed rate of infusion results in "rebound" hypoglycemia caused by delayed pancreatic reaction to change in insulin requirements.

Category: Implementation/Physiological Integrity/Pharmalogical and Parenteral Therapies

(1) Prepare to change the central line dressing—dressing might be removed later to further assess the situation, but this is not the most important action

(2) Verify that the client is on antibiotics—no evidence of line infection

(3) Place the client's head lower than his feet—CORRECT: indicates a break in the line, which places client at risk for air embolism; turn client on left side and place head lower than feet; notify physician

(4) Secure the Y-port where the lipids are infusing—leakage is occurring at the IV site, not the Y site

36.   The Answer is 2

A 46-year-old man is admitted to the hospital with a fractured right femur. He is placed in balanced suspension traction with a Thomas splint and Pearson attachment. During the first 48 hours, the nurse should assess the client for which of the following complications?

Reworded Question: What complication of a fracture is seen in the first 48 hours?

Strategy: Be careful! They are asking for the complication that occurs during the first 48 hours. Later complications may be included as answer choices.

Needed Info: Complications of fractures: (1) compartment syndrome (increased pressure externally [casts, dressings] or internally [bleeding, edema]

resulting in compromised circulation); Signs/Symptoms (S/S): pallor, weak pulse, numbness, pain; (2) shock: bone is vascular; (3) fat embolism; (4) deep vein thrombosis; (5) infection, avascular necrosis; (6) delayed union, nonunion, malunion.

Category: Assessment/Physiological Integrity/Physiological Adaptation

(1) Pulmonary embolism—obstruction of pulmonary system by thrombus from venous system or right side of heart; seen 2–3 days to several weeks after fracture

(2) Fat embolism—CORRECT: fat moves into bloodstream from fracture; formed by alteration in lipids in blood; fat combines with platelets to form emboli; S/S: abnormal behavior due to cerebral anoxia (confusion, agitation, delirium, coma), abnormal ABGs (pO_2 below 60 mm Hg), increased resp; chest pain, dyspnea, pallor, hypertension, petechiae on chest, upper arms, abdomen; treatment: high Fowler's, high concentration O_2, ventilation with PEEP (positive end expiratory pressure) to decrease pulmonary edema, IVs, steroids, Dextran to prevent shock

(3) Avascular necrosis—(seen later than 48 hrs) bone loses blood supply and dies; seen with chronic renal disease or prolonged steroid use; treatment: bone graft, joint fusion, prosthetic replacement

(4) Malunion—bone fragments heal in deformed position as a result of inadequate reduction and immobilization; treatment: surgical or manual manipulation to realign

37.   The Answer is 1

The nurse is helping an NAP provide a bed bath to a comatose client who is incontinent. The nurse should intervene if which of the following actions is noted?

Reworded Question: What is an incorrect action?

Strategy: "Should intervene" indicates that you are looking for something wrong.

Needed Info: Standard precautions (barrier) used with all clients: primary strategy for nosocomial infection control. Most important way to reduce transmission of pathogens. Gloves: use clean, non-sterile when touching blood, body fluids, secretions, excretions, contaminated articles; remove promptly after use, before touching items and environmental surfaces.

Category: Evaluation/Safe and Effective Care Environment/Safety and Infection Control

(1) The NAP answers the phone while wearing gloves—CORRECT: contaminated gloves should be removed before answering the phone

(2) The NAP log-rolls the client to provide back care—correct way to roll a client to maintain proper alignment

(3) The NAP places an incontinence diaper under the client—appropriate to use incontinence diapers for this client

(4) The NAP positions the client on the left side, head elevated—appropriate position to prevent aspiration and protect the airway

---

38. The Answer is 3

A 70-year-old woman is brought to the emergency room for treatment after being found on the floor by her daughter. X-rays reveal a displaced subcapital fracture of the left hip and osteoarthritis. When comparing the legs, the nurse would most likely make which of the following observations?

Reworded Question: What is a symptom of a hip fracture?

Strategy: Think about each answer choice.

Needed Info: Symptoms of fracture: swelling, pallor, ecchymosis; loss of sensation to other body parts; deformity; pain/acute tenderness; muscle spasms; loss of function, abnormal mobility; crepitus (grating sound on movement); shortening of affected limb; decreased or absent pulses distal to injury; affected extremity colder than contralateral part. Emergency nursing care: immobilize joint above and below fracture by use of splints before client is moved; in open fracture, cover the wound with sterile dressings or cleanest material available, control bleeding by direct pressure; check temp, color, sensation, capillary refill distal to fracture; in emergency

room, give narcotic adequate to relieve pain (except in presence of head injury).

Category: Assessment/Physiological Integrity/Physiological Adaptation

(1) The client's left leg is longer than the right leg and externally rotated—leg is shorter due to contraction of muscles attached above and below fracture site

(2) The client's left leg is shorter than the right leg and internally rotated—leg is usually externally rotated

(3) The client's left leg is shorter than the right leg and adducted—CORRECT: extremity shortens due to contraction of muscles attached above and below fracture site, fragments overlap by 1–2 inches

(4) The client's left leg is longer than the right leg and is abducted—extremity shortens and externally rotates

---

39. The Answer is 3

The nurse is caring for a client with a cast on the left leg. The nurse would be *MOST* concerned if which of the following is observed?

Reworded Question: What is a complication of a cast?

Strategy: "*MOST* concerned" indicates a complication.

Needed Info: Immediate nursing care for plaster cast: don't cover cast until dry (48 hours), handle with palms not fingertips; don't rest on hard surfaces; elevate affected limb above heart on soft surface until dry; don't use head lamp; check for blueness or paleness, pain, numbness, tingling (if present, elevate area; if it persists, contact physician); client should remain inactive while cast is drying. Intermediate nursing care: mobilize client, isometric exercises; check for break in cast or foul odor; tell client not to scratch skin under cast and not to put anything underneath cast; if fiberglass cast gets wet, dry with hair dryer on cool setting. After-cast nursing care: wash skin gently, apply baby powder/cornstarch/baby oil; have client gradually adjust to movement without support of cast; swelling is common, elevate limb and apply elastic bandage.

Category: Analysis/Physiological Integrity/Physiological Adaptation

(1) Capillary refill time is less than 3 seconds—capillary refill time is within normal limits

(2) Client complains of discomfort and itching—a casted extremity may itch or feel uncomfortable due to prolonged immobility

(3) Client complains of tightness and pain—CORRECT: client with a pressure ulcer usually reports pain and tightness in the area; infection or necrosis will result in feeling of warmth and a foul odor

(4) Client's foot is elevated on a pillow—newly casted extremity may be slightly elevated to help relieve edema; should remain in correct anatomical position and below heart level to allow sufficient arterial perfusion

40. The Answer is 2

The nurse is discharging a client from an inpatient alcohol treatment unit. Which of the following statements by the client's wife indicates to the nurse that the family is coping adaptively?

Reworded Question: What indicates that the client's family is coping with the client's alcoholism?

Strategy: Think about what each statement means.

Needed Info: Nursing care for chronic alcohol dependence: safety; monitor for withdrawal; reality orientation; increase self-esteem and coping skills; balanced diet; abstinence from alcohol; identify problems related to drinking in family relationships, work, etc.; help client to see/admit problem; confront denial with slow persistence; maintain relationship with client; establish control of problem drinking; provide support; Alcoholics Anonymous; disulfiram (Antabuse): drug used to maintain sobriety, based on behavioral therapy.

Category: Analysis/Psychosocial Integrity

(1) "My husband will do well as long as I keep him engaged in activities that he likes."—wife is accepting responsibility, codependent behavior

(2) "My focus is learning how to live my life."—CORRECT: wife is working to change codependent patterns

(3) "I am so glad that our problems are behind us."—unrealistic; discharge is not the final step of treatment

(4) "I'll make sure that the children don't give my husband any problems."—wife is accepting responsibility, codependent behavior

41. The Answer is 3

A nurse is caring for clients in the mental health clinic. A woman comes to the clinic complaining of insomnia and anorexia. The client tearfully tells the nurse that she was laid off from a job that she had held for 15 years. Which of the following responses by the nurse would be *MOST* appropriate?

Reworded Question: What is the most therapeutic response?

Strategy: Remember therapeutic communication.

Needed Info: Nursing considerations, explore client's understanding of the problem: focus on the present; emphasize client's strengths; avoid blaming; determine how client handled similar situations; provide support; mobilize client's coping strategies.

Category: Implementation/Psychosocial Integrity

(1) "Did your company give you a severance package?"—yes/no question, nontherapeutic

(2) "Focus on the fact that you have a healthy, happy family."—gives advice, false assurance

(3) "Tell me what happened."—CORRECT: explores situation; allows client to verbalize

(4) "Losing a job is common nowadays."—dismisses the client's concern

42. The Answer is 1

A client with a history of alcoholism is brought to the emergency room in an agitated state. He is vomiting and diaphoretic. He says he had his last drink 5 hours ago. The nurse would expect to administer which of the following medications?

Reworded Question: What is the best medication to treat acute alcohol withdrawal?

Strategy: Think about the action of each drug.

Needed Info: Alcohol sedates the central nervous system; rebound during withdrawal. Early symptoms occur 4–6 hours after last drink. Symptoms: tremors; easily startled; insomnia; anxiety; anorexia; alcoholic hallucinosis (48 hours after last drink). Nursing care: administer sedation as needed, usually benzodiazepines; monitor vital signs, particularly pulse; take seizure precautions; provide quiet, well-lit environment; orient client frequently; don't leave hallucinating, confused client alone; administer anticonvulsants as needed, thiamine IV or IM, and IV glucose.

Category: Planning/Psychosocial Integrity

(1) Chlordiazepoxide hydrochloride (Librium)— CORRECT: antianxiety; used to treat symptoms of acute alcohol withdrawal; Side effects (S/E): lethargy, hangover, agranulocytosis

(2) Disulfiram (Antabuse)—used as a deterrent to compulsive drinking; contraindicated if client drank alcohol in previous 12 hours

(3) Methadone hydrochloride (Dolophine)—opioid analgesic; used to treat narcotic withdrawal; syndrome, S/E: seizures, respiratory depression

(4) Naloxone hydrochloride (Narcan)—narcotic antagonist used to reverse narcotic-induced respiratory depression; S/E: ventricular fibrillation, seizures, pulmonary edema

---

43. The Answer is 1

An elderly client is admitted to the nursing home setting. The client is occasionally confused and her gait is often unsteady. Which of the following actions by the nurse would be *MOST* appropriate?

Reworded Question: What are visual cues for a client who is confused?

Strategy: Determine the outcome of each answer choice.

Needed Info: Nursing care for Alzheimer's disease: provide calm, predictable environment with regular routine; give clear and simple explanations; display clock and calendar; color-code objects and areas; monitor medications and food intake; secure doors leading from house/unit; gently distract and redirect during wandering behavior; avoid restraints (increases combativeness); organize daily activities into short, achievable steps; discourage long naps during the day. If client experiences catastrophic reaction, remain calm and stay with client; provide distraction such as music, rocking, stroking.

Category: Implementation/Psychosocial Integrity

(1) Ask the woman's family to provide personal items such as photos or mementos—CORRECT: provides visual stimulation to reduce sensory deprivation

(2) Select a room with a bed by the door so the woman can look down the hall—provides only occasional stimulation

(3) Suggest the woman eat her meals in the room with her roommate—needs to eat in the dining hall with others for stimulation

(4) Encourage the woman to ambulate in the halls twice a day—unsafe due to unsteady gait and confusion

---

44. The Answer is 2

The nurse teaches an elderly client how to use a standard aluminum walker. Which of the following behaviors by the client indicates that the nurse's teaching was effective?

Reworded Question: What is the correct technique when ambulating with a walker?

Strategy: Determine the outcome of each answer choice.

Needed Info: Elbows flexed at 20–30-degree angle when standing with hands on grips. Lift and move walker forward 8–10 inches. With partial or non-weight-bearing, put weight on wrists and arms and step forward with affected leg, supporting self on arms, and follow with good leg. Nurse should stand behind client, hold onto gait belt at waist as needed for balance. Sit down by grasping armrest on affected side, shift weight to good leg and hand, lower self into chair. Client should wear sturdy shoes.

Category: Evaluation/Physiological Integrity/Basic Care and Comfort

(1) The client slowly pushes the walker forward 12 inches, then takes small steps forward while leaning on the walker—should not push the walker

(2) The client lifts the walker, moves it forward 10 inches, and then takes several small steps forward—CORRECT: walker needs to be picked up, placed down on all legs

(3) The client supports his weight on the walker while advancing it forward, then takes small steps while balancing on the walker—should not support weight on walker while trying to move it

(4) The client slides the walker 18 inches forward, then takes small steps while holding onto the walker for balance—walker should be picked up, not slid forward

45. The Answer is 2

A nurse is supervising a group of elderly clients in a residential home setting. The nurse knows that the elderly are at greater risk of developing sensory deprivation for which of the following reasons?

Reworded Question: Why do the elderly have sensory deprivation?

Strategy: Think about each answer choice.

Needed Info: Plan/Implementation: assist clients with adjusting to lifestyle changes; allow clients to verbalize concerns; prevent isolation; provide assistance as required.

Category: Analysis/Psychosocial Integrity

(1) Increased sensitivity to the side effects of medications—many medications alter GI functioning but do not cause decreased vision, hearing, or taste

(2) Decreased visual, auditory, and gustatory abilities—CORRECT: gradual loss of sight, hearing, and taste interferes with normal functioning

(3) Isolation from their families and familiar surroundings—clients are in contact with other residents and staff who provide stimulation

(4) Decreased musculoskeletal function and mobility—clients can be placed in wheelchairs and moved

46. The Answer is 1

After receiving report, the nurse should see which of the following clients *FIRST?*

Reworded Question: Who is the priority client?

Strategy: Think ABCs.

Needed Info: Consider the following factors: chief complaint; age of client; medical history; potential for life-threatening event

Category: Analysis/Safe and Effective Care Environment/Management of Care

(1) A 14-year-old client in sickle-cell crisis with an infiltrated IV—CORRECT: IV fluids are critical to reduce clotting and pain

(2) A 59-year-old client with leukemia who has received half of a packed red blood cell transfusion—no indication that client is unstable

(3) A 68-year-old client scheduled for a bronchoscopy—stable client

(4) A 74-year-old client complaining of a leaky colostomy bag—stable client

47. The Answer is 3

The home care nurse is visiting a client with a diagnosis of hepatitis of unknown etiology. The nurse knows that teaching has been successful if the client makes which of the following statements?

Reworded Question: What is a correct statement about hepatitis?

Strategy: Determine the outcome of each statement.

Needed Info: Hepatitis A (HAV): high risk groups include young children, institutions for custodial care, international travelers; transmission by fecal/oral, poor sanitation; nursing considerations include prevention, improved sanitation, treat with gamma globulin early postexposure, no preparation of food. Hepatitis B (HBV): high risk groups include drug addicts, fetuses from infected mothers, homosexually active men, transfusions, health care workers; transmission by parenteral, sexual contact, blood/

body fluids; nursing considerations include vaccine (Heptavax-B, Recombivax HB), immune globulin (HBLg) postexposure, chronic carriers (potential for chronicity 5–10%). Hepatitis C (HVC): high risk groups include transfusions, international travelers; transmission by blood/body fluids; nursing considerations include great potential for chronicity. Delta hepatitis: high risk groups same as for HBV; transmission coinfects with HBV, close personal contact.

Category: Evaluation/Physiological Integrity/Reduction of Risk Potential

(1) "I am so sad that I am not able to hold my baby."—hepatitis not spread by casual contact

(2) "I will eat after my family eats."—can eat with family; cannot share eating utensils

(3) "I will make sure that my children don't use my eating utensils or drinking glasses."—CORRECT: to prevent transmission, families should not share eating utensils or drinking glasses; wash hands before eating and after using toilet

(4) "I'm glad that I don't have to get help taking care of my children."—need to alternate rest and activity to promote hepatic healing; mothers of young children will need help

48. The Answer is 2

The nurse calculates the IV flow rate for a postoperative client. The client is to receive 3,000 mL of Ringer's lactate solution IV to run over 24 hours. The IV infusion set has a drop factor of 10 drops per milliliter. The nurse should regulate the client's IV to deliver how many drops per minute?

Reworded Question: What is the IV flow rate?

Strategy: Remember the formula to calculate IV flow rate: Total volume × drop factor divided by the time in minutes.

Needed Info: Ringer's lactate: electrolyte solution used to expand extracellular fluid volume, and reduce blood viscosity.

Category: Implementation/Physiological Integrity/Pharmacological and Parenteral Therapies

(1) 18—incorrect

(2) 21—CORRECT: (3,000 × 10) divided by (24 × 60) = 30,000 divided by 1,440 = 20.8 = 21

(3) 35—incorrect

(4) 40—incorrect

49. The Answer is 1

A client with emphysema becomes restless and confused. Which of the following actions should the nurse take next?

Reworded Question: What should the nurse do to raise the oxygen levels of a client with emphysema?

Strategy: Determine the outcome of each answer choice.

Needed Info: Emphysema: overinflation of alveoli resulting in destruction of alveoli walls; predisposing factors include smoking, chronic infections, environmental pollution. Teaching includes breathing exercises; stop smoking; avoid hot/cold air or allergens; instructions regarding medications; avoid crowds or close contact with persons who have colds or flu; adequate rest and nutrition; oral hygiene; prophylactic flu vaccines; observe sputum for indications of infection.

Category: Implementation/Physiological Integrity/Reduction of Risk Potential

(1) Encourage the client to perform pursed-lip breathing—CORRECT: prevents collapse of lung unit and helps client control rate and depth of breathing

(2) Check the client's temperature—confusion is probably due to decreased oxygenation

(3) Assess the client's potassium level—confusion is probably due to decreased oxygenation, not electrolyte imbalance

(4) Increase the client's oxygen flow rate to 5 L/min—should receive low flow oxygen to prevent carbon dioxide narcosis

50. The Answer is 2

The nurse is caring for a client 1 day after an abdominal-perineal resection for cancer of the rectum. The nurse should question which of the following orders?

Reworded Question: What is an incorrect behavior?

Strategy: Determine the outcome of each answer choice.

Needed Info: Skin care for stoma: effect on skin depends on composition, quality, consistency of drainage, medication, location of stoma, frequency of removal of appliance adhesive. Principles of skin protection: use skin sealant under all tapes; use skin barrier to protect skin around stoma; cleanse skin gently and pat dry, not rub; change appliance immediately when seal breaks.

Category: Analysis/Physiological Integrity/Basic Care and Comfort

(1) Discontinue the nasogastric tube when bowel sounds are heard—this usually means peristalsis has occurred and the physician will also order a clear liquid diet, then advance as tolerated

(2) Irrigate the colostomy—CORRECT: colostomy begins to function 3–6 days after surgery

(3) Place petrolatum gauze over the stoma—done if no pouch in place; keeps stoma moist; cover with dry, sterile dressing

(4) Administer meperidine (Demerol) 50 mg IM for pain—prevents post-op pain

51. The Answer is 4

The nurse is caring for a client 4 hours after intracranial surgery. Which of the following actions should the nurse take immediately?

Reworded Question: What is a priority after intracranial surgery?

Strategy: Determine the outcome of each answer choice.

Needed Info: Monitor vital signs hourly. Elevate head 15–30 degrees to promote venous drainage from brain. Avoid neck flexion and head rotation (support in cervical collar or neck rolls). Reduce environmental stimuli. Prevent the Valsalva maneuver; teach client to exhale while turning or moving in bed. Administer stool softeners. Restrict fluids to 1,200–1,500 mL/day. Administer medications: osmotic diuretics, corticosteroid therapy, anticonvulsant meds.

Category: Implementation/Physiological Integrity/ Reduction of Risk Potential

(1) Turn, cough, and deep-breathe the client— coughing is discouraged, can increase intracranial pressure

(2) Place the client with the neck flexed and head turned to the side—will increase ICP; keep head in a neutral position

(3) Perform passive range-of-motion exercises— changes in client's position can increase intracranial pressure

(4) Move the client to the head of the bed using a turning sheet—CORRECT: client's body should be moved as a unit to prevent increased ICP; prevent disruption of the ICP monitoring system

52. The Answer is 2

A 6-year-old child with a congenital heart disorder is admitted with congestive heart failure. Digoxin (Lanoxin) 0.12 mg is ordered for the child. The bottle of Lanoxin contains 0.05 mg of Lanoxin in 1 mL of solution. Which of the following amounts should the nurse administer to the child?

Reworded Question: How much of the medication should you give?

Strategy: Remember how to calculate dosages. Be careful and don't make math errors.

Needed Info: Formula: dose on hand over 1 mL = dose desired.

Category: Implementation/Physiological Integrity/ Pharmacological and Parenteral Therapies

(1) 1.2 mL—inaccurate

(2) 2.4 mL—CORRECT: 0.05 mg/1 mL = 0.12 mg/x mL, 0.05x = 0.12, x = 2.4 mL

(3) 3.5 mL—inaccurate

(4) 4.2 mL—inaccurate

53. The Answer is 3

The nurse is caring for a client with chest pain in the Emergency Department. Which of the following laboratory findings would *MOST* concern the nurse?

Reworded Question: What is the most significant lab value for an MI?

Strategy: "*MOST* concerned" indicates that you are looking for a problem.

Needed Info: Special tests are ordered for clients suspected of having an myocardial infarction (MI). Creatine phosphokinase (CK-MB) is usually ordered along with total CK in a client with chest pain to determine whether the pain is due to a heart attack. It may also be ordered in a client with a high total CK to determine whether damage is to the heart or other muscles. Increased CK-MB can usually be detected in heart attack patients about 3–4 hours after onset of chest pain. The concentration of CK-MB peaks in 18–24 hours and then returns to normal within 72 hours.

Category: Analysis/Physiological Integrity/Reduction of Risk Potential

(1) Erythrocyte sedimentation rate (ESR): 10 mm/hr—rate at which RBCs settle out of unclotted blood in 1 hour; indicates inflammation/neurosis; normal: men 1–15 mm/hr, women 1–20 mm/hr

(2) Hematocrit (Hct): 42%—relative volume of plasma to RBC; increased with dehydration; decreased with fluid volume excess; normal: men 40–45%, women 37–45%

(3) Creatine phosphokinase (CK-MB): 4 ng/mL—CORRECT: enzyme specific to myocardium; indicates tissue necrosis or injury to heart muscle; normal: 0–3 ng/mL

(4) Serum glucose: 100 mg/dL—indicates insulin production; normal: 60–110 mg/dL

54. The Answer is 3

The nurse is caring for a client with cervical cancer. The nurse notes that the radium implant has become dislodged. Which of the following actions should the nurse take *FIRST*?

Reworded Question: What is the best action when a radium implant becomes dislodged?

Strategy: Think about the outcome of each answer choice.

Needed Info: Limit radioactive exposure: assign client to private room; place "Caution: Radioactive Material" sign on door; wear dosimeter film badge at all times when interacting with client (measures amount of exposure); do not assign pregnant nurse to client; rotate staff caring for client; organize tasks so limited time is spent in client's room; limit visitors; encourage client to do own care; provide shield in room. Client care: use antiemetics for nausea; consider body image; provide comfort measures; provide good nutrition.

Category: Implementation/Safe and Effective Care Environment/Safety and Infection Control

(1) Grasp the implant with a sterile hemostat and carefully reinsert it into the client—the implant should be picked up with long-handled forceps, not a hemostat, and deposited into a lead container in the room, not reinserted into the client

(2) Wrap the implant in a blanket and place it behind a lead shield—the implant should be picked up with long-handled forceps and put into a lead container in the room

(3) Ensure the implant is picked up with long-handled forceps and placed in a lead container—CORRECT: the priority is to secure the implant to prevent unwanted and dangerous radiation exposure; the implant should be picked up with long-handled forceps and then placed in a lead container; this equipment should be kept in the room of any client receiving this therapy so that it is readily available; institutional guidelines and procedures for managing dislodgement should be followed; radiology is usually involved as soon as dislodgement occurs

(4) Obtain a dosimeter reading on the client and report it to the physician—the priority is to secure the implant and place it into a lead container

55. The Answer is 3

The nurse in a primary care clinic is caring for a 68-year-old man. History reveals that the client has smoked 1 pack of cigarettes per day for 45 years and drinks 2 beers per day. He is complaining of a nonproductive cough, chest discomfort, and dyspnea. The nurse hears isolated wheezing in the right middle lobe. It would be *MOST* important for the nurse to complete which of the following orders?

Reworded Question: Which order should the nurse complete first?

Strategy: "*MOST* important" indicates the possibility of more than one good answer.

Needed Info: Symptoms to look for: cough; change in a chronic cough; wheezing; recurring fever.

Category: Analysis/Physiological Integrity/Reduction of Risk Potential

(1) Pulmonary function tests—evaluates lung capacity; done for constrictive disease such as asthma

(2) Echocardiogram—determines cardiac structure

(3) Chest x-ray—CORRECT: client's symptoms, smoking history, and age are suspicious of lung cancer; wheezing caused by constrictive airways

(4) Sputum culture—determines if infection is present; crackles present with infections

56. The Answer is 3

The nurse is caring for a client with pernicious anemia. The nurse knows that her teaching has been successful if the client makes which of the following statements?

Reworded Question: What is true about pernicious anemia?

Strategy: Determine the outcome of each answer choice.

Needed Info: Pernicious anemia is caused by failure to absorb vitamin B_{12} because of a deficiency of intrinsic factor from the gastric mucosa. Symptoms: pallor, slight jaundice, glossitis, fatigue, weight loss, paresthesias of hands and feet, disturbances of balance and gait. Treatment: vitamin B_{12} IM monthly.

Category: Evaluation/Physiological Integrity/Physiological Adaptation

(1) "In order to get better, I will take iron pills."—pernicious anemia is due to vitamin B deficiency

(2) "I am going to attend smoking cessation classes."—no direct link to smoking

(3) "I will learn how to perform IM injections."—CORRECT: many clients are instructed how to give monthly IM B_{12} injection

(4) "I will increase my intake of carbohydrates."—pernicious anemia is caused by faulty absorption of vitamin B_{12}

57. The Answer is 2

The nurse is caring for clients in the Emergency Department of an acute care facility. Four clients have been admitted in the last 20 minutes. Which of the following admissions should the nurse see *FIRST*?

Reworded Question: Who is the priority client?

Strategy: Think ABCs.

Needed Info: Factors to consider: chief complaint; age of client; medical history; potential for life-threatening event.

Category: Analysis/Physiological Integrity/Reduction of Risk Potential

(1) A client complaining of chest pain that is unrelieved by nitroglycerin—airway issue takes priority

(2) A client with third-degree burns to the face—CORRECT: face, neck, chest, or abdominal burns result in severe edema, causing airway restriction

(3) A client with a fractured left hip—airway issue takes priority

(4) A client complaining of epigastric pain—airway issue takes priority

58. The Answer is 4

The nurse is caring for a client with a diagnosis of COPD, bronchitis-type, in the long-term care facility. The client is wheezing, and his oxygen saturation is 85%. Four hours ago, the oxygen saturation was 88%. It is *MOST* important for the nurse to take which of the following actions?

Reworded Question: What is the best action for a client with COPD?

Strategy: Determine the outcome of each answer choice.

Needed Info: Emphysema: overinflation of alveoli resulting in destruction of alveoli walls; predisposing factors include smoking, chronic infections, environmental pollution. Teaching includes breathing exercises; stop smoking; avoid hot/cold air or allergens; instructions regarding medications; avoid crowds or close contact with persons who have colds or flu; adequate rest and nutrition; oral hygiene;

prophylactic flu vaccines; observe sputum for indications of infection.

Category: Implementation/Physiological Integrity/ Pharmacological and Parenteral Therapies

(1) Administer beclomethasone (Vanceril), 2 puffs per metered-dose inhaler—administer brochodilator first to open passageways

(2) Listen to breath sounds—situation does not require further assessment

(3) Increase oxygen to 4 L per mask—increased oxygen levels in client's blood may lead to respiratory depression

(4) Administer albuterol (Proventil), 2 puffs per metered-dose inhaler—CORRECT: brochodilator, relaxes bronchial smooth muscles

59. The Answer is 4

The nurse is caring for a client hospitalized for observation after a fall. The client states, "My friend fell last year, and no one thought anything was wrong. She died 2 days later!" Which of the following responses by the nurse is *BEST*?

Reworded Question: What is the most therapeutic response?

Strategy: Remember therapeutic communication.

Needed Info: Therapeutic communication: using silence allows client time to think and reflect; conveys acceptance; allows client to take lead in conversation; using general leads or broad openings (encourages client to talk, indicates interest in client); clarification (encourages description of feelings and details of particular experience; makes sure nurse understands client); reflecting (paraphrases what client says; reflects what client says, especially feelings conveyed).

Category: Implementation/Psychosocial Integrity

(1) "This happens to quite a few people."—nontherapeutic; doesn't address client's concerns

(2) 'We are monitoring you, so you'll be okay."—nontherapeutic; "don't worry" response

(3) "Don't you think I'm taking good care of you?"—nontherapeutic; focus is on the nurse

(4) "You're concerned that it might happen to you?"—CORRECT: reflects client's feelings

60. The Answer is 2

The nurse is caring for clients on the pediatric unit. An 8-year-old client with second- and third-degree burns on the right thigh is being admitted. The nurse should assign the new client to which of the following roommates?

Reworded Question: Who is the appropriate roommate for a client with burns?

Strategy: Think about the transmission of diseases.

Needed Info: Droplet precautions: used with pathogens transmitted by infectious droplets; involves contact of conjunctivae or mucous membranes of nose or mouth, or during coughing, sneezing, talking, or procedures such as suctioning or bronchoscopy; private room or with client with same infection; spatial separation of 3 feet between infected client and visitors or other clients; door may remain open; place mask on client during transportation.

Category: Implementation/Safe and Effective Care Environment/Safety and Infection Control

(1) A 2-year-old with chickenpox—infectious disease

(2) A 4-year-old with asthma—CORRECT: client not infectious; lowest risk of cross-contamination

(3) A 9-year-old with acute diarrhea—requires contact precautions

(4) A 10-year-old with methicillin-resistant *Staphylococcus aureus* (MRSA)—requires contact isolation

61. The Answer is 4

The nurse teaches a client about elastic stockings. Which of the following statements by the client indicates to the nurse that teaching was successful?

Reworded Question: What is a correct statement about elastic stockings?

Strategy: Determine the outcome of each answer choice.

Needed Info: Maintain pressure on muscles of the lower extremities. Don't use if there are any skin lesions or gangrenous areas. Remove and reapply at least twice per day. Stockings should be clean and dry.

Category: Evaluation/Physiological Integrity/Basic Care and Comfort

(1) "I will wear the stockings until the physician tells me to remove them."—remove daily for bathing and inspection of the extremities

(2) "I should wear the stockings even when I am asleep."—elastic stockings promote venous return; not necessary during prolonged periods of sleep

(3) "Every 4 hours I should remove the stockings for a half-hour."—stockings should be worn when client is up to promote venous return

(4) "I should put on the stockings before getting out of bed in the morning."—CORRECT: promote venous return by applying external pressure on veins

62. The Answer is 3

The nurse is teaching a client who is scheduled for a paracentesis. Which of the following statements by the client to the nurse indicates that teaching has been successful?

Reworded Question: What is a correct statement about paracentesis?

Strategy: Determine the outcome of each answer choice.

Needed Info: Paracentesis: removal of fluid from the peritoneal cavity; 2–3 liters may be removed. Prep: informed consent; void, take vital signs; measure abdominal girth; weigh client. During procedure: take vital signs q 15 minutes. After procedure: document amount, color, characteristics of drainage obtained; assess pressure dressing for drainage; position in bed until vital signs are stable.

Category: Evaluation/Physiological Integrity/ Reduction of Risk Potential

(1) "I will be in surgery for less than an hour."—not a surgical procedure

(2) "I must not void prior to the procedure."—bladder is emptied prior to the procedure to prevent puncture

(3) "The physician will remove 2 to 3 liters of fluid."—CORRECT: fluid removed slowly to decrease ascites; can remove up to 4–6 liters in severe cases

(4) "I will lie on my back and breathe slowly."—positioned in an upright position with feet supported

63. The Answer is 2

The home care nurse is performing chest physiotherapy on an elderly client with chronic airflow limitations (CAL). Which of the following actions should the nurse take *FIRST*?

Reworded Question: What should the nurse do prior to beginning chest physiotherapy?

Strategy: Determine whether to assess or implement.

Needed Info: Postural drainage: uses gravity to facilitate removal of bronchial secretions; client is placed in a variety of positions to facilitate drainage into larger airways; secretions may be removed by coughing or suctioning. Percussion and vibration: usually performed during postural drainage to augment the effect of gravity drainage; percussion: rhythmic striking of chest wall with cupped hands over areas where secretions are retained; vibration: hand and arm muscles of person doing vibration are tensed, and a vibrating pressure is applied to chest as client exhales.

Category: Assessment/Physiological Integrity/ Reduction of Risk Potential

(1) Perform chest physiotherapy prior to meals—prevents nausea, vomiting, aspiration

(2) Auscultate the chest prior to beginning the procedure—CORRECT: identify areas of the lung that require drainage; auscultate chest at end of procedure to determine effectiveness

(3) Administer bronchiodilators after the procedure—given before chest physiotherapy to dilate the bronchioles and to liquify secretions

(4) Percuss each lobe prior to asking the client to cough—may cause fractures of the ribs; percussion helps loosen thick secretions

64. The Answer is 3

A client is admitted to the hospital with a diagnosis of chronic bronchitis. He has a 10-year history of emphysema. The nurse should place him in which of the following positions?

Reworded Question: What is the best position for a client with a respiratory problem?

Strategy: Picture the client as described.

Needed Info: Fowler's position: 45–60 degrees. High Fowler's position: 80–90 degrees. Used to promote cardiac and respiratory function. Chronic bronchitis S/S: productive cough, wheezing, shortness of breath (SOB), exercise intolerance. Treatment: bronchodilators, antihistamines, steroids, antibiotics, expectorants. Theophylline: bronchodilator. Side effects: restlessness, dizziness, palpitations, tachycardia, anorexia. Emphysema S/S: marked dyspnea on exertion that proceed to dyspnea at rest, use of accessory muscles for breathing, barrel chest, "pink puffer" (normal O_2 level and dyspnea). Treatment: low-flow O_2 (1–3 L/min), CO_2 resp stimulus obliterated.

Category: Implementation/Physiological Integrity/Basic Care and Comfort

(1) Side-lying—diaphragm against abdominal organs

(2) Supine—can't breathe

(3) High Fowler's—CORRECT: head of bed elevated 60–90 degrees; gravity displaces abdominal organs

(4) Semi-Fowler's—head of bed elevated 30–45 degrees

65. The Answer is 2

A client is to receive 1,000 mL of 5% dextrose in 0.45 NaCl intravenous solution in an 8-hour period. The intravenous set delivers 15 drops per milliliter. The nurse should regulate the flow rate so it delivers how many drops of fluid per minute?

Reworded Question: What is the correct IV flow rate?

Strategy: Use the correct formula and be careful not to make math errors.

Needed Info: Formula: total volume × drip factor divided by the total time in minutes.

Category: Planning/Physiological Integrity/Pharmacological and Parenteral Therapies

(1) 15—incorrect

(2) 31—CORRECT: (1,000 × 15) divided by (8 × 60)

(3) 45—incorrect

(4) 60—incorrect

66. The Answer is 2

The nurse knows the plan of care for a client with severe liver disease should include which of the following actions?

Reworded Question: What is included in the plan of care?

Strategy: Determine the outcome of each answer choice.

Needed Info: Nutrition—Early stages: high-protein, high-carb diet; advanced stages: fiber, protein, fat, and sodium restrictions; small, frequent feedings; fluid restriction; avoid alcohol. Administer blood products; observe vital signs for shock; monitor abdominal girth; maintain skin integrity; assess degree of jaundice; promote rest; promote adequate respiratory function; reduce exposure to infection; reduce ascites (sodium and fluid restrictions, diuretics).

Category: Implementation/Physiological Integrity/Basic Care and Comfort

(1) Administer Kayexelate enemas—decreases serum potassium levels

(2) Offer a low-protein, high-carbohydrate diet—CORRECT: hepatic coma caused by increased levels of ammonia from breakdown of protein

(3) Insert a Sengsteken-Blakemore tube—applies pressure against bleeding esophageal varices

(4) Administer salt-poor albumin IV—balances osmotic pressure

67. The Answer is 2

A client with a diagnosis of delirium is admitted to the hospital. To evaluate the cause of a client's delirium, blood is sent to the laboratory for analysis. The results are as follows: NA^+ 156, Cl^- 100, K^+ 4.0, HCO_3 21, BUN 86, glucose 100. Based on these laboratory results, the nurse should record which of the following nursing diagnoses on the client's care plan?

Reworded Question: What nursing diagnosis is appropriate?

Strategy: Determine if each lab value is normal or abnormal. Decide what the abnormal lab values indicate about the client and how it would influence your development of appropriate nursing diagnoses for that client.

Needed Info: Normal Na$^+$: 135–145 mEq/L. Hypernatremia: dehydration and insufficient water intake. Normal Cl: 95–105 mEq/L. Normal K: 3.5–5.0 mEq/L. Normal HCO$_3$: 22–26 mEq/L. Decreased levels seen with starvation, renal failure, diarrhea. Normal BUN (blood, urea, nitrogen): 6–20 mg/100 mL. Elevated levels indicate rapid protein catabolism, kidney dysfunction, dehydration. Normal glucose: 70–100 mg/dL.

Category: Analysis/Physiological Integrity/Reduction of Risk Potential

(1) Alteration in patterns of urinary elimination—would have altered K$^+$

(2) Fluid volume deficit—CORRECT: elevated Na$^+$, decreased CO$_2$, elevated BUN, other values are normal; elevated Na$^+$ and BUN seen with dehydration

(3) Nutritional deficit: less than body requirements—seen with decreased CO$_2$, but would have altered K$^+$

(4) Self-care deficit: feeding—no information to support this

68. The Answer is 3

A client is to receive 3,000 mL of 0.9% NaCl IV in 24 hours. The intravenous set delivers 15 drops per milliliter. The nurse should regulate the flow rate so that the client receives how many drops of fluid per minute?

Reworded Question: How should you regulate the IV flow rate?

Strategy: Use the formula and avoid making math errors.

Needed Info: Formula: total volume × the drop factor divided by the total time in minutes

Category: Planning/Physiological Integrity/Pharmacological and Parenteral Therapies

(1) 21—inaccurate

(2) 28—inaccurate

(3) 31—CORRECT: (3,000 × 15) divided by (24 × 60)

(4) 42—inaccurate

69. The Answer is 3

The nurse is supervising care of a client receiving TPN through a single-lumen percutaneous central catheter. The nurse would be *MOST* concerned if which of the following was observed?

Reworded Question: What is an incorrect action?

Strategy: "*MOST* concerned" indicates that you are looking for an incorrect intervention.

Needed Info: TPN: method of supplying nutrients to the body by the IV route. Nursing care: site of catheter changed every 4 weeks, change IV tubing and filters every 24 hours, dressing changed 2–3 times a week and PRN; initial rate of infusion 50 mL/hr and gradually increased (100–125 mL/hr) as client's fluid and electrolyte tolerance permits; increased rate of infusion causes hyperosmolar state (headache, nausea, fever, chills, malaise); slowed rate of infusion results in "rebound" hypoglycemia caused by delayed pancreatic reaction to change in insulin requirements.

Category: Evaluation/Physiological Integrity/Pharmacological and Parenteral Therapies

(1) The client receives insulin through the single-lumen—insulin compatible with TPN solution

(2) A mask is placed on the client when changing the client's dressing—decreases chance of airborne contamination; nurse also wears mask when changing dressing

(3) The client's dressing is changed daily using sterile technique—CORRECT: dressing changed 1–2 times per week and PRN

(4) The client is weighed 2–3 times per week—assess fluid balance

70. The Answer is 2

The nurse is caring for clients in the outpatient clinic. A client tells the nurse that he developed weakness and numbness in the legs the previous day and now his body feels the same way. The client's vital signs are: BP 120/60, pulse 86, and resp 20. The client denies any pain but appears anxious to the nurse. It would be *MOST* important for the nurse to ask which of the following questions?

Reworded Question: What is a possible cause of Guillain-Barré syndrome (GBS)?

Strategy: Determine the relationship between the answers and Guillain-Barré syndrome (GBS).

Needed Info: GBS Plan/Implementation: intervention is symptomatic; steroids in acute phase; plasmapheresis; aggressive respiratory care; prevent hazards of immobility; maintain adequate nutrition; physical therapy; pain-reducing measures; eye care; prevention of complications (UTI, aspiration); psychosocial support.

Category: Assessment/Physiological Integrity/Physiological Adaptation

(1) "Have you recently fallen or had some other type of physical injury?"—symptoms consistent with GBS; not related to injury

(2) "Have you recently had a viral infection, such as a cold?"—CORRECT: GBS often preceded by a viral infection as well as immunizations/vaccinations

(3) "Have you recently taken any over-the-counter medication?"—no association with symptoms; appropriate question for health history

(4) "Have you recently experienced headaches?"—GBS affects peripheral, not central nervous system

71. The Answer is 1

The nurse is admitting a client who is jaundiced due to pancreatic cancer. The nurse should give the *HIGHEST* priority to which of the following needs?

Reworded Question: What is the highest priority for a client with pancreatic cancer?

Strategy: Remember Maslow.

Needed Info: Medical treatment: high-calorie, bland, low-fat diet; small, frequent feedings; avoid alcohol; anticholinergics; antineoplastic chemotherapy

Category: Planning/Physiological Integrity/Reduction of Risk Potential

(1) Nutrition—CORRECT: profound weight loss and anorexia occur with pancreatic cancer

(2) Self-image—jaundiced clients are concerned about how they look, but physiological needs take priority

(3) Skin integrity—jaundice causes dry skin and pruritis; scratching can lead to skin breakdown

(4) Urinary elimination—urine is dark due to obstructive process; kidney function is not affected

72. The Answer is 1

Which of the following statements by a client during a group therapy session would the nurse identify as reflecting a client's narcissistic personality disorder?

Reworded Question: Which statement would a client with narcissistic personality disorder be most likely to make?

Strategy: Think about each answer choice.

Needed Info: Clients with narcissistic personality disorder display grandiosity about their self-importance and achievements. These clients overvalue themselves and are indifferent to others' criticism; the feelings of others are not understood or considered. They have a sense of entitlement and expect special treatment, and also use rationalization to blame others, make excuses, and provide alibis for self-focused behaviors.

Category: Analysis/Psychosocial Integrity

(1) "I'm sick of hearing about all your life tragedies."—CORRECT: lack of empathy is the main characteristic of a narcissistic personality disorder

(2) "I know I'm interrupting others. So what?"—prominent behavior in an antisocial personality disorder

(3) "I just can't stop wanting to slash myself."—characteristic of a borderline personality disorder

(4) "I just have no hope for the future."—characteristic of depression

73. The Answer is 4

A teenage client is admitted to the hospital with anorexia nervosa. Which of the following statements by the client requires immediate follow-up by the nurse?

Reworded Question: Which problem has the highest priority for this client?

Strategy: Remember Maslow's hierarchy of needs.

Needed Info: Anorexia nervosa: a disorder characterized by restrictive eating resulting in emaciation, disturbance in body image, and an intense fear of being obese. Physical needs must be met first in order to keep the client in stable condition. A difficult area to maintain is that of appropriate hydration and fluid and electrolyte balance.

Category: Planning/Psychosocial Integrity

(1) "My gums were bleeding this morning."—vitamin deficiencies occur in anorectic clients, but not the highest priority

(2) "I'm getting fatter every day."—body image disturbance is a perceptual problem with anorectics, but not the highest priority; this is a psychosocial need

(3) "Nobody likes me because I'm so ugly."—chronic low self-esteem is a psychodynamic factor, but not the highest priority; this is a psychosocial need

(4) "I'm feeling dizzy and weak today."—CORRECT: fluid volume deficit is client's highest priority; dehydration is common and could lead to irreversible renal damage and vital sign alterations

74. The Answer is 4

A client is admitted to the hospital for treatment of *Pneumocystis jiroveci* pneumonia and Kaposi's sarcoma. The client tells the nurse that he has been considering organ donation when he dies. Which of the following responses by the nurse is *BEST*?

Reworded Question: Can this client be an organ donor?

Strategy: Think about each answer choice.

Needed Info: Criteria for organ/tissue donation: no history of significant disease process in organ/tissue to be donated; no untreated sepsis; brain death of donor; no history of extracranial malignancy; relative hemodynamic stability; blood group compatibility; newborn donors must be full-term (more than 200 g); only absolute restriction to organ donation is documented case of HIV infection. Family members can give consent. Nurse can discuss organ donation

with other death-related topics (funeral home to be used, autopsy request).

Category: Implementation/Physiological Integrity/Physiological Adaptation

(1) "What does your family think about your decision?"—client has the right to make the decision

(2) "You will help many people by donating your organs."—clients with documented HIV are prohibited from donating organs

(3) "Would you like to speak to the organ donor representative?"—passing the responsibility

(4) "That is not possible based on your illness."—CORRECT: clients with documented HIV are prohibited from donating organs

75. The Answer is 3

The nurse is caring for a client 5 hours after a pancreatectomy for cancer of the pancreas. On assessment, the nurse notes that there is minimal drainage from the nasogastric (NG) tube. It is *MOST* important for the nurse to take which of the following actions?

Reworded Question: What is the best action when an NG tube is not draining?

Strategy: Determine whether it is appropriate to assess or implement.

Needed Info: Insertion of Levin/Salem sump: measure distance from tip of nose to earlobe, plus distance from earlobe to bottom of xyphoid process. Mark distance on tube with tape and lubricate end of tube. Insert tube through nose to stomach. Offer sips of water and advance tube gently; bend head forward. Observe for respiratory distress. Secure with hypoallergenic tape. Verify tube position initially and before feeding. Aspirate for gastric contents and check pH. Inject approx. 15 mL of air into stomach while listening over epigastric area (not always accurate).

Category: Assessment/Physiological Integrity/Basic Care and Comfort

(1) Notify the physician—should assess first

(2) Monitor vital signs q 15 minutes—does not address lack of drainage

(3) Check the tubing for kinks—CORRECT: assess prior to implementing; maintain tubing in a dependent position

(4) Replace the NG tube—assess before implementing

76. The Answer is 4

When collecting a 24-hour urine specimen for creatinine clearance, it is *MOST* important for the nurse to do which of the following?

Reworded Question: What is the correct procedure for a 24-hour urine analysis?

Strategy: "*MOST* important" indicates there may be more than one response that appears correct.

Needed Info: Hydrate client before test. Encourage hourly intake of water during test. Have client void and discard urine; note the time; save all urine for specified time. Do not contaminate specimen with feces or toilet paper.

Category: Implementation/Physiological Integrity/Reduction of Risk Potential

(1) Obtain an order from the physician for insertion of a Foley catheter—not necessary unless client is incontinent

(2) Obtain the client's weight prior to beginning the urine collection—not necessary

(3) Discard the last voided specimen prior to ending the collection—collect all urine voided during the time period

(4) Ask if a preservative is present in the container—CORRECT: save all urine in a container with no preservatives; refrigerate or keep on ice

77. The Answer is 1

The nurse is planning discharge teaching for a client with Parkinson's disease. To maintain safety, the nurse should make which of the following suggestions to the family?

Reworded Question: What is a correct client teaching for Parkinson's disease?

Strategy: Determine the outcome of each answer choice.

Needed Info: Symptoms: tremors, akinesia, rigidity, weakness, "motorized propulsive gait, slurred monotonous speech, dysphagia, drooling, mask-like expression. Nursing care: Encourage finger exercises. Administer Artane, Cogentin, L-dopa, Parlodel, Sinemet, Symmetrel. Teach client ambulation modification. Promote family understanding of the disease (intellect/sight/hearing not impaired, disease progressive but slow, doesn't lead to paralysis). Refer for speech therapy, potential stereotactic surgery.

Category: Implementation/Physiological Integrity/Basic Care and Comfort

(1) Install a raised toilet seat—CORRECT: helps client to be independent; slightly elevate the back leg of chairs

(2) Obtain a hospital bed—no indications that this is needed

(3) Instruct the client to hold his arms in a dependent position when ambulating—should swing arms to assist in balance when walking

(4) Perform an exercise program during the late afternoon—activities should be scheduled for late morning when energy level is highest and client won't be rushed

78. The Answer is 3

The nurse is performing discharge teaching for a client with chronic pancreatitis. Which of the following statements by the client to the nurse indicates that further teaching is necessary?

Reworded Question: What is an incorrect statement about pancreatitis?

Strategy: This is a negative question; you are looking for incorrect information.

Needed Info: Plan/Implementation: NPO, gastric decompression. Meds: antacids, analgesics, antibiotics, anticholinergics. Maintain fluid/electrolyte balance. Monitor for signs of infection. Cough and deep breathe; semi-Fowler's position. Monitor for shock and hyperglycemia. TPN. Treatment of exocrine insufficiency: meds containing amylase, lipase, trypsin to aid digestion. Long-term: avoid alcohol; low-fat, bland diet; small, frequent meals. Monitor S/S of diabetes mellitus.

Category: Evaluation/Physiological Integrity/ Reduction of Risk Potential

(1) "I do not have to restrict my physical activity."— no specific restrictions on activity

(2) "I should take pancrelipase (Viokase) before meals."—pancreatic enzyme replacement; take before or with meals

(3) "I will eat 3 meals per day."—CORRECT: small, frequent feedings are most beneficial

(4) "I am not allowed to drink any alcoholic beverages."—complete abstinence from alcohol required

79. The Answer is 3

After a laparoscopic cholecystectomy, the client complains of abdominal pain and bloating. Which of the following responses by the nurse is *BEST*?

Reworded Question: What is the best intervention for a client complaining of free air pain?

Strategy: "*BEST*" indicates there may be more than one response that appears correct.

Needed Info: Cholecystectomy: removal of gallbladder. T-tube inserted to ensure drainage of bile from common bile duct until edema diminishes. Check amount of drainage (usually 500–1,000 mL/ day, decreases as fluid begins to drain into duodenum). Protect skin around incision from bile drainage irritation (use zinc oxide or water-soluble lubricant). Keep drainage bag at same level as gallbladder. Maintain client in semi-Fowler's position after T-tube is removed; observe dressing for bile; notify physician if there is significant drainage. Evaluate pain to check for other problems. Monitor for S/S of K^+ and Na^+ loss; flattened or inverted T waves on EKG; muscle weakness; abdominal distension; headache; apathy; nausea or vomiting; jaundice.

Category: Implementation/Physiological Integrity/ Physiological Adaptation

(1) "Increase your intake of fresh fruits and vegetables."—no indication of constipation

(2) "I'll give you the prescribed pain medication."— less pain medication needed with laparoscopic procedure

(3) "Why don't you take a walk in the hallway."— CORRECT: "free air" pain caused by CO_2; ambulation will increase absorption

(4) "You may need an indwelling catheter."—pain due to retention of CO_2

80. The Answer is 2

The nurse in an outpatient clinic is supervising student nurses administering influenza vaccinations. The nurse should question the administration of the vaccine to which of the following clients?

Reworded Question: What is a contraindication to receiving flu vaccine?

Strategy: Think about what each answer choice means.

Needed Info: Influenza vaccine: given yearly, preferably Oct.–Nov.; recommended for people age 65 or older; people under 65 with heart disease, lung disease, diabetes, immunosuppression; chronic care facility residents

Category: Assessment/Health Promotion and Maintenance

(1) A 45-year-old male who is allergic to shellfish— allergy to eggs is a contraindication

(2) A 60-year-old female who says she has a sore throat—CORRECT: vaccine deferred in presence of acute respiratory disease

(3) A 66-year-old female who lives in a group home—vaccine deferred only if client has an active immunization

(4) A 70-year-old female with congestive heart failure—no contraindication

81. The Answer is 2

An arterial blood gas is ordered for a man after a myocardial infarction. After obtaining the specimen, it would be *MOST* appropriate for the nurse to take which of the following actions?

Reworded Question: What is the priority action after an ABG?

Strategy: Take care of the client first.

Needed Info: ABG: measurement of partial pressure of oxygen, CO_2, and pH of blood; assessment of acid-base status of body. Use a heparinized syringe. Needle inserted 45–60 degrees to skin surface and advanced into radial artery. Apply pressure after needle is removed. Put specimen on ice.

Category: Implementation/Physiological Integrity/Reduction of Risk Potential

(1) Obtain ice for the specimen—should be done, but not the most important

(2) Apply direct pressure to the site—CORRECT: prevents bleeding, hematoma; maintain for 5 minutes, 15 minutes if on anticoagulant

(3) Apply a sterile dressing to the site—Band-Aid is applied

(4) Observe the site for hematoma formation—more important to prevent hematoma

82. The Answer is 1

The nurse is caring for a man who was involved in an auto accident the previous day. The client has a double-lumen tracheostomy tube with a cuff. Which of the following actions should the nurse perform?

Reworded Question: What is a correct action when caring for a tracheostomy?

Strategy: Determine the outcome of each answer choice.

Needed Info: Cuffed tracheostomy tube permits mechanical ventilation and seals off lower airways. Inject air with a syringe into one-way valve in pilot line. Nursing responsibilities: change client's position frequently, provide humidification and hydration, suction as necessary.

Category: Implementation/Physiological Integrity/Basic Care and Comfort

(1) Change the tracheostomy dressing every 8 hours and PRN—CORRECT: prevents infection; use pre-cut gauze pads

(2) Change the tracheostomy ties every 48 hours—change PRN; keep old ties on until new ties are in place; 1 finger space between tie and neck

(3) Keep the inner cannula of the tracheostomy in place at all times—remove and clean q 8 hours and PRN using H_2O

(4) Push the outer cannula back in if it accidentally "blows out"—maintain open airway and contact physician

83. The Answer is 3

The nurse performs discharge teaching with a client with emphysema. Which statement by the client indicates that teaching was successful?

Reworded Question: What is true about emphysema?

Strategy: Determine the outcome of each answer choice.

Needed Info: Emphysema: chronic progressive respiratory disease caused by destruction of alveolar walls. Complications: acute respiratory infections, cardiac failure or cor pulmonale, cardiac dysrhythmias. Symptoms: cough, dyspnea, wheezing, barrel chest, use of accessory muscles to breathe. Treatment: bronchodilators, corticosteroids, cromolyn sodium, oxygen, diaphragmatic and pursed-lip breathing maneuvers, energy conservation, diet therapy.

Category: Evaluation/Physiological Integrity/Physiological Adaptation

(1) "Cold weather will help my breathing problems."—will exacerbate breathing problems by causing bronchospasms

(2) "I should eat 3 balanced meals but limit my fluid intake."—need small, frequent feedings to increase caloric intake, limit SOB caused by eating; hydration will liquify secretions

(3) "My outside activity should be limited when pollution levels are high."—CORRECT: pollution will act as irritant by causing bronchospasms

(4) "An intensive exercise program is important in regaining my strength."—unable to tolerate intensive exercise; conditioning program to conserve and increase pulmonary ventilation

84. The Answer is 1

The nurse assists the physician with the removal of a chest tube. Before the physician removes the chest tube, which instruction should the nurse give to the client?

Reworded Question: What should the client do when a chest tube is removed?

Strategy: Determine the outcome of each answer choice.

Needed Info: Pneumothorax: air in pleural space causes collapse of lung. Chest tubes: used with Pleur-evac 3-chamber system to restore negative pressure in pleural space. Removal: chest tube is clamped, client does Valsalva maneuver; apply petroleum gauze dressing sealed with tape.

Category: Implementation/Physiological Integrity/ Reduction of Risk Potential

(1) "Exhale and bear down."—CORRECT: Valsalva maneuver; increased intrathoracic pressure; occlusive dressing applied

(2) "Hold your breath for 5 seconds."—unnecessary

(3) "Inhale and exhale rapidly."—unsafe

(4) "Cough as hard as you can."—unnecessary

85.   The Answer is 2

A client comes into the emergency room with complaints of sudden onset of severe right flank pain. While tests are being performed, it is *MOST* important for the nurse to take which of the following actions?

Reworded Question: What is the priority action for a client with suspected renal calculi?

Strategy: "*MOST* important" indicates a priority question.

Needed Info: Symptoms of renal calculi: pain (depends on location of stone), diaphoresis, nausea and vomiting, fever and chills, hematuria. Nursing care: monitor intake and outake (I & O) and temp; force fluids; strain urine and check pH of urine; administer analgesics. Diet for prevention of stones (most stones contain calcium, phosphorus, and/or oxalate): consume foods low in calcium, sodium, and oxalates; avoid vitamin D–enriched foods; decrease purine sources; to make urine alkaline, restrict citrus fruits, milk, potatoes; to acidify urine, increase consumption of eggs, fish, cranberries.

Category: Implementation/Physiological Integrity/ Physiological Adaptation

(1) Make sure that he does not eat or drink anything—not most important

(2) Strain all his urine through several layers of gauze—CORRECT: symptoms suggestive of urinary calculi, should strain urine for passage of stone

(3) Check his grip strength and pupil reactivity— symptoms suggestive of urinary calculi, not neurological

(4) Send blood and urine specimens to the lab for analysis—not most important if urinary calculi is suspected

86.   The Answer is 4

The nurse is preparing discharge teaching for a client with a new colostomy. The nurse knows teaching was successful when the client chooses which of the following menu options?

Reworded Question: What is the appropriate diet for a client with a colostomy?

Strategy: Recall the type of diet required and then select the menu that is appropriate.

Needed Info: Diet: a low-residue diet for 4–6 weeks post-op, avoiding gas-forming, odor-producing, or excessively laxative/constipating foods.

Category: Evaluation/Physiological Integrity/Basic Care and Comfort

(1) Sausage, sauerkraut, baked potato, and fresh fruit—sausage and sauerkraut are gas-producing and should be avoided with a new colostomy

(2) Cheese omelet with bran muffin and fresh pineapple—bran muffin and fresh fruit are high-fiber (residue)

(3) Pork chop, mashed potatoes, turnips, and salad—turnips are odor-causing and salad is high-residue

(4) Baked chicken, boiled potato, cooked carrots, and yogurt—CORRECT: provides balanced nutrition, high-protein, low-residue, low-fat, and non-irritating foods

87. The Answer is 4

A client is seen in the outpatient clinic to rule out acute renal failure. The nurse would be *MOST* concerned if the client made which of the following statements?

Reworded Question: What is a symptom of acute renal failure?

Strategy: "*MOST* concerned" indicates you are looking for a symptom of acute renal failure.

Needed Info: Symptoms of oliguric phase of acute renal failure: urinary output less than 400 mL/day; irritability, drowsiness, confusion, coma; restlessness, twitching, seizures; increased serum K+, BUN, creatinine, Ca+, Na+, pH; anemia; pulmonary edema, CHF, hypertension. Symptoms of diuretic or recovery phase: urinary output of 4–5 L/day; increased serum BUN; Na+ and K+ loss in urine; increased mental and physical activity.

Category: Assessment/Physiological Integrity/Physiological Adaptation

(1) "My urine is often pink-tinged."—seen with urinary tract infections or trauma; hematuria not usually a symptom of acute renal failure

(2) "It is hard for me to start the flow of urine."—urinary hesitancy not usually seen with acute renal failure

(3) "It is quite painful for me to urinate."—dysuria seen with urinary tract infections, not with acute renal failure

(4) "I urinate in the morning and again before dinner."—CORRECT: symptoms of acute renal failure include decreased urinary output (anuria or ologuria), hypotension, tachycardia, lethargy; normal output 1,200–1,500 mL/day or 50–63 mL/hr, normal voiding pattern 5–6 times/day and once at night

88. The Answer is 2

The nurse is teaching a new mother how to breastfeed her newborn. The nurse knows that teaching has been successful if the client makes which of the following statements?

Reworded Question: What indicates that a newborn is receiving adequate nutrition when breastfeeding?

Strategy: Think about each statement. Is it true?

Needed Info: Breastfeeding is recommended for the first 6–12 months of life; human milk is considered ideal food. Colostrum is secreted at first; clear and colorless; contains protective antibodies; high in protein and minerals. Milk is secreted after 2–4 days; milky white appearance; contains more fat and lactose than colostrum.

Category: Evaluation/Health Promotion and Maintenance

(1) "My baby's weight should equal her birthweight in 5 to 7 days."—breastfeeding infants should surpass birthweight in 10–14 days

(2) "My baby should have at least 6 to 8 wet diapers per day."—CORRECT: indicates newborn is ingesting an adequate amount of nutrition; should have at least 2 bowel movements per day

(3) "My baby will sleep at least 6 hours between feedings."—newborns feed approximately every 2–3 hours during the day and every 4 hours at night

(4) "My baby will feed for about 10 minutes per feeding."—should feed for approx. 15–20 minutes per breast

89. The Answer is 2

A man is admitted to the telemetry unit for evaluation of complaints of chest pain. Eight hours after admission, the client goes into ventricular fibrillation. The physician defibrillates the client. The nurse understands that the purpose of defibrillation is to do which of the following?

Reworded Question: Why is a client defibrillated?

Strategy: Think about each answer choice.

Needed Info: Defibrillation: produces asystole of heart to provide opportunity for natural pacemaker (SA node) to resume as pacer of heart activity

Category: Analysis/Physiological Integrity/Physiological Adaptation

(1) Increase cardiac contractility and cardiac output—inaccurate

(2) Cause asystole so the normal pacemaker can recapture—CORRECT: allows SA node to resume as pacer of heart activity

(3) Reduce cardiac ischemia and acidosis—inaccurate

(4) Provide energy for depleted myocardial cells—inaccurate

90. The Answer is 3

A man is brought to the emergency room complaining of chest pain. The nurse performs an assessment of the client. Which of the following symptoms would be *MOST* characteristic of an acute myocardial infarction?

Reworded Question: What type of pain is characteristic in an MI?

Strategy: Think about the cause of each type of pain.

Needed Info: MI signs and symptoms: chest pain radiating to neck, jaw, shoulder, back, or left arm; unrelieved by nitroglycerin. Also fever, apprehension, dizziness, diaphoresis, palpitations, shortness of breath.

Category: Assessment/Physiological Integrity /Physiological Adaptation

(1) Colic-like epigastric pain—indicates GI disorder

(2) Sharp, well-localized, unilateral chest pain—symptom of pneumothorax

(3) Severe substernal pain radiating down the left arm—CORRECT: crushing; may radiate; unrelated to emotion or exercise

(4) Sharp, burning chest pain moving from place to place—anxiety state

91. The Answer is 3

The nurse is caring for clients on the medical unit. A client is admitted with a diagnosis of deep vein thrombosis (DVT). Admission orders include heparin 2,000 units per hour in 5% dextrose in water. The nurse should have which of the following available?

Reworded Question: What is an antidote for heparin?

Strategy: Think about the action of each medication.

Needed Info: Heparin: anticoagulant. Side effects: hemorrhage, thrombocytopenia. Antidote: protamine sulfate.

Category: Planning/Physiological Integrity/Pharmacological and Parenteral Therapies

(1) Propranolol (Inderal)—beta-blocker; reduces myocardial oxygen consumption

(2) Protamine zinc—long-acting insulin

(3) Protamine sulfate—CORRECT: antidote, acts as base to neutralize heparin; give IV over 3 minutes

(4) Vitamin K—antidote to Coumadin

92. The Answer is 2

A client returns to the clinic 2 weeks after discharge from the hospital. He is taking warfarin sodium (Coumadin) 2 mg PO daily. Which of the following statements by the client to the nurse indicates that further teaching is necessary?

Reworded Question: What is contraindicated for Coumadin?

Strategy: Think about what each statement means and how it relates to Coumadin.

Needed Info: Coumadin: anticoagulant. Side effects: hemorrhage, fever, rash. Prothrombin time (PT) used to monitor effectiveness; PT usually maintained at 1.5–2 times normal. Antidote: vitamin K (aquamephyton). Nursing responsibilities: check for bleeding gums, bruises, nosebleeds, petechiae, melena, tarry stools, hematuria. Use electric razor, soft toothbrush; green leafy vegetables (contain vitamin K).

Category: Evaluation/Physiological Integrity/Pharmacological and Parenteral Therapies

(1) "I have been taking an antihistamine before bed."—no contraindication

(2) "I take aspirin when I have a headache."—CORRECT: inhibits platelet aggregation; effect lasts 3–8 days

(3) "I use sunscreen when I go outside."—correct behavior

(4) "I take Mylanta if my stomach gets upset."—correct information

93. The Answer is 3

To enhance the percutaneous absorption of nitro-glycerine ointment, it would be *MOST* important for the nurse to select a site that is which of the following?

Reworded Question: What is the best site for nitro-glycerin ointment?

Strategy: Think about each site.

Needed Info: Nitroglycerin: used in treatment of angina pectoris to reduce ischemia and relieve pain by decreasing myocardial oxygen consumption; dilates veins and arteries. Side effects: throbbing headache, flushing, hypotension, tachycardia. Nursing responsibilities: teach appropriate administration, storage, expected pain relief, side effects. Ointment applied to skin; sites rotated to avoid skin irritation. Prolonged effect up to 24 hours.

Category: Implementation/Physiological Integrity/Pharmacological and Parenteral Therapies

(1) Muscular—not most important

(2) Near the heart—not most important

(3) Non-hairy—CORRECT: skin site free of hair will increase absorption; avoid distal part of extremities due to less than maximal absorption

(4) Over a bony prominence—most important is that the site be non-hairy

94. The Answer is 3

A client with chronic alcohol abuse has been admitted to a rehabilitation unit. The nurse knows that the client is denying alcoholism when he makes which of the following statements?

Reworded Question: Which statement signifies denial?

Strategy: What are the defense mechanisms and how are they manifested?

Needed Info: Defense mechanisms include: repression, denial, suppression, rationalization, intellectualization, identification, introjection, compensation, reaction formation, sublimation, displacement, projection, conversion, undoing, dissociation, regression.

Category: Analysis/Psychosocial Integrity

(1) "My brother did this to me."—projection: blaming someone else for one's difficulties

(2) "Drinking always calms my nerves."—rationalization: the attempt to prove that one's feelings or behavior are justifiable

(3) "I can stop drinking anytime I feel like it."—CORRECT: denial is the unconscious refusal to admit an unacceptable idea or behavior

(4) "Let's all plan to play cards tonight."—suppression: the voluntary exclusion from awareness of feelings, ideas, or situations that produce anxiety

95. The Answer is 4

During the acute phase of a cerebrovascular accident (CVA), the nurse should maintain the client in which of the following positions?

Reworded Question: What is the best way to position a client during the acute phase of a CVA?

Strategy: Remember the positioning strategy.

Needed Info: Nursing responsibilities during acute phase: maintain client airway; monitor vital signs; neurological assessment (Glasgow coma scale); passive ROM exercises; NPO for 24–48 hours; tube feedings.

Category: Implementation/Physiological Integrity/Physiological Adaptation

(1) Semi-prone with the head of the bed elevated 60–90 degrees—on left side with legs flexed on abdomen, hip flexion increases intrathoracic pressure

(2) Lateral, with the head of the bed flat—helps with drainage of secretions, but not the best

(3) Prone, with the head of the bed flat—interferes with respiration

(4) Supine, with the head of the bed elevated 30–45 degrees—CORRECT: facilitates venous drainage from brain; reduces intracranial pressure; keeps head in midline

96. The Answer is 4

Which of the following statements by a client during a group therapy session requires immediate follow-up by the nurse?

Reworded Question: Which statement indicates the possibility of impending danger?

Strategy: Think about which statement would make you question the client's intentions.

Needed Info: In *Tarasoff v. The Regents of the University of California* (1976), the court established a duty to warn of threats of harm to others. Failure to warn, coupled with subsequent injury to the threatened person, exposes the mental health professional to civil damages for malpractice. Based on this and other rulings in many states, the mental health caregiver must take responsibility to warn society of potential danger.

Category: Implementation/Psychosocial Integrity

(1) "I know I'm a chronically compulsive liar, but I can't help it."—this statement is revealing, but does not indicate impending threat

(2) "I don't ever want to go home; I feel safer here."—this statement is a response to anxiety or fear, but does not indicate immediate danger

(3) "I don't really care if I ever see my girlfriend again."—this statement does not imply a threat or impending violence

(4) "I'll make sure that doctor is sorry for what he said."—CORRECT: under the Tarasoff Act, a threatened person, including health professionals, must be warned about threats or potential threats to personal safety

97. The Answer is 4

A client newly diagnosed with Alzheimer's disease is admitted to the unit. Which of the following actions by the nurse is *BEST?*

Reworded Question: What is the best assessment?

Strategy: Determine whether to assess or implement.

Needed Info: Alzheimer's disease (senile dementia): chronic, progressive, degenerative, resulting in cerebral atrophy. S/S: changes in memory, confusion, disorientation, change in personality; most common after age 65. Nursing responsibilities: reorient as needed; speak slowly; place clocks and calendars in room; place bed in low position with side rails up.

Category: Assessment/Psychosocial Integrity

(1) Place the client in a private room away from the nurses' station—should be in a semiprivate room near nurses' station; needs frequent assessment

(2) Ask the family to wait in the waiting room while the nurse admits the client—familiar people decrease confusion of unfamiliar environment

(3) Assign a different nurse daily to care for the client—consistency is important

(4) Ask the client to state today's date—CORRECT: assessment is the first step in planning care

98. The Answer is 3

A female client visits the clinic with complaints of right calf tenderness and pain. It would be *MOST* important for the nurse to ask which of the following questions?

Reworded Question: What is a predisposing factor to developing venous thrombosis (VT)?

Strategy: Determine why you would ask each question.

Needed Info: Thrombophlebitis (phlebitis, phlebothrombosis, or deep vein thrombosis [DVT]): clot formation in a vein secondary to inflammation of vein or partial vein obstruction. Risk factors: history of varicose veins, hypercoagulation, cardiovascular disease, pregnancy, oral contraceptives, immobility, recent surgery or injury.

Category: Assessment/Physiological Integrity/Pharmacological and Parenteral Therapies

(1) "Do you exercise excessively?"—could cause shin splints

(2) "Have you had any fractures in the last year?"—not relevant to client's complaints

(3) "What type of birth control do you use?"—CORRECT: increased risk of DVT with oral contraceptives

(4) "Are you under a lot of stress?"—should be concerned about possibility of DVT

99. The Answer is 3

A mother calls the well-baby clinic to report that her 4-month-old son has an upper respiratory infection (URI) with a temperature of 104° F (40° C). The infant is scheduled to receive his DPT and TOPV immunizations later that day. The mother asks the nurse if she should bring him in for his scheduled immunizations. Which of the following responses by the nurse would be *MOST* appropriate?

Reworded Question: Is a URI and elevated temp contraindication for routine immunization?

Strategy: Picture the client as described.

Needed Info: URI: acute rhinitis (cold), pharyngitis, tonsillitis. Nursing responsibilities: liquid to soft diet, cool mist vaporizer, analgesics, antipyretics, antibiotics. Contraindications for immunizations: moderate to severe febrile illness, severe anaphylactic reaction from previous immunization, congenital disorders of immune system, immunosuppressive therapy, anaphylactic egg hypersensitivity for MMR and OPV.

Category: Implementation/Safe and Effective Care Environment/Safety and Infection Control

(1) "Keep him at home. We'll give him a double dose next time."—immunization not given, schedule resumed when infant well

(2) "Bring him in. His illness will not interfere with his immunizations."—febrile illness contraindication for all immunizations

(3) "Keep him at home until his temperature and infection resolve."—CORRECT: immunization contraindicated during infectious or inflammatory state, pre-existing symptoms could mask adverse or allergic reaction

(4) "Bring him in. We'll give some antibiotics with the immunizations."—involves giving immunization with febrile illness

100. The Answer is 2

The nurse in the postpartum unit cares for a client who delivered her first child the previous day. During her assessment of the client, the nurse notes multiple varicosities on the client's lower extremities. Which of the following actions should the nurse perform?

Reworded Question: What is the best way to prevent thrombophlebitis?

Strategy: Think about what causes thrombophlebitis.

Needed Info: High risk of developing thrombophlebitis during pregnancy and immediate postpartum period. Thrombophlebitis: inflammation of vein associated with formation of a thrombus or blood clot. Other risk factors: prolonged immobility, use of oral contraceptives, sepsis, smoking, dehydration, and CHF. S/S: pain in the calf, localized edema of one extremity, positive Homan's sign (pain in calf when foot is dorsiflexed). Treatment: bed rest and elevation of extremity, anticoagulant (heparin).

Category: Planning/Health Promotion and Maintenance

(1) Teach the client to rest in bed when the baby sleeps—not preventive; bed rest can cause thrombophlebitis

(2) Encourage early and frequent ambulation—CORRECT: facilitates emptying of blood vessels in lower extremities

(3) Apply warm soaks for 20 minutes every 4 hours—not a preventive measure but an intervention used to treat; must be ordered by physician; can be intermittent or continuous

(4) Perform passive range-of-motion (ROM) exercises 3 times daily—early ambulation more effective; passive ROM retains joint function, maintains circulation; passive exercises: no assistance from client

101. The Answer is 2

A man fractures his left femur in a bicycle accident. A cast is applied. The nurse knows that which of the following exercises would be *MOST* beneficial for this client?

Reworded Question: What exercise is best for a client in a cast?

Strategy: Picture the client as described. Imagine client performing each type of exercise. Also think about the key words "MOST beneficial."

Needed Info: Fracture: break in continuity of bone. Complications: hemorrhage (bone vascular), shock, fat embolism (long bones), sepsis, peripheral nerve damage, delayed union, nonunion. Treatment: reduction (closed or open), immobilization (cast, traction, splints, internal and external fixation). Cast allows early mobility. Nursing responsibilities: teach isometric exercises.

Category: Planning/Physiological Integrity/Reduction of Risk Potential

(1) Passive exercise of the affected limb—nurse moves extremity; unable to do

(2) Quadriceps setting of the affected limb—CORRECT: isometric exercise: contraction of muscle without movement of joint; maintains strength

(3) Active ROM exercises of the unaffected limb—not best

(4) Passive exercise of the upper extremities—need strengthening, not passive exercises

102. The Answer is 1

The nurse plans care for a client receiving electroconvulsive treatments (ECT). Immediately after a treatment, the nurse should take which of the following actions?

Reworded Question: What should you do right after a client has ECT?

Strategy: Picture the client as described in the question.

Needed Info: ECT: stimulation of convulsions similar to grand mal seizures as treatment for depression. Requires 6–12 treatments. Preparation: NPO 4 hrs, informed consent, void, remove jewelry, atropine 30 min before to reduce secretions. During: short-acting IV anesthesia and muscle relaxant, O_2, suction available. After: confusion and memory loss for recent events, stay with client and orient, check vital signs.

Category: Implementation/Psychosocial Integrity

(1) Orient the client to time and place—CORRECT: short-term memory loss common side effect

(2) Talk about events prior to the client's hospitalization—long-term memory not affected

(3) Restrict fluid intake and encourage the client to ambulate—should encourage fluids, rest

(4) Initiate comfort measures to relieve vertigo—dizziness not common side effect

103. The Answer is 3

A client is to receive 35 mg/hr of intravenous aminophylline. The nurse mixes 350 mg of aminophylline in 500 mL D_5W. At which of the following rates should the nurse infuse this solution?

Reworded Question: What is the IV flow rate?

Strategy: Set up a ratio and solve for x. If you miss this, review your nursing math.

Needed Info: Formula: med on hand over volume on hand = desired med over x. Solve for x.

Category: Implementation/Physiological Integrity/Pharmacological and Parenteral Therapies

(1) 20 mL/hr—incorrect

(2) 35 mL/hr—incorrect

(3) 50 mL/hr—CORRECT: 350 mg/500 mL = 35 mg/x, $350x = 17,500$, $x = 50$

(4) 70 mL/hr—incorrect

104. The Answer is 3

The nurse prepares an adult client for instillation of eardrops. The nurse should use which of the following methods to administer the eardrops?

Reworded Question: How are eardrops given?

Strategy: Picture yourself doing the procedure. Picture an arrow pointing upward for a "tall" adult to straighten ear canal.

Needed Info: Pull earlobe up and back for adult. Pull earlobe down and back for child.

Category: Implementation/Safe and Effective Care Environment/Safety and Infection Control

(1) Cool the solution for better absorption. Drop the medication directly into the auditory canal—stimulates acoustic nerve reflex, may cause nausea and vomiting

(2) Warm the solution. Flush the medication rapidly into the ear—causes pressure against tympanic membrane, possible rupture

(3) Warm the solution. Drop the medication along the side of the ear canal—CORRECT: prevents acoustic nerve reflex and dizziness; will not damage tympanic membrane

(4) Warm the solution to 104° F (40° C). Drop the medication slowly into the ear canal—too hot, 95–98.6° F (35–37° C)

105. The Answer is 2

The nurse is inserting an IV catheter into a client's left arm. Suddenly the client exclaims, "It feels like an electric shock is going all the way down my arm and into my hand!" What is the *FIRST* action the nurse should take?

Reworded Question: What should the nurse do if a nerve is struck when inserting an IV?

Strategy: Determine the outcome of each answer. Is it appropriate?

Needed Info: When choosing location to insert peripheral IV, consider the condition of vein, type of fluid/med to be infused, duration of therapy, and client's age, size, and status.

Category: Implementation/Physiological Integrity/Reduction of Risk Potential

(1) Instruct the client to take slow, deep breaths—incorrect action; will cause harm to the client

(2) Remove the needle from the client's arm—CORRECT: electric shock sensation indicates needle point is touching a nerve; remove needle immediately to prevent permanent nerve injury; can also occur with blood draws

(3) Tell the client this is a common response to IV insertion—it does sometimes happen; important to remove needle immediately

(4) Withdraw the needle slightly and then push it forward—action can damage the nerve

106. The Answer is 3

A client comes to the emergency room with complaints of nausea, vomiting, and abdominal pain. He is a type 1 diabetic (IDDM). Four days earlier, he reduced his insulin dose when flu symptoms prevented him from eating. The nurse performs an assessment of the client that reveals poor skin turgor, dry mucous membranes, and fruity breath odor. The nurse should be alert for which of the following problems?

Reworded Question: What do these symptoms indicate?

Strategy: Think about each answer.

Needed Info: Diabetes mellitus: disorder of carbohydrate metabolism: insufficient insulin to meet metabolic needs. Type 1 (juvenile): insulin dependent, prone to ketoacidosis. Type 2 (adult onset): controlled by diet and oral agents, non–ketosis prone. In ketoacidosis, the body becomes dehydrated from osmotic diuresis. The fruity breath odor develops from acetone, a component of ketone bodies. Rate and depth of resp increase (Kussmaul) in attempt to blow off excess carbonic acid. Difference between ketoacidosis and hyperglycemic hyperosmolar non-ketonic syndrome (HHNKS)—lack of ketonuria.

Category: Planning/Physiological Integrity/Reduction of Risk Potential

(1) Hypoglycemia—cause: too much insulin; blood sugar below 60 mg; S/S: tachycardia, perspiration, confusion, lethargy, numb lips, anxiety, hunger

(2) Viral illness—not best answer

(3) Ketoacidosis—CORRECT: cause: insufficient insulin; S/S: polyuria, polydipsia, nausea, vomiting, dry mucous membranes, weight loss, abdominal pain, hypotension, shock, coma

(4) Hyperglycemic hyperosmolar nonketotic coma—(HHNK) extreme hyperglycemia (800–2,000 mg/dL) with absence of acidosis; some insulin production so don't mobilize fats for energy or form ketones; usually seen in type 2; cause: infections, stress, meds (steroids, thiazide diuretics), TPN; S/S: polyphagia, polyuria, polydipsia, glycosuria, dehydration, abdominal discomfort, hyperpyrexia, changes in level of consciousness (LOC), hypotension, shock; treatment: fluid replacement (2 L 0.45% NaCl over 2 hrs), K^+, Na^+, Cl^-, phosphates, insulin given IV

107. The Answer is 1

The nurse knows that it is *MOST* important for which of the following clients to receive their scheduled medication on time?

Reworded Question: Which medication, if given late, might cause harm to the client?

Strategy: Think about each answer.

Needed Info: Myasthenia gravis is deficiency of acetylcholine at myoneural junction; symptoms include muscular weakness produced by repeated movements that soon disappears following rest, diplopia, ptosis, impaired speech, and dysphagia

Category: Analysis/Physiological Integrity/Pharmacological and Parenteral Therapies

(1) A client diagnosed with myasthenia gravis receiving pyridostigmine bromide (Mestinon)—CORRECT: Mestinon is a cholinesterase inhibitor which increases acetylcholine concentration at the neuromuscular junction; early administration can precipitate a cholinergic crisis; late administration can precipitate myasthenic crisis

(2) A client diagnosed with bipolar disorder receiving lithium carbonate (Lithobid)—Lithobid is a mood stabilizer; targeted blood level = 1–1.5 mEq/L

(3) A client diagnosed with tuberculosis receiving isonicotinic acid hydrazide (INH)—INH is given in a single daily dose; side effects include hepatitis, peripheral neuritis, rash, and fever

(4) A client diagnosed with Parkinson's disease receiving levodopa (L-dopa)—L-dopa is thought to restore dopamine levels in extrapyramidal centers; sudden withdrawal can cause parkinsonian crisis; priority is to administer Mestinon

108.   The Answer is 3

An 11-year-old boy is admitted to the hospital for evaluation for a kidney transplant. During the initial assessment, the nurse learns that the client received hemodialysis for 3 years due to renal failure. The nurse knows that his illness can interfere with this client's achievement of which of the following?

Reworded Question: What developmental stage is altered in a client due to this chronic disease?

Strategy: Picture the person described in the question. Think about his activities and interests. This helps eliminate incorrect answer choices. An 11-year-old is usually in grade school thinking about homework, doing chores at home.

Needed Info: Eric Erikson developed a theory of the stages of personality development that progressed in predictable stages from birth to death. Other stages:

autonomy versus shame and doubt (task of 1–3 yrs); initiative versus guilt (task of 3–6 yrs).

Category: Analysis/Health Promotion and Maintenance

(1) Intimacy—young adult: 20–40 yrs; achieving sexual and loving relationship with another; alternative: isolation

(2) Trust—infancy; results from consistent care by a loving caretaker; teaches that basic needs will be met; alternative: mistrust

(3) Industry—CORRECT: 6–12 yrs; aspires to be the best; learns social skills, how to finish tasks; sensitive about school expectations; may be impaired due to absences from school, growth retardation, and emotional difficulties

(4) Identity—adolescence; peer groups important; used to define identity, establish body image, form new relationships; alternative: role diffusion

109.   The Answer is 4

The nurse assesses a client with a history of Addison's disease who has received steroid therapy for several years. The nurse could expect the client to exhibit which of the following changes in appearance?

Reworded Question: What changes are seen in a client after taking steroids long-term?

Strategy: All the options in an answer choice must be correct for the option to be right.

Needed Info: Meds: cortisone and hydrocortisone usually given in divided doses: 2/3rds in morning and 1/3rd in late afternoon with food to decrease GI irritation. Teach to report S/S of excessive drug therapy (rapid weight gain, round face, fluid retention).

Category: Assessment/Physiological Integrity/Physiological Adaptation

(1) Buffalo hump, girdle-obesity, gaunt facial appearance—hump and girdle-obesity true; gaunt face seen with lack of steroids

(2) Tanning of the skin, discoloration of the mucous membranes, alopecia, weight loss—tanning and weight loss seen with lack of steroids; rest not seen

(3) Emaciation, nervousness, breast engorgement, hirsutism—nothing to do with steroids; hirsutism: excessive growth of hair

(4) Truncal obesity, purple striations on the skin, moon face—CORRECT: due to excess glucocorticoids

110.   The Answer is 2

Haloperidol (Haldol) 5 mg tid is ordered for a client with schizophrenia. Two days later, the client complains of "tight jaws and a stiff neck." The nurse should recognize that these complaints are which of the following?

Reworded Question: Why does the client taking Haldol have these symptoms?

Strategy: Think about each answer and how it relates to Haldol.

Needed Info: Haldol is a medication used in the treatment of psychotic disorders. High incidence of extrapyramidal reactions: pseudoparkinsonism (rigidity and tremors), akathisia (motor restlessness), dystonia (involuntary jerking, uncoordinated body movements), tardive dyskinesia (abnormal movements of lips, jaws, tongue). Schizophrenia: retreat from reality, flat affect, suspiciousness, hallucinations, delusions, loose associations, psychomotor retardation or hyperactivity, regression. Nursing responsibilities: maintain safety, meet physical needs, decrease sensory stimuli. Treatment: antipsychotic meds, individual therapy.

Category: Analysis/Psychosocial Integrity

(1) Common side effects of antipsychotic medications that will diminish over time—gets worse; untreated, life-threatening

(2) Early symptoms of extrapyramidal reactions to the medication—CORRECT: dystonic reaction, airway may become obstructed

(3) Psychosomatic complaints resulting from a delusional system—not accurate

(4) Permanent side effects of Haldol—reversible when treated with IV Benadryl

111.   The Answer is 3

The nurse is caring for a woman who states she was beaten and sexually assaulted by a male friend. Which of the following should the nurse do *FIRST*?

Reworded Question: What is the *MOST* important initial nursing action to take with a sexual assault victim?

Strategy: Discriminate between what is appropriate and inappropriate nursing behavior.

Needed Info: Nursing care for crime victims must address both physical and emotional needs. The nurse must be cautious not to disturb or eliminate any evidence until the victim has been examined by a physician. The nurse must document all evidence found during the nursing assessment. After the client has been examined and a course of action determined, the nurse can begin to address the expressed needs of the client, such as contacting legal counsel or the chaplain.

Category: Implementation/Psychosocial Integrity

(1) Encourage the client to call her family lawyer—not the first action the nurse should take with this client

(2) Ask for a psychiatry consult—nurse should not initiate a psychiatry consult

(3) Stay with the client during the physical exam—CORRECT: provide consistent emotional and physical support for the client

(4) Wash and dress the client's wounds before the physical exam—contraindicated; eradicates potential evidence

112.   The Answer is 4

The nurse cares for a client after surgery for removal of a cataract in her right eye. The client complains of severe eye pain in her right eye. The nurse knows this symptom is which of the following?

Reworded Question: Is pain after cataract surgery normal?

Strategy: Think about each answer and how it relates to cataract surgery.

Needed Info: Cataract: change in the transparency of crystalline lens of eye. Causes: aging, trauma, congenital, systemic disease. S/S: blurred vision, decrease in color perception, photophobia. Treated by removal of lens under local anesthesia with sedation. Intraocular lens implantation, eyeglasses, or contact lenses after surgery. Complications: glaucoma, infection, bleeding, retinal detachment.

Category: Analysis/Physiological Integrity/Physiological Adaptation

(1) Expected; the nurse should administer analgesic to the client—severe pain not expected; mild discomfort treated with analgesics

(2) Expected; the nurse should maintain the client on bed rest—activity restrictions: no coughing, bending at waist, vomiting, sneezing, lifting more than 15 lb., squeezing eyelid, straining at stool, lying on affected side; these increase intraocular pressure; however client need not remain on bed rest

(3) Unexpected and may signify a detached retina—lens was removed during surgery

(4) Unexpected and may signify hemorrhage—CORRECT: ruptured blood vessel or suture causing hemorrhage or increased intraocular pressure; notify physician if restless, increased pulse, drainage on dressing

113. The Answer is 3

A client returns to his room after a lower GI series. When he is assessed by the nurse, he complains of weakness. Which of the following nursing diagnoses should receive priority in planning his care?

Reworded Question: What is most important for a client after a GI series?

Strategy: Establish priorities.

Needed Info: Upper GI series (barium swallow): radiologic visualization of esophagus, stomach, duodenum, jejunum. Lower GI series (barium enema): visualize colon. Prep for test: NPO 6–8 hrs, enemas, laxatives, fluid restriction. Post-test: laxatives to remove barium. Nursing responsibilities after test: check abdomen for distention, encourage fluids. Initially stool is white from barium. Should return to normal color in 72 hrs.

Category: Analysis/Physiological Integrity/Physiological Adaptation

(1) Alteration in sensation-perception, gustatory—not highest priority; gustatory: pertaining to sense of taste

(2) Constipation, colonic—not highest priority

(3) High risk for fluid-volume deficit—CORRECT: prep for test: low-residue or clear liquid diet 2 days, NPO midnight, enemas, laxatives; post-test: laxatives to remove barium

(4) Nutrition, less than body requirements—not highest priority

114. The Answer is 2

A client hospitalized with a gastric ulcer is scheduled for discharge. The nurse teaches the client about an anti-ulcer diet. Which of the following statements by the client indicates to the nurse that dietary teaching was successful?

Reworded Question: What statement is true about an anti-ulcer diet?

Strategy: "Dietary teaching was successful" means you are looking for correct information.

Needed Info: Gastric ulcers form within 1 inch of the pylorus of the stomach usually caused by break in mucosa. Onset 45–54 years old, men twice as often as women, pain increased by food, relieved by vomiting, hematemesis common. Treatment: antacids (Amphojel), H2 receptor antagonists (Tagamet), anticholinergics (Bentyl), mucosal barrier fortifiers (Carafate).

Category: Evaluation/Physiological Integrity/Basic Care and Comfort

(1) "I must eat bland foods to help my stomach heal."—transitional diet used for severe inflammation; not speed healing

(2) "I can eat most foods, as long as they don't bother my stomach."—CORRECT: not severely restricted; small, frequent feedings; avoid foods known to increase gastric acidity: coffee, alcohol, seasonings, milk

(3) "I cannot eat fruits and vegetables because they cause too much gas."—restricted only if they bother stomach

(4) "I should eat a low-fiber diet to delay gastric emptying."—used with acute diverticulitis,

ulcerative colitis; foods with fiber: cereals, whole grains products, fruits, vegetables

115. The Answer is 2

A 6-year-old boy is returned to his room after a tonsillectomy. He remains sleepy from the anesthesia but is easily awakened. The nurse should place the child in which of the following positions?

Reworded Question: What is the best position after tonsillectomy to help with drainage of oral secretions?

Strategy: Picture the client as described.

Category: Implementation/Safe and Effective Care Environment/Safety and Infection Control

(1) Sims'—on side with top knee flexed, thigh drawn up to chest, and lower knee less sharply flexed: used for vaginal or rectal examination

(2) Side-lying—CORRECT: most effective to facilitate drainage of secretions from the mouth and pharynx; reduces possibility of airway obstruction

(3) Supine—increased risk for aspiration, would not facilitate drainage of oral secretions

(4) Prone—risk for airway obstruction and aspiration, unable to observe the child for signs of bleeding such as increased swallowing

116. The Answer is 1

A client is preparing to take her 1-day-old infant home from the hospital. The nurse discusses the test for phenylketonuria (PKU) with the mother. The nurse's teaching should be based on an understanding that the test is *MOST* reliable after which of the following?

Reworded Question: When is the PKU test most reliable?

Strategy: Focus on the key words in the question. Think about what you know about the PKU test.

Needed Info: PKU: genetic disorder caused by a deficiency in liver enzyme phenylalanine hydroxylase. Body can't metabolize essential amino acid phenylalanine, allows phenyl acids to accumulate in the blood. If not recognized, resultant high levels of phenylketone in the brain cause mental retardation.

Guthrie test: screening for PKU. Treatment: dietary restriction of foods containing phenylalanine. Blood levels of phenylalanine monitored to evaluate the effectiveness of the dietary restrictions.

Category: Analysis/Health Promotion and Maintenance

(1) A source of protein has been ingested—CORRECT: recommended to be performed before newborns leave hospital; if initial blood sample is obtained within first 24 hrs recommended to be repeated at 3 weeks

(2) The meconium has been excreted—no relationship; dark-green, tarry stool passed within first 48 hrs of birth

(3) The danger of hyperbilirubinemia has passed—no relationship; excessive accumulation of bilirubin in blood; S/S: jaundice (yellow discoloration of skin); common finding in newborn; not cause for concern

(4) The effects of delivery have subsided—no relationship

117. The Answer is 4

The nurse is completing a client's preoperative checklist prior to an early morning surgery. The nurse obtains the client's vital signs: temperature 97.4° F (36° C), radial pulse 84 strong and regular, respirations 16 and unlabored, and blood pressure 132/74. Which of the following actions should the nurse take *FIRST*?

Reworded Question: What should you do for a client with normal vital signs?

Strategy: Identify normal serum electrolyte values.

Needed Info: Normal electrolyte values (range may vary by laboratory): Na$^+$ (sodium) 135–145 mEq/L, K$^+$ (potassium) 3.6–5.4, Cl$^-$ (chloride) 96–106 mEq/L, mEq/L = milliequivalents per liter.

Category: Assessment/Physiological Integrity/Reduction of Risk Potential

(1) Notify the physician of the client's vital signs—most physicians do not want to be notified about normal values

(2) Obtain orthostatic blood pressures lying and standing—there is no information to support this action

(3) Lower the side rails and place the bed in its lowest position—bed side rails should be raised, not lowered

(4) Record the data on the client's preoperative checklist—CORRECT: the vital signs are normal and should be recorded in the client's medical record

118. The Answer is 2

A woman is hospitalized with a diagnosis of bipolar disorder. While she is in the client activities room on the psychiatric unit, she flirts with male clients and disrupts unit activities. Which of the following approaches would be *MOST* appropriate for the nurse to take at this time?

Reworded Question: How should you deal with a client with bipolar disorder who is disruptive?

Strategy: Determine the outcome of each answer. Is it desirable?

Needed Info: Nursing responsibilities: accompany client to room when hyperactivity escalates, set limits, remain nonjudgmental.

Category: Planning/Psychosocial Integrity

(1) Set limits on the client's behavior and remind her of the rules—too confrontational

(2) Distract the client and escort her back to her room—CORRECT: clients are easily distracted, nonthreatening action

(3) Instruct the other clients to ignore this client's behavior—does not ensure safety

(4) Tell the client that she is behaving inappropriately and send her to her room—too confrontational, may agitate

119. The Answer is 1

A client is brought to the emergency room bleeding profusely from a stab wound in the left chest area. The nurse's assessment reveals a blood pressure of 80/50, pulse of 110, and respirations of 28. The nurse should expect which of the following potential problems?

Reworded Question: What type of shock is described?

Strategy: Form a mental image of the person described.

Needed Info: Symptoms of hypovolemic shock: tachycardia, reduced output, irritability. Treatment: O_2, IV fluids to restore volume, Adrenaline, Apresoline. Nursing responsibilities: check airway, vital signs, insert IV, check blood gases, CVP measurements, insert catheter, hourly I & O, position flat with legs elevated, keep warm.

Category: Planning/Physiological Integrity/Physiological Adaptation

(1) Hypovolemic shock—CORRECT: loss of circulating volume

(2) Cardiogenic shock—decrease in cardiac output; cause: cardiac dysfunction, MI, CHF

(3) Neurogenic shock—increase in vascular bed; cause: spinal anesthesia, spinal cord injury

(4) Septic shock—decreased cardiac output, hypotension; cause: gram+ or gram– bacteria

120. The Answer is 3

A client is admitted to the hospital for surgical repair of a detached retina in the right eye. In planning care for this client postoperatively, the nurse should encourage the client to do which of the following?

Reworded Question: What should you do after surgery for detached retina?

Strategy: Picture the client as described.

Needed Info: Detached retina: separation of retina from pigmented epithelium. S/S: curtain falling across field of vision, black spots, flashes of light, sudden onset. Treatment: surgical repair (photocoagulation, electrodiathermy, cryosurgery, scleral buckling). Complications: infection, redetachment, increased intraocular pressure. Nursing responsibilities post-op: check eye patch for drainage, position with detached area dependent; no rapid eye movement (reading, sewing); no coughing, vomiting, sneezing.

Category: Planning/Physiological Integrity/Reduction of Risk Potential

(1) Perform self-care activities—activity restrictions depend on location and size of tear

(2) Maintain patches over both eyes—only affected eye covered

(3) Limit movement of both eyes—CORRECT: bed rest with eye patch or shield

(4) Refrain from excessive talking—no restriction

121.   The Answer is 2

The nurse cares for a client receiving a balanced complete food by tube feeding. The nurse knows that the *MOST* common complication of a tube feeding is which of the following?

Reworded Question: What is a common complication of a tube feeding?

Strategy: Focus on the words "MOST common" which means there may be more than one answer. And in this situation there is—(4) is a complication —but not common.

Needed Info: Tube feedings are used with clients unable to tolerate the oral route but who have a functioning GI tract. May be given by intermittent or continuous infusion. Elevate head of bed 30–45 degrees. Give at room temp. Check for placement and residual before feeding or every 4–8 hrs (should be less than 50% of previous hour's intake). Replace residual to prevent fluid and electrolyte imbalances unless it appears abnormal (coffee ground–like material). Don't hang solution more than 6 hrs. Flush tubing with 20–30 mL water every 4 hrs. Change feeding set every 24 hrs. Balanced compete food product/ supplement containing intact protein.

Category: Evaluation/Physiological Integrity/Basic Care and Comfort

(1) Edema—not frequently seen; if present, physician may change formula to contain less Na+

(2) Diarrhea—CORRECT: intolerance to solution, rate; give slowly; other symptoms of intolerance: nausea, vomiting, aspiration, glycosuria, diaphoresis

(3) Hypokalemia—normal potassium 3.5–5.0 mEq/L; not commonly seen; common causes: diuretics, diarrhea, GI drainage

(4) Vomiting—can happen with rapid increase in rate; give feeding slowly

122.   The Answer is 4

A 6-week-old infant is brought to the hospital for treatment of pyloric stenosis. The nurse enters the following nursing diagnosis on the infant's care plan: "fluid volume deficit related to vomiting." Which of the following assessments supports this diagnosis?

Reworded Question: What would indicate volume deficit?

Strategy: Think about each answer and how it relates to fluid volume deficit.

Needed Info: Pyloric stenosis: obstruction of the sphincter between stomach and duodenum. Onset: within 2 months of birth. S/S: vomiting that becomes projectile. Treatment: surgery. Nursing responsibilities: small frequent feedings with glucose water or electrolyte solutions 4–6 hrs post-op. Small frequent feedings with formula 24 hrs post-op.

Category: Analysis/Physiological Integrity/Physiological Adaptation

(1) The infant eagerly accepts feedings—may vomit after eating

(2) The infant vomited once since admission—don't assume will continue to vomit

(3) The infant's skin is warm and moist—normal; would be cool and dry with fluid volume deficit

(4) The infant's anterior fontanelle is depressed— CORRECT: indicates dehydration

123.   The Answer is 2

A client is diagnosed with thrombocytopenia due to acute lymphocytic leukemia. She is admitted to the hospital for treatment. To which of the following should the nurse assign the client?

Reworded Question: What are the needs of a client with acute lymphocytic leukemia and thrombocytopenia?

Strategy: What is the highest priority for this client?

Needed Info: Lymphocytic leukemia, disease characterized by proliferation of immature WBCs. Immature cells unable to fight infection as competently as mature white cells. Treatment: chemotherapy, antibiotics, blood transfusions, bone marrow transplantation. Nursing responsibilities: private room, no raw fruits or vegetables, small frequent meals, O_2, good skin care.

Category: Planning/Safe and Effective Care Environment/Management of Care

(1) To a private room so she will not infect other clients and health care workers—poses little or no threat

(2) To a private room so she will not be infected by other clients and health care workers—CORRECT: protects client from exogenous bacteria, risk for developing infection from others due to depressed WBC count, alters ability to fight infection

(3) To a semiprivate room so she will have stimulation during her hospitalization—should be placed in a room alone

(4) To a semiprivate room so she will have the opportunity to express her feelings about her illness—ensure that client is provided with opportunities to express feelings about illness

124. The Answer is 2

A woman comes to the clinic because she thinks she is pregnant. Tests are performed and the pregnancy is confirmed. The client's last menstrual period began on September 8 and lasted for 6 days. The nurse calculates that her expected date of confinement (EDC) is which of the following?

Reworded Question: How do you calculate the EDC?

Strategy: Perform the calculation required and check for math errors!

Needed Info: EDC or estimated date of delivery (EDD): calculated according to Nägele's rule (first day of the last normal menstrual period minus 3 months plus 7 days and 1 year). Assumes that every woman has a 28-day cycle and pregnancy occurred on 14th day. Most women deliver within a period extending from 7 days before to 7 days after the EDC.

Category: Implementation/Health Promotion and Maintenance

(1) May 15—too early

(2) June 15—CORRECT: September 8 minus 3 months = June 8 + 7 days plus 1 year = June 15 of next year

(3) June 21—EDC is calculated from first, not last, day of last normal menstrual period

(4) July 8—not accurate

125. The Answer is 3

A 2-month-old infant is brought to the pediatrician's office for a well-baby visit. During the examination, congenital subluxation of the left hip is suspected. The nurse would expect to see which of the following symptoms?

Reworded Question: What will you see with congenital hip dislocation?

Strategy: Form a mental image of the deformity.

Needed Info: Subluxation: most common type of congenital hip dislocation. Head of femur remains in contact with acetabulum but is partially displaced. Diagnosed in infant less than 4 weeks old. S/S: unlevel gluteal folds, limited abduction of hip, shortened femur affected side, Ortolani's sign (click). Treatment: abduction splint, hip spica cast, Bryant's traction, open reduction.

Category: Assessment/Health Promotion and Maintenance

(1) Lengthening of the limb on the affected side—inaccurate

(2) Deformities of the foot and ankle—inaccurate

(3) Asymmetry of the gluteal and thigh folds—CORRECT: restricted movement on affected side

(4) Plantar flexion of the foot—seen with clubfoot

126. The Answer is 3

After 2 weeks of receiving lithium therapy, a client in the psychiatric unit becomes depressed. Which of the following evaluations of the client's behavior by the nurse would be *MOST* accurate?

Reworded Question: Is the depression normal, or something to be concerned about?

Strategy: Think about each answer and how it relates to lithium therapy.

Needed Info: Lithium is used to control manic episodes of bipolar psychosis; nursing care includes monitor blood levels 2–3 times a week when started and monthly while on maintenance. Need fluid intake of 2,500–3,000 mL/day and adequate salt intake. Side effects include dizziness, hand tremors, impaired vision.

Category: Evaluation/Psychosocial Integrity

(1) The treatment plan is not effective; the client requires a larger dose of lithium—not accurate

(2) This is a normal response to lithium therapy; the client should continue with the current treatment plan—does not address safety needs

(3) This is a normal response to lithium therapy; the client should be monitored for suicidal behavior—CORRECT: delay of 1–3 wks before med benefits seen

(4) The treatment plan is not effective; the client requires an antidepressant—normal response

127. The Answer is 1

A client is admitted for treatment of pulmonary edema. During the admission interview, she states she has a 6-year history of congestive heart failure (CHF). The nurse performs an initial assessment. When the nurse auscultates the breath sounds, the nurse should expect to hear which of the following?

Reworded Question: What will you hear when listening to the breath sounds for a client with CHF?

Strategy: Picture the situation as described.

Needed Info: Use diaphragm of stethoscope to listen to breath sounds. Normal breath sounds: (1) vesicular: low-pitched, swishing sounds heard at bases of lungs, (2) bronchial: loud, high-pitched, hollow sounds heard over large tracheal airways during expiration, (3) bronchovesicular: breeze sound heard over central large airways.

Category: Assessment/Physiological Integrity/Physiological Adaptation

(1) Crackling—CORRECT: rales; air passes over fluid; heard during inspiration; found with pulmonary edema, pneumonia

(2) Wheezing—passage of air through narrowed airway; heard during inspiration and expiration; found with asthma

(3) Whistling—noisy respirations; air through obstructed larynx

(4) Absent breath sounds—pneumothorax; collapse of lung

128. The Answer is 2

A man is diagnosed with cancer of the larynx and comes to the hospital for a total laryngectomy. When admitting this client, the nurse should assess laryngeal nerve function by doing which of the following?

Reworded Question: How do you assess normal functioning of the laryngeal nerve? What functions are controlled by the laryngeal nerve?

Strategy: Think about each answer and how it relates to laryngeal nerve function.

Needed Info: Risk factors: smoking, chronic bronchitis, polluted air, alcohol abuse. S/S: chronic hoarseness, lump in neck, difficulty swallowing, persistent sore throat. Treatment: radiation therapy, surgical removal. Total laryngectomy: loss of voice. Nursing responsibilities post-op: position semi-Fowler's to high Fowler's, care for cuffed tracheostomy tube, chest physiotherapy, assess drainage on dressing or Hemovac container. Teach use of artificial larynx or esophageal speech.

Category: Assessment/Physiological Integrity/Reduction of Risk Potential

(1) Assess the extent of neck edema—not accurate

(2) Check his ability to swallow—CORRECT

(3) Observe for excessive drooling—seen with facial paralysis, Bell's palsy

(4) Tap the side of his neck gently and observe for facial twitching—Chvostek's sign: test for hypocalcemia and tetany, tap over facial nerve on side of face, if mouth twitches, indicates tetany

129. The Answer is 4

The nurse supervises care at an adult day-care center. Four meal choices are available to the residents. The nurse should ensure that a resident on a low-cholesterol diet receives which of the following meals?

Reworded Question: What should a client on a low-cholesterol diet eat?

Strategy: Think about each answer.

Needed Info: Low-cholesterol diet should reduce total fat to 20–25% of total calories and reduce the ingestion of saturated fat. Carbohydrates (especially complex carbohydrates) should be 55–60% of calories. High-cholesterol foods: eggs, dairy products, meat, fish, shellfish, poultry.

Category: Implementation/Physiological Integrity/Basic Care and Comfort

(1) Egg custard and boiled liver—high amounts of cholesterol

(2) Fried chicken and potatoes—avoid fried foods

(3) Hamburger and french fries—avoid fried foods

(4) Grilled flounder and green beans—CORRECT: fish instead of meat, increase vegetables

130. The Answer is 1

The nurse cares for a client with a possible bowel obstruction. A nasogastric (NG) tube is to be inserted. Before inserting the tube, the nurse explains its purpose to the client. Which of the following explanations by the nurse is *MOST* accurate?

Reworded Question: What is the purpose of an NG tube?

Strategy: Think about how an NG tube works.

Needed Info: Gastric tubes can also be used for tube feedings. Decompression relieves pressure caused by GI contents and gases that remain in stomach due to obstruction.

Category: Implementation/Physiological Integrity/Basic Care and Comfort

(1) "It empties the stomach of fluids and gas."—CORRECT: used for decompression, gavage, lavage, gastric analysis

(2) "It prevents spasms of the sphincter of Oddi."—controls release of pancreatic juices and bile into duodenum

(3) "It prevents air from forming in the small and large intestine."—goes only to duodenum

(4) "It removes bile from the gallbladder."—action of T-tube

131. The Answer is 2

The nurse cares for a client diagnosed with cholecystitis. The client says to the nurse, "I don't understand why my right shoulder hurts, when the gallbladder is not near my shoulder!" Which of the following responses by the nurse is *BEST*?

Reworded Question: Why does the client's shoulder hurt?

Strategy: "*BEST*" indicates discrimination is required to answer the question.

Needed Info: Cholecystitis is inflammation of the gallbladder; indications include intolerance to fatty foods, indigestion, severe pain in upper right quadrant of abdomen radiating to back and right shoulder; leukocytosis, and diaphoresis.

Category: Implementation/Physiological Integrity/Physiological Adaptation

(1) "Sometimes small pieces of the gallstones break off and travel to other parts of the body."—gallstones do not become emboli

(2) "There is an invisible connection between the gallbladder and the right shoulder."—CORRECT: describes referred pain; when visceral branch of a pain receptor fiber is stimulated, vasodilation and pain may occur in a distant body area; right shoulder or scapula is the referred-pain site for gallbladder

(3) "The gallbladder is on the right side of the body and so is that shoulder."—anatomically correct but is not the best explanation

(4) "Your shoulder became tense because you were guarding against the gallbladder pain."—possible; not the best explanation

132. The Answer is 3

The nurse teaches a primigravid woman how to measure the frequency of uterine contractions. The nurse should explain to the client that the frequency of uterine contractions is determined by which of the following?

Reworded Question: How do you determine the frequency of uterine contractions?

Strategy: Think about each answer.

Needed Info: There must be at least 3 contractions to establish frequency.

Category: Implementation/Health Promotion and Maintenance

(1) By timing from the beginning of one contraction to the end of the next contraction—not accurate

(2) By timing from the beginning of one contraction to the end of the same contraction—defines duration

(3) By the number of contractions that occur within a given period of time—CORRECT

(4) By the strength of the contraction at its peak—describes intensity

133. The Answer is 2

The nurse is teaching a woman who is receiving estrogen replacement therapy. Which of the following statements by the nurse indicates that the nurse is aware of the possible complications of estrogen therapy?

Reworded Question: What complications are seen with the use of estrogen therapy?

Strategy: Think about each answer and the effects of estrogen therapy.

Needed Info: Estrogen therapy predisposes to cancer of reproductive organs. Other side effects are nausea, skin rashes, pruritis, breast secretion, and thromboembolic disorders. Used cautiously with family history of breast or genital tract cancer.

Category: Implementation/Health Promotion and Maintenance

(1) "Take an analgesic before you take estrogen, because estrogen may cause discomfort."—not accurate; may cause nausea, weight gain, lethargy

(2) "Make sure you keep your clinic appointments, especially your gynecologic checkup."—CORRECT: have checkup at 6 months

(3) "Limit your fluid intake, because estrogen promotes the retention of fluids."—causes fluid retention and edema; monitor weight; restrict Na^+ intake; don't limit fluids

(4) "Increase roughage in your diet to avoid constipation."—not a complication of estrogen therapy

134. The Answer is 3

Several days after being admitted for depression, a man is observed sitting alone in the clients' dining room. The nurse notes that the client has not finished his meal. Which of the following nursing measures would be *MOST* appropriate?

Reworded Question: How would you meet this client's needs?

Strategy: Determine the outcome of each answer. Is it desired?

Needed Info: Symptoms of depression: withdrawn, regressive behavior, psychomotor retardation.

Category: Planning/Psychosocial Integrity

(1) Allow the client to eat in his room until he becomes more comfortable eating with other clients—social isolation, reinforces depression

(2) Ask the client's family to bring foods that he likes to eat—does not address problem

(3) Order small, frequent meals and sit with the client while he eats in the dining room—CORRECT: diminished appetite, prevents social isolation

(4) Do not focus on eating behaviors because his appetite will improve over time—does not meet nutritional needs

135. The Answer is 3

A client is being treated for injuries sustained in an automobile accident. The client has a central venous pressure (CVP) line in place. The nurse recognizes that CVP measurement reflects which of the following?

Reworded Question: What does CVP measure?

Strategy: Think about CVP and cardiac function.

Needed Info: CVP: central venous line placed in superior vena cava. To obtain a reading: client placed supine, 0 on manometer placed at level of right atrium (midaxillary line at 4th intercostal space), turn stopcock to allow manometer to fill with fluid, turn to allow fluid to go into client. Fluid will fluctuate with resp. When stabilizes take reading at highest level of fluctuation. Normal: 4–10 cm/H_2O. Elevated: hypervolemia, CHF, pericarditis. Low: hypovolemia.

Category: Analysis/Physiological Integrity/Reduction of Risk Potential

(1) Cardiac output—Swan-Ganz line

(2) Pressure in the left ventricle—Swan-Ganz line

(3) Pressure in the right atrium—CORRECT: determined by blood volume, vascular tone, action of right side of heart

(4) Pressure in the pulmonary artery—Swan-Ganz line: 4-lumen, balloon-tipped, flow-directed catheter

136. The Answer is 2

A mother brings her 4-year-old daughter to the pediatrician for treatment of chronic otitis media. The mother asks the nurse how she can prevent her child from getting ear infections so often. The nurse's response should be based on an understanding that the recurrence of otitis media can be decreased by which of the following?

Reworded Question: What will prevent the development of otitis media? What causes otitis media?

Strategy: Think about the causes of otitis media.

Needed Info: Otitis media: frequently follows respiratory infection. Reduce occurrences: holding child upright for feedings, encourage gentle nose-blowing, teach modified Valsava maneuver (pinch nose, close lips, and force air up through eustachian tubes), blow up balloons or chew gum, eliminate tobacco smoke or known allergens.

Category: Analysis/Health Promotion and Maintenance

(1) Covering the child's ears while bathing—not preventive

(2) Treating upper respiratory infections quickly—CORRECT: respiratory fluids are a medium for bacteria; antihistamines used

(3) Administering nose drops at bedtime—not preventive

(4) Isolating her child from other children—too extreme a measure

137. The Answer is 3

A client receives 10 units of NPH insulin every morning at 8 A.M. At 4 P.M., the nurse observes that the client is diaphoretic and slightly confused. The nurse should take which of the following actions *FIRST*?

Reworded Question: What is the cause of these symptoms? What is the first thing you should do?

Strategy: "*FIRST*" indicates that this is a priority question.

Needed Info: NPH insulin: intermediate-acting preparation: onset 1–4 hrs, peak 2–15 hrs, duration 12–28 hrs. S/S hypoglycemia: confusion, tremors, hypotension, cool clammy skin, diaphoresis. Treatment: if conscious, liquids containing sugar; dextrose 50% IV if unconscious; client education.

Category: Planning/Physiological Integrity/Pharmacological and Parenteral Therapies

(1) Check vital signs—not first action; should recognize S/S hypoglycemia

(2) Check urine for glucose and ketones—indicates only hyperglycemia, no information about hypoglycemia; should recognize S/S hypoglycemia

(3) Give 6 oz. of skim milk—CORRECT: S/S of hypoglycemia; give fast-acting sugar and protein; recheck blood sugar in 15 min

(4) Call the physician—not necessary; unless hypoglycemia is not corrected

138. The Answer is 2

Prior to the client undergoing a scheduled intravenous pyelogram (IVP), the nurse reviews the client's health history. It would be *MOST* important for the nurse to obtain the answer to which of the following questions?

Reworded Question: What do you need to know before an IVP?

Strategy: Think about each answer and how it relates to an IVP.

Needed Info: IVP: radiopaque dye that contains iodine injected into the body and is filtered through the kidneys and excreted by the urinary tract. Visualizes kidneys, ureters, and bladder. Preparation: NPO midnight, cathartics evening before test. Injection of dye causes flushing of face, nausea, salty taste in mouth.

Category: Assessment/Physiological Integrity/ Reduction in Risk Potential

(1) Does the client have difficulty voiding?—not most important

(2) Does the client have any allergies to shellfish or iodine?—CORRECT: anaphylactic reaction; itching, hives, wheezing; treatment: antihistamines, O_2, CPR, epinephrine, vasopressor

(3) Does the client have a history of constipation? —not essential info

(4) Does the client have frequent headaches?—not most important

139. The Answer is 1

A child with chickenpox (varicella) is brought by her parents to the physician for evaluation. The nurse knows the rash characteristic of chickenpox can be described as which of the following?

Reworded Question: What does the rash from chickenpox look like?

Strategy: Form a mental image of client with characteristic rash.

Needed Info: Chickenpox transmission: direct contact, droplet. Incubation period: 13–17 days. Treatment: Zovirax, Benadryl, and/or calamine lotion for itching, good skin care to prevent secondary infection, bathe daily, change clothes and linens, strict isolation in hospital, at home isolate until vesicles have dried (usually 1 week after onset), short fingernails, avoid use of aspirin due to Reye's syndrome. Measles transmission: direct contact, droplets. Incubation period: 10–20 days. Symptoms: fever, cough, conjunctivitis, erythematous maculopapular rash on face. Treatment: bed rest, antipyretics, antibiotics to prevent secondary infection. Isolate until 5th day of rash, cool mist vaporizer, good skin care, dim lights.

Category: Assessment/Health Promotion and Maintenance

(1) Maculopapular—CORRECT: prodromal stage: slight fever, malaise and anorexia, maculopapular rash, becomes vesicular: fluid-filled vesicles form crusts, or scabs, communicable from 1 day before eruption of lesions (during prodromal

stage) up to 6 days after first crop of vesicles appear and crusts form

(2) Small, irregular red spots with minute bluish-white centers—Koplik spots: prodromal stage of measles, first seen on buccal mucosa 2 days before rash

(3) Round or oval erythematous scaling patches— psoriasis: treatment: exposure to sunlight/ultraviolet light, topical corticosteroids, coal-tar derivates

(4) Petechiae—pinpoint, nonraised, perfectly round purplish red spots caused by intradermal or submucosal hemorrhage, seen in severe sepsis with disseminated intravascular coagulation (DIC), Rocky Mountain spotted fever, and subacute bacterial endocarditis (SBE)

140. The Answer is 2

A primigravid woman at 28 weeks' gestation takes a 3-hour glucose tolerance test. The results indicate a fasting blood sugar of 100 mg/dL and a 2-hour post-load blood sugar of 300 mg/dL. Which of the following nursing diagnoses should be considered the *HIGHEST* priority at this time?

Reworded Question: What is most important for a newly diagnosed client with gestational diabetes mellitus (GDM)?

Strategy: Use Maslow's hierarchy of needs to establish priorities. Remember to first meet physical needs before addressing other concerns.

Needed Info: GDM: carbohydrate intolerance that occurs during pregnancy in women with no prior history of diabetes. May exhibit the classic symptoms of diabetes: polyuria (excessive urination), polydipsia (excessive thirst), and polyphagia (hunger). Half the women are asymptomatic. Diagnosed: 3-hr glucose tolerance test (GTT) (administer a high glucose load to fasting pt; blood glucose levels are measured fasting, and at 1-hr intervals for 3 hrs; test is positive if 2 or more of the blood sugars are elevated). Normal: fasting, 60–110 mg/dL; 1 hr—190; 2 hrs—165; 3 hrs—145.

Category: Analysis/Physiological Integrity/Physiological Adaptation

(1) Potential impaired family coping related to diagnosis of GDM—not highest priority; psychosocial need

(2) Potential noncompliance related to lack of knowledge or lack of adequate support system—CORRECT: client may not be able to meet physical needs because of lack of knowledge

(3) Potential for altered parenting related to disappointment—psychosocial need; not highest priority

(4) Ineffective family coping related to anticipatory grieving—psychosocial need

141. The Answer is 3

The nurse cares for a client admitted for a possible herniated intervertebral disk. Ibuprofen (Motrin), propoxyphene hydrochloride (Darvon), and cyclobenzaprine hydrochloride (Flexeril) are ordered PRN. Several hours after admission, the client complains of pain. Which of the following actions should the nurse do *FIRST*?

Reworded Question: What should you do first?

Strategy: Set priorities. Compare the answers to the steps in the nursing process.

Needed Info: Herniated disk: knifelike pain aggravated by sneezing, coughing, straining.

Category: Planning/Physiological Integrity/Pharmacological and Parenteral Therapies

(1) Administer Motrin—implementation; not first step

(2) Call the physician to determine which medication should be given—assess before implementing

(3) Gather more information from the client about the complaint—CORRECT: assess; first step in nursing process

(4) Allow the client some time to rest and see if the pain subsides—implementation; not first step

142. The Answer is 2

When planning care for a client hospitalized with depression, the nurse includes measures to increase his self-esteem. Which of the following actions should the nurse take to meet this goal?

Reworded Question: How do you increase the self-esteem of a depressed client?

Strategy: Think about each answer in relation to depression.

Needed Info: Increase self-esteem: warm, supportive environment, consistent daily care.

Category: Implementation/Psychosocial Integrity

(1) Encourage him to accept leadership responsibilities in milieu activities—too demanding

(2) Set simple, realistic goals with him to help him experience success—CORRECT: sense of accomplishment

(3) Help him to accept his illness and the adjustments that are required—does not help feelings of hopelessness

(4) Assure him that when he is discharged, he will be able to resume his previous activities—false reassurance

143. The Answer is 3

The nurse finds a visitor unconscious on the floor of a client's room during visiting hours at the hospital. Which of the following nursing assessments is consistent with cardiopulmonary arrest?

Reworded Question: What are the signs of cardiopulmonary arrest?

Strategy: Think about the steps you would take to evaluate an unconscious client.

Needed Info: Cardiopulmonary arrest: heart, circulation and respirations cease. CPR: (1) determine unresponsiveness, (2) open airway (head tip–chin lift maneuver or jaw thrust), (3) determine breathlessness (look, listen, feel), (4) perform rescue breathing (2 slow breaths, chest rise 1–2 in.), (5) determine pulselessness (check carotid pulse 5–10 sec), (6) provide circulation (chest compressions 1.5–2 in.).

Category: Assessment/Physiological Integrity/Physiological Adaptation

(1) Absent pulse, fixed dilated pupils—not accurate

(2) Absent respirations, fixed and dilated pupils—not accurate

(3) Absent pulse and respirations—CORRECT: no palpable pulse; no breath sounds; ashen color

(4) Thready pulse and pupillary changes—not accurate

144. The Answer is 4

A client is transferred to an extended care facility after a cerebrovascular accident (CVA). The client has right-sided paralysis and has been experiencing dysphagia. The nurse observes an aide preparing the client to eat lunch. Which of the following situations would require an intervention by the nurse?

Reworded Question: Which option is wrong?

Strategy: This is a negative question. Make sure you know if you are looking for a correct situation or a problematic situation.

Needed Info: Dysphagia: difficulty swallowing. Provide support if necessary for the head, have the client upright, feed the client slowly in small amounts, place food on unaffected side of mouth. Maintain upright position for 30–45 minutes after eating. Good oral care after eating.

Category: Evaluation/Physiological Integrity/ Reduction of Risk Potential

(1) The client is in bed in high Fowler's position—correct positioning, or may sit in chair

(2) The client's head and neck are positioned slightly forward—correct positioning; helps client chew and swallow

(3) The aide puts the food in the back of the client's mouth on the unaffected side—helps client handle food

(4) The aide waters down the pudding to help the client swallow—CORRECT: requires intervention, usually able to better handle soft or semi-soft foods; difficulty with liquids

145. The Answer is 3

The home care nurse plans care for a client with pernicious anemia. A monthly intramuscular injection is ordered for the client. The nurse knows that in an adult, the best muscle to administer an intramuscular injection is which of the following?

Reworded Question: Where should you give an IM injection in an adult?

Strategy: Think about each answer in relation to anatomy and physiology.

Needed Info: Pernicious anemia: lack of intrinsic factor from stomach leading to decreased absorption of vitamin B_{12}. S/S: low hemoglobin and hematocrit. Diagnosed: Schilling test (measures absorption of orally administered radioactive B_{12} by amount of radioactive B_{12} excreted in urine in 24 hrs). Treatment: lifelong B_{12} injections, iron supplements. Factors to consider when selecting site for injection: amount of muscle mass and condition, amount and character of med, type of med, frequency of injections.

Category: Implementation/Physiological Integrity/ Pharmacological and Parenteral Therapies

(1) Gluteus maximus—possible injury to sciatic nerve

(2) Deltoid—not well developed in some adults, especially elderly; possible injury to brachial artery; can only use for small amount of med

(3) Vastus lateralis—CORRECT: no major nerves or blood vessels; to locate, palpate greater trochanter and knee joint; divide distance between them into quadrants; inject into middle of upper quadrant

(4) Dorsogluteal—possible injury to sciatic nerve

146. The Answer is 2

A man comes to the emergency room complaining of nausea, vomiting, and severe right upper quadrant pain. His temperature is 101.3° F (38.5° C) and an abdominal x-ray reveals an enlarged gallbladder. He is given a diagnosis of acute cholecystitis and is scheduled for surgery. After administering an analgesic to the client, the nurse recognizes that which of the following actions is the *HIGHEST* priority?

Reworded Question: What should you do after giving an analgesic to the client?

Strategy: Establish priorities. Remember Maslow's hierarchy of needs. Meet physical needs first.

Needed Info: S/S: pain in upper midline area radiating around to back, jaundice, nausea, vomiting, flatulence, bloating, belching, intolerance to fatty foods. Treatment: cholecystectomy (removal of gallbladder). Post-op: T-tube inserted for drainage from bile duct. Complications: hemorrhage, pneumonia, thrombophlebitis, urinary retention, ileus. Preop nursing responsibilities: Demerol for pain (morphine contraindicated; causes spasms for sphincter of Oddi), nitroglycerin to relax smooth muscle, NG tube for decompression, IVs. Post-op nursing responsibilities: change position every 2 hrs, check breath sounds and vital signs every 4 hrs, I & O, anti-embolitic stockings.

Category: Planning/Physiological Integrity/Physiological Adaptation

(1) Assessing the client's need for dietary teaching—not highest priority

(2) Assessing the client's fluid and electrolyte status—CORRECT: hypokalemia and hypomagnesemia common *from vomiting & diarrhea*

(3) Examining the client's health history for allergies to antibiotics—not highest priority

(4) Determining whether the client has signed consent for surgery—not highest priority

147. The Answer is 3

A mother with 4 children calls the clinic for advice on how to care for her oldest child, who has developed chickenpox. Which of the following statements by the mother indicates a need for further teaching?

Reworded Question: What teaching is necessary for parent of child with chickenpox?

Strategy: Be careful! This is a negative question. You are looking for incorrect info.

Needed Info: Teaching: calamine lotion for itching, good skin care to prevent secondary infection, bathe daily, change clothes and linens, isolate until vesicles have dried (usually 1 week after onset), short fingernails, avoid use of aspirin due to Reye's syndrome.

Category: Evaluation/Safe and Effective Care Environment/Safety and Infection Control

(1) "I should keep my child home from school until the vesicles are crusted."—correct information; chickenpox transmitted by direct contact with droplets of infected person; communicable period: 2 days before rash until vesicles crusted (scabbed), then child may interact with siblings and others

(2) "I can use calamine lotion if needed."—correct information, used to treat itching

(3) "I should remove the crusts so the skin can heal."—CORRECT: indicates need for further

teaching; good skin care important; crusts usually not removed, can cause scarring

(4) "I can use mittens if scratching becomes a problem."—rash itches; mittens used to prevent scratching

148. The Answer is 4

The nurse is teaching a woman who comes to the clinic at 32 weeks' gestation with a diagnosis of pregnancy-induced hypertension (PIH). Which of the following statements by the client indicates to to the nurse that further teaching is required?

Reworded Question: What is not accurate about the care of a woman with PIH?

Strategy: This is a negative question. It can be reworded to say, "All of the following are true *EXCEPT.*"

Needed Info: PIH, preeclampsia, toxemia: development of hypertension (increase 30 mmHg systolic or 15 mmHg diastolic) with proteinuria and/or edema (dependent or facial) after 20 weeks' gestation. Risk factors: parity (first-time mothers), age (younger than 20 or older than 35), geographic location (southern or western U.S.), multifetal gestation, hydatidiform mole, hypertension, and diabetes. Prevention: early prenatal care, identify high risk clients, recognize S/S early; bed rest lying on left side, daily weights. Treatment: urine checks for proteinuria; diet (increased protein and decreased Na+). Can develop into eclampsia (convulsions or coma).

Category: Evaluation/Health Promotion and Maintenance

(1) "Lying in bed on my left side is likely to increase my urinary output."—true; bed rest promotes good perfusion of blood to uterus; decreases BP and promotes diuresis

(2) "If the bed rest works, I may lose a pound or two in the next few days."—true; causes diuresis; results in reduction of retained fluids; instruct to monitor weight daily and notify physician if notices abrupt increase even after resting in bed for 12 hrs

(3) "I should be sure to maintain a diet that has a good amount of protein."—true; replaces protein lost in urine; increases plasma colloid osmotic

pressure; avoid salty foods; avoid alcohol; drink 8 glasses of water daily; eat foods high in roughage

(4) "I will have to keep my room darkened and not watch much television."—CORRECT: incorrect info, not necessary; diversional activities helpful

149. The Answer is 2

The nurse evaluates the care provided to a client hospitalized for treatment of adrenal crisis. Which of the following changes would indicate to the nurse that the client is responding favorably to medical and nursing treatment?

Reworded Question: What shows a positive response to treatment for adrenal crisis?

Strategy: Think about each answer.

Needed Info: In adrenal crisis the required adrenal hormones exceed the supply available. Usually precipitated by stress, surgery, trauma, or infection. S/S: hypotension, cool pale skin, increased urinary output, dehydration.

Category: Evaluation/Physiological Integrity/Physiological Adaptation

(1) The client's urinary output has increased—indicates continuing lack of hormones; will decrease with treatment

(2) The client's blood pressure has increased—CORRECT: hypotension S/S of adrenal insufficiency; without treatment Na^+ level falls, resulting in volume depletion and hypotension; K^+ rises, resulting in cardiac dysrhythmias

(3) The client has lost weight—indicates continuing loss of water and continuing lack of hormones

(4) The client's peripheral edema has decreased—edema not seen with adrenal crises

150. The Answer is 4

After completing an assessment, the nurse determines that a client is exhibiting early symptoms of a dystonic reaction related to the use of an antipsychotic medication. Which of the following actions by the nurse would be *MOST* appropriate?

Reworded Question: What is the first thing you do for a client with a dystonic reaction?

Strategy: Set priorities. Remember Maslow's hierarchy of needs.

Needed Info: Dystonic reaction: muscle tightness in throat, neck, tongue, mouth, eyes, neck, and back; difficulty talking and swallowing. Treatment: IM or IV Benadryl or Cogentin.

Category: Implementation/Psychosocial Integrity

(1) Reality-test with the client and assure her that her physical symptoms are not real—real symptoms, not delusions

(2) Teach the client about common side effects of antipsychotic medications—physical needs are highest priority

(3) Explain to the client that there is no treatment that will relieve these symptoms—Benadryl used IM or IV

(4) Notify the physician and obtain an order for IM Benadryl—CORRECT: emergency situation, can occlude airway

151. The Answer is 2

The physician orders heparin for a client. In order to evaluate the effectiveness of the client's heparin therapy, the nurse should monitor which of the following laboratory values?

Reworded Question: What blood work is done to monitor heparin therapy?

Strategy: Think about each answer.

Needed Info: Heparin: anticoagulant. Side effects: hemorrhage, thrombocytopenia. Antidote: Protamine sulfate. When given subcutaneously, inject slowly; leave needle in place 10 seconds, then withdraw; don't massage site; rotate sites. Nursing responsibilities: check for bleeding gums, bruises, nosebleeds, petechiae, melena, tarry stools, hematuria; use electric razor and soft toothbrush.

Category: Assessment/Physiological Integrity/Reduction of Risk Potential

(1) Platelet count—evaluates platelet production; not altered

(2) Clotting time—CORRECT: or partial thromboplastin time (PTT); 1.5–2 times control, clotting time 2–3 times control

(3) Bleeding time—duration of bleeding after small puncture wound; detects platelet and vascular problems; not altered

(4) Prothrombin time—PT used to monitor Coumadin therapy

152. The Answer is 3

A client comes to the clinic for evaluation of acute onset of seizures. A thorough history and physical examination is performed. The nurse would expect which of the following diagnostic tests to be performed *FIRST*?

Reworded Question: What test is used to diagnose seizure disorders?

Strategy: Consider the purpose of each test.

Needed Info: EEG: recording of electrical activity of brain. Electrodes attached to scalp, waveforms recorded. Checked relaxing, hyperventilating, sleeping, with lights flickering. Prep: kept awake night before, shampoo hair. Stimulants (tea, coffee, alcohol, cola, cigarettes), antidepressants, tranquilizers, anticonvulsants withheld 24–48 hours before test. After test, seizure precautions and wash hair. Seizure: uncontrolled discharge of electrical activity from brain.

Category: Planning/Physiological Integrity/Reduction of Risk Potential

(1) Magnetic resonance imaging (MRI)—uses magnetic fields to get detailed pictures; prep: remove jewelry, metal objects, lie still, may feel claustrophobic; not first choice for diagnosing seizure disorders

(2) Cerebral angiography—dye injected into catheter in femoral artery, x-rays taken; prep: check sensitivity to dye; post-test: pressure on insertion site; not first choice for diagnosing seizure disorders

(3) Electroencephalogram (EEG)—CORRECT

(4) Electromyogram (EMG)—evaluates activity of muscles; electrodes placed in nerves, small amount of electricity applied

153. The Answer is 1

The nurse performs dietary teaching with a client on a low-protein diet. The nurse knows that teaching has been successful if the client identifies which of the following meals as lowest in protein?

Reworded Question: Which foods are the *LOWEST* in protein?

Strategy: Consider each meal and eliminate those with high-protein components.

Needed Info: Avoid high-protein foods: eggs, milk products, meat, beans, nuts, cereals.

Category: Evaluation/Physiological Integrity/Basic Care and Comfort

(1) Cranberries and broiled chicken—CORRECT: cranberries, no protein; chicken, 7 g/oz.

(2) Tomatoes and flounder—tomato, 2 g/oz.; flounder, 8 g/oz.

(3) Broccoli and veal—broccoli, 2 g/oz.; veal, 7 g/oz.

(4) Spinach and tofu—spinach, 2 g/serving; tofu, 7 g/oz.

154. The Answer is 1

A client has a vagotomy with antrectomy to treat a duodenal ulcer. Postoperatively, the client develops dumping syndrome. Which of the following statements by the client indicates to the nurse that further dietary teaching is necessary?

Reworded Question: What is contraindicated for the client with dumping syndrome?

Strategy: Be careful! You are looking for incorrect information.

Needed Info: Antrectomy: surgery to reduce acid-secreting portions of stomach. Delays or eliminates gastric phase of digestion. Dumping syndrome occurs in clients after a gastric resection. It occurs after eating and is related to the reduced capacity of the stomach. Undigested food is dumped into the jejunum, resulting in distention, cramping, pain, diarrhea 15–30 min after eating. Subsides in 6–12 months. S/S 5–30 min after eating: vertigo, tachycardia, syncope, diarrhea, nausea. Treatment: sedatives, antispasmodics; high-protein, high-fat, low-carbohydrate, dry diet. Eat in semirecumbent position, lying down after eating.

Category: Evaluation/Physiological Integrity/Basic Care and Comfort

(1) "I should eat bread with each meal."—CORRECT: incorrect info; should decrease intake of carbohydrates

(2) "I should eat smaller meals more frequently."—true; 5–6 small meals per day

(3) "I should lie down after eating."—true; delays gastric emptying time

(4) "I should avoid drinking fluids with my meals."—true; no fluids 1 hr before, with, or 2 hrs after meal

155.   The Answer is 2

A man is admitted to the hospital with a diagnosis of acquired immunodeficiency syndrome (AIDS). He is being treated for *Pneumocystis jiroveci* pneumonia. The nurse evaluates the care provided to this client by other members of the health care team. The nurse should intervene in which of the following situations?

Reworded Question: Which situation describes an unsafe or inappropriate practice?

Strategy: Picture each situation as described in the question.

Category: Evaluation/Safe and Effective Care Environment/Safety and Infection Control

(1) A housekeeper cleans up spilled blood with a bleach solution—appropriate activity, solution of 1:10 sodium hypochlorite, or bleach with water, kills AIDS virus

(2) A nursing student takes the client's blood pressure wearing a mask and gloves—CORRECT: inappropriate practice; mask and gloves necessary only when possibility of contact with blood and body fluids; when taking a BP, very low risk for contact with blood and body fluids; behavior insensitive to client's feelings, does not promote trust

(3) A technician wears gloves to perform a venipuncture—safe practice, barrier precaution used to prevent skin and mucous-membrane exposure if contact with blood or other body fluids of any client anticipated

(4) A nurse attendant allows visitors to enter his room without masks—appropriate activity: visitors do not need masks, PCP parasite found in lungs of healthy people, thought to cause subclinical pulmonary infection worldwide, only dangerous to immunosuppressed clients; sick people not permitted to visit client

156.   The Answer is 2

A woman comes to the physician's office for a routine prenatal checkup at 34 weeks' gestation. Abdominal palpation reveals the fetal position as right occipital anterior (ROA). At which of the following sites would the nurse expect to find the fetal heart tone?

Reworded Question: The fetus is ROA. Where should the nurse listen for the FHT?

Strategy: Picture the situation described. It may be helpful for you to draw this out so that you can imagine where the heartbeat would be found.

Needed Info: Describing fetal position: practice of defining position of baby relative to mother's pelvis. The point of maximum intensity (PMI) of the fetus: point on mother's abdomen where FHT is the loudest, usually over the fetal back. Divide mother's pelvis into 4 parts or quadrants: right and left anterior (front), and right and left posterior (back). Abbreviated: R and L for right and left, and A and P for anterior and posterior. The head, particularly the occiput, is the most common presenting part, and is abbreviated O. LOA is most common fetal presentation and FHT heard on left side. In a vertex presentation, FHT is heard below the umbilicus. In a breech presentation, FHT is heard above umbilicus.

Category: Assessment/Health Promotion and Maintenance

(1) Below the umbilicus, on the mother's left side—found on right, not left, side

(2) Below the umbilicus, on the mother's right side—CORRECT: occiput and back are pressing against right side of mother's abdomen; FHT would be heard below umbilicus on right side

(3) Above the umbilicus, on the mother's left side—found in breech presentation

(4) Above the umbilicus, on the mother's right side—found in breech presentation

157. The Answer is 3

A client is admitted to the hospital with complaints of seizures and a high fever. A brain scan is ordered. Before the scan, the client asks the nurse what position he will be in while the procedure is being done. Which of the following statements by the nurse is *MOST* accurate?

Reworded Question: What is the proper position for a brain scan?

Strategy: Think about each answer.

Needed Info: Brain scan: measures amount of uptake by the brain of radioactive isotopes. Damaged tissue absorbs more than normal tissue. Nursing care before: withhold medications (antihypertensives, vasoconstrictors, vasodilators for 24 hrs). During the test, client will need to change position while pictures of the brain are taken. Test is painless. After test, force fluids to promote excretion of isotopes. Urine doesn't need special handling.

Category: Implementation/Physiological Integrity/ Reduction of Risk Potential

(1) "You will be in a side-lying position with the foot of the bed elevated."—incorrect

(2) "You will be in a semi-upright sitting position with your knees flexed."—incorrect

(3) "You will be lying supine with a small pillow under your head."—CORRECT

(4) "You will be flat on your back, with your feet higher than your head."—incorrect

158. The Answer is 3

A man is admitted to the psychiatric hospital with a diagnosis of obsessive-compulsive disorder. He is unable to stay employed because his ritualistic behavior causes him to be late for work. Which of the following interpretations by the nurse of the client's behavior is *MOST* accurate?

Reworded Question: Why does the client perform ritualistic behavior?

Strategy: Think about each answer in relation to compulsive activity.

Needed Info: Obsession: recurrent or persistent thought, image, or impulse. Compulsion: repetitive, purposeful, or intentional behavior performed in a stereotypical manner. Nursing responsibilities: accept ritualistic behavior, structure environment, meet physical needs, minimize choices. Anafranil: tricyclic antidepressant. Side effects: dizziness, libido change, nervousness, dry mouth, sweating, urine retention, constipation, photosensitivity.

Category: Analysis/Psychosocial Integrity

(1) He is responding to auditory hallucinations and trying to gain control over his behavior—hallucinations: false sensory perceptions in the absence of external stimuli, associated with schizophrenia

(2) He is fulfilling an unconscious desire to punish himself—not accurate

(3) He is attempting to reduce anxiety by taking control of the environment—CORRECT: unconscious attempt to reduce anxiety

(4) He is malingering in order to avoid responsibilities at work—conscious feigning of illness to promote secondary gain, conscious effort to manipulate

159. The Answer is 4

A client diagnosed with chronic lymphocytic leukemia is admitted to the hospital for treatment of hemolytic anemia. Which of the following measures incorporated into the nursing care plan *BEST* addresses the client's needs?

Reworded Question: What should you do for a client with anemia?

Strategy: Although the client has leukemia, he is admitted with anemia. You must focus on the anemia.

Needed Info: Lymphocytic leukemia: characterized by proliferation of lymphocytes. S/S: fatigue, weakness, headache, easy bruising, bleeding gums, epistaxis, fever, generalized pain. Diagnostic tests: CBC, bone marrow aspiration, lumbar puncture, x-rays, lymph node biopsy. Treatment: total body irradiation or radiation to spleen, chemotherapy. Nursing responsibilities: low-bacteria diet (no raw fruits or vegetables), institute bleeding precautions (soft toothbrush, don't floss, no injections, no aspirin, pad bed rails, use air mattress, use paper tape), antiemetics, comfort measures. Hemolytic anemia

S/S: jaundice, splenomegaly, hepatomegaly, fatigue, weakness. Treatment: O_2, blood transfusions, corticosteroids.

Category: Planning/Physiological Integrity/Basic Care and Comfort

(1) Encourage activities with other clients in the dayroom—does not meet need for rest

(2) Isolate the client from visitors and clients to avoid infection—no info given about WBC or reverse isolation; on reverse isolation if neutrophil count is less than 500/mm³

(3) Provide a diet high in vitamin C—needed for wound healing and resistance to infection; not best choice

(4) Provide a quiet environment to promote adequate rest—CORRECT: primary problem activity intolerance due to fatigue

160. The Answer is 1

The nurse plans morning care for a client hospitalized after a cerebrovascular accident (CVA) resulting in left-sided paralysis and homonymous hemianopia. During morning care, the nurse should do which of the following?

Reworded Question: What should you do for morning care for this client?

Strategy: Think about the outcome of each answer choice.

Needed Info: Homonymous hemianopia: blindness in half of each visual field caused by damage to brain. Client cannot see past midline toward the side opposite the lesion without turning the head toward that side. Approach client from side that is not visually impaired. Reduce noise and complexity of decision-making.

Category: Implementation/Physiological Integrity/Physiological Adaptation

(1) Provide care from the client's right side—CORRECT: approach from side with intact vision

(2) Speak loudly and distinctly when talking with the client—no hearing loss

(3) Reduce the level of lighting in the client's room to prevent glare—increase light to assist with vision

(4) Provide all of the client's care to reduce his energy expenditure—encourage independence

161. The Answer is 2

The nurse prepares for the admission of a client with a perforated duodenal ulcer. Which of the following should the nurse expect to observe as the primary initial symptom?

Reworded Question: What symptom is seen first with a perforated abdominal ulcer?

Strategy: Discrimination is required to answer the question.

Needed Info: Perforation of ulcer: medical emergency. Gastroduodenal contents empty into peritoneal cavity resulting in peritonitis, paralytic ileus, septicemia, and shock. S/S: sudden, sharp pain; abdomen becomes tender, rigid. Treatment: fluids, electrolytes, antibiotics, NG suction, vagotomy, hemigastrectomy. S/S of duodenal ulcer: 25–30 years old, male-female 4:1, blood type O, pain 2–3 hrs after meal and hs, food intake relieves pain. Treatment: small frequent feedings; avoid coffee, alcohol, seasonings; antacids (Maalox) 1 hr before or after meals; anticholinergics (Probanthine), take 30 minutes before meals; histamine receptor site antagonists (Tagamet), take with meals.

Category: Assessment/Physiological Integrity/Physiological Adaptation

(1) Fever—later with peritonitis (S/S: pain, nausea, vomiting, rigid abdomen, low-grade fever, absent bowel sounds, shallow respirations)

(2) Pain—CORRECT: sudden, sharp, begins mid-epigastric; boardlike abdomen

(3) Dizziness—later with shock (S/S: hypotension, tachycardia, tachypnea, decreased urinary output, decreased LOC)

(4) Vomiting—seen with peritonitis

162. The Answer is 3

A 3-week-old boy is admitted with a diagnosis of pyloric stenosis. The mother tells the nurse that this is her first child and asks if there is anything she can do to prevent this from happening to her next child.

Which of the following statements by the nurse *BEST* addresses her concern?

Reworded Question: What should you say to the mother about the possibility of this happening in the future?

Strategy: Remember your therapeutic communication techniques.

Category: Implementation/Psychosocial Integrity

(1) "This type of thing generally happens to first children"—inaccurate

(2) "When you have your second child, at least you'll know what signs to look for"—invalidates concerns

(3) "This is a structural problem; it is not a reflection of your parenting skills"—CORRECT: provides acknowledgment; contains facts

(4) "This is an inherited condition; it is not your fault"—does not acknowledge feelings

163.   The Answer is 3

The nurse cares for a client diagnosed with bipolar disorder. The client paces endlessly in the halls and makes hostile comments to other clients. The client resists the nurse's attempts to move him to a room in the unit. Which of the following actions by the nurse is *MOST* important?

Reworded Question: What is priority for the client who is experiencing mania?

Strategy: "*MOST* important" indicates priority.

Needed Info: Bipolar disorder is a chronic mood syndrome that causes mania, hypomania, and depression; during mania, client is hyperactive, anxious, and unable to meet physical needs; also see flight of ideas, inappropriate dress, and a lack of inhibitions.

Category: Planning/Psychosocial Integrity

(1) Offer the client fluids every hour—appropriate action; at risk for cardiac collapse due to dehydration; first give medication to decrease hyperactivity

(2) Inform the client about the unit rules—inappropriate; administer medication, reduce environmental stimuli

(3) Administer haloperidol (Haldol) IM—CORRECT: decrease hyperactive behavior so client can take fluids and food

(4) Encourage the client to rest—important; first decrease hyperactive behavior

164.   The Answer is 3

The nurse is caring for an Rh-negative mother who has delivered an Rh-positive child. The mother states, "The doctor told me about RhoGAM, but I'm still a little confused." Which of the following responses by the nurse is *MOST* appropriate?

Reworded Question: What is RhoGAM and why is it used?

Strategy: Remember what you know about RhoGAM.

Needed Info: RhoGAM: given to unsensitized Rh-negative (Rh–) mother after delivery or abortion of an Rh-positive (Rh+) infant or fetus to prevent development of sensitization. Rh– mother produces antibodies in response to the Rh+ RBCs of fetus. If occurs during pregnancy, fetus is affected. If occurs during delivery, later pregnancies may be affected. An indirect Coombs test is performed on the mother during pregnancy, and a direct Coombs test is done on cord blood after delivery. If both are negative and the neonate is Rh+, the mother is given RhoGAM to prevent sensitization. RhoGAM is usually given to unsensitized mothers within 72 hrs of delivery, but may be effective when given 3–4 weeks after delivery. To be effective, RhoGAM must be given after the first delivery and repeated after each subsequent delivery. RhoGAM is ineffective against Rh+ antibodies that are already present in the maternal circulation. The administration of RhoGAM at 26–28 weeks' gestation is also recommended.

Category: Implementation/Health Promotion and Maintenance

(1) "RhoGAM is given to your child to prevent the development of antibodies."—not given to neonate

(2) "RhoGAM is given to your child to supply the necessary antibodies."—not given to neonate

(3) "RhoGAM is given to you to prevent the formation of antibodies."—CORRECT: prevents maternal circulation from developing antibodies

(4) "RhoGAM is given to you to encourage the production of antibodies."—not accurate; given to discourage antibody production

165. The Answer is 3

The nurse performs client teaching for a woman with osteoarthritis. The client asks what she can do to effectively decrease pain and stiffness in her joints before beginning her daily routine. The nurse should instruct the client to do which of the following?

Reworded Question: What should the client with osteoarthritis do first thing in the morning?

Strategy: Which answer would reduce an osteoarthritic client's pain?

Category: Implementation/Physiological Integrity/Basic Care and Comfort

(1) "Perform isometric exercises for 10 minutes."—done to preserve muscle strength; tighten muscle, hold for few seconds, then relax without moving joint

(2) "Do range-of-motion exercises then apply ointment to your joints."—done after ointment applied; ROM does not reduce pain

(3) "Take a warm bath and rest for a few minutes."—CORRECT: heat reduces pain, spasms, stiffness in joints

(4) "Stretch all muscle groups."—would be painful

166. The Answer is 2

The nurse cares for a client receiving paroxetine (Paxil). It is *MOST* important for the nurse to report which of the following to the physician?

Reworded Question: What is a potential drug interaction?

Strategy: "*MOST* important" indicates priority.

Needed Info: Paxil is a selective serotinin reuptake inhibitor (SSRI) used to treat depression, panic disorder, obsessive-compulsive disorder; side effects include palpitations, bradycardia, nausea and vomiting, and decreased appetite.

Category: Evaluation/Physiological Integrity/Pharmacological and Parenteral Therapies

(1) The client states there is no change in her appetite—causes anorexia; monitor weight and nutritional intake; report continued weight loss

(2) The client states she has started taking digoxin (Lanoxin)—CORRECT: may decrease effectiveness of digoxin

(3) The client states she applies sunscreen before going outside—appropriate action; prevents photosensitivity reactions

(4) The client states she drives her car to work—driving is acceptable after determining client's response to drugs

167. The Answer is 2

A client returns to his room after a cardiac catheterization. Which of the following assessments by the nurse would justify calling the physician?

Reworded Question: What is the most serious complication that can occur after a cardiac catheterization? How would you know it occurred?

Strategy: Think about each answer. Recognize and eliminate expected outcomes.

Needed Info: Cardiac catheterization prep: may feel palpitations as catheter is passed and feelings of heat and desire to cough as dye is injected (check allergies to iodine and shellfish). Obtain consent. No solid food for 6–8 hrs or liquids 4 hrs before test. Mark peripheral pulses. Post-test: check vital signs every 30 min for 2 hrs. Keep extremity of insertion site straight 4–6 hrs. If femoral artery used, bed rest 6–12 hrs with bed flat. Check pressure dressing for drainage. Check pulses, color, warmth, sensation every 30 min. Monitor cardiac rhythm. Encourage fluids.

Category: Evaluation/Physiological Integrity/Reduction of Risk Potential

(1) Pain at the site of catheter insertion—expected; pain med given

(2) Absence of a pulse distal to the catheter insertion site—CORRECT: decrease in blood supply; report change in sensation, color, pulses to physician immediately

(3) Drainage on the dressing covering the catheter insertion site—some expected; pressure dressing applied; may have sandbag applied 4–6 hrs

(4) Redness at the catheter insertion site—some expected

168. The Answer is 1

An 8-year-old boy is seen in a clinic for treatment of attention-deficit/hyperactivity disorder (ADHD). Medication has been prescribed for the child along with family counseling. The nurse teaches the parents about the medication and discusses parenting strategies. Which of the following statements by the parents indicates that further teaching is necessary?

Reworded Question: What information is wrong for child with ADHD?

Strategy: Be careful! You are looking for incorrect info.

Needed Info: ADHD: developmentally inappropriate inattention, impulsivity, hyperactivity. Treatment: medication (Ritalin), family counseling, remedial education, environmental manipulation (decrease external stimuli), psychotherapy.

Category: Evaluation/Psychosocial Integrity

(1) "We will give the medication at night so it doesn't decrease his appetite."—CORRECT: incorrect info; stimulants (Ritalin) used; side effects: insomnia, palpitations, growth suppression, nervousness, decreased appetite; give 6 hrs before bedtime

(2) "We will provide a regular routine for sleeping, eating, working, and playing."—true

(3) "We will establish firm but reasonable limits on his behavior."—true

(4) "We will reduce distractions and external stimuli to help him concentrate."—true

169. The Answer is 3

A client has been taking aluminum hydroxide (Amphojel) daily for 3 weeks. The nurse should be alert for which of the following side effects?

Reworded Question: What is a side effect of Amphojel?

Strategy: Think about each answer.

Needed Info: Aluminum hydroxide (Amphojel): antacid that reduces the total amount of acid in the GI tract and elevates the gastric pH level. May cause hypophosphatemia. Shake suspension well and give with milk or water.

Category: Assessment/Physiological Integrity/Pharmacological and Parenteral Therapies

(1) Nausea—not common

(2) Hypercalcemia—seen with calcium-containing antacids (Tums); normal Ca 8.5–10.5 mg/dL

(3) Constipation—CORRECT: may need laxatives or stool softeners

(4) Anorexia—not common

170. The Answer is 3

A client recovering from a laparoscopic laser cholecystectomy says to the nurse, "I hate the thought of eating a low-fat diet for the rest of my life." Which of the following responses by the nurse is *MOST* appropriate?

Reworded Question: Is a low-fat diet required indefinitely?

Strategy: "*MOST* appropriate" indicates discrimination may be required to answer the question.

Needed Info: Laparoscopic laser cholecystectomy is removal of the gallbladder by laser through a laparoscope; monitor T-tube if present; observe for jaundice; monitor intake and output; monitor for pain and encourage early ambulation to rid the body of carbon dioxide.

Category: Implementation/Physiological Integrity/Physiological Adaptation

(1) "I will ask the dietician to come talk to you."—passing the responsibility; nurse should respond to the client

(2) "What do you think is so bad about following a low-fat diet?"—does not respond directly to the client's statement

(3) "It may not be necessary for you to follow a low-fat diet for that long."—CORRECT: fat restriction is usually lifted as the client tolerates fat; biliary ducts dilate sufficiently to accommodate bile volume that was held by the gallbladder

(4) "At least you will be alive and not suffering that pain."—nontherapeutic and judgmental

171. The Answer is 1

A client returns to his room after a transurethral resection of the prostate (TURP) for benign prostatic hypertrophy (BPH). Which of the following would cause the nurse to suspect postoperative hemorrhage?

Reworded Question: What are the signs of post-op hemorrhage?

Strategy: The entire answer choice must be correct for the answer to be correct. Read each one carefully.

Needed Info: Symptoms of hemorrhage: restlessness, dizziness, pallor, cool and clammy skin, dyspnea, rapid thready pulse, fall in BP, decrease in level of consciousness. Treatment: elevate legs 45 degrees, knees straight, trunk flat, head slightly elevated, IV fluids (Ringer's lactate, normal saline, D_5W, dextran), packed cells, vasoactive meds (Levophed, Nipride).

Category: Assessment/Physiological Integrity/Physiological Adaptation

(1) Decreased blood pressure, increased pulse, increased respirations—CORRECT: caused by decreased blood volume, as intravascular volume decreases and BP falls, heart rate increases in attempt to maintain cardiac output, respirations increase in attempt to increase oxygenation

(2) Fluctuating blood pressure, decreased pulse, rapid respirations—pulse rate will increase, not decrease

(3) Increased blood pressure, bounding pulse, irregular respirations—BP drops, pulse increases to compensate for decreased cardiac output

(4) Increased blood pressure, irregular pulse, shallow respirations—BP drops, heart rate increases to maintain cardiac output

172. The Answer is 4

The home care nurse screens a group of residents in a dependent living facility for risk factors to pneumonia. The nurse determines that which of the following clients is *MOST* at risk to develop pneumonia?

Reworded Question: Who is most likely to develop pneumonia?

Strategy: Think about each answer.

Needed Info: Pneumonia is an inflammatory process that results in edema of lung tissues and extravasion of fluid into alveoli, causing hypoxia; symptoms include fever, leukocytosis, productive cough, dyspnea, and pleuritic pain.

Category: Evaluation/Health Promotion and Maintenance

(1) A 72-year-old female who has left-sided hemiparesis after a cerebrovascular accident—advanced age is a risk factor

(2) A 76-year-old male who has a history of hypertension and type 2 diabetes—age is a risk factor

(3) An 80-year-old female who walks 1 mile every day and has a history of depression—age is a risk factor

(4) An 87-year-old male who smokes and has a history of lung cancer—CORRECT: advanced age, smoking, underlying lung disease, malnutrition, and bedridden status are risk factors for development of pneumonia

173. The Answer is 1

The nurse performs teaching with a client undergoing a paracentesis for treatment of cirrhosis. The client asks what position he will be in for the procedure. The nurse's reply should be based on an understanding that the *MOST* appropriate position for the client is which of the following?

Reworded Question: What is the correct position for a paracentesis?

Strategy: Visualize the procedure.

Needed Info: Paracentesis: removal of fluid from abdominal or peritoneal cavity. Can be used for diagnostic purposes, to remove ascitic fluid, to prepare for peritoneal dialysis. Preparation: have client void, take vital signs, weigh client, measure abdominal girth. During procedure: check vital signs every 15 min. Measure and document amount of drainage (2–3 L can be removed), characteristics. After procedure: apply pressure dressing, check for leakage. Bed rest until vital signs stable. Complications: hypovolemia and shock. Cirrhosis: degenerative liver disease;

tissue is replaced by scar tissue. Causes: alcoholism, hepatic inflammation or necrosis, chronic bilary obstruction. S/S: ascites, lower-leg edema, jaundice, esophageal varices, hemorrhoids, bleeding tendencies, pruritis, dark urine, clay-colored stools. Nursing responsibilities: high-protein, high-carbohydrate, low-Na+ diet, good skin care, promote rest, reduce exposure to infection.

Category: Analysis/Physiological Integrity /Reduction of Risk Potential

(1) Sitting with his lower extremities well supported—CORRECT: Fowler's position or sitting on side of bed with feet on stool; easy access to abdominal area; allows intestines to float to prevent laceration

(2) Side-lying with a pillow between his knees—not accurate

(3) Prone with his head turned to the left side—not accurate

(4) Dorsal-recumbent with a pillow at the back of his head—not accurate

174.   The Answer is 2

A man calls the Suicide Prevention Hotline and states that he is going to kill himself. Which of the following questions should the nurse ask *FIRST?*

Reworded Question: What is most important to know about a client who has threatened to kill himself?

Strategy: "*FIRST*" indicates priority.

Needed Info: Signs of suicide: symptoms of depression, client gives away possessions, gets finances in order, has a means, makes direct or indirect statements, leaves notes, has increased energy. Predisposing factors: male over age 50, age 15–19, poor social attachments, client with previous attempts, client with auditory hallucinations, overwhelming precipitating events (terminal disease, death or loss of loved one, failure at school, job).

Category: Assessment/Psychosocial Integrity

(1) "What has happened to cause you to want to end your life?"—does not determine immediate need for safety

(2) "How have you planned to kill yourself?"—CORRECT: lets you prioritize interventions to. assure safety

(3) "When did you start to feel as though you wanted to die?"—does not determine immediate need for safety

(4) "Do you want me to prevent you from killing yourself?"—yes/no question, closed

175.   The Answer is 4

A man is admitted for treatment of heart failure. The physician orders an IV of 125 mL of normal saline per hour and central venous pressure (CVP) readings every 4 hours. Sixteen hours after admission, the client's CVP reading is 3 cm/H_2O. Which of the following evaluations of the client's fluid status by the nurse would be *MOST* accurate?

Reworded Question: What does this CVP reading indicate?

Strategy: Consider each answer and remember normal CVP reading values.

Needed Info: CVP: central venous line placed in superior vena cava. To obtain a reading: client placed supine, 0 on manometer placed at level of right atrium (midaxillary line at 4th intercostal space), turn stopcock to allow manometer to fill with fluid, turn to allow fluid to go into client. Fluid will fluctuate with respirations. When stabilized, take reading at highest level of fluctuation. Normal: 4–10 cm/H_2O. Elevated: hypervolemia, CHF, pericarditis. Low: hypovolemia.

Category: Evaluation/Physiological Integrity/ Reduction of Risk Potential

(1) The client has received enough fluid—inaccurate

(2) The client's fluid status remains unaltered—nothing to compare to

(3) The client has received too much fluid—inaccurate

(4) The client needs more fluid—CORRECT: normal 4–10 cm/H_2O; indicates hypovolemia

176. The Answer is 4

An agitated client throws a chair across the dayroom on the psychiatry floor and threatens the other clients with physical harm. Which of the following should the nurse do *FIRST*?

Reworded Question: What is the nurse's first action?

Strategy: Use Maslow. Safety first—the client must be removed from the situation.

Needed Info: The nurse can initiate seclusion procedures in an escalating situation per hospital policy. The principle of seclusion is containment, to avoid injury, and to prevent anticipated violence. Violence must be prevented to ensure the safety of other clients and staff.

Category: Implementation/Psychosocial Integrity

(1) Tell the client that his wife will be called to the hospital—calling wife will not solve the immediate problem and may complicate the situation

(2) Ask the client why he is so angry—asking client for causes of anger is inappropriate when the client's behavior is escalating

(3) Remove the other clients from the dayroom—allowing client to determine disposition of other clients gives client control over staff and other clients

(4) Assemble staff and put the client in preventive seclusion—CORRECT: seclusion may be used alone or in conjunction with medication to de-escalate a potentially dangerous situation; nurse can initiate and terminate client seclusion based on established protocols

177. The Answer is 4

The nurse is caring for a depressed client who spends most of the day sitting at a window, and is about to implement a physical activity plan for him. The nurse knows that the purpose of this plan is to do which of the following?

Reworded Question: What is the purpose of the different plans typically implemented for clients with mental illness?

Strategy: Consider the rationales for plans typically used for clients with mental illness.

Needed Info: Physical and mental health are linked. A level of fitness enhances a sense of mental well-being. Withdrawn clients have decreased motivation to exercise. Physical exercise can also distract clients from stressful thoughts, and helps clients focus on things other than themselves.

Category: Planning/Psychosocial Integrity

(1) Help the client understand the problems creating the depression—purpose of physical activity is not to provide insight into one's problems

(2) Reduce the client's risk for obesity and diabetes—this would not necessarily reduce the risk for obesity and diabetes

(3) Transform self-destructive impulses into positive behaviors—physical activity may channel energy differently, but does not guarantee to change self-destructiveness

(4) Encourage socialization and improve self-esteem—CORRECT: purpose of physical activity is to promote focused socialization with clients and staff and to increase a sense of self-esteem

178. The Answer is 2

The nurse is caring for a client with bipolar disorder. Which of the following behaviors by the client indicates to the nurse that a manic episode is subsiding?

Reworded Question: What indicates normalizing behavior?

Strategy: Think about the behaviors that indicate mania.

Needed Info: Manic clients may tease, talk, and joke excessively. They usually cannot sit to eat and may need to carry fluids and food around in order to eat. Manic clients often try to take a leadership position in an environment, and try to engage others.

Category: Assessment/Psychosocial Integrity

(1) The client tells several jokes at a group meeting—reflects an elated mood and no real participation in the meeting; manic clients may tease, talk, and joke excessively

(2) The client sits and talks with other clients at mealtimes—CORRECT: manic clients have difficulty socializing because of flight of ideas and

intrusiveness; usually cannot sit to eat and will carry fluids and food around

(3) The client begins to write a book about his life—manic clients often write voluminously; may help to express feelings, but does not reflect improvement, especially if thoughts are grandiose

(4) The client initiates an effort to start a radio station on the unit—manic clients often try to take a leadership position in an environment and try to recruit others

179.   The Answer is 1

A client hospitalized for treatment of delusions tells the nurse that he is really the head of the hospital system and that his "cover" is being a client to get information on client abuse. Which of the following statements by the nurse is *BEST* initially?

Reworded Question: How would you handle a client with delusions?

Strategy: Know when further assessment is needed and what the appropriate communication techniques are to use with delusional clients.

Needed Info: The initial approach to delusions is to clarify meanings. After clarification, the delusions should not be discussed as this could reinforce them. Arguing with a client about delusions may also reinforce them. Delusions that entail injury or death should be addressed immediately, and client protections put into place.

Category: Assessment/Psychosocial Integrity

(1) "Tell me what you mean about being head of the hospital system and getting client abuse information."—CORRECT: initial approach is to further assess by clarifying the meaning of the delusion to the client

(2) "I think you should share this story with the other clients at dinnertime and see what they say."—could cause disruption among other clients and embarrass the client

(3) "You are not the head of the hospital system, you are an accountant under treatment for a mental disorder."—arguing with client about delusion is ineffective and inappropriate and may strengthen the client's belief in it

(4) "It worries me when you say these things; it means you are not responding to the medication."—nurse is communicating disappointment to the client and treating the delusion as though it were a behavior under the client's control

180.   The Answer is 1

The nurse is caring for a client in labor. The nurse palpates a firm, round form in the uterine fundus, small parts on the woman's right side, and a long, smooth, curved section on the left side. Based on these findings, the nurse should anticipate auscultating the fetal heart in which of the following locations?

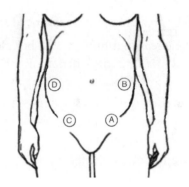

Reworded Question: If a fetus is LOA, where should the nurse listen for the fetal heart tone?

Strategy: Examine the diagram carefully. Know the woman's right from left.

Needed Info: Fetal reference point: vertex presentation—dependent upon degree of flexion of fetal head on chest; full flexion/occiput (O), full extension chin (M), moderate extension (military) brow (B). Breech presentation—sacrum (S). Shoulder presentation—scapula (SC). Maternal pelvis is designated per her right/left and anterior/posterior. Position = relationship of fetal reference point to mother's pelvis; expressed as standard 3-letter abbreviation: LOA (left occiput anterior) (most common), LOP (left occiput posterior), ROA (right occiput anterior), ROP (right occiput posterior), LOT (left occiput transverse), ROT (right occiput transverse).

Category: Planning/Health Promotion and Maintenance

(1) A—CORRECT: point of maximum intensity for fetal heart with fetus in LOA position

(2) B—PMI location for fetus in LOP position

(3) C—PMI location for fetus in ROA position

(4) D—PMI location for fetus in ROP position

181. The Answer is 1

A 69-year-old female client admitted with pneumonia is receiving gentamicin (Garamycin). For this client, which of the following laboratory values would be *MOST* important for the nurse to monitor?

Reworded Question: What are the adverse effects of Garamycin?

Strategy: Use the process of elimination, noting the key words "*MOST* important," which indicates that more than one answer choice may be correct.

Needed Info: Garamycin is a broad-spectrum antibiotic used to treat bacterial infections, particularly those caused by gram–negative bacteria. Side effects: neuromuscular blockage, ototoxic to the eighth cranial nerve (tinnitus, vertigo, hearing loss), nephrotoxicity; less commonly, may cause anemia and hypokalemia. Blood should be drawn for peak levels 1 hour after IM and 30 minutes; 1 hour after IV infusion and for trough just before next dose.

Category: Implementation/ Physiological Integrity/ Reduction of Risk Potential

(1) BUN and creatinine—CORRECT: Garamycin is nephrotoxic; proteinuria, oliguria, hematuria, thirst, increased BUN, decreased creatinine clearance

(2) Hemoglobin and hematocrit—Garamycin can cause anemia but is less common

(3) Sodium and potassium—hypokalemia is an infrequent problem

(4) Platelet count and clotting time—these do not usually change

182. The Answer is 2

The nurse is preparing a client newly diagnosed with Addison's disease for discharge. Which of the following statements by the client indicates a need for further instruction from the nurse?

Reworded Question: Which instruction about Addison's disease does the client not understand?

Strategy: Use the process of elimination, noting the key words "need for further instruction." Be careful: you are looking for an answer choice that contains incorrect information. If you had trouble with this question, review client teaching for Addison's disease.

Needed Info: Addison's disease is the most common form of adrenal hypofunction. It occurs when more than 90 percent of the adrenal gland is destroyed. Early diagnosis and adequate hydrocortisone replacement therapy indicate a good prognosis. Acute adrenal insufficiency, or adrenal crisis, is a medical emergency requiring immediate treatment. Corticosteroid replacement is the primary lifelong treatment for clients with primary or secondary adrenal hypofunction. An adrenal crisis usually subsides quickly with proper treatment, and subsequent oral maintenance doses of hydrocortisone preserve stability.

Category: Analysis/Physiological Integrity/Reduction of Risk Potential

(1) "I understand that I will need lifelong cortisone replacement therapy."—indicates the client understands the discharge teaching; clients with Addison's disease require lifelong cortisone replacement therapy

(2) "During times of stress, I will need to decrease my medication."—CORRECT: indicates the client does not understand discharge teaching and requires further instructions; during times of stress, clients with Addison's disease need to *increase* the medication dosage, not decrease it

(3) "I must be careful not to injure myself."—indicates the client understands the discharge teaching; clients with Addison's disease should be warned that infection, injury, or profuse sweating in hot weather may precipitate a crisis

(4) "I should always carry a medical identification card."—indicates the client understands the discharge teaching; clients with Addison's disease should always carry a medical identification card and wear a bracelet stating the name and dosage of the steroid the client takes

183. The Answer is 2

The nurse suspects a client has meningitis. The nurse places the client in a dorsal recumbent position, puts her hands behind the client's neck, and bends it forward. The nurse knows that pain and resistance may indicate neck injury or arthritis, but if the client also flexes the hips and knees, this positive response is which of the following?

Reworded Question: A positive response to which sign helps establish a diagnosis of meningitis?

Strategy: Knowledge regarding each of these tests is needed to answer this question. Review these tests to determine which positive response is a sign of meningitis if you had difficulty with this question.

Needed Info: Meningitis is an infection that causes inflammation of the brain and spinal meninges that can involve the meningeal membranes. When a client is placed in a dorsal recumbent position and the nurse puts her hands behind the client's neck and bends it forward, pain and resistance may indicate neck injury or arthritis. However, if the client also flexes the hips and knees, chances are that he has meningeal irritation and inflammation, which is a sign of meningitis.

Category: Assessment/Physiological Integrity/Reduction of Risk Potential

(1) Trousseau's sign—this is for clients who have suspected hypocalcemia. The nurse places a blood pressure cuff on the client's arm and inflates it above the client's systolic pressure. If it is positive, the client will exhibit carpal spasm (ventral contraction of the thumb and digits) within 3 minutes

(2) Brudzinki's sign—CORRECT: a positive response to this test is a sign of meningitis

(3) Homans' sign—discomfort behind the knee on forced dorsiflexion of the foot, due to thrombosis in calf veins

(4) Chvostek's sign—spasm of the facial muscles elicited by tapping the facial nerve in the region of the parotid gland; seen in tetany and is a sign of hypocalcemia

184. The Answer is 2 and 4

The nurse is assessing a client newly diagnosed with initial-stage chronic glomerulonephritis. Which of the following findings should the nurse expect to see? **Select all that apply.**

Reworded Question: What are the signs/symptoms of initial-stage chronic glomerulonephritis?

Strategy: Focus on the key words "Select all that apply." This indicates there is more than one correct answer. Think about the signs and symptoms of initial-stage chronic glomerulonephritis as opposed to late-stage findings.

Needed Info: Chronic glomerulonephritis is a slowly progressive, noninfectious disease characterized by inflammation of the renal glomeruli. By the time it produces symptoms, it is usually irreversible and eventually results in renal failure. Symptoms of the initial stage are nephrotic syndrome, hypertension, proteinuria, and hematuria. Late-stage findings include azotemia, nausea, vomiting, pruritus, dyspnea, malaise, fatigability, mild to severe anemia, and severe hypertension.

Category: Assessment/Physiological Integrity/Physiological Adaptation

(1) Hypotension—initial-stage findings include hypertension; late-stage symptoms include severe hypertension

(2) Proteinuria—CORRECT: this is an initial-stage finding

(3) Severe anemia—this is a late-stage finding

(4) Hematuria—CORRECT: this is an initial-stage finding

(5) Azotemia—this is a late-stage finding

(6) Nausea—this is a late-stage finding

185. The Answer is 4

A 56-year-old male client with a history of myocardial infarction is admitted for evaluation of chest pain. Several hours later, the client goes into ventricular fibrillation and a code blue is called. The Emergency Department physician defibrillates the client. The nurse knows that the purpose of defibrillation is to do which of the following?

Reworded Question: Why is a client defibrillated?

Strategy: Think about each answer choice. What does defibrillation do?

Needed Info: The goal of defibrillation is to temporarily depolarize the irregularly beating heart and allow more coordinated contractile activity to resume. Defibrillation depolarizes the myocardium and produces temporary asystole to provide the opportunity for the natural pacemaker of the heart to resume normal activity.

Category: Implementation/Physiological Integrity/Physiological Adaptation

(1) Energize myocardial cells—this is inaccurate

(2) Improve left ventricular function—this is inaccurate

(3) Increase cardiac output—this is inaccurate

(4) Produce momentary asystole to allow the natural pacemaker to resume activity—CORRECT: defibrillation produces momentary asystole

186. The Answer is 4

The physician orders 0.25 mg digoxin (Lanoxin) for a client diagnosed with heart failure. The client's pulse is 86 prior to administration of the prescribed dose. The nurse should do which of the following?

Reworded Question: What are the side effects of Lanoxin?

Strategy: Think about each answer choice and the action of Lanoxin.

Needed Info: Lanoxin is an antiarrhythmic prescribed for atrial fibrillation and heart failure. The apical pulse should be monitored for 1 full minute before administering, and the dose withheld and the physician notified if the pulse rate is less than 60 per minute in an adult.

Category: Analysis/Physiological Integrity/Pharmacological and Parenteral Therapies

(1) Give half of the prescribed dose (0.125)—you would need a physician order to change the dose if warranted (only a physician can make that determination)

(2) Delay the dose until the pulse is below 60—inaccurate; the dose would be held with a pulse below 60

(3) Omit the dose, and record the pulse rate as the reason—inaccurate

(4) Give the full dose as ordered—CORRECT: the dose should be given as prescribed

187. The Answer is 1

The nurse knows that the atorvastatin (Lipitor) administered to a client is effective when there is a reduction in which of the following?

Reworded Question: What are the indications for use of Lipitor?

Strategy: Think about each answer choice and what Lipitor is prescribed for.

Needed Info: Lipitor belongs to a group of drugs called "statins." Therapeutic effects of Lipitor include decreased LDLs, triglycerides, and cholesterol, when used along with a proper diet.

Category: Evaluation/Physiological Integrity/Pharmacological and Parenteral Therapies

(1) Triglycerides—CORRECT: Lipitor lowers LDLs, cholesterol, and triglycerides

(2) Chest pain—Lipitor is not prescribed to reduce chest pain

(3) Blood pressure—Lipitor is not prescribed for high blood pressure

(4) PTT—Lipitor is not prescribed to reduce PTT; a PTT is ordered when a client has unexplained bleeding or clotting, and also ordered at intervals to monitor unfractionated heparin anticoagulant therapy

188. The Answer is 4

A 37-year-old female has been prescribed sumatriptan (Imitrex) for severe migraines. The nurse explains that the client should watch for which of the following adverse drug effects?

Reworded Question: What are the adverse effects of Imitrex?

Strategy: Use the process of elimination.

Needed Info: Imitrex works by narrowing the blood vessels around the brain. It can cause serious side effects on the heart, including heart attack or stroke. Adverse side effects include chest pain; pain spreading to arm or shoulder; sudden numbness or weakness; confusion; problems with vision, speech, or balance; nausea and bloody diarrhea; convulsions; numbness or tingling in fingers or toes; and sudden numbness or weakness, especially on one side of the body.

Category: Planning/Physiological Integrity/Pharmacological and Parenteral Therapies

(1) Constipation—adverse effects of Imitrex include bloody diarrhea, not constipation

(2) Bradycardia—adverse effects of Imitrex include tachycardia, not bradycardia

(3) Somnolence—adverse effects of Imitrex include agitation, not somnolence

(4) Sudden numbness or weakness—CORRECT: adverse effects of Imitrex include sudden numbness or weakness, especially on one side of the body

189. The Answer is 3

The client is resuming a diet after undergoing a Billroth II procedure. To minimize complications from eating, the nurse instructs the client to do which of the following?

Reworded Question: How does a client avoid dumping syndrome, a complication of this surgical procedure?

Strategy: Focus on the surgical procedure and recall that dumping syndrome is a complication of this surgery. If you had difficulty with this question, review the prevention and management of complications of gastric surgery.

Needed Info: The client who has had a Billroth II procedure is at risk for dumping syndrome. The client should eat small, frequent meals evenly spaced throughout the day; chew food thoroughly and drink fluids between meals rather than with them; decrease intake of carbohydrates and salt while increasing fat and protein. After meals, the client should lie down for 20–30 minutes.

Category: Implementation/Physiological Integrity/ Basic Care and Comfort

(1) Drink fluids with meals—client should drink fluids between meals, not with meals

(2) Increase intake of carbohydrates and salt—client should decrease intake of carbohydrates and salt

(3) Increase fat and protein—CORRECT: client should increase fat and protein

(4) Eat 3 large meals a day—client should eat small, frequent meals evenly spaced throughout the day

190. The Answer is 4

The nurse is caring for a client who is having difficulty eating due to mouth sores from chemotherapy treatments. Which of the following interventions is *MOST* appropriate to promote basic comfort and nutrition?

Reworded Question: What are the side effects of chemotherapy?

Strategy: Focus on the issue: promoting basic care and nutrition for a client having pain due to mouth sores. If you had difficulty with this question, review the side effects of chemotherapy and appropriate nursing interventions.

Needed Info: Mouth sores are a side effect of chemotherapy and can cause discomfort when eating and swallowing. Mouth sores occur because chemotherapy destroys cells in the mouth and esophagus, as well as cancer cells.

Category: Implementation/Physiological Integrity/ Basic Care and Comfort

(1) Obtain an order for TPN—only used when oral intake is not possible

(2) Keep the client NPO—would not promote nutrition but increase nutritional risk

(3) Administer a stool softener as ordered—is used when constipation is present

(4) Provide frequent oral hygiene—CORRECT: aids in providing temporary relief of pain from mouth sores so that a client can eat

191. The Answer is 2

The nurse is caring for an adult male client who has just undergone spinal fusion for a herniated intervertebral disk. To promote comfort and minimize complications, the nurse tells the client to avoid which of the following?

Reworded Question: What should the client avoid after having undergone spinal fusion?

Strategy: Note the key word "avoid" in the question stem. Focus on the surgical procedure and recall that activity and positioning should not cause discomfort or unnecessary strain on the back.

Needed Info: To avoid complications and promote comfort after spinal fusion, the client should be advised to bend at the knees when lifting (never at the waist); lie down when tired and sleep on his side with a pillow between his knees. Lying on the stomach causes strain on the back; use a firm mattress to reduce tension on the spine. Choose a firm, hardback chair for sitting, no longer than 20 minutes at a time.

Category: Implementation/Physiological Integrity/ Basic Care and Comfort

(1) Bending the knees when lying on one side—will decrease the strain on the shoulders, neck, and arms

(2) Sitting for longer than 20 minutes at a time— CORRECT: puts strain on the back; is better to walk around or lie down to rest

(3) Using an extra-firm mattress—reduces tension on the spine

(4) Sitting in a hardback chair—provides support for the back

192. The Answer is 4

The nurse is preparing a client for surgery. When obtaining informed consent, the nurse should *INITIALLY* do which of the following?

Reworded Question: What are the elements of informed consent and what are the nurse's responsibilities?

Strategy: Think about the elements of informed consent and the responsibilities of the physician and nurse. *"INITIALLY"* indicates there may be more than one correct response.

Needed Info: Informed consent is more than simply getting a client to sign a written consent form. It is a process of communication between a client and physician that results in the client's authorization or agreement to undergo a specific medical intervention. The client should have an opportunity to

ask questions to elicit a better understanding of the treatment/procedure and make an informed decision to proceed or refuse.

Category: Assessment/Safe and Effective Care Environment/Management of Care

(1) Explain the risks, benefits, and alternatives of the procedure—this is the responsibility of the practitioner performing the procedure, not of the nurse

(2) Tell the client that obtaining the signature is routine for all surgeries—although this is true, it does not determine the client's ability to give informed consent

(3) Witness the client's signature—this is true; however, the nurse should first assess the client's knowledge of the procedure

(4) Assess whether the client's understanding of the procedure is sufficient to give consent—CORRECT: informed consent means the client must understand and comprehend the risks, benefits, and alternatives of the procedure to be performed

193. The Answer is 3

The nurse is preparing to administer heparin sodium to a client diagnosed with thrombophlebitis. The nurse should ensure that which of the following is available if the client develops a significant bleeding problem?

Reworded Question: What is the antidote for heparin sodium?

Strategy: Focus on the name of the medication administered and remember that the antidote for heparin sodium is protamine sulfate. Review antidotes for commonly administered medications.

Needed Info: Heparin sodium is indicated for prophylaxis and treatment of venous thrombosis, pulmonary embolism, and atrial fibrillation with embolization. Heparin prevents formation of clots. Its antidote is protamine sulfate.

Category: Planning/Safe and Effective Care Environment/Management of Care

(1) Phytonadione (vitamin K)—is the antidote for warfarin (Coumadin)

(2) Fresh frozen plasma (FFP)—can also be used for bleeding associated with warfarin (Coumadin) therapy

(3) Protamine sulfate—CORRECT: is the antidote for heparin sodium

(4) Reteplase (Retavase)—a thrombolytic that breaks up blood clots, does not prevent formation of clots and is not an antidote

194. The Answer is 2

A client is being admitted to the hospital for elective surgery. During the admission assessment, the nurse asks the client if he has an advance directive. The nurse knows that clients have the right to play an active role in their care and treatment, and this is guaranteed by which of the following?

Reworded Question: Which act guarantees clients the right to make their own care and treatment decisions?

Strategy: Recall the provisions of each federal act. Use the process of elimination. Review the different federal acts if you had difficulty with this question.

Needed Info: The Client Self-Determination Act requires that, upon admission to hospitals, long-term care facilities, and home health agencies, clients be informed that they have the right to accept or refuse medical care, and the right to refuse treatment.

Category: Analysis/Safe and Effective Care Environment/Management of Care

(1) The Health Insurance Portability and Accountability Act (HIPAA)—provides for the rights and protections for participants and beneficiaries in group health plans; protects personally identifying information, and information about diagnosis and treatment

(2) The Client Self-Determination Act—CORRECT: guarantees clients the right to make their own care and treatment decisions

(3) The Civil Rights Act—prohibits employment discrimination on the basis of race, color, religion, sex, or national origin

(4) The Americans with Disabilities Act—recognizes and protects the civil rights of people with disabilities

195. The Answer is 3

The nurse enters a client's hospital room to find the client sitting on the bathroom floor. The nurse assesses the client, obtains assistance, and assists the client back to bed. The nurse notifies the physician and completes an incident report. Which of the following is the *MOST* appropriate nursing action?

Reworded Question: What is the nurse's responsibility related to incident reporting?

Strategy: Use the process of elimination.

Needed Info: Incident reports are confidential and privileged information. They should not be placed in a client's chart, copied, or referenced in the chart. The person who witnesses the incident should write the report. An objective entry of the incident should be documented in the client's chart.

Category: Implementation/Safe and Effective Care Environment/Management of Care

(1) Document in the client's chart that an incident report has been completed—reference to incident reports should not be documented in a client's chart

(2) Make a copy of the incident report for the nurse manager—incident reports should never be copied

(3) Document the incident in the client's chart—CORRECT: objective details of the incident should be documented in the client's chart

(4) Place the incident report in the client's chart—incident reports should not be placed in a client's chart but routed to the hospital's risk management or legal department according to hospital policy

196. The Answer is 3

The nurse is performing an initial postoperative assessment on a client who has just returned from surgery with a chest tube and water seal drainage system. The nurse should immediately intervene if she makes which of the following observations?

Reworded Question: Which observation of chest tube and water seal drainage system requires immediate attention?

Strategy: Use the process of elimination. Three of the answer choices need no intervention.

Needed Info: A chest tube with water seal drainage allows air and fluid to be removed from the intrapleural space. The underwater seal drainage to which the chest tube is connected prevents backflow into the pleural space. The chest tube is attached to a valve mechanism designed to allow air or fluid to drain out of, but not into, the chest cavity. There should be no dependent loops or kinks in the tube, and the tube should be unclamped, including during transport and ambulation, unless ordered by the physician. The fluid level in the water seal should be at 2 cm.

Category: Assessment/Safe and Effective Care Environment/Management of Care

(1) There are no dependent loops in the chest tube—no need to intervene because this is correct

(2) The chest tube is not clamped—no need to intervene; chest tube should be unclamped

(3) The chest tube and drainage system is above the client's chest—CORRECT: chest tube and drainage system should be *below* the client's chest

(4) The fluid level in the water seal is at 2 cm—no need to intervene; this is the correct fluid level

197. The Answer is 3

The nurse is present during an informed consent discussion between the client and the physician regarding recommended surgery. The physician discusses the risks, benefits, and alternatives of the procedure with the client. The nurse knows that the client's decision whether or not to have the surgery is based on which of the following ethical principles?

Reworded Question: Which principle defines the right of individuals to make their own decisions?

Strategy: Use the process of elimination. If you had difficulty with this question, review ethical principles of clinical practice.

Needed Info: Ethics help the nurse determine whether an action is right or wrong and guide professional practice. Nonmaleficence is the nurse's duty to do no harm. Beneficence is a nurse's duty to do what is in

the best interest of the client. Autonomy is the right of individuals to make their own decisions regarding care and treatment. Capacity is a client's ability to make medical decisions.

Category: Analysis/Safe and Effective Care Environment/Management of Care

(1) Nonmaleficence—is the nurse's duty to do no harm

(2) Beneficence—is the nurse's duty to do what is in the best interest of the client

(3) Autonomy—CORRECT: is the right of individuals to make their own medical decisions

(4) Capacity—is the client's *ability* to make medical decisions

198. The Answer is 2

The nurse is caring for a terminal cancer client at home. The nurse knows that which of the following ethical principles *BEST* supports keeping client and family care consistent with the nurse's professional code of ethics?

Reworded Question: Keeping client and family care consistent with the nurse's professional code of ethics is the definition of which principle?

Strategy: Think about the definition of each principle. Review ethical principles if you had trouble with this question.

Needed Info: A nurse should be able to identify ethical issues that affect client care. If ethical issues arise, the nurse must be able to handle them according to ethical principles.

Category: Analysis/Safe and Effective Care Environment/Management of Care

(1) Virtues—refers to compassion, trustworthiness, integrity, and veracity

(2) Fidelity—CORRECT: refers to keeping faithful to ethical principles and the American Nurses Association Code of Ethics for Nurses

(3) Beneficence—refers to a nurse's duty to do what is in the best interest of the client

(4) Justice—refers to a fair, equitable, and appropriate treatment

199. The Answer is 3

The nurse is caring for a client receiving intravenous therapy through a peripherally inserted central catheter (PICC). Which of the following actions implemented by the nurse will decrease the risk of infection?

Reworded Question: What should the nurse know about preventing infection with intravenous therapy?

Strategy: Note the key words "decrease the risk of infection." Use the process of elimination.

Needed Info: Although PICC-related complications are low, those caring for PICC lines must know how to prevent and manage them. After the PICC line is inserted using sterile technique, the goal is to monitor for signs of infection and maintain sterile technique throughout care.

Category: Planning/Safe and Effective Care Environment/Safety and Infection Control

(1) Assess vital signs every 4 hours—will detect signs of infection but is not associated with prevention

(2) Ask the physician for an order for antibiotics—are administered to treat, not prevent, infection

(3) Maintain sterile technique during all phases of PICC care—CORRECT: during all phases of PICC care, there should be meticulous attention to cleanliness and aseptic technique

(4) Administer acetaminophen (Tylenol) before dressing changes—is not related to decreasing the risk of infection

200. The Answer is 1

The nurse is caring for a client with chronic obstructive pulmonary disease (COPD) and is planning to obtain an arterial blood gas (ABG). Which of the following should the nurse plan to do to prevent bleeding following the procedure?

Reworded Question: What do you do to prevent bleeding after an arterial puncture?

Strategy: Use the process of elimination and focus on the issue, which is preventing bleeding.

Needed Info: After a blood sample is obtained for an ABG, pressure should be applied to the puncture site for 5 minutes and then a gauze pad should be taped in place. Monitor the site for bleeding and check the arm for signs of complications (swelling, pain, numbness, tingling).

Category: Planning/Safe and Effective Care Environment/Safety and Infection Control

(1) Apply 2 × 2 gauze to the puncture site and hold pressure for 5 minutes—CORRECT: pressure should be applied to the arterial puncture site for 5 minutes to prevent bleeding

(2) Have the client hold the puncture site in a dependent position for 5 minutes—promotes bleeding

(3) Apply a warm compress to the puncture site for 15 minutes—promotes bleeding

(4) Encourage the client to open and close the hand rapidly for several minutes—promotes bleeding

201. The Answer is 3

The nurse is caring for a client diagnosed with acute myocardial infarction (MI) and a history of severe uncontrolled hypertension. The nurse should question which of the following physician orders?

Reworded Question: What is not an appropriate order for this client?

Strategy: Think about the combination of MI and severe uncontrolled hypertension. Use the process of elimination.

Needed Info: Limiting physical activity, IV nitroglycerin, thrombolytic therapy, and oxygen therapy are all appropriate treatments for a client with an MI. However, severe uncontrolled hypertension is one of the many contraindications of thrombolytic therapy.

Category: Planning/Safe and Effective Care Environment/Safety and Infection Control

(1) Limit physical activity for the first 12 hours—this is an appropriate order

(2) IV nitroglycerin—this is an appropriate order

(3) Thrombolytic therapy—CORRECT: thrombolytic therapy is contraindicated in severe uncontrolled hypertension

(4) Oxygen therapy—this is an appropriate order

202. The Answer is 2

The nurse is preparing to administer warfarin (Coumadin) to a client diagnosed with atrial fibrillation. The nurse knows that which of the following nursing diagnoses takes priority?

Reworded Question: Which nursing diagnosis is appropriate for anticoagulant therapy?

Strategy: Think safety, and use the process of elimination.

Needed Info: Anticoagulants inhibit clot formation by blocking the action of clotting factors or platelets. Coumadin is prescribed for the prophylaxis and/or treatment of complications associated with atrial fibrillation. Bleeding is a major risk.

Category: Planning/Safe and Effective Care Environment/Safety and Infection Control

(1) Risk for imbalanced fluid volume—is not associated with anticoagulant therapy

(2) Risk for injury—CORRECT: clients on anticoagulant therapy are at risk for injury

(3) Constipation—is not associated with anticoagulant therapy

(4) Risk for unstable blood glucose—is not associated with anticoagulant therapy

203. The Answer is 4

Prior to administering a tuberculin (Mantoux) skin test, the nurse in an outpatient clinic is educating a client suspected of having tuberculosis (TB). The nurse determines that the client understands the teaching when the client states which of the following?

Reworded Question: What is the purpose of the Mantoux skin test?

Strategy: Use the process of elimination.

Needed Info: A Mantoux skin test is performed to see if a client has ever had TB. It is done by putting a small amount of TB protein under the top layer of skin on the inner forearm. If a client has ever been exposed to the bacteria, the skin will react to the antigens by developing a firm red bump at the site within 2 days. A TB skin test cannot tell how long a person has been infected with TB or if the infection is inactive or active and can be passed to others.

Category: Assessment/Safe and Effective Care Environment/Safety and Infection Control

(1) "I know the test will tell me how long I've been infected with TB."—tuberculin test cannot tell how long a client has been infected with TB

(2) "This test will tell me if I am contagious."—tuberculin test cannot tell if a client is contagious

(3) "I will need to come back and have a nurse look at the site in a week."—site of the skin test must be read within 48–72 hours

(4) "The test will tell us if I've ever been infected with TB bacteria."—CORRECT: tuberculin skin test is done to see if a client has ever had TB

204. The Answer is 3

The nurse is preparing to enter the private, well-ventilated isolation room of a client with active tuberculosis (TB). Which of the following actions should the nurse take before entering the room?

Reworded Question: What precautions should the nurse take before entering the room of a client with active TB?

Strategy: Use the process of elimination. Note the client's diagnosis and the need for respiratory precautions.

Needed Info: TB is caused by germs that are spread from person to person through the air. The germs are put into the air when a person with TB disease of the lungs or throat coughs, sneezes, speaks, or sings. The germs can stay in the air for several hours depending on the environment. Persons who breathe in the air containing these TB germs can become infected. Persons entering areas of high risk exposure should use respiratory protective equipment.

Category: Implementation/Safe and Effective Care Environment/Safety and Infection Control

(1) Wash her hands and wear gown and gloves—this action is incomplete and incorrect

(2) Wash her hands—this action is incomplete

(3) Wash her hands and place a particulate filter respirator over her nose and mouth—CORRECT: a particulate filter respirator should be placed over the nose and mouth in areas of high risk exposure

(4) Ask the client to don a mask—this action is incorrect

205. The Answer is 3

The nurse is preparing a female client for a cardiac catheterization with the femoral approach. The nurse should do which of the following when the client returns to her room after the procedure?

Reworded Question: After cardiac catheterization, how should the client be positioned?

Strategy: Visualize the approach used during the procedure. Use the process of elimination.

Needed Info: During cardiac catheterization with the femoral approach, access to the coronary arteries is gained through the femoral artery in the right or left groin. Upon completion of the procedure, the sheath is removed and pressure is held over the site for approximately 20 minutes until hemostasis is achieved. A pressure dressing is applied and the client is instructed to lie on her back and keep the procedural leg straight for 12 hours to avoid bleeding and possible hematoma.

Category: Implementation/Safe and Effective Care Environment/Safety and Infection Control

(1) Elevate the head of the bed 45 degrees—should be elevated no more than 30 degrees

(2) Keep the client's arm immobilized for the first 24 hours—arm is immobilized if the brachial approach is used

(3) Keep the client's leg immobilized for the first 12 hours—CORRECT: affected leg is immobilized for the first 12 hours

(4) Tell the client to lie on the procedural side for 2 hours—client is instructed to lie on her back for the first 12 hours

206. The Answer is 2

A 65-year-old woman with metastatic breast cancer has been admitted to the hospital with neutropenic fever. She informs the nurse that she does not want CPR or artificial ventilation to be performed under any circumstances. The nurse explains that this information can be outlined in an advance directive. The nurse understands that which of the following

addresses the client's right to identify treatment desires in advance?

Reworded Question: What ensures that clients are informed of their right to create advance directives?

Strategy: Knowledge regarding each of these choices is required to answer this question. If you had difficulty with this question, review the Patient's Bill of Rights, the Patient Self-Determination Act, the Health Insurance Portability and Accountability Act (HIPAA), and the Americans with Disabilities Act to be sure you understand the objective of each.

Needed Info: The Patient Self-Determination Act outlines the requirements for informing clients they have right to refuse medical treatment and to specify their wishes for treatment through advance directives.

Category: Analysis/Safe and Effective Care Environment/Management of Care

(1) The Patient's Bill of Rights—does not address advance directives

(2) The Patient Self-Determination Act—CORRECT: ensures that patients are informed of their right to refuse medical treatment and (in advance directives) to specify their wishes for treatment

(3) The Health Insurance Portability and Accountability Act (HIPAA)—does not address advance directives

(4) The Americans with Disabilities Act— does not address advance directives

207. The Answer is 1

After receiving morning report on a medical/surgical unit, which of the following clients should the nurse address *FIRST*?

Reworded Question: Which client requires immediate attention?

Strategy: Focus on the key word "*FIRST.*" This indicates the need to prioritize, or triage, the clients based on the need for nursing intervention.

Needed Info: Pulmonary embolism (PE) occurs when the pulmonary artery becomes occluded by a blood clot. PE can lead to death if not diagnosed and treated promptly. Although symptoms may be nonspecific, hemoptysis (blood in sputum) in the postoperative client is suspicious for PE.

Category: Analysis/Safe and Effective Care Environment/Management of Care

(1) A 36-year-old man who underwent surgery to repair multiple fractures in his left leg after an automobile accident reports coughing up blood—CORRECT: hemoptysis in a postoperative trauma client is suspicious for PE, requires immediate intervention

(2) A 56-year-old woman newly diagnosed with diabetes has a fasting blood sugar of 83 mg/dL—fasting blood sugar of 83 mg/dL is considered within normal limits; does not require intervention

(3) A 68-year-old man with head and neck cancer receiving a continuous 5-fluorouracil infusion reports feeling nauseated—nausea is a side effect of 5-fluorouracil treatment; although it should be addressed, not the first priority

(4) A 28-year-old woman with sickle cell anemia reports a pain level of 6 on a scale of 1–10—pain is frequently associated with sickle cell anemia; although the nurse should assess and intervene to alleviate client's pain, not the first priority

208. The Answer is 1

A 58-year-old Spanish-speaking woman is being discharged after having a central venous access device placed. Which of the following *BEST* describes the nurse's role in advocating for her client?

Reworded Question: Which answer best characterizes advocacy?

Strategy: Think about the definition of nurse advocacy. Focus on the key word "*BEST*," which may indicate there is more than one correct response. Consider each answer and select the action that is most representative of a nurse advocating for her client.

Needed Info: Advocacy: the act of promoting a client's rights and interests.

Category: Implementation/Safe and Effective Care Environment/Management of Care

(1) The nurse uses a translator when she provides the client with discharge instructions—CORRECT:

using a translator is the best example of an act of advocacy that promotes the client's rights and interests

(2) The nurse provides both written and verbal discharge instructions—providing written and verbal instructions may benefit the client, but is not the best example of advocacy

(3) The nurse ensures the client has transportation home upon discharge—asking the client if she has a ride home is appropriate, but not the best example of advocacy

(4) The nurse provides discharge instructions in a private room—providing discharge instructions in way that maintains privacy is important, but not the best example of advocacy

209. The Answer is 2

A 26-year-old man being admitted for an emergency appendectomy asks the nurse why she is asking about his medications and history of previous illnesses. In addition to explaining why it is relevant to the care of the client, the nurse knows this client responsibility has been outlined in which of the following?

Reworded Question: Which of the choices defines providing information about medications and past illness as a client's responsibility?

Strategy: Be familiar with the Americans with Disabilities Act, the Patient's Bill of Rights, Nursing Scope and Standards of Practice, and the Health Insurance Portability and Accountability Act (HIPAA).

Needed Info: The Patient's Bill of Rights was adopted to boost confidence in the health care system, emphasize the need for strong patient/provider relationship, and to define rights and responsibilities for patients and providers. Included was the need for patients to take responsibility for their health care by, among other things, providing information on medications and past health history to providers.

Category: Analysis/Safe and Effective Care Environment/Management of Care

(1) The Americans with Disabilities Act—does not define these responsibilities

(2) The Patient's Bill of Rights—CORRECT: includes a provision that the client is responsible

for providing information about medications and past illnesses

(3) Nursing Scope and Standards of Practice—does not define these responsibilities

(4) The Health Insurance Portability and Accountability Act (HIPAA)—does not define these responsibilities

210. The Answer is 2

A nurse is working on the medical/surgical unit. The nurse knows that which of the following tasks should *NOT* be delegated to nursing assistive personnel (NAP)?

Reworded Question: Which task is outside the scope of NAPs and should not be delegated?

Strategy: Focus on the key words "should *NOT*." Think about the skill level required in each scenario, and use the process of elimination to select which task is not appropriate for an NAP.

Needed Info: Nurses should not delegate tasks to NAPs related to assessment, diagnosis, or intervention that requires professional knowledge and skill.

Category: Implementation/Safe and Effective Care Environment/Management of Care

(1) Setting up a meal tray for a 75-year-old client with Alzheimer's disease— appropriate to delegate

(2) Assessing a newly postoperative client's pain level—CORRECT: best example of task that should not be delegated

(3) Setting up a water basin for a 45-year-old client who wishes to shave at the bedside—appropriate to delegate

(4) Transferring a 70-year-old client awaiting discharge from the bed to a wheelchair—appropriate to delegate

211. The Answer is 4

A nurse receives a phone call from a family member asking for health-related information on a client being treated for suspected myocardial infarction in the Emergency Department. The nurse explains she cannot disclose personal information about the client without the client's consent. The nurse knows

this represents which of the following ethical principles?

Reworded Question: Which ethical principle relates to maintaining a client's privacy?

Strategy: Use the process of elimination. Review ethical principles of clinical practice.

Needed Info: Accountability: responsibility for one's actions. Autonomy: right to make one's own decisions. Beneficence: duty to do what is in the best interests of the client. Confidentiality: maintaining privacy by not disclosing personal information.

Category: Analysis/Safe and Effective Care Environment/Management of Care

(1) Accountability—does not relate to client privacy

(2) Autonomy—does not relate to client privacy

(3) Beneficence—does not relate to client privacy

(4) Confidentiality—CORRECT: not disclosing personal information represents confidentiality

212. The Answer is 2

A nurse is caring for a 48-year-old man with a new colostomy. Which of the following activities *BEST* describes the nurse's role as an advocate for the client?

Reworded Question: Which task best advocates for the client?

Strategy: Focus on the key word "*BEST*." This indicates there may be more than one correct response. Consider each option and select the action that best advocates for the client.

Needed Info: Nurse advocacy is based on the premise that a nurse acts to protect the best interests of the client as well as to protect a client's right to make decisions. Nurse advocacy includes empowering a client through education.

Category: Implementation/Safe and Effective Care Environment/Management of Care

(1) Ensuring the skin is dry before re-adhering the pouch—proper procedure, but does not provide client with education needed to care for his own ostomy

(2) Teaching the client how to change and care for the ostomy pouch—CORRECT: best represents

nurse's role as client advocate; educating client about how to care for himself empowers him to self-advocate

(3) Providing the client's wife with a list of foods to avoid—may be important to client in terms of dietary choices, but does not teach client directly how to manage his ostomy

(4) Explaining to the client that psychological adjustment to an ostomy can take time—likely useful to client, but does not teach client directly how to manage ostomy

213.   The Answer is 3

A client who has scabies has been admitted to the medical/surgical unit. The nurse knows he should use which of the following precautions when caring for this client?

Reworded Question: What type of precautions should be initiated for a client with scabies?

Strategy: Consider the method by which scabies is transmitted and correlate that with the type of precaution required to prevention its transmission.

Needed Info: Be familiar with the way in which scabies is transmitted from person to person (contact) and identify the corresponding type of precaution the nurse should take (contact).

Category: Implementation/Safe and Effective Care Environment/Safety and Infection Control

(1) Droplet precautions—scabies not transferred via droplets, so droplet precautions not required

(2) Airborne precautions—scabies not transferred via the air, so airborne precautions not required

(3) Contact precautions—CORRECT: mites from scabies can be transferred via contact; contact precautions should be initiated

(4) Precautions are not necessary with this client— at a minimum, standard precautions should be used with all clients, regardless of health status

214.   The Answer is 2

A client who has a localized herpes simplex virus (HSV) infection is admitted to the maternity unit. The nurse knows the client should *IDEALLY* be placed in which of the following?

Reworded Question: What type of room should a client with HSV be assigned?

Strategy: Consider how localized HSV infections are transmitted. Focus on the key word "*IDEALLY*." This may mean more than one choice is acceptable. Use the process of elimination to determine the best choice.

Needed Info: A nurse caring for a client with a localized HSV infection should use contact precautions. To minimize the likelihood of infecting another client with HSV, the ideal room placement for this client is a single, unoccupied room.

Category: Implementation/Safe and Effective Care Environment/Safety and Infection Control

(1) Any available room—contact precautions should be initiated for a client with a localized HSV infection; consideration should be given to ideal room placement

(2) A single, unoccupied room—CORRECT: best choice for this client, who, based on her localized HSV infection, should be placed on contact precautions

(3) A double room with a client who underwent a cesarean section 3 days prior—client with an active HSV infection should not share a room with a client who underwent a cesarean section 3 days prior

(4) A double room with a curtain divider—not the ideal room for a client requiring contact precautions

215.   The Answer is 1

A 38-year-old client with breast cancer will be self-administering filgrastim (Neupogen) subcutaneously. The nurse knows that teaching should include which of the following?

Reworded Question: What instructions should the nurse give the client related to self-injections of Neupogen?

Strategy: Consider each option and, using the process of elimination, select elements of teaching the nurse should include.

Needed Info: Neupogen is a drug used to boost white blood cell counts in individuals undergoing chemotherapy treatment. It's not classified as a hazardous medication, so chemotherapy-resistant gloves are not required. Safe administration of injections requires the client to understand that needles should not be recapped or reused, and that they should be placed in a puncture-resistant container.

Category: Implementation/Safe and Effective Care Environment/Safety and Infection Control

(1) Dispose of needles in a puncture-resistant container—CORRECT: needles should not be recapped or bent, and should always be disposed of in a puncture-resistant container

(2) Wear chemotherapy-resistant gloves—not required with Neupogen, as it is not classified as a hazardous agent

(3) Recap the needles for reuse—needles should never be recapped or reused

(4) Neupogen has been prescribed to boost platelets—is prescribed to increase white blood cell count

216. The Answer is 1, 2, 4, and 5

A 76-year-old woman has been admitted to a rehabilitation center after a hip replacement. During an episode of confusion in which she became a danger to herself, the client was placed in a vest restraint. The nurse knows that which of the following are also considered types of restraints? **Select all that apply.**

Reworded Question: What are examples of restraints?

Strategy: Consider each response.

Needed Info: Know the definition of medical restraints and be able to provide examples.

Category: Analysis/Safe and Effective Care Environment/Safety and Infection Control

(1) Administering a haloperidol (Haldol) injection—CORRECT: a chemical restraint

(2) Raising 4 bed side rails—CORRECT: a mechanical restraint

(3) Assigning a nurse's aide to sit and observer the client—non-restraint effort to protect the client

(4) Applying wrist cuffs and tying them to the bed—CORRECT: a mechanical restraint

(5) Clipping a tray across the front of the client's wheelchair—CORRECT: trays that clip across the front of a wheelchair so that the client can't fall out easily are a form of mechanical restraint

217. The Answer is 1

A physician has written an order for escitalopram oxalate (Lexapro) 10 mg PO daily for a 15-year-old client with depression. After performing an initial assessment, the nurse calls the physician to verify the order. Which of the following *BEST* explains the nurse's concern about the safety of the order?

Reworded Question: What are contraindications to Lexapro therapy?

Strategy: Using the process of elimination, determine when Lexapro may not be appropriate to administer.

Needed Info: Know indications/contraindications and recommended dose ranges for Lexapro.

Category: Assessment/Safe and Effective Care Environment/Safety and Infection Control

(1) The client reported a history of facial swelling and difficulty breathing while on citalopram (Celexa)—CORRECT: facial swelling, difficulty breathing characteristic of allergic reaction; individuals who have experienced allergic reactions to Celexa should not take Lexapro

(2) The drug has not been approved for use in the client's age group—Lexapro approved for acute and maintenance treatment for major depressive disorder in adults and in adolescents aged 12–17 years

(3) The ordered dose is higher than the suggested range—typical starting dose for Lexapro is 10 mg PO daily

(4) The ordered dose is lower than the suggested range—typical starting dose for Lexapro is 10 mg PO daily

218. The Answer is 3 and 4

A 75-year-old client has an unsteady gait and requires assistance with ambulation. The nurse decides to use a gait belt. The nurse knows she should do which of the following when using a gait belt? **Select all that apply.**

Reworded Question: Which of the following are correct when using a gait belt?

Strategy: Focus on the key words "Select all that apply." More than one response may be correct. Think about elements of proper gait belt use, and use the process of elimination to rule out the incorrect responses.

Needed Info: Know proper technique for gait belt use.

Category: Implementation/Safe and Effective Care Environment/Safety and Infection Control

(1) Secure the gait belt loosely around the client's waist—the gait belt should fit snugly, with room for the nurse's fingers between the belt and client

(2) Twist her upper body to position the client—the nurse should keep her back straight to practice proper body mechanics and prevent injury

(3) Remove the gait belt after use—CORRECT: gait belts should be removed after use

(4) Place the gait belt over the client's clothes with the clip in front—CORRECT: allows for easier adjustment

(5) Use the gait belt to help lift the client from a sitting into a standing position—should never be used to lift a client.

219. The Answer is 2

After receiving report at the start of a night shift, the nurse finds an elderly client lying on the floor with the bedrails down. When documenting findings, which of the following *BEST* describes what the nurse should do?

Reworded Question: What is the proper way to complete incident reports?

Strategy: Consider each response. Focus on the key word "*BEST.*"

Needed Info: Know proper procedure for completing incident reports, including who should fill them out and when they should be filled out.

Category: Analysis/Safe and Effective Care Environment/Safety and Infection Control

(1) Complete an incident report at the end of his shift, when he is less busy—the incident report should be completed as soon as possible

(2) Complete an incident report using clear, concise, and factual language—CORRECT: the incident report should be completed using clear, concise, and factual language

(3) Complete an incident report and place a copy of it in the client's medical record—incident reports should not be filed in the client's medical record

(4) Ask the evening shift nurse to complete an incident report because the fall occurred on her shift—an incident report should be completed by the individual who identified the problem, in this case, the night shift nurse

220. The Answer is 1

A nurse is caring for an 8-year-old girl with urinary retention. The nurse is preparing to insert a Foley catheter. Which of the following catheter sizes is most appropriate for this client?

Reworded Question: What size Foley catheter should be used for pediatric clients?

Strategy: Consider how Foley catheters are sized and select the best choice for a pediatric client.

Needed Info: Foley catheters are sized according to the French scale, abbreviated Fr. Each unit corresponds with a diameter of approximately 0.33 mm. So, an 18 Fr catheter equals a diameter of about 6 mm. The larger the number, the larger the catheter size. For a smaller pediatric client, the smaller size is the best choice.

Category: Implementation/Physiological Integrity/Basic Care and Comfort

(1) Number 8 French—CORRECT: the number 8 French catheter is the smallest of the choices, and is the right answer; typically, number 8 Fr or number 10 Fr catheters are used in children

(2) Number 16 French—number 16 Fr is usually used for adult women

(3) Number 20 French—number 20 Fr is usually used for adult men

(4) Number 22 French—number 22 Fr is usually used for adult men

221. The Answer is 4

A 42-year-old male client weighs 196 lbs. (89.1 kg) and is 65 inches (1.65 meters) tall. Based on the client's body mass index (BMI), the nurse knows this client would fall into which of the following categories?

Reworded Question: What is this client's BMI and weight status?

Strategy: Calculate the BMI and determine the corresponding weight status.

Needed Info: The formula for calculating a BMI is $[wt \times 703 / (ht)^2]$, or $[196 \times 703 / (65)^2] = 32.6$. BMI interpretation is the same for male and female adults over the age of 20. BMI below 18.5, underweight; 18.5–24.9, normal; 25.0–29.9, overweight; 30.0 and above, obese

Category: Assessment/Physiological Integrity

(1) Underweight—a BMI below 18.5 indicates a weight status of underweight

(2) Normal weight—a BMI of 18.5–24.9 indicates a normal weight status

(3) Overweight—a BMI of 25.0–29.9 indicates a weight status of overweight

(4) Obese—CORRECT: a BMI of 30.0 or more indicates a weight status of obese

222. The Answer is 2

A 10-year-old girl is being seen in the Pediatric Emergency Department following a motor vehicle accident. She has been stabilized but reports a pain level of 8 on a scale of 1 to 10. The nurse is preparing to transfer the client to x-ray. The nurse knows that which nonpharmacologic intervention should *NOT* be used to help reduce pain in this client?

Reworded Question: Which nonpharmacologic intervention is not appropriate?

Strategy: Consider each response, and using the process of elimination, select the intervention that should not be used.

Needed Info: Pain is individualized and can be affected by coping skills, emotional state, temperament, and past experiences. Nonpharmacologic interventions can be effective in managing pain

and should be implemented in an age-appropriate manner. For school-aged children, the following examples of nonpharmacologic interventions may be useful: providing complete explanations, encouraging participation in decision making, allowing choices if feasible, using distraction, using relaxation and using imagery.

Category: Implementation/Physiological Integrity/Basic Care and Comfort

(1) Offer choices when possible—it is appropriate to offer choices when possible

(2) Reassure the client that the procedure will not hurt—CORRECT: client should be given age-appropriate but truthful explanations about any procedures

(3) Provide complete explanations about what is going to happen: this is appropriate

(4) Use distraction, relaxation, and imagery—this is appropriate

223. The Answer is 2

In preparation for doxorubicin (Adriamycin) administration, the nurse is assessing a client's arm to determine where to attempt venipuncture. The nurse knows which of the following veins is the *BEST* choice to start the IV?

Reworded Question: Which is the best choice of venipuncture sites to administer Adriamycin?

Strategy: Focus on the key word "*BEST*." This indicates there may be more than one acceptable choice. Consider ways to prevent complications associated with intravenous chemotherapy administration.

Needed Info: Adriamycin is an antitumor antibiotic used in the treatment of cancer. It is a vesicant, which means that it can cause blistering if it extravasates during administration. Proper vein selection is critical in preventing this complication. The antecubital fossa and wrist are not the ideal sites for vesicant administration because movement may increase the likelihood of dislodging the IV and causing extravasation. In addition, extravasations are more difficult to identify in the antecubital fossa. Sites distal to previous venipunctures should not be used.

Category: Implementation/Physiological Integrity/ Pharmacological and Parenteral Therapies

(1) The non-dominant antecubital fossa—not the best choice

(2) The distal forearm—CORRECT: the distal forearm is the best venipuncture site because the soft tissue present in that location limits the potential for harm to nerves and tendons should extravasation occur

(3) The wrist—not the best choice

(4) A vein used for venipuncture within the previous 24 hours—not the best choice

224. The Answer is 4

A 24-year-old client with anorexia has had a nasogastric (NG) tube placed in preparation for intermittent enteral feedings. The nurse knows to do which of the following when administering medications via an NG tube?

Reworded Question: What is the appropriate way to administer medications via an NG tube?

Strategy: Consider the proper technique for administering medications via an NG tube. Review each response and use the process of elimination to determine the correct choice.

Needed Info: Know the procedure for administering medications via an NG tube. Enteric coated aspirin should not be crushed because this action removes the protective coating and potentially clogs the tube. Medications should not be mixed with the client's feeding formula. The feeding should be stopped, the tube should be flushed, and then medications should be administered. A minimum of a 30-mL syringe should be used to flush or irrigate the tube. Each medication should be administered separately; medications should not be mixed and administered together.

Category: Implementation/Physiological Integrity/ Pharmacological and Parenteral Therapies

(1) Crush the enteric coated aspirin—enteric coated medications should not be crushed

(2) Mix the medications with the client's feeding formula—medications should not be mixed with the client's feeding formula

(3) Flush the tube using a 15-mL syringe—tube should be flushed using a minimum of a 30-mL oral syringe

(4) Administer each medication separately—CORRECT: medications should not be combined and administered together

225. The Answer is 3

A 3-year-old client with acute otitis media has been prescribed ofloxacin (Floxin) ear drops. The nurse knows that which of the following statements by the father demonstrates that he understands how to properly administer the ear drops?

Reworded Question: What is the proper way to administer ear drops?

Strategy: Consider each of the statements. Using the process of elimination, select the statement that best reflects the technique that should be used to administer ear drops to a pediatric client.

Needed Info: Ear drop medication technique: warm the drops to body temperature to prevent pain and dizziness; lie the client down with affected ear facing up; place drops on the wall of the ear canal to allow air to escape and the medication to flow into the ear; give the medication as prescribed.

Category: Implementation/Physiological Integrity/ Pharmacological and Parenteral Therapies

(1) "I can stop giving the ear drops as soon as my daughter's fever is gone."—medication should be administered as prescribed and should not be discontinued based on the presence or absence of a fever

(2) "I should give the drops directly on the eardrum to help get rid of the infection quickly."—drops should not be administered directly on the eardrum

(3) "I should warm the ear drops before giving them by wrapping the bottle in my hand."— CORRECT: temperature should be between 95–98.6° F (35–37° C)

(4) "My daughter should lie flat while I give the drops."—client should lie on her side with the affected ear facing upwards

226. The Answer is 1

A 68-year-old woman recently diagnosed with hypertension has started taking furosemide (Lasix) 40 mg PO twice daily. During a clinic appointment, she reports new onset muscle weakness and abdominal cramping. Lab tests are performed. The nurse knows which of the following results is the best explanation for the symptoms experienced by the client?

Reworded Question: What is the most likely reason for the client's symptoms?

Strategy: Consider the side effects of Lasix. What effects does the drug have on potassium levels? What symptoms might be seen with this side effect?

Needed Info: Lasix is a diuretic that can lead to electrolyte imbalances. The normal range for potassium is 3.5 to 5 mEq/L. Symptoms associated with hypokalemia include abdominal cramping and muscle weakness.

Category: Analysis/Physiological Integrity/Reduction of Risk Potential

(1) Potassium 3.0 mEq/L—CORRECT: a potassium level of 3.0 mEq/L is below the normal range and may be associated with symptoms such as abdominal cramping and muscle weakness

(2) Creatinine 1.5 mg/dL—this is a normal range value and is not the correct response

(3) Fasting glucose 145 mg/dL—this is a normal range value and is not the correct response

(4) Total calcium 10.0 mg/dL—this is a normal range value and is not the correct response

227. The Answer is 2

A 64-year-old man with heart failure has recently been told by his physician to increase his digoxin (Lanoxin) dose to 0.25 mg. He has 125 mcg tablets on hand. Which of the following statements by the client to the home health nurse indicates the client has understood the teaching provided about the medication?

Reworded Question: Which statement is correct?

Strategy: Recall how to calculate Lanoxin dosages, as well as the side effects of the drug. Consider the consequence of each action, and eliminate the incorrect statements.

Needed Info: A Lanoxin 125 mcg tablet is equivalent to 0.125 mg. GI disturbances may be associated with Lanoxin toxicity. Regular follow-up and blood work monitoring is required for clients taking Lanoxin. Over-the-counter medications can interfere with Lanoxin therapy and should not be taken without physician approval.

Category: Assessment/Physiological Integrity/Reduction of Risk Potential

(1) "I should take one tablet."—client should take 2 tablets

(2) "I should notify my doctor if I experience diarrhea."—CORRECT: client should notify his physician if he experiences GI disturbances including diarrhea

(3) "I don't need to follow up with my doctor unless I'm having a problem."—routine follow-up and monitoring is required

(4) "I can take over-the-counter medications without the approval of my physician."—over-the-counter medications should not be taken without physician approval

228. The Answer is 3

The nurse is preparing to administer a tuberculin skin test to a pregnant 26-year-old client. The nurse knows which of the following statements about tuberculin skin testing is *TRUE*?

Reworded Question: How are tuberculin skin tests correctly administered?

Strategy: Consider proper techniques associated with tuberculin skin test administration. Using the process of elimination, select the correct answer.

Needed Info: Mantoux tuberculin skin testing is used to determine whether a client is infected with *Mycobacterium tuberculosis*. Tuberculin skin tests may be administered during pregnancy. They should be read 48 to 72 hours after administration. The reaction is measured in millimeters of the induration. The test should be administered into the inner surface of the forearm.

Category: Implementation/Physiological Integrity/Reduction of Risk Potential

(1) The test should not be administered during pregnancy—test may be administered during pregnancy

(2) The test should be read between 24 and 48 hours after administration—test should be read between 48 and 72 hours after administration

(3) The reaction is measured in millimeters of the induration—CORRECT: reaction is measured in millimeters of the induration

(4) The test should be administered into the outer surface of the forearm—test should be administered into the inner surface of the forearm

229. The Answer is 1, 3, and 5

The nurse takes report on a client who underwent a thyroidectomy 24 hours ago. The nurse understands that the client is at risk for hypocalcemia. Which of the following assessment findings indicate the client may be hypocalcemic? **Select all that apply.**

Reworded Question: Which findings are associated with hypocalcemia?

Strategy: Note the instruction to "select all that apply." More than one response may be correct. Consider the signs and symptoms associated with hypocalcemia. Use the process of elimination to determine which response or responses are correct.

Needed Info: Hypocalcemia is a risk associated with thyroidectomy and is most common 24 to 48 hours after surgery. Signs and symptoms of hypocalcemia in a client who has undergone thyroidectomy may include positive Trousseau's sign, positive Chvostek's sign, periorbital numbness, mental status changes, tetany, seizures, EKG changes, and cardiac arrest.

Category: Assessment/Physiological Integrity/Physiological Adaptation

(1) Positive Trousseau's sign—CORRECT: positive Trousseau's sign may be associated with hypocalcemia

(2) Negative Chvostek's sign—incorrect

(3) Numbness around the mouth—CORRECT: may be associated with hypocalcemia

(4) Positive Moro reflex test—incorrect

(5) "Pins and needles" sensation in client's feet—CORRECT: an early symptom of hypocalcemia

230. The Answer is 2

A 58-year-old client is receiving the monoclonal antibody rituximab (Rituxan) and develops an infusion reaction manifested by chest pain and dyspnea. The nurse should do which of the following *FIRST*?

Reworded Question: What should the nurse do *FIRST* during an infusion reaction?

Strategy: Focus on the key word "*FIRST*." This indicates there may be more than one correct answer. Select the intervention that must be performed first.

Needed Info: The nurse should assess frequently for reactions during monoclonal antibody infusions. When an infusion reaction is suspected, the nurse should immediately stop the infusion but maintain vascular access with a normal saline infusion. After that, it is appropriate for the nurse to assess the client, and prepare emergency equipment and medication. Depending on the situation, it may be appropriate to restart the infusion at a slower rate.

Category: Implementation/Physiological Integrity/Physiological Adaptation

(1) Assess the client's airway—not the intervention that should be performed first

(2) Stop the infusion—CORRECT: the infusion should be stopped *FIRST*

(3) Slow down the rate of infusion—not the intervention that should be performed first

(4) Administer epinephrine—not the intervention that should be performed first

231. The Answer is 4

The nurse is assigned as the team leader on a busy medical/surgical unit. Which of the following *BEST* describes the "rights" of delegation the nurse must consider when assigning tasks to other members of the health care team?

Reworded Question: What are the five principles of delegation when assigning tasks to the health care peers on your shift?

Strategy: Apply your knowledge of the topic—delegation of tasks. Eliminate the answer choices that are incorrect first.

Needed Info: Delegation is an important skill. The nurse should identify the right person to do the specific task, explain or give clear directions regarding the task, choose the right task for the appropriate person, and keep the client in mind. Is the client able to tolerate the task being performed by the person chosen?

Category: Analysis/Safe and Effective Care Management/Management of Care

(1) Right task, right timing, right client, right person, and right date—right client refers to the five rights of dispensing medications

(2) Right task, right client, right direction, right supervision, and right date—right client and right date refer to medications

(3) Right client, right direction, right day, right medication, and right unit—right day, right medication, and right unit do not refer to the delegation of tasks

(4) Right task, right circumstance, right person, right direction, and right supervision—CORRECT: these are the five rights of delegation; when delegating, the charge nurse must make certain of the following regarding the task: (1) it can be safely delegated; (2) the client is stable and a good outcome is anticipated; (3) the task is being delegated to the right person; (4) there is clear communication; (5) the charge nurse is responsible for supervision

232. The Answer is 4

Which of the following pediatric clients should the nurse provide assessment and intervention for *FIRST*?

Reworded Question: Which client requires immediate intervention?

Strategy: Think ABCs and airway.

Needed Info: Understand the ABCs framework of prioritizing airway, breathing, and circulation in order of importance. Always assess the client before checking alarms.

Category: Assessment/Safe and Effective Care Environment/Management of Care

(1) A 15-month-old who has developed hives—no indication that the infant with hives is in immediate distress; requires an assessment but is not the priority

(2) A 2-year-old who is ventilated but stable—no indication that an alarm is sounding; client requires an assessment but not immediately

(3) A 12-year-old recovering from surgical repair of a fractured femur — no indication of immediate distress

(4) The 2-month-old infant whose apnea monitor is sounding with an oxygen saturation reading of 82%—CORRECT: reading below normal on the oxygen saturation must be assessed immediately; a 2-month-old cannot tell you what is wrong and has little room for compensation when oxygen levels drop; it is imperative that this infant is assessed and an intervention initiated; it may be simple repositioning, suctioning, or readjusting the probe, but apnea alarms should not be ignored

233. The Answer is 2

The nurse knows that she would *NOT* be required to use airborne precautions for which of the following clients?

Reworded Question: Which pathogen is not spread by small airborne droplets traveling more than 3 feet?

Strategy: Think about the transmission of pathogens.

Needed Info: Transmission-based precautions help to limit the spread of germs. Small germ-infected drops that travel far require airborne precautions. Droplet precautions are for those germs found in droplets of secretions when a client coughs or sneezes. Contact precautions are for germs spread by hand-to-skin touching or from germs on an object to skin.

Category: Implementation/Safe and Effective Care Environment/Safety and Infection Control

(1) A young adult with possible tuberculosis who is also HIV positive—tuberculosis is carried in small airborne droplets over 3 feet and requires airborne precautions

(2) A middle-aged adult with herpes simplex— CORRECT: herpes simplex is spread from hand to skin or object to skin; requires contact not airborne precautions

(3) A teenager with chicken pox and a sore throat—chicken pox is spread by small airborne droplets so airborne precautions are appropriate

(4) A college student with possible rubella—rubella is an airborne pathogen requiring airborne precautions until a diagnosis is confirmed

234. The Answer is 3

The nurse is caring for an elderly female with dementia. The nurse knows that which of the following should be the priority for care for this client?

Reworded Question: What is an important health risk when caring for an elderly adult with dementia?

Strategy: Think client safety.

Needed Info: You should know the health risks to consider for any elderly adult regardless of medical diagnosis. Elderly clients have slower reflexes, decreasing ability to adapt to new environments especially with dementia, and balance issues leading to falls.

Category: Implementation/Safe and Effective Care Environment/Management of Care

(1) Nutrition—factored into the nursing care plan but is in the category of basic needs and comfort

(2) Hygiene—in the category of basic needs and comfort

(3) Fall risk—CORRECT: in the category of safety or safe and effective care, and should be part of any care plan for an elderly adult with or without dementia

(4) Cardiac care—particular to clients who have symptoms or a history of heart disease and would not necessarily be included in this care plan

235. The Answer is 2

The nurse is planning the care of an elderly male client with very poor oral hygiene and gum disease. The nurse knows that the teeth and gums can be which of the following in the chain of infection?

Reworded Question: Which element in the chain of infection would the mouth, teeth, and gums of an older adult with gum disease be considered?

Strategy: Think about the six elements in the chain of infection.

Needed Info: A pathogen has the potential to cause infection under the right conditions including environment, portal of exit, transmission mode, a way to enter, and a susceptible host.

Category: Analysis/Safe and Effective Care Management/Safety and Infection Control

(1) The method of transmission for bacteria—direct, indirect, or airborne contact; the teeth most often are not the mode of transmission

(2) The portal of entry for bacteria—CORRECT: unhealthy gums generally are red, swollen, and bleed with brushing, offering the portal of entry; bacteria enters and can easily spread through the blood stream due to poor oral hygiene and gum disease

(3) The pathogen—the teeth alone are not the pathogen

(4) A portal of exit—the teeth and gums are not a portal of exit

236. The Answer is 2

In the event of a fire, the nurse should do which of the following *FIRST*?

Reworded Question: Which should the nurse do *FIRST* in the event of a fire?

Strategy: Think about what you know about the steps involved in fire safety in a hospital setting.

Needed Info: If a fire occurs, the first step is to get clients out of danger, then work to contain the fire, and then to determine the order in which clients should be evacuated.

Category: Implementation/Safe and Effective Care Management/Safety and Infection Control

(1) Leave the building—the nurse should not leave the building without attempting to remove clients from danger

(2) Attempt to get clients out of immediate danger—CORRECT: this is the first step the nurse should take in the event of fire

(3) Work to contain the fire—the first thing the nurse should do is attempt to get clients out of immediate danger

(4) Determine the order in which to evacuate clients—not the first step

237. The Answer is 1

The nurse knows that which of the following *BEST* describes the role of a nursing supervisor?

Reworded Question: What do you expect from a supervisor?

Strategy: Think authority, guidance, and follow-up responsibilities.

Needed Info: The role of a nursing supervisor is one of authority. The nursing supervisor implements different ideas assisting in the safe and effective management of care for the clients in the facility. The nursing supervisor also manages the professional employees to ensure tasks are done efficiently and correctly.

Category: Implementation/Safe and Effective Care Environment/Management of Care

(1) Chooses and implements interventions—CORRECT: a nursing supervisor chooses strategies and interventions that may be necessary to ensure timely and efficient tasks are completed

(2) Attends meetings to keep staff up to date—although a nursing supervisor does attend meetings, her role is to help to implement ideas when staff members require guidance

(3) Does not require special skills to oversee other professionals—a nursing supervisor should have special skills like active listening, good communication skills, ability to solve problems, and knowledge about the clients and staff being supervised

(4) Is friendly and can make contributions to an employee evaluation—a nursing supervisor should be friendly and not intimidating but friendliness does not make a nurse qualified to supervise others; supervisors may directly contribute information to an employee evaluation

238. The Answer is 2

The nurse is conversing with a young adult client regarding an ordered blood transfusion. It is clear to the nurse that the client does not understand the risks involved with the procedure. Which of the following statements *BEST* describes the nurse's role regarding informed consent for this procedure?

Reworded Question: What is the role of the nurse regarding informed consent?

Strategy: Think about the process of informed consent and whose responsibility it is to obtain informed consent.

Needed Info: The practitioner ordering the procedure is responsible for explaining the risks, benefits, and alternatives to the client. The nurse may witness the signing of the consent but should only sign if he is confident that the client does indeed understand and wants the procedure. The nurse should also be familiar with the ethics of decision making for any client.

Category: Implementation/Safe and Effective Care Environment/Management of Care

(1) The nurse tells the client not to worry because blood transfusions are very common—telling the client not to worry leaves the client without the information required to make an informed consent

(2) The nurse informs the ordering physician that the client does not understand the risks and will need further explanation—CORRECT: the nurse should advocate for the client and call the practitioner who ordered the procedure to come offer further information

(3) The nurse has someone else witness the signature on the consent—the nurse should not have someone else witness the signature on the consent especially if he knows the client does not fully understand the risks involved

(4) The nurse describes alternative treatments—the nurse's role is not to provide alternative treatment choices; physicians are the ones to discuss alternative treatments

239. The Answer is 3

The nurse is caring for a famous basketball player who may have sustained a career-changing injury. When asked by coworkers about the status of the client, she responds that she is not able to discuss her client. Which of the following ethical principles *BEST* supports her statement?

Reworded Question: Which ethical principle should the nurse use when asked about a client by other staff not caring for the client?

Strategy: Think about ethical practice and the Code of Ethics for Nurses.

Needed Info: Understand the ethical principles that determine what is right and wrong when caring for clients. You should be able to define and review outcomes and interventions to promote ethical practice. Justice, nonmaleficence, fidelity, confidentiality, and accountability are some of the ethical principles that a nurse should understand and practice.

Category: Implementation/Safe and Effective Care Environment/Management of Care

(1) Justice—providing fair and appropriate treatment

(2) Beneficence—doing what is in the best interest of the client

(3) Confidentiality—CORRECT: maintaining the client's privacy and supporting what the nurse's role is by not talking to her coworkers about her client

(4) Accountability—being responsible for one's actions

240. The Answer is 3

The nurse is on duty on a busy cardiac telemetry unit. Which of the following situations requires the nurse's immediate attention?

Reworded Question: Which scenario needs the immediate attention of the nurse?

Strategy: Think triage, establishing priorities, and ABCs.

Needed Info: You must understand priorities and symptoms of cardiac compromise. The nurse should know the basics for recognizing a sudden change in the level of consciousness or a reduced heart rate and its importance. Know normal vital signs and symptoms of respiratory compromise such as snoring and being unable to arouse a client. A client sleeping soundly with a normal heart rate would not be as worrisome.

Category: Analysis/Safe and Effective Care and Environment/Management of Care

(1) The wife of a cardiac client states that his IV pump is alarming and he is not receiving the pain medication dose due to the pump malfunctioning—can wait, not life-threatening

(2) The daughter of an elderly client states that her mother is uncomfortable and that her electrodes have come off—can wait, not life-threatening

(3) The new CNA reports that she cannot wake her elderly client to take his blood pressure because he is sleeping soundly and snoring, but she obtained his pulse and it is 30. She wants you to come to see if you can wake him—CORRECT: a new CNA may not have enough experience to recognize the difference between sleeping and an unconscious state in this elderly client; this client should be assessed immediately with a heart rate of 30 and nursing interventions should be initiated; if the client is really sleeping soundly, arousing him to increase his heart rate might be appropriate; if the client cannot be aroused, cardio pulmonary resuscitation efforts should be initiated by calling for help and following the ABCs of resuscitation

(4) The new admission from earlier today is complaining that he has not been assessed in over an hour and he would like to order dinner—the new admission requires assessment but is not as much of a priority as the client in answer choice 3

241. The Answer is 4

The nurse knows that which of the following terms *BEST* defines the multidisciplinary care planning for a young adult with breast cancer?

Reworded Question: What is the term for multidisciplinary team meetings to plan client care?

Strategy: Think about reaching common goals, reviewing client information, and communication.

Needed Info: You should understand the definition of terms surrounding multidisciplinary team interaction and the purpose for collaboration versus case management.

Category: Planning/Safe and Effective Care Environment/Management of Care

(1) Team work—refers to peers working together to complete tasks; does not define multidisciplinary actions for the benefit of the client's plan of care

(2) Team building—refers to a working relationship between peers for a variety of reasons, not always client related

(3) Case management—coordinates the care, improves outcomes, and reduces cost but does not initially plan the care of the client

(4) Collaboration—CORRECT: defines the multidisciplinary team approach to building a plan of care for the client

---

242. The Answer is 1, 3, 4, and 5

The charge RN is preparing assignments on a busy medical unit. For this shift, there are several LPNs, several RNs, and one CNA. Which of the following assignments by the charge RN is appropriate? **Select all that apply.**

Reworded Question: Which tasks are within the scope of practice for the RN, the LPN, and the CNA?

Strategy: Eliminate the choices that are out of the scope of practice for the professional assigned to the task.

Needed Info: Think through which tasks can be appropriately delegated to trained personnel. You also should review the principles of delegation, the Nurse Practice Act, and know what it means to supervise those who have been assigned tasks.

Category: Analysis/Safe and Effective Care Environment/Management of Care

(1) The CNA is assigned to give morning baths—CORRECT: giving a bath is within the scope of practice for a CNA

(2) An LPN is assigned to perform an initial assessment on a newly admitted client—LPNs do not perform initial client assessments

(3) An LPN is assigned to clients who are prescribed oral medications, and will do vital signs on those clients—CORRECT: LPNs may administer oral medications and do vital signs

(4) The clients with IV medications are divided among the RNs—CORRECT: RNs administer IV medications

(5) AN LPN is assigned to insert a urinary cathether—CORRECT: inserting a urinary cathether is within the scope of practice of an LPN

---

243. The Answer is 4

The nurse is educating new nursing staff members about safety on the pediatric unit. Which of the following comments by one of the new staff members *BEST* demonstrates that teaching has been successful?

Reworded Question: Which statement is correct about childhood safety practices in and out of the hospital setting?

Strategy: Think prevention and safety with children.

Needed Info: Begin by reviewing pediatric growth and development including age-related safety regulations for each age group. Review prevention strategies for children including car seat safety, poison prevention, fall risks, and preventing injuries.

Category: Evaluation/Safe and Effective Care Environment/Safety and Infection Control

(1) "A toddler may be taken to the car in a wheelchair when discharged and, after that, the hospital is not responsible for how the child is transported in the family car."—toddler should not be discharged to parents if they do not have an appropriate car seat; laws state that toddler must be in child-appropriate car seat and the hospital should be held accountable for making certain that when a child is discharged it is with the proper car restraint

(2) "School-aged children do not require booster seats if they are less than 80 pounds, and they do not require bicycle helmets when they are more than 80 pounds."—school-aged children less than 80 pounds should still be in an appropriate booster seat or car restraint until they reach 4 foot 8 inches and weigh over 80 pounds; children of all ages and sizes should wear bicycle helmets

(3) "Medications can be left at the bedside for pediatric clients, and the parent will dispense when

needed."—medications should not be left at the bedside of any client

(4) "All medications and cleaning supplies must be locked in a child-proof cabinet on the pediatric unit at all times."—CORRECT: all medications and cleaning supplies should be locked in a child-proof cabinet

244. The Answer is 2

The nurse knows that which of the following is the *MOST* appropriate infection control method when caring for clients on a surgical unit?

Reworded Question: How can staff members prevent the spread of infection to a fresh surgical client?

Strategy: The word *MOST* indicates there may be more than one possibility but that only one is the best choice.

Needed Info: Review how infection is spread, the elements of the chain of infection, and universal precautions.

Category: Implementation/Safe and Effective Care Environment/Safety and Infection Control

(1) Hand hygiene before charting or using the keyboard—appropriate but not the most effective directly related to the surgical client

(2) Handwashing before and after contact with each client—CORRECT: washing hands before entering the room and after contact with the client is the most effective way to prevent infection

(3) Use of gloves—using gloves is helpful but does not take the place of handwashing

(4) Use of gowns with each client—gowns may be appropriate for certain bacteria but do not take the place of proper handwashing

245. The Answer is 1

The nurse on the adult medical unit assesses an elderly client with vertigo. Which of the following interventions demonstrates that the nurse understands the symptoms of vertigo?

Reworded Question: What actions can the nurse take to make this client safe?

Strategy: Think safety risks for the elderly.

Needed Info: You should know the definition of vertigo and a basic understanding of the head-spinning feeling that this client may be experiencing. Basic safety for fall prevention is helpful, and knowing that vertigo originates in the inner ear will help guide your critical thinking skills.

Category: Implementation/Safe and Effective Care Environment/Safety and Infection Control

(1) The nurse recognizes this client as at risk for falls and relays this to the other team members—CORRECT: the nurse should alert staff and the multidisciplinary team about fall risk precautions to help prevent injury during a vertigo episode with this client

(2) The nurse allows the client to ambulate alone—an elderly client with vertigo should not ambulate alone and should be instructed to call for assistance to avoid falling

(3) The nurse encourages the client to sit up quickly before standing—instructing a client to sit up quickly can make the vertigo worse; encourage the client to sit up slowly and maintain that position until the vertigo subsides

(4) The nurse makes no change in routine precautions because vertigo is an expected symptom for this age group—making no change in the care of a client with vertigo is reckless and could lead to injury

246. The Answer is 2

The nurse is preparing to change a sterile surgical dressing. While repositioning herself, the client touches a sterile sponge. Which of the following is the *BEST* nursing intervention to promote and maintain surgical asepsis?

Reworded Question: What is the best way to handle the situation when a sterile field has been contaminated?

Strategy: Think about the principles of surgical asepsis.

Needed Info: You must understand the basis for surgical asepsis and how to set up and maintain a sterile field.

Category: Implementation/Safe and Effective Care Environment/Safety and Infection Control

(1) Reassure the client and continue with the dressing change—if the sterile field has been contaminated, a new sterile field must be set up

(2) Reassure the client but instruct her to keep her hands free from the sterile field. Clear the contaminated area, rewash hands, and assemble another sterile field to start over—CORRECT: reassurance and education for the client can be done while setting up a new sterile field; it is for the safety of the client and to prevent infection

(3) Have the client sterilize her hands so the episode is not repeated—skin cannot be sterilized, but the client should cleanse her hands for her own protection

(4) Continue with the dressing change, avoiding the items that came in contact with the client's hands—if the sterile field has been contaminated, a new sterile field must be set up

247. The Answer is 3

The nurse is caring for a client who has just undergone an open laparotomy with ileostomy. The nurse knows that client education should include which of the following topics?

Reworded Question: What are the principles that nursing care focuses on with ileostomy care?

Strategy: Think about stoma and wound care.

Needed Info: An ileostomy is an opening at the distal end of the small intestine. Stool will be loose and acidic and can be irritating to the skin. Skin care, hygiene, diet, and fluid intake will be educational topics.

Category: Planning/Physiological Integrity: Basic Care and Comfort

(1) Constipation management—will not be an important topic to discuss because it is rare with an ileostomy

(2) Limited activity—activity should not be limited after healing from the surgery; education should

center on returning to normal activity with the ileostomy

(3) Stoma care and skin care—CORRECT: education should include stoma care, skin care, diet, fluid intake, and how to safely remove a food blockage from the stoma

(4) Urinary incontinence—not a symptom associated with an ileostomy

248. The Answer is 1

The nurse is assessing a client who has multiple sclerosis and can no longer live alone due to immobility. Which of the following statements by the nurse demonstrates her understanding of this client's impaired physical mobility?

Reworded Question: What are some of the complications of immobility?

Strategy: Think about how multiple sclerosis (MS) affects each body system and prioritize.

Needed Info: Understand the effects of immobility caused by neuromuscular disorders. Apply that knowledge to the systems of the body. Look first at the cause of the immobility and the length of time it has occurred, and then look for complications and symptoms.

Category: Assessment/Physiological Integrity/Basic Care and Comfort

(1) "Do you have any areas of pain, pressure, or open ulcers on your legs, ankles, or hips?"—CORRECT: an assessment of a client with MS should include looking for pressure areas and skin breakdown; look for areas of injury due to falls and potential areas of open wounds for sources of infection; look for bruising, atrophy, and signs of thrombosis

(2) "They do make motor wheelchairs. Maybe we can look into that."—although a motor chair may increase mobility, it may not be enough to allow the client to live alone; this would be determined by a complete physical assessment and home visit

(3) "How often do you have episodes of diarrhea?"—clients with MS are prone to constipation due to sluggish peristalsis, not diarrhea

(4) "What kinds of meals would you like prepared while in the hospital?"—meal preparation would not be the first priority in an assessment

249. The Answer is 3

The nurse is educating a client who is scheduled for surgery in the near future about autologous blood donation. Which of the following statements by the client indicates the teaching has been successful?

Reworded Question: What are the criteria for autologous blood donations prior to surgery?

Strategy: Think client's own blood.

Needed Info: Know the criteria for blood donation and the different blood types. Understand transfusion reactions and the life cycle of the red blood cell. Know the proper procedures for both blood transfusion and donation.

Category: Assessment/Physiological Integrity/Pharmacological and Parenteral Therapies

(1) "I cannot donate blood for myself because of my age."—not a true statement

(2) "I will not need a transfusion after major surgery."—you cannot assume that blood won't be needed during or after a major surgical procedure

(3) "I can be an autologous blood donor 6 weeks before my surgery in the event that I may need a transfusion."—CORRECT: to be an autologous donor (donating your own blood), donation should be done 4–6 weeks before your surgery and when blood counts are within normal limits

(4) "I cannot get a transfusion reaction with my own blood."—blood transfusion reactions are rare with one's own blood but they are possible and the risks should be discussed with the client

250. The Answer is 4

The RN is providing education to the LPN about administrating oral medications. Which of the following statements demonstrates to the RN that the LPN understands the teaching?

Reworded Question: Which statement provides correct information about administering oral medication?

Strategy: Think about what extended-release tablets are designed to do and the effects of crushing them. Know the responsibility of administering oral medication in the proper dose.

Needed Info: Know your medications and the actions, length of effect, and the purpose for each type of medication.

Category: Analysis/Physiological Integrity/Pharmacological and Parenteral Therapies

(1) "Giving oral medications is simple and requires little training."—statement indicates a lack of knowledge regarding the training and responsibility of administering medication

(2) "If the client can't swallow a time-released tablet, I will crush it."—time-released medications should not be crushed; if a client cannot take a medication prescribed, the nurse should call the practitioner and discuss the possibility of a different medication

(3) "It is okay to crush the client's extended-release tablet to put it in applesauce."—extended-release tablets should not be crushed

(4) "I can break this scored tablet for the partial dose ordered for the client."—CORRECT: scored tablets can be broken for a partial dose

251. The Answer is 2

The nurse is reviewing the lab work of a pediatric client admitted for chemotherapy treatment. For which of the following laboratory values should the nurse call the physician?

Reworded Question: Which laboratory values are most affected by chemotherapy?

Strategy: Think anemia.

Needed Info: Be familiar with the normal ranges of routine laboratory values. WBC ranges from 5–10 although chemotherapy will reduce the level to almost zero between doses. Hemoglobin levels are lower in anemia, which decreases the ability for blood to carry oxygen to tissue. If the doses are too low, transfusions may be ordered before chemotherapy. Chemotherapy destroys both good blood cells and cancerous cells, so blood counts are important when evaluating the risks of chemo and the ability for the client to tolerate the next round.

Category: Analysis/Physiological Integrity/Reduction of Risk Potential

(1) BUN 5, creatinine 0.7—these BUN and creatinine values are normal; would not postpone chemotherapy

(2) WBC 0, hemoglobin 2—CORRECT: a zero white blood cell count and a hemoglobin level of 2 would most likely postpone chemotherapy due to the severity of the anemia

(3) Hemoglobin 9.5, WBC 14—a normal hemoglobin level and an elevated WBC would be expected when taking chemotherapy and would not be a reason to postpone the dose unless the client was experiencing other symptoms of sepsis

(4) Magnesium 2—this is a normal magnesium value

252. The Answer is 2

The nurse is doing a follow-up telephone call with a new mother regarding her newborn. The mother states the baby's eyes look yellow. Which of the following is the *MOST* appropriate response by the nurse?

Reworded Question: What are the causes of newborn jaundice after discharge from the hospital?

Strategy: Think breastfeeding and hydration. The phrase *"MOST* appropriate" indicates that more than one answer may be correct.

Needed Info: You should have a basic understanding of newborn feeding and care, breastfeeding issues for the new mom, and the significance of jaundice in the newborn. Breastfeeding moms need to maintain good hydration and pay attention to how much milk they are producing for their newborn. You should understand the risks of dehydration for the infant and jaundice if it remains a long-term issue.

Category: Assessment/Physiological Integrity/Reduction of Risk Potential

(1) "How often are you nursing your baby?"—this should be the second question after finding out how the baby is being fed

(2) "Are you breastfeeding or bottle feeding?"—CORRECT: it is important to know how the baby is being fed; breastfed babies may have jaundice for a few days due to lack of milk production or not nursing well; bottle-fed infants who are taking the appropriate amount of formula tend to not be as jaundiced after discharge; determining how the infant is fed is important to assess the risk for dehydration

(3) "Do you know what your baby's bilirubin level was before discharge?"—the mother may know the bilirubin level at discharge but this is not the most important question; it may be part of the conversation, but the most important information is about the way the baby is being fed

(4) "Has your baby been seen by the pediatrician?"—the next pediatrician appointment is important but not before finding out how the baby eats and the hydration state of the infant

253. The Answer is 1

The nurse is assessing a young adult client who begins to have a grand mal seizure for the first time. Which of the following actions should the nurse do *FIRST*?

Reworded Question: What is the nurse's first response to a client having a seizure?

Strategy: Think ABCs and priority—this suggests that all the answers may be correct; however, one takes precedence.

Needed Info: Seizures can be life threatening if the airway becomes obstructed. Know the types of seizures, treatments, and the emergency care of a client who seizes. Understanding the causes of seizures can assist you in planning for the follow-up care of a client who has a seizure. First-time seizures often require a neurological workup including a CT scan or MRI of the brain. A seizing client must be protected from aspiration and choking by placing the client on her side or turning her head.

Category: Implementation/Physiological Integrity/Physiological Adaptation

(1) Protect the client's airway—CORRECT: the priority is to protect the client's airway and prevent aspiration; you can turn her head to the side or turn the client on her side

(2) Restrain the client—attempts to retrain can cause injury; it is better to move objects away,

lower the client to the floor, or protect the client from hitting the side rails if in bed

(3) Record the length of the seizure—you must record the length of the seizure but timing can be done while you protect the airway; airway always comes first

(4) Report this to the physician—you must report the seizure, but you would not leave a seizing client to report it; you may call others for help; someone else may call the physician, but the first responder stays with the client to protect the airway

254. The Answer is 3

The nurse is educating a client with a history of hyponatremia on diet choices. Which of the following statements by the client *BEST* indicates the teaching was successful?

Reworded Question: What foods promote adequate sodium retention?

Strategy: Think about nutrition and the food pyramid.

Needed Info: Know the symptoms of hyponatremia. Know the food sources best offering those nutrients. Helping a client to understand the symptoms and risks of low sodium may encourage the client to be more compliant with diet choices.

Category: Planning and Implementation/Physiological Integrity/Physiological Adaptation

(1) "I should maintain a low-sodium diet."—a low-sodium diet is not indicated for a client with a history of hyponatremia

(2) "I can drink as much beer as I want to."—beer is a diuretic beverage whose consumption should be limited by a client with a history of hyponatremia

(3) "I should avoid caffeine."—CORRECT: caffeine is a diuretic that a client with a history of hyponatremia should avoid

(4) "I should drink a lot of water."—excess water consumption increases risk of hyponatremia

255. The Answer is 2

The nurse is caring for an alert and oriented teen with a head injury who complains of a slight headache. Which of the following symptoms exhibited by the client would require immediate intervention by the nurse?

Reworded Question: What are the symptoms of increased intracranial pressure?

Strategy: Think of the risks of a brain hemorrhage, Glasgow coma scale, and intracranial pressure signs and symptoms.

Needed Info: Understand the symptoms of a mild concussion and more severe head injuries. Amnesia may be part of a mild head injury, but even mild injuries can be a risk for intracranial bleeding. Know the types of brain bleeding that can occur and what to look for.

Category: Assessment/Physiological Integrity/Physiological Adaptation

(1) The client complains of a continued headache and becomes drowsy—headache and drowsiness are common with a minor head injury

(2) The headache becomes worse and the client shows a decrease in the level of consciousness—CORRECT: an increase in headache and a decrease in level of consciousness requires medical intervention; choices are repeating CT scans, giving steroids to help with brain tissue swelling, inserting an ICP monitor, among other choices

(3) The client vomits one time and continues to have a slight headache—vomiting once or twice is a normal response to a minor head injury

(4) The client has no headache but has little memory of the incident—amnesia affects are normal with a minor head injury

256. The Answer is 3

The nurse is admitting a client to the neurology unit at the medical center. The nurse has arrived at the advance directive section of the initial nursing assessment flowsheet. The nurse assisting with the admission would intervene if the primary admitting nurse made which of the following statements to the client?

Reworded Question: What are the nurse's responsibilities when asking clients about advance directives?

Strategy: Think about each statement. Does it describe an inappropriate statement made by the nurse regarding advance directives?

Needed Info: The Centers for Medicare and Medicaid (CMS) require that clients are asked about their wishes regarding advance directives upon admission to an inpatient hospital setting.

Category: Implementation/Safe and Effective Care Environment/Management of Care

(1) "Do you have someone who would be a surrogate decision maker for you if you were unable to make decisions for yourself?"—this is an appropriate statement by the nurse

(2) "Are you familiar with what an advance directive is?"—this is an appropriate statement by the nurse

(3) "I should find out if you want an advance directive, but you seem tired and confused so I will ask you later."—CORRECT: this is an inappropriate statement by the nurse; unless the client is unable to comprehend due to a lack of capacity, the client should be asked about advance directives upon admission

(4) "Let me tell you a little bit about what an advance directive is so that you can decide if you want one set up."—this is an appropriate statement by the nurse

257. The Answer is 4

The nurse is caring for a client on the medical/surgical unit who is receiving an intravenous insulin drip due to severe uncontrollable episodic hyperglycemia. After several hours of administering the insulin and monitoring blood glucose levels regularly, the glucose levels are normalizing. The physician orders the nurse to maintain the IV insulin drip despite the nurse's concerns. Which of the following actions by the nurse is the *MOST* appropriate?

Reworded Question: What is a correct behavior?

Strategy: Think about the consequences of each action.

Needed Info: Nurses have a duty and ethical obligation to advocate for their clients even if they are in disagreement with the physician about a client's clinical status. The ultimate obligation is to the client and to providing appropriate and safe care. A physician's order alone will not protect a nurse's license or integrity.

Category: Implementation/Safe and Effective Care Environment/Management of Care

(1) The nurse should explain the procedure of administering the insulin intravenously to the client—this is good practice by the nurse but not the best answer given the circumstances of the scenario; this should be done *before* administering the drug

(2) The nurse should maintain the intravenous medication according to the physician's orders—the nurse still has an obligation to advocate for her client if her clinical judgment differs from that of the physician's; a physician's order alone is not enough reason to maintain a medication

(3) The nurse should wait until the next blood glucose level check is due and make a decision then about next steps—this is an inappropriate action because the client's blood glucose could dramatically drop in this time period

(4) The nurse should contact the nursing supervisor and possibly the supervisor of the physician who ordered the medication—CORRECT: this is an appropriate action by the nurse to prevent the client's blood glucose levels from dropping dramatically

258. The Answer is 1

The home care nurse is caring for an elderly client who lives alone. The nurse notices that the client is beginning to show signs of failure to thrive at home and has no family to assist him. The nurse is unsure how long this client will be able to remain in his home alone. Which of the following is the next step the nurse should take based on this assessment?

Reworded Question: What is the appropriate action by the nurse?

Strategy: Think about each response.

Needed Info: The home care nurse has other resources available to assist with the care of clients.

Home care agencies typically employ case managers, social workers, physical therapists, and other health care providers to assist their clients with their activities of daily living and care needs. Case managers can assist with proper placement of clients who require alternative levels of care and support. Case managers are aware of services available in communities and long-term care or rehabilitation facilities.

Category: Planning/Safe and Effective Care Environment/Management of Care

(1) The nurse should consult with the case manager employed by the home care agency—CORRECT: the nurse should utilize the resources available within the home care agency

(2) The nurse should call 911 for an emergency response due to concerns for safety—this is not the best action because the nurse is not concerned about an immediate risk of safety

(3) The nurse should call the client's community center for advice—this is not the best action; case managers specialize in this

(4) The nurse should call the client's neighbors to ask them to look in on the client—this is not the best action by the nurse due to confidentiality

259. The Answer is 1

The new staff nurse working on the intensive care unit is concerned about her client's status. The client has continued to decline throughout the shift. The client's blood pressure, heart rate, and oxygen saturation have progressively dropped in a relatively short period of time. The nurse inquires with the charge nurse assigned to that shift. The charge nurse says "Don't worry, the client will be fine, he always does that." Which of the following actions should the nurse take?

Reworded Question: What is the *most* appropriate action for the nurse to take?

Strategy: Determine the outcome of each answer choice.

Needed Info: The nurse caring for the client has the ultimate responsibility and ethical obligation to act on behalf of the client. If the new nurse is concerned for the client's status, and the charge nurse is not inducing actions that support the appropriate

provision of care that the client needs, the new nurse must escalate up the chain of command to enlist the support of supervisors and leadership to help the client.

Category: Implementation/Safe and Effective Care Environment/Management of Care

(1) The nurse should call the nursing supervisor on duty to assist—CORRECT: the nurse should escalate up the chain of command to advocate for the client

(2) The nurse should wait and see how the client does—this is incorrect because the client is exhibiting serious symptoms that could represent a grave diagnosis

(3) The nurse should agree with the charge nurse because that nurse has more experience—this is incorrect because the nurse must trust her own clinical judgment even if it is in conflict with a more senior nurse

(4) The nurse should discuss this with other nurses on the unit—this might be an appropriate strategy, but a supervisor can provide more immediate assistance

260. The Answer is 3

The nurse on a busy surgical unit has just received report from the previous shift on the clients assigned to that shift. Which of the following clients should the nurse see *FIRST*?

Reworded Question: Which client is least stable?

Strategy: Think ABCs.

Needed Info: The most unstable client should be seen first. The most urgent client needs should be attended to first.

Category: Analysis/Safe and Effective Care Environment/Management of Care

(1) A young adult client who fractured his arm while playing football, had surgical repair of the fracture, and is awaiting discharge—client is stable

(2) A middle-aged client recovering from a knee replacement who is currently on the continuous passive motion machine with the physical therapist—client is stable and not the first priority

(3) A middle-aged client recovering from abdominal surgery who is complaining of wheezing and has a new oxygen requirement—CORRECT: a new oxygen requirement is concerning postoperatively and could indicate a complication of the surgery

(4) An elderly client 1-day post-op for a hip replacement whose blood pressure is elevated—you would want to attend to the blood pressure, but based on the facts given, it is not as urgent as the client recovering from abdominal surgery

261. The Answer is 2

On a medical/surgical unit, each nurse is paired with nursing assistive personnel (NAP) for the night shift. The nurse should assign which of the following clients to the NAP?

Reworded Question: Which client is an appropriate assignment for the NAP?

Strategy: Think about the skill level involved in each client's care.

Needed Info: NAPs are considered unlicensed assistive personnel. They assist clients with activities of daily living (ADL). They cannot perform activities that require nursing judgment or assessment.

Category: Planning/Safe and Effective Care Environment/Management of Care

(1) A middle-aged client receiving chemotherapy and complaining of nausea and vomiting—requires nursing judgment/assessment

(2) A middle-aged client who is an unstable diabetic requiring a blood glucose level check—CORRECT: although the client is considered unstable, the check can be done by the NAP; the nurse can then subsequently make a decision about how to react to the level appropriately

(3) An elderly client complaining of pain from restless leg syndrome—this requires a nurse to assess the pain

(4) A young adult client recovering from a drug overdose requesting to leave the unit against medical advice—not an appropriate assignment for the NAP

262. The Answer is 1

The nurse is working on a state-of-the-art nursing unit with completely electronic medical records. The rooms are semi-private, with two clients to a room, and equipped with a computer for each client. Which of the following actions by the nurse is the *MOST* appropriate?

Reworded Question: What behavior is acceptable?

Strategy: Consider each answer.

Needed Info: Although electronic medical records offer certain amounts of protection of protected health information (PHI), the Health Insurance Portability and Accountability Act (HIPAA) mandates that other necessary safeguards be put in place.

Category: Analysis/Safe and Effective Care Environment/Management of Care

(1) After each use of the computer and upon leaving the client room, log off from the computer—CORRECT: this is the most appropriate answer because the rooms are not completely private and leave the information vulnerable to be seen by others

(2) After each use of the computer and upon leaving the client room, face the computer away from where visitors would be able to see the screen—this is not the most appropriate action because it is still possible for visitors to see PHI

(3) The nurse should not be concerned about the security of the information because there is a single computer for each client and therefore no risk of the information being seen—not enough security

(4) The nurse should pull the curtain to cover the computer screen so that visitors cannot view it—not enough security

263. The Answer is 2

The nurse is working on a unit that is equipped with electronic medication administration processes. This includes a computer at the bedside that allows for scanning a bar code on the medication order, the medication label, and the client's identification band. Which of the following is the *BEST* method for the nurse to practice regularly?

Reworded Question: What is a best practice for nurses who work with medication administration bar-coding?

Strategy: Consider each answer.

Needed Info: Electronic medication administration programs such as scanners that use bar-coding encourage safer practices and promote the reduction of errors in the medication administration process. However, a machine does not take the place of nursing clinical judgment. Appropriate nursing judgment and practices are paramount.

Category: Analysis/Safe and Effective Care Environment/Management of Care

(1) The nurse should rely solely on the bar-coding scanner because it promotes safer medication administration practices—although bar-coding scanners promote safer medication administration practices, they do not replace the judgment of the nurse

(2) The nurse should rely on a combination of nursing judgment and decision-making along with the computerized system—CORRECT: computers do not take the place of nursing judgment

(3) The nurse should never give a medication that a bar-coding system scans as "incorrect medication"—this is not true; computerized systems can have glitches and improper codes inadvertently in the system; the nurse should confirm the order, the medication, and the client, and then make the decision to administer or not based on nursing judgment

(4) The nurse should override any medication that the machine scans as "incorrect medication" and administer it—this may be true in certain situations, but there is not enough information provided to determine if that is the case

264. The Answer is 3

The nurse is administering medications to a client on an inpatient psychiatric unit. The client states "I don't usually take a pink pill" when the nurse gives a cup holding 4 different pills to the client. Which of the following is the *MOST* appropriate response by the nurse?

Reworded Question: How should a nurse handle a client's concerns about medications?

Strategy: Consider each answer.

Needed Info: The Joint Commission (TJC) promotes the practice of medication reconciliation, safety of using medications, and involving the client as a partner in the client's care. The Institute of Medicine (IOM) also promotes partnering with clients.

Category: Implementation/Safe and Effective Care Environment/Safety and Infection Control

(1) The nurse checks the medication administration record, determines it is correct, and tells the client to take the medication—not an appropriate response; the nurse is not including the client as a partner in the client's care

(2) The nurse discounts the client's concern because he is a psychiatric client and doesn't know any better—being a psychiatric client does not automatically make the client unable to participate in his or her own care

(3) The nurse asks the client for a list of medications he routinely takes, and tells the client that she will review and confirm the order with the physician—CORRECT: best response, validates client's concern

(4) The nurse tells the client that sometimes drugs come in different colors depending on what pharmacy they come from—not an appropriate response even though it may be true; still need to confirm it is the appropriate drug and alleviate the client's concerns

265. The Answer is 4

The nurse is working at a skilled nursing facility. The nurse enters the client's room and sees the client attempting to pull himself up from a sitting position on the floor. The nurse inquires with the client as to what happened. The client responds "I fell." Which of the following should the nurse document in the incident report?

Reworded Question: How does a nurse report an event?

Strategy: Determine the outcome of each answer choice.

Needed Info: As a measure of tracking and of preventing future events, the nurse is required to report events or injuries that are not expected with the typical provision of care. When reporting, the nurse should state events factually and objectively.

Category: Implementation/Safe and Effective Care Environment/Safety and Infection Control

(1) The nurse should file an incident report stating "Client fell, no injury noted."—not an appropriate answer because the nurse did not witness the client fall

(2) The nurse should file an incident report stating "Client fell on floor."—not an appropriate answer because the nurse did not witness the client fall

(3) The nurse should document the event only in the client's medical record and not in an incident report—although the event should be documented in the client's medical record, the event should be documented in an incident report as well

(4) The nurse should file an incident report stating "Client found on floor. Client stated "I fell." Assessment completed, no injury noted, physician notified."—CORRECT: this is the best answer that states the facts objectively

PART 4

THE LICENSURE PROCESS

CHAPTER 12

APPLICATION, REGISTRATION, AND SCHEDULING

The process of obtaining an American nursing license requires a definite sequence of actions by the candidate. Because this may be your first experience with the RN licensure process, and because there are no established test dates, you may have difficulty knowing exactly how to complete the paperwork and go through the process. This chapter will give you a checklist to follow when planning to take the NCLEX-RN® exam. This is a general list, so you must individualize it according to the requirements for the state in which you wish to become licensed; see Appendix D, State Licensing Requirements, for information on individual state requirements. We will outline the questions that you need to ask and the steps you need to take to complete the licensure process.

HOW TO APPLY FOR THE NCLEX-RN® EXAM

During your last semester of nursing school, you will be given the following applications:

(1) Application for licensure that goes to your state board of nursing

(2) Application for the NCLEX-RN® exam that goes to Pearson VUE

On a predetermined date, you will submit the completed forms and the required licensure fees to your nursing school.

Application Fees

- The NCLEX-RN® exam fee is $200. Additional licensure fees are determined by each state nursing board; see Appendix D, State Licensing Requirements, to determine your state's fee.

- You are responsible for submitting the completed test application and the $200 fee to Pearson VUE. Starting January 1, 2014, all applications will be processed by phone or online; applications by mail will no longer be accepted.

The Registration Process

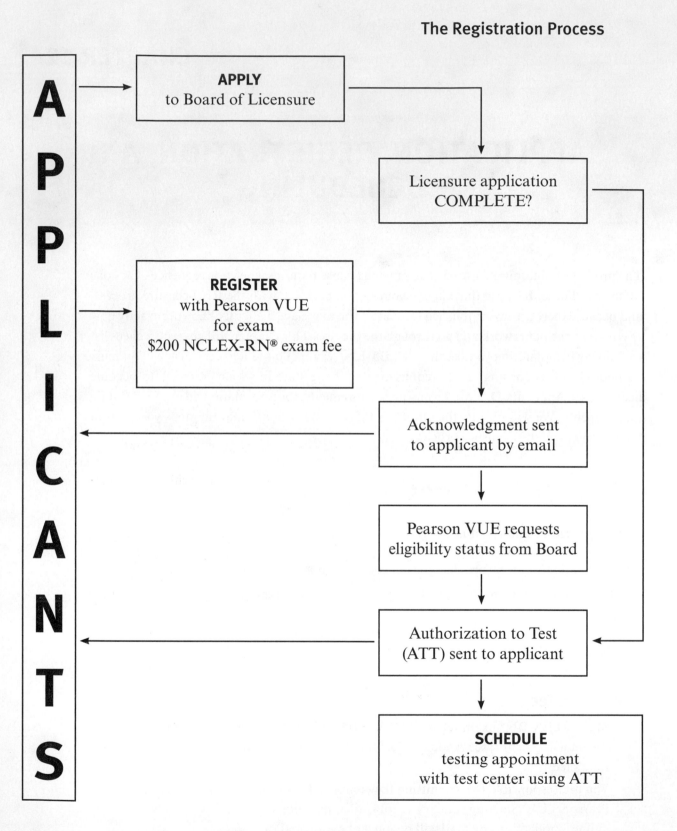

APPLICANTS

APPLY
to Board of Licensure

Licensure application
COMPLETE?

REGISTER
with Pearson VUE
for exam
$200 NCLEX-RN® exam fee

Acknowledgment sent
to applicant by email

Pearson VUE requests
eligibility status from Board

Authorization to Test
(ATT) sent to applicant

SCHEDULE
testing appointment
with test center using ATT

Applicant must APPLY, REGISTER, and SCHEDULE

Registration

You can register for the NCLEX-RN® exam with Pearson VUE using either of the following two methods:

(1) *Internet Registration:* To register online, go to *pearsonvue.com/nclex* (the NCLEX® candidate website). There are two general payment options: credit or debit card (using VISA, MasterCard or American Express) or money order, cashier's check, or certified check. If you choose the latter, upon completion of the registration information, you will be provided with directions to print a confirmation document that should be mailed with a certified check, cashier's check, or money order (made payable to the National Council of State Boards of Nursing) in U.S. currency drawn on a bank in the United States to:

> NCLEX Operations
> P.O. Box 64950
> St. Paul, MN 55164-0950

(2) *Telephone Registration:* Call VUE NCLEX Candidate Services at 1-866-496-2539 (1-866-49-NCLEX). To register by phone, you must pay using a VISA, MasterCard, or American Express credit or debit card. Even if you register by phone, you must provide an email address to receive communications from Pearson VUE about your registration.

As of January 1, 2014, Pearson VUE no longer accepts registrations submitted by mail.

Some states require that the testing application form and fee be sent along with the licensure application and fee.

For more information, visit *ncsbn.org* and download the *2014 NCLEX-RN® Examination Candidate Bulletin*. For questions regarding registering to take the NCLEX® exam, your Authorization to Test (ATT), a lost ATT, acceptable forms of identification, or comments about the test center, visit the NCLEX® candidate website (*pearsonvue.com/nclex*) or contact:

> NCLEX® Candidate Services
> 1-866-496-2539 (1-866-49-NCLEX)
>
> NCLEX-RN® Examination Program
> Pearson Professional Testing
> 5601 Green Valley Drive
> Bloomington, MN 55437-1099
> *pvamericascustomerservice@pearson.com*

How Do You Know Your Application Has Been Received?

You will receive a card from your state board stating that all of your information has been received.

Potential Problems with Licensure Application

Some states require that your permanent transcript be mailed with your application.

Here is a checklist to help avoid problems with your application:

- Have you met all requirements for graduation? Do you have any electives still outstanding?
- Has your nursing school received a permanent transcript for any credits that you transferred from another institution?
- Do you owe any fines or have any unpaid parking tickets? (This can delay the release of your permanent transcript. Check at your nursing school office, just to be sure.)
- Some states require that a statement be sent from your nursing school stating that you have met all requirements for graduation.
- Did you change your mind about the state in which you want to apply for licensure? If so, you must apply to a new state—and forfeit the original application fee.

What If You Want to Apply for Licensure in a Different State?

If you plan to apply for licensure in a different state from the one in which you are attending nursing school, contact the state board of nursing in the state in which you wish to become licensed (refer to Appendix D, State Licensing Requirements).

Here's a checklist for obtaining a license in another state:

- Call or write the state board of nursing of that state and find out what their requirements are for licensure.
- Find out what their fees are.
- Request a new candidate application for licensure.

After you pass the NCLEX-RN® exam, you will receive your nursing license from the state in which you applied for licensure regardless of where you took your exam. For example, if you applied for licensure in Michigan, you can take the test in Florida, if you wish. You would then receive a license to practice as an RN in Michigan because that is where you applied for licensure.

When Can You Schedule Your NCLEX-RN® Exam?

Pearson VUE will send you a document entitled "Authorization to Test" (ATT). The ATT will be sent to you via email at the email address you provided when you registered. You will be unable to schedule your test date until you receive this form.

On the ATT is your assigned candidate number; you will need to refer to this when scheduling your exam. Your ATT is valid for a time determined by the individual state board of nursing, and you must test before your ATT expires. If you don't, you will need to reapply to take the exam and pay the testing fees again. With your ATT, you will receive a list of test centers (see Appendix E for a current listing). You can schedule your NCLEX-RN® exam using the following procedures:

- Log on to the NCLEX® Candidate Website at *pearsonvue.com/nclex*
- Call NCLEX® Candidate Services
  - United States: 1-866-496-2539 (1-866-49-NCLEX) (toll-free)
  - Asia Pacific Region: +603-8314-9605 (pay number)
  - Europe, Middle East, Africa (EMEA): +44-161-855-7445 (pay number)
  - India: 91-120-439-7837 (pay number)
  - All other countries not listed above: 1-952-905-7403 (pay number)

Candidates with hearing impairments who use a Telecommunications Device for the Deaf (TDD) can call the U.S.A. Relay Service at 1-800-627-3529 (toll-free) or the Canada & International Inbound relay service at 1-605-224-1837 (pay number).

Those with special testing requests, such as persons with disabilities, must call the NCLEX-RN® Program Coordinator at NCLEX® Candidate Services at one of the numbers listed above. If you require special accommodations, you cannot schedule your exam through the NCLEX® Candidate Website.

There is a space on the ATT for you to record the date and time of your scheduled exam. You will also receive confirmation of your scheduled date and time.

Potential Rescheduling Problems

- You must test prior to the expiration date of your ATT. If you miss your appointment, you forfeit your testing fees and must reapply to both the state board of nursing and Pearson VUE.
- If you wish to change your appointment, you must notify Pearson VUE during business hours, at least 24 hours prior to your scheduled appointment. Call one of the numbers listed above or go the NCLEX® candidate website (*pearsonvue.com/nclex*). If your test date is on Saturday, Sunday, or Monday, make sure to call on or before Friday.

Do not call the test site directly or leave a message on an answering machine if you are unable to take your test on the scheduled date. You must follow the procedure listed above.

When Will You Take the Exam?

The earliest date on which you can take the NCLEX-RN® exam varies depending on your state, but the majority of students test approximately 45 days after the date of their graduation. Variables include: when you submit the applications and fees, the length of time the ATT is valid, personal factors (weddings, births, vacations), and job requirements. Each state determines the requirements for graduate nurses, licensure pending. If you are working as a graduate nurse, you must be knowledgeable about the rules in your state.

TAKING THE EXAM

What Happens on the Day of My NCLEX-RN® Exam?

Arrive at the test center at least 30 minutes before your scheduled test time. Wear layered clothing—the rooms may be cool in the morning but can warm up as the day progresses.

Here's a checklist of things to bring on the day of the exam:

- Your Authorization to Test (ATT).
- One form of signed identification that includes a picture. If you have changed your hair color, lost weight, or grown a beard, have a new picture ID made before test day. The name on your ID must match exactly the name on your ATT. Acceptable forms of identification include driver's license, state/province identification, passport, and U.S. military ID.
- A snack and something to drink.
- Do not bring any study materials to the test center.

Check-in procedure:

- Present your ATT.
- Present your picture ID.
- Sign in.
- A computer picture will be taken of you.
- You will be fingerprinted and may have your palm vein pattern scanned.
- All of your belongings will be placed in a locker outside the testing room.
- Earplugs are available on request. Request them, in case you find yourself distracted by background noise.

Where Will I Take My Test?

You will be in a room separate from the rest of the test center. Many testing sites consist of a room with 10–15 computers placed around the outside walls. Each computer sits on a full-size desk, with an adjustable chair for you to sit on. There are dividers between desks, but you will be able to see the person sitting next to you. There is a picture window from which the proctor will observe each person testing. There are also video cameras and sound sensors mounted on the walls to monitor each candidate.

What Will the Computer Screen Look Like?

The number of the question you are answering is located in the lower-right side of your computer screen. In the upper-right corner is a digital clock that counts down from 6:00—representing the six hours you have to complete the short tutorial that begins the exam, the exam itself, and all breaks.

If the question is a traditional four-option, text-based, multiple-choice question, the question stem is located in the top half of the screen and the four answer choices are located in the lower half of the screen (Figure 1). Radio buttons are in front of each answer choice.

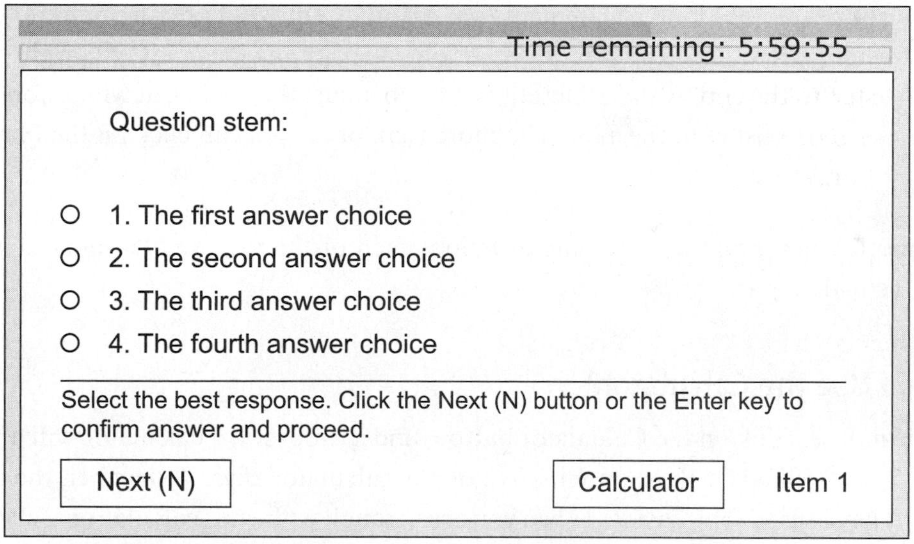

```
                                    Time remaining: 5:59:55

    Question stem:

    O   1. The first answer choice
    O   2. The second answer choice
    O   3. The third answer choice
    O   4. The fourth answer choice

    ──────────────────────────────────────────────────
    Select the best response. Click the Next (N) button or the Enter key to
    confirm answer and proceed.

    [  Next (N)  ]                    [  Calculator  ]     Item 1
```

Figure 1

You will notice that there are two buttons at the bottom of the computer screen. You use the Next (N) button to confirm your answer selection and move to the next question. Click the Calculator button to display a drop-down calculator that can be used to perform computations.

If the question is an alternate question that may have more than one correct answer, you will see the phrase, "Select all that apply" between the stem of the question and five or six answer choices. A small box is in front of each answer choice. The Next (N) button and Calculator button are at the bottom of the computer screen.

If the question is a hot spot alternate question, the screen will contain a graphic or a picture. The Next (N) button and Calculator button are at the bottom of the computer screen.

If the question is a fill-in-the-blank alternate question, a text box will be under the question. The Next (N) button and Calculator button are at the bottom of the computer screen.

If the question is a drag-and-drop/ordered response alternate question, the unordered options will be under the question and to the left. The space for the ordered response will be to the right of the unordered options. The Next (N) button and Calculator button are at the bottom of the screen.

If the question is a chart/exhibit alternate question, it will include the following prompt after the question stem: "Click on the exhibit button below for additional client information." The Exhibit button is located in the bottom of the computer screen between the Next (N) button and the Calculator button. Click on the Exhibit button to display a pop-up box containing 3 tabs. Click on each of the tabs to display information needed to answer the question.

If the question is an audio alternate question, the question will contain an audio clip that you must listen to in order to answer the question. Click on the Play button (a right-pointing arrow) to listen to the clip. A slider bar allows you to adjust the volume at which you hear the clip. If you want to listen to the audio clip more than once, you can click on the Play button again.

If the question is a graphics alternate question, each of the four answer choices will be a graphic instead of text.

How Do I Use the Calculator?

Using the mouse, click on the Calculator button, and a drop-down calculator will appear on the computer screen. Use the mouse to click on the calculator keys. Remember, the diagonal or slash (/) key is used for division. When you are through with your calculations, click on the Calculator button again, and the calculator will disappear.

How Do I Select an Answer Choice for Traditional, Four-Option, Multiple-Choice Questions?

You will use a two-step process to answer each question. Read the question and select an answer by using the mouse to click on the radio button preceding your answer choice. Your answer is now highlighted. When you are certain of your answer, click on the Next (N) button or the Enter key to confirm your answer. Your answer is now locked in and a new question will appear on the screen. *You are not able to change your answer after clicking on the Next (N) button or pressing the Enter key, so be certain of your answer before doing so.*

After your answer is entered into the computer, the computer selects a new question for you based on the accuracy of your previous answer and the components of the NCLEX-RN® exam test plan. If you answer a question correctly, the next question selected by the computer is more difficult. If you answer a question incorrectly, the next question selected by the computer is easier.

What If I Want to Change the Answer That I Have Highlighted?

If you want to change the highlighted answer, click on a different answer choice. Your answer is not locked in until you click on the Next (N) button or press the Enter key.

Even if you've never used a computer before, don't panic. You will be given instructions at the beginning of the test, and you will have to answer three tutorial questions before your test begins. These questions allow you to practice using the mouse to select an answer.

How Do I Select an Answer Choice for Select All That Apply Questions?

Read the question and click on the small box in front of the answer choice you want. A small check will appear in the box. Click on each answer choice that answers the question.

What If I Want to Change an Answer That I Have Checked?

If you change your mind and don't want an answer choice that you have selected, just click again on the small box in front of that answer choice and the check will disappear. When you are certain of your answer, click on the Next (N) button or press the Enter key to confirm your answer. Your answer is now locked in and a new question appears on the screen.

How Do I Select an Answer Choice for Hot Spot Questions?

To answer a hot spot alternate question, just click on the area of the graphic or picture that answers the question.

What If I Want to Change the Area That I Have Selected?

If you change your mind and want to select another area of the graphic or picture, just use your mouse to click on the area that you want and the original selection disappears. When you are certain of your answer, click on the Next (N) button or press the Enter key to confirm your answer. Your answer is now locked in and a new question appears on the screen.

How Do I Enter an Answer Choice for Fill-in-the-Blank Questions?

To enter an answer for a fill-in-the-blank question, just use the keyboard to select the numbers or letters you want. If a unit of measurement already appears next to the answer box on the screen, be sure you enter *numbers* only into the answer box; adding a unit of measurement may cause your answer to be wrong.

What If I Want to Change What I Have Entered in the Text Box?

If you change your mind and want to enter another answer in the text box, just backspace over the answer you entered and then use the keyboard to enter another answer. When you are certain of your answer, click on the Next (N) button or press the Enter key to confirm your answer. Your answer is now locked in and a new question appears on the screen.

How Do I Select Options for Drag-and-Drop/Ordered Response Questions?

To put the responses in the correct order, click on the option you think should come first, hold down the button on the mouse, and drag the option over to the box on the right side of the screen. You may also highlight the option in the box on the left side and then click the arrow key that points to the box on the right side to move the option. Do the same with each response in the proper order.

What If I Want to Change the Order of My Responses?

If you change your mind about a response, click on it with the mouse and drag it back to the left side of the screen or use the arrow key as described above. To complete the question, you must move all options from the box on the left side of the screen to the box on the right side. When you are certain of your answer, click on the Next (N) button or press the Enter key to confirm your answer. Your answer is now locked in and a new question appears on the screen.

How Do I Enter or Change an Answer Choice for Chart/Exhibit, Audio, and Graphics Alternate Questions?

Chart/exhibit, audio, and graphics alternate questions all use a four-option, multiple-choice format, so you can enter or change your answer choices just as you would for traditional text-based, four-option, multiple-choice questions.

Do I Get Any Breaks?

You will receive an optional break at the end of two hours of testing. There will be a pre-programmed prompt offering you a break. Leave the testing room, stretch your legs and eat your snack. Take some deep, cleansing breaths and get yourself ready to go back into the testing room. The computer will offer you another optional break after 3½ hours of testing. We recommend that you take it unless you feel you're on a roll.

You may take a break at any time during your test, but the time that you spend away from your computer is counted as a part of your six hours of total testing time. Kaplan recommends that you take a short (2–5 minute) break if you are having trouble concentrating. Take time to go to the restroom, eat your snack, or get a drink. This will enable you to maintain or regain your concentration for the test. Remember, every question counts! If you need to take a break, raise your hand to notify the test administrator. You must leave the testing room, and you will be required to take a palm vein scan before you are allowed to resume your test.

How Will I Know When My Test Ends?

A screen will appear on your computer that states, "Your test is concluded." You will then be required to answer several exit questions. These are a few multiple-choice questions about your impression of the examination experience. They do not count toward your results.

How Long Will It Take to Receive My Results?

Your results are sent to you by your state board of nursing. Each state board determines when the NCLEX-RN® exam results are released. In the following jurisdictions, you may access your "unofficial" results two business days after taking your examination via the NCLEX® candidate website (for a $7.95 fee):

> Alaska, Arizona, Colorado, Connecticut, District of Columbia, Florida, Georgia, Hawaii, Idaho, Illinois, Indiana, Iowa, Kansas, Kentucky, Louisiana, Maine, Maryland, Massachusetts, Michigan, Minnesota, Mississippi, Missouri, Montana, Nebraska, Nevada, New Jersey, New Mexico, New York, North Carolina, North Dakota, Ohio, Oklahoma, Oregon, Pennsylvania, Rhode Island, South Carolina, South Dakota, Tennessee, Texas, U.S. Virgin Islands, Utah, Vermont, Washington, Wisconsin, Wyoming

For most states, you will receive your official results approximately one month after your test date.

CHAPTER 13

TAKING THE TEST MORE THAN ONCE

Some people may never have to read this chapter, but it's a certainty that others will. The most important advice we can give to repeat test takers is: Don't despair. There is hope. We can get you through the NCLEX-RN® exam.

YOU ARE NOT ALONE

Think about that awful day when the big brown envelope arrived. You just couldn't believe it. You had to tell family, friends, your supervisor, and coworkers that you didn't pass the NCLEX-RN® exam. When this happens, each unsuccessful candidate feels like he or she is the only person who has failed the exam.

HOW TO INTERPRET UNSUCCESSFUL TEST RESULTS

Most unsuccessful candidates on the NCLEX-RN® exam will usually say, "I almost passed." Some of you did almost pass, and some of you weren't very close. If you fail the exam, you will receive a diagnostic profile from NCSBN. In this profile, you will be told how many questions you answered on the exam. The more questions you answered, the closer you came to passing. The only way you will continue to get questions after you answer the first 75 is if you are answering questions close to the level of difficulty needed to pass the exam. If you are answering questions far above the level needed to pass or far below the level needed to pass, your exam will end at 75 questions.

Figure 1 on the next page shows a representation of what happens when a candidate fails in 75 questions. This student does not come close to passing. In 75 questions, this student demonstrates an inability to consistently answer questions correctly at or above the level of difficulty needed to pass the exam. This usually indicates a lack of nursing knowledge, considerable difficulties with taking a standardized test, or a deficiency in critical thinking skills.

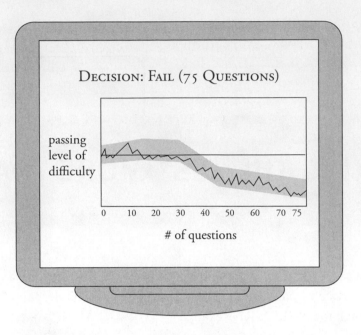

Figure 1

Figure 2 shows what happens when a candidate takes all 265 questions and fails. This candidate "almost passed." The candidate answers question 264 and the computer does not make a determination when it selects the last question. If the last question is below the level of difficulty needed to pass, the candidate fails.

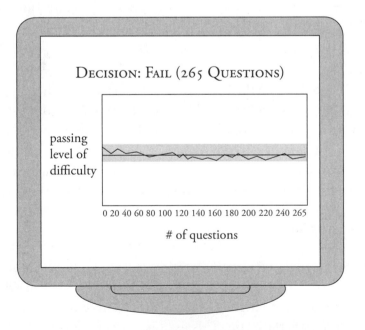

Figure 2

If the last question is above the level of difficulty needed to pass, the candidate passes. If you took a test longer than 75 questions and failed, you were probably familiar with most of the content you saw on the exam but you may have difficulty using critical thinking skills or taking standardized tests.

The information contained on the diagnostic profile helps you identify your strengths and weaknesses on this particular NCLEX-RN® exam. This knowledge will help you identify where to concentrate your study when you prepare to retake the NCLEX-RN® exam.

SHOULD YOU TEST AGAIN?

Absolutely! You completed your nursing education to become an RN. The initial response of many unsuccessful candidates is to declare, "I'm never going back! That was the worst experience of my life! What do I do now?"

When you first received your results, you went through a period of grieving—the same stages that you learned about in nursing school. Three to four weeks later, you find that you want to begin preparing to retake the NCLEX-RN® exam.

HOW SHOULD YOU BEGIN?

You should prepare in a different way this time. Whatever you did to prepare last time didn't work well enough. The most common mistake that candidates who failed make is to assume that they did not study hard enough or learn enough content. For some of you, that's true. But for the majority of you, memorizing more content does not mean more right answers. It could simply mean more frustration for you.

The first step in preparing for your next exam is to make a commitment that you will test again. Decide when you want to schedule your test and allow yourself enough time to prepare. Mark this test date on your calendar. You can do all of this before you send in your fees and receive your authorization to test. Remember, you cannot retake the NCLEX-RN® exam for 45 to 90 days, depending on your state board of nursing, so you may as well use this time wisely.

The next step is to figure out why you failed the NCLEX-RN® exam. Check off any reasons that pertain to you:

- ☐ I didn't know the nursing content.
- ☐ I memorized facts without understanding the principles of client care.
- ☐ I had unrealistic expectations about the NCLEX-RN® exam test questions.
- ☐ I had difficulty correctly identifying THE REWORDED QUESTION.

☐ I had difficulty staying focused on THE REWORDED QUESTION.

☐ I found myself predicting answer choices.

☐ I did not carefully consider each answer choice.

☐ I am not good at choosing answers that require me to establish priorities of care.

☐ I answered questions based on my real-world experiences.

☐ I did not cope well with the computer-adaptive test experience.

☐ I thought I would complete the exam in 75 questions.

☐ When I got to question 200, I totally lost my concentration and just answered questions to get through the rest of the exam.

After determining why you failed, the next step is to establish a plan of action for your next test. Remember, you should prepare differently this time. Consider the following when setting up your new plan of study.

You've seen the test.

You may wish that you didn't have to walk back into the testing center again, but if you want to be a registered professional nurse, you must go back. This time you have an advantage over the first-time test taker: you've seen the test! You know exactly what you are preparing for, and there are no unknowns. The computer will remember what questions you took before, and you will not be given any of the same questions. However, the content of the question, the style of the question, and the kinds of answer choices will not change. You will not be surprised this time.

Study both content and test questions.

By the time you retest, you will be out of nursing school for 6 months or longer. Remember that old saying, "What you are not learning, you are forgetting"? Because this is a content-based test about safe and effective nursing care, you must remember all you can about nursing theory in order to select correct answers. You must study content that is integrated and organized like the NCLEX-RN® exam.

You must also master exam-style test questions. It is essential that you be able to correctly identify what each question is asking. You will *not* predict answers. You will *think* about each and every answer choice to decide if it answers the reworded question. In order to master test questions, you must practice answering them. We recommend that you answer hundreds of exam-style test questions, especially at the application level of difficulty.

Know all of the words and their meanings.

Some students who have to learn a great deal of material in a short period of time have trouble learning the extensive vocabulary of the discipline. For example, difficulty with terminology is a problem for many good students who study history. They enjoy the concepts but find it hard to memorize all of the names and dates to allow them to do well on history tests. If you have trouble memorizing terms, you may find it useful to review a list of the terminology that you must know to pass the NCLEX-RN® exam. There is a list of those words at the end of this book.

Practice test-taking strategies.

There is no substitute for mastering the nursing content. This knowledge, combined with test-taking strategies, will help you to select a greater number of correct answers. For many students, the strategies mean the difference between a passing test and a failing test. Using strategies effectively can also determine whether you take a short test (75 questions) or a longer test (up to 265 questions).

Evaluate your testing experience.

Some students attribute their failure to the testing experience. Comments we have heard include:

> *"I didn't like answering questions on the computer."*
>
> *"I found the background noise distracting. I should have taken the earplugs!"*
>
> *"I looked up every time the door opened."*
>
> *"I should have taken a snack. I got so hungry!"*
>
> *"After 2½ hours I didn't care what I answered. I just wanted the computer to shut off!"*
>
> *"I didn't expect to be there for four hours!"*
>
> *"I should have rescheduled my test, but I just wanted to get it over with!"*
>
> *"I wish I had taken aspirin with me. I had such a headache before it was over!"*

Do any of these comments sound familiar? It is important for you to take charge of your testing experience. Here's how:

- Choose a familiar testing site.
- Select the time of day that you test your best. (Are you a morning person or an afternoon person?)
- Accept the earplugs when offered.
- Take a snack and a drink for your break.
- Take a break if you become distracted or fatigued during the test.
- Contact the proctors at the test site if something bothers you during the test.
- Plan on testing for six hours. Then, if you get out early, it's a pleasant surprise.
- Say to yourself every day, "I will pass the NCLEX-RN® exam."

CHAPTER 14

ESSENTIALS FOR INTERNATIONAL NURSES

Many of you have years of nursing experience in your home country. Now you are preparing for the NCLEX-RN® exam so you can be licensed to practice your profession in the United States. Because of Kaplan's extensive experience preparing nurses educated in other countries, we are very aware of the special issues that you face when trying to pass the NCLEX-RN® exam. Your special concerns will be discussed in this chapter.

Many nurses educated outside of the United States have not had the experience of taking an objective multiple-choice test as well as answering alternate question types, including those that require you to select more than one response, fill-in-the-blank questions, and pictures and graphs that require you to identify a "hot spot" or specific area on an image. Your testing experience may have been limited to oral exams or writing answers to essay and short answer questions. Multiple-choice tests are used in the United States because they measure knowledge more objectively and are easier to administer to large groups of people. In order to pass the NCLEX-RN® exam, you must demonstrate that you are a safe and effective nurse by correctly answering a predominantly multiple-choice test as well as the alternate question types.

NCLEX-RN® EXAM ADMINISTRATION ABROAD

NCSBN administers the NCLEX-RN® exam in selected international locations, including Australia, Canada, the United Kingdom, Hong Kong, India, Japan, Mexico, the Philippines, Puerto Rico, and Taiwan. (Testing is temporarily unavailable in Germany.) Please see *ncsbn. org* for details and *pearsonvue.com/nclex* to locate a test center near you.

These sites provide greater convenience for international nurses to take the NCLEX-RN® exam. The international administration does not circumvent any regulations posed by the state boards of nursing, and the test sites are subject to the same security and procedures followed in U.S. test sites. If you choose to take the test at one of these sites, you must pay an additional $150 international scheduling fee plus a Value Added Tax (VAT) where applicable.

THE CGFNS® CERTIFICATE

Before considering applications for licensure as a registered nurse in the United States, many U.S. state boards of nursing require internationally educated nurses to obtain a certificate from the Commission on Graduates of Foreign Nursing Schools (CGFNS®). Some states require applicants to complete this process before taking the NCLEX-RN® exam. The process of obtaining a CGFNS® certificate involves: (1) a review of your secondary and nursing education credentials and original nursing program, (2) passing the CGFNS® exam that tests nursing knowledge, and (3) obtaining a minimum score on a designated English language proficiency exam.

The CGFNS® exam is a two-part test of nursing knowledge. Nurses who pass this exam have been shown to be more likely to pass the NCLEX-RN® exam on the first try than nurses who have not. The CGFNS® exam can be taken overseas at a number of international testing sites run by CGFNS® or at selected sites in the United States.

Applications for the CGFNS® exam are free, and you may apply online at *cgfns.org*. Effective January 1, 2011, only online applications for the CGFNS® Certification Program are accepted. On the CGFNS® website, you will also find application deadlines and test dates. With an online application, you can submit your educational and professional documentation, choose a location and date for your exam, and pay fees by credit card. The online CGFNS Qualifying Exam® is administered in March, July, September, and November during a five-day testing window in each of these months.

To find out about a particular state's requirements for international nurses, contact that state's board of nursing and request an application packet for initial licensure as an internationally educated nurse. You can also visit your chosen state's website using the key words "Board of Nursing" and the state name. The phone numbers and addresses for each of the state boards of nursing in the United States are listed in Appendix D.

For detailed information regarding the CGFNS® English proficiency requirements, go to *cgfns.org*. The following information will help you register for the appropriate exams. Remember that these exam results are usually only valid for two years, so plan accordingly to avoid retakes. To learn more about preparing for these exams, see the Kaplan English Programs section at the end of this chapter.

> TOEFL®, TWE®, and TSE®
> Educational Testing Service
> P.O. Box 6151
> Princeton, NJ 08541-6151
> 1-800-468-6335 (United States, U.S. Territories, Canada)
> 1-443-751-4862 (all other locations)
> Fax: 1-610-290-8972
> Website: *www.ets.org/toefl*

TOEIC® Testing Program
Educational Testing Service
Rosedale Road
Princeton, NJ 08541
Phone: 1-609-771-7170
Fax: 1-610-628-3722
Email: *toeic@ets.org*
Website: *www.ets.org/toeic*

IELTS® International
825 Colorado Boulevard, Suite 201
Los Angeles, CA 90041
Phone 1-323-255-2771
Fax 1-323-255-1261
Website: *www.ielts.org*

WORK VISAS

For the most current information on visa requirements, contact the nearest U.S. embassy or consulate in your home country or the nearest regional office of the U.S. Citizenship and Immigration Services if you already live in the United States. You can also contact the CGFNS® by telephone at 1-215-222-8454, by mail at 3600 Market Street, Suite 400, Philadelphia, PA 19104-2665, or through its website at *cgfns.org*.

NURSING PRACTICE IN THE UNITED STATES

Some international nurses find nursing in the United States similar to nursing as they learned it in their country. For others, nursing in the United States is very different from what they learned or experienced in their country. The NCLEX-RN® exam may ask you questions about procedures that are unfamiliar to you. You may be asked questions about diets and foods that are new to you. In order to be successful on the NCLEX-RN® exam, you must be able to correctly answer questions about nursing as it is practiced in the United States.

Here is an overview of services and skills that U.S. nurses are expected to perform:

- Nurses are involved with prevention, early detection, and treatment of illness for people of all ages.
- Nurses care for the whole person, not just an illness. Their focus is on client needs; that is, how a client will respond to an illness.

- Nurses are professionals who are responsible for their actions.
- Nurses must communicate with clients and all the members of the health care team: other nurses, nursing assistive personnel, physicians, dietitians, pharmacists, therapists, technicians, and social workers.
- Nurses serve as clients' advocates; that is, they counsel clients and make sure their rights are protected.
- Nurses help clients understand the health care system, and assist clients to make decisions about their health care.
- Nurses are assertive and ask questions of health care professionals when necessary, including physicians. Their style of communication is polite and professional but very direct.
- Nurses are responsible for meeting the needs of clients whose care involves high-tech equipment.
- Nurses are responsible for basing their actions on knowledge and acceptable nursing practice.
- Nurses, not families, are responsible for all the hands-on nursing care for clients in the hospital setting.
- Nurses are responsible for teaching clients and their families how to manage their health care needs.

U.S.-STYLE NURSING COMMUNICATION

An issue of special concern for international nurses is therapeutic communication. Correctly answering the questions about communication can be difficult for some nurses educated in the United States. These questions become a special challenge to test takers for whom English is a second language, or for test takers who do not yet fully understand American-style communication.

Key features of U.S.-style communication in nursing:

- *Validate the client's experience and feelings by responding to the client verbally.* Ask questions that relate directly to what the client says.
- *Direct the client's behavior to promote comfort and well-being.* Do not patronize or reject the client by imposing a value judgment.
- *Maintain eye contact with the client, especially during conversation.* Lean forward to face the client. Nod, smile, or frown to demonstrate agreement or disagreement while listening.

Responses used in U.S. nursing are based on an assessment of the client's needs and are designed to foster growth and establish mutually formulated goals.

NCLEX-RN® exam questions concerning communication are best answered by:

- Conveying *respect* and *warmth*, making the client feel accepted and respected as an individual regardless of his or her words, actions, or behavior. This means that the nurse:

- Assumes that all client behavior is purposeful and has meaning even though it may not make sense to others
- Defines the social, physical, and emotional boundaries of the nurse-client relationship
- Develops a contract with the client
- Structures time to develop a nurse-client relationship
- Creates a safe and secure environment
- Accepts the dependency needs of the client while encouraging, assisting, and supporting movement toward health and independence
- Intervenes when a client behaves inappropriately to directly reject the behavior but not the client
- Intervenes directly to respond to the client, not to reinforce an inappropriate behavior

- Demonstrating active *listening* and *genuineness*. This means that the nurse:
  - Asks questions that relate directly to what the client says
  - Maintains good eye contact
  - Leans forward in the chair to face the client
  - Nods, smiles, or frowns to show agreement or disagreement
  - Understands that the personal feelings and past experiences of the nurse can negatively or positively affect relationships with clients

- Communicating *interest* and *empathy* by allowing the client to comfortably communicate concerns and behave in new ways. This means that the nurse:
  - Focuses conversation on the client's feelings
  - Understands that clients respond to the behavioral expectations of the nursing staff
  - Validates the client's feelings
  - Analyzes both verbal and nonverbal behavioral clues
  - Anticipates that there might be some difficulty as the client learns new behaviors

Nurses create barriers in the communication process when they demonstrate a poor understanding of the basics in therapeutic communication. They must convey respect, warmth, and genuineness through active listening and communicating interest and empathy about the concerns of clients, families, and/or staff.

Examples of barriers to communication:

- Minimizing concerns
- Giving false reassurance
- Giving approval
- Rejecting the person, not the behavior
- Choosing sides with the client, family member, or staff member in a conflict
- Blaming the external environment for the situation

- Disagreeing or arguing with the client or family member
- Offering advice about a situation
- Pressuring the client or family member for an explanation
- Defending one's own actions or behavior
- Belittling client, family member, or staff concerns
- Giving one-word responses to questions
- Using denial
- Interpreting or analyzing both verbal and nonverbal behavioral clues in the situation to the client
- Shifting the focus of the conversation away from the client, family member, or staff concerns
- Using jargon or medical terminology without explanation in conversation with the client and/or family
- Invalidating the client's, family member's, or staff's feelings
- Offering unrealistic hope for the future
- Ignoring client clues to help the client set appropriate limits on his or her behavior

The following are some questions that will allow you to practice the right approach.

SAMPLE QUESTIONS

Directions: Carefully read the question and all answer choices. Examine each answer choice and determine whether it is an appropriate response. Indicate your decision in the column labeled Correct/Incorrect and give the reason for your choice.

QUESTION	CORRECT/INCORRECT	REASON
1. A client has been hospitalized for 2 days for treatment of hepatitis A. When the nurse enters the client's room, he asks the nurse to leave him alone and stop bothering him. Which of the following responses by the nurse would be *MOST* appropriate? (1) "I understand and will leave you alone for now." (2) "Why are you angry with me?" (3) "Are you upset because you do not feel better?" (4) "You seem upset this morning."		
2. A client states she is afraid to have her cast removed from her fractured arm. Which of the following would be the *MOST* appropriate response by the nurse? (1) "I know it is unpleasant. Try not to be afraid. I will help you." (2) "You seem very anxious. I will stay with you while the cast is removed." (3) "I don't blame you. I'd be afraid also." (4) "My aunt just had a cast removed and she's just fine."		

QUESTION	CORRECT/ INCORRECT	REASON

3. A client comes to the clinic because she thinks she is pregnant. She tells the nurse that she wants the pregnancy terminated because she and her husband do not want to have children, and then begins to cry. Which of the following statements by the nurse would be the *MOST* appropriate?

   (1) "Are you upset because you forgot to use birth control?"

   (2) "Why are you so upset? You're married. There's no reason not to have the baby."

   (3) "If you're so upset, why don't you have the baby and put it up for adoption?"

   (4) "You seem upset. Let's talk about how you're feeling."

4. A client is in the terminal stages of carcinoma of the lung. A family member asks the nurse, "How much longer will it be?" Which of the following responses by the nurse would be *MOST* appropriate?

   (1) "I cannot say exactly. What are your concerns at this time?"

   (2) "I don't know. I'll call the doctor."

   (3) "This must be a terrible situation for you."

   (4) "Don't worry, it will be very soon."

	QUESTION	CORRECT/ INCORRECT	REASON

5. A client is admitted to the hospital with a diagnosis of manic-depressive disorder. The man approaches the nurse and says, "Hi, baby," and opens his robe, under which he is naked. Which of the following comments by the nurse would be *MOST* appropriate?

   (1) "This is inappropriate behavior. Please close your robe and return to your room."

   (2) "Please dress in your clothes and then join us for lunch in the dining room."

   (3) "I am offended by your behavior and will have to report you."

   (4) "Do you need some assistance dressing today?"

6. A client is placed in Buck's traction. The nurse assigned to her prepares to assist her with a bath. The woman says, "You're too young to know how to do this. Get me somebody who knows what they're doing." Which of the following responses by the nurse would be *MOST* appropriate?

   (1) "I am young, but I graduated from nursing school."

   (2) "If I don't bathe you now, you'll have to wait until I'm finished with my other clients."

   (3) "Can you be more specific about your concerns?"

   (4) "Your concerns are unnecessary. I know what I'm doing."

	QUESTION	CORRECT/ INCORRECT	REASON
7.	A client is admitted to the hospital with an abdominal mass and is scheduled for an exploratory laparotomy. She asks the nurse admitting her, "Do you think I have cancer?" Which of the following responses by the nurse would be *MOST* appropriate?		
	(1) "Would you like me to call your doctor so that you can discuss your specific concerns?"		
	(2) "Your tests show a mass. It must be hard not knowing what is wrong."		
	(3) "It sounds like you are afraid that you are going to die from cancer."		
	(4) "Don't worry about it now; I'm sure you have many healthy years ahead of you."		
8.	A client is admitted to the postpartum unit following a miscarriage. The next day the nurse finds the woman crying while looking at the babies in the newborn nursery. Which of the following approaches by the nurse would be *MOST* appropriate?		
	(1) Assure the woman that the loss was "for the best."		
	(2) Explain to her that she is young enough to have more children.		
	(3) Ask her why she is looking at the babies.		
	(4) Acknowledge the loss and be supportive.		

	QUESTION	CORRECT/ INCORRECT	REASON
9.	An elderly client is hospitalized with Alzheimer's disease. His daughter tells the nurse that caring for him is too hard, but that she feels guilty placing him in a nursing home. Which of the following statements by the nurse would be *MOST* appropriate? (1) "It is hard to be caught between taking care of your needs and your father's needs." (2) "Would you like me to help you find a nursing home?" (3) "Don't feel guilty. The only solution is to place your father in a nursing home." (4) "I think I would feel guilty too if I had to place my father in a nursing home."		

Read the explanations to these questions and make sure that the American approach to these communications questions is understandable to you. It will help you to choose the right answer on the NCLEX-RN® exam.

ANSWERS TO SAMPLE QUESTIONS

1. (4) **"You seem upset this morning,"** is the correct answer choice because the nurse seeks to verbally validate the client's behavior rather than simply respond to the behavior. This response promotes the nurse-client relationship by encouraging the client to share his feelings with the nurse.

   (1) *"I understand and will leave you alone for now,"* is not the best approach because it does not promote further communication between the nurse and the client about how the client is feeling. In order to interpret this client's behavior, the nurse must first validate it with the client.

   (2) *"Why are you angry with me?"* is incorrect. The nurse is drawing a conclusion about the client's behavior. This type of action is too confrontational. "Why" questions are considered nontherapeutic.

   (3) *"Are you upset because you do not feel better?"* is not the best choice. The nurse is drawing a conclusion about the client's behavior without validating it first. This type of response may also belittle the client's actual concerns.

2. (2) **"You seem very anxious. I will stay with you while the cast is removed,"** is the best response because the nurse responds to the client's feelings of fear. This is consistent with therapeutic communication used in American nursing. This response also provides an additional opportunity for the nurse to remain with the client in a supportive capacity, enhancing the nurse-client relationship.

   (1) *"I know it is unpleasant. Try not to be afraid. I will help you,"* is not the best response. It is not clear what concerns the client has about this procedure. The nurse should establish this before responding. The nurse falsely reassures the client by saying, "I will help you." Because you do not know the nature of the client's concerns, you cannot honestly offer help.

   (3) *"I don't blame you. I'd be afraid also,"* is not the correct response because the nurse shifts the focus of the conversation from the client to the nurse. This sets up a barrier to further communication. The nurse concedes the issue too quickly, leaving the source of the client's fear unknown.

   (4) *"My aunt just had a cast removed and she's just fine,"* is not the best choice. The focus of the conversation is shifted from the client to the nurse's aunt, who is of no concern to the client. This response fails to explore the source of the client's anxiety and sets up a block to further communication.

3. (4) **"You seem upset. Let's talk about how you're feeling,"** is the best answer to this question. This promotes the nurse-client relationship and illustrates therapeutic

communication used in American nursing. The nurse responds to the client's feelings in a nonjudgmental empathetic way.

(1) *"Are you upset because you forgot to use birth control?"* is inappropriate because it places blame on the client. The nurse should not assume that the client "forgot" to do something. This response also fails to respond to the client's feelings and does not encourage the client to discuss her concerns.

(2) *"Why are you so upset? You're married. There's no reason not to have the baby"* is inappropriate in terms of American therapeutic communication. This response is harsh, presumptive, and assumes that the purpose of every marriage is to have children. This is not always the case in American culture. With this response, the nurse does not attempt to verify the reason for the client's tears, thereby discouraging further conversation about what the client is actually experiencing.

(3) *"If you're so upset, why don't you have the baby and put it up for adoption?"* is also inappropriate. This is a value-laden assumption placing positive value on adoption. Again, the nurse fails to explore with the client the reason for the client's tears, thereby discouraging further communication. The nurse is also offering advice.

4. (1) **"I cannot say exactly. What are your concerns at this time?"** is the most appropriate response because it is unclear why the family member has approached the nurse at this point. Perhaps the client is in pain and the family member wants to discuss it with the nurse. This response allows for that possibility. This response is also direct and factually correct.

(2) *"I don't know. I'll call the doctor,"* is not the most appropriate response. It shifts the focus of responsibility from the nurse to the physician, which prevents a nurse-family member relationship from developing.

(3) *"This must be a terrible situation for you,"* is not the most appropriate response. It is a value-laden statement that fails to explore the family member's reason for approaching the nurse.

(4) *"Don't worry, it will be very soon,"* is inappropriate because the nurse offers the family member false reassurance. It also offers advice by telling the family member not to worry. This statement is demeaning and may sound as if the nurse is too busy to discuss the family member's concerns.

5. (1) **"This is inappropriate behavior. Please close your robe and return to your room,"** is the correct answer choice. This statement by the nurse responds to the client's behavior, sets limits on the behavior, and directs the client toward more appropriate social behavior in the milieu. This statement rejects the client's behavior, not the client as a person.

(2) *"Please dress in your clothes and then join us for lunch in the dining room,"* is incorrect. It ignores the behavior of the client exposing himself. Instead it directs the client to dress and report to the dining room for lunch as though nothing has happened. This is inappropriate and nontherapeutic.

(3) *"I am offended by your behavior and will have to report you,"* is incorrect. It shifts the focus from the client to the nurse and the nurse's feelings. The nurse's personal feelings are irrelevant. Also, the nurse goes on to threaten the client by reporting him. This is nontherapeutic.

(4) *"Do you need some assistance dressing today?"* is incorrect. This question fails to respond to the client's behavior. It is also a yes/no question, which is nontherapeutic.

6. (3) **"Can you be more specific about your concerns?"** is the correct answer. This is the best answer choice because it seeks to validate the client's message. It is direct, not defensive, and allows the client to express her point of view.

(1) *"I am young, but I graduated from nursing school,"* is incorrect. It responds to only part of the message that the client sent to the nurse. It assumes that the nurse knows what the client's concerns are and agrees that there is some problem associated with being too young. Further clarification is necessary in this situation.

(2) *"If I don't bathe you now, you'll have to wait until I'm finished with my other clients,"* is a nontherapeutic response. It fails to explore the client's concerns about the nurse. It is an uncaring and punitive statement by the nurse that is inappropriate in a nurse-client relationship.

(4) *"Your concerns are unnecessary. I know what I'm doing,"* is incorrect. The nurse dismisses the client's concerns by telling her that she shouldn't be concerned. The nurse should not tell a client how the client should be feeling. It may sound as if the nurse is trying to reassure the client by telling her that the nurse knows what he or she is doing; however, the nurse has yet to validate the concerns that underlie the client's statement.

7. (2) **"Your tests show a mass. It must be hard not knowing what is wrong,"** is the correct answer choice. This is the best answer choice because it responds to the client's feelings. It allows the client to continue to identify and express her concerns regarding surgery, hospitalization, and the possibility of having a potentially life-threatening illness. The nurse validates that the client has appropriate concerns and invites her to elaborate on them.

(1) *"Would you like me to call your doctor so that you can discuss your specific concerns?"* This response is incorrect because it shifts the focus of responsibility from the nurse to the doctor, thereby reducing the possibility of developing an ongoing nurse-client relationship.

(3) *"It sounds like you are afraid that you are going to die from cancer,"* is inappropriate. It fails to validate with the client that "dying from cancer" is in fact the issue. The nurse inappropriately concludes this on the basis of a brief statement made by the client without giving the client a chance to elaborate.

(4) *"Don't worry about it now; I'm sure that you have many healthy years ahead of you,"* is inappropriate. The nurse is telling the client how she should feel, and then goes

on to offer false reassurance. This response fails to address or explore the actual concerns of the client.

8. (4) **"Acknowledge the loss and be supportive,"** is the best answer choice. It promotes the nurse-client relationship, and allows for the identification of feelings and the expression of sadness. The client is in an acute stage of grief. This type of response addresses this issue.

   (1) *"Assure the woman that the loss was 'for the best,'"* is incorrect. This statement is insensitive to the client, offers false reassurance, and belittles the client's most immediate concerns.

   (2) *"Explain to her that she is young enough to have more children,"* is inappropriate because it is insensitive to the grief that the client is experiencing. The nurse offers false reassurance by telling the woman that she can have other children.

   (3) *"Ask her why she is looking at the babies,"* is also incorrect. This is inappropriate because it is a "why" question and because the woman may become defensive when answering such a question. This response also fails to respond to the client's immediate grief.

9. (1) **"It is hard to be caught between taking care of your needs and your father's needs,"** is the correct response. This is the most therapeutic response as it allows for continued development of a relationship with the family member of the client. This response allows the nurse to explore and validate the daughter's feelings about the nursing home placement.

   (2) *"Would you like me to help you find a nursing home?"* is not the best answer choice. It is a yes/no question and doesn't encourage discussion of the daughter's feelings.

   (3) *"Don't feel guilty. The only solution is to place your father in a nursing home,"* is not the best therapeutic response. The daughter's concerns are minimized when the nurse tells the daughter not to worry. Although it may be true that the daughter has done all that she can, this response cuts off an opportunity for further conversation with the nurse.

   (4) *"I think I would feel guilty too if I had to place my father in a nursing home,"* is also incorrect. This statement is value-laden and judgmental, and blocks any further communication between the nurse and the client's daughter. It is not important what the nurse thinks about the daughter's decision, nor is it the nurse's role to make the daughter feel more guilty about her decision.

LANGUAGE

English is the predominant language spoken and written in the United States, and the NCLEX-RN® exam is administered only in English. With the exception of the medical terminology, the reading level of the NCLEX-RN® exam is that of a junior in an American high school (11th grade). In order to be successful on the NCLEX-RN® exam, you must understand English—and the terminology—as it is used in the United States.

Vocabulary

Vocabulary can be a challenge for international nurses on the NCLEX-RN® exam. Not only must you know what each word means, but sometimes a word may have more than one meaning. You need to be able to correctly identify words as they are used in context. Refer to the NCLEX-RN® Exam Resources section in the back of this book for some of the commonly found words on the NCLEX-RN® exam. Some other ways to increase your vocabulary and learn how the words are used in everyday English include:

- Talking with Americans
- Watching American movies and television
- Reading American newspapers and magazines

Abbreviations

Many of you are unfamiliar with the abbreviations used in the United States. When studying, always look up unknown words in a medical dictionary. Consult the NCLEX-RN® Exam Resources section in the back of this book for a list of abbreviations used by nurses in American health care settings.

As an internationally educated nurse, you face special challenges in preparing for the NCLEX-RN® exam. Following the tips and guidelines outlined in this book will increase your chances of passing the NCLEX-RN® exam and will allow you to reach your career goals.

KAPLAN PROGRAMS FOR INTERNATIONAL NURSES

Knowing something about U.S. culture and how U.S. nurses fit into the overall health care industry is important for nurses trained outside the United States. If you are not from the United States, but are interested in learning more about U.S nursing, wish to practice in the United States, or are exploring the possibilities of attending a U.S. nursing school for graduate study, Kaplan is able to help you.

CGFNS® (Commission on Graduates of Foreign Nursing Schools) Preparation for International Nurses

Many U.S. state boards of nursing require internationally educated nurses to obtain a CGFNS® certificate before applying for initial licensure as a registered nurse. The certification process requires that a candidate pass a two-part test of nursing knowledge and demonstrate English language proficiency on the TOEFL® exam. Kaplan offers a comprehensive course of study to help you earn your CGFNS®certificate. To obtain information, please call 1-800-527-8378. Outside the United States, please call 1-212-997-5883 or log on to the website at *kaplannursing.com*.

Preparation for the NCLEX-RN® (National Council Licensure Examination) Examination for International Nurses

An internationally educated nurse must pass the NCLEX-RN® exam in order to obtain a license to practice as a registered nurse in the United States. Kaplan has a comprehensive course and review products to help international nurses pass this exam. To obtain information, please call 1-800-527-8378. Outside the United States, please call 1-212-997-5883 or log on to the website at *kaplannursing.com*.

Kaplan English Programs

In addition to Kaplan Nursing programs, Kaplan also offers English programs to help you improve your English skills and score on the TOEFL®. Kaplan's English Programs were designed to help students and professionals from outside the United States meet their educational and career goals. At locations throughout the United States, international students take advantage of Kaplan's programs to help them improve their academic and conversational English skills, raise their scores on the TOEFL® and other standardized exams, and gain admission to the schools of their choice. Our staff and instructors give international students the individualized instruction they need to succeed. The following sections provide brief descriptions of some of Kaplan's programs for non-native English speakers.

English Language Programs

Kaplan offers a wide range of English language programs to help you improve your English quickly and effectively, regardless of your current level. Each of our programs has a special focus, allowing you to direct your study in a way that suits your particular language needs. All of the essential language skills are covered, and your fluency and confidence will increase rapidly thanks to Kaplan's communicative teaching method.

TOEFL® and Academic English

Kaplan's world-famous TOEFL® course prepares students for the TOEFL® iBT. Designed for high-intermediate to advanced-level English speakers, our course focuses on the academic English skills you will need to succeed on the test. The course includes TOEFL®-focused reading, writing, listening, and speaking instruction and hundreds of practice items similar to those on the exam. Kaplan's expert instructors help you prepare for the four sections of the TOEFL® iBT, including the Speaking section. Our simulated online TOEFL® tests help you monitor your progress and provide you with feedback on areas where you require improvement. We will teach you how to get a higher score!

Other Kaplan Programs

Since 1938, more than 3 million students have come to Kaplan to advance their studies, prepare for entry to American universities, and further their careers. In addition to the above programs, Kaplan offers courses to prepare for the SAT®, ACT®, GMAT®, GRE®, LSAT®, MCAT®, DAT®, USMLE®, and other standardized exams at locations throughout the United States.

Applying to Kaplan English Programs*

To get more information, or to apply for admission to any of Kaplan's programs for non-native English speakers, contact us at:

Kaplan English Programs
21 East Victoria Street, Suite 300
Santa Barbara, CA 93101
USA
Phone: 1-800-818-9128
Fax: 1-805-884-9464
Website: *kaplaninternational.com*
Email: *northamerica@kaplaninternational.com*

*Kaplan is authorized under federal law to enroll nonimmigrant alien students.
Test names are registered trademarks of their respective owners.

FREE Services for International Students

Kaplan now offers international students many services online—free of charge! Students may assess their TOEFL® skills and gain valuable feedback on their English language proficiency in just a few hours with Kaplan's TOEFL® Skills Assessment. Log on to *kaplaninternational.com* today.

PART 5

NCLEX-RN®
EXAM RESOURCES

SUMMARY OF CRITICAL THINKING PATHS

The 10 charts below illustrate different paths you must choose from in order to correctly answer NCLEX-RN® exam questions. The stepping stones stand for steps that you must follow in order to find the correct answer for that question type. Use the chart to refresh your memory with respect to the various steps for each type of question. Tear out this page and refer to it to practice using this book's strategies when answering practice NCLEX-RN® exam-style questions.

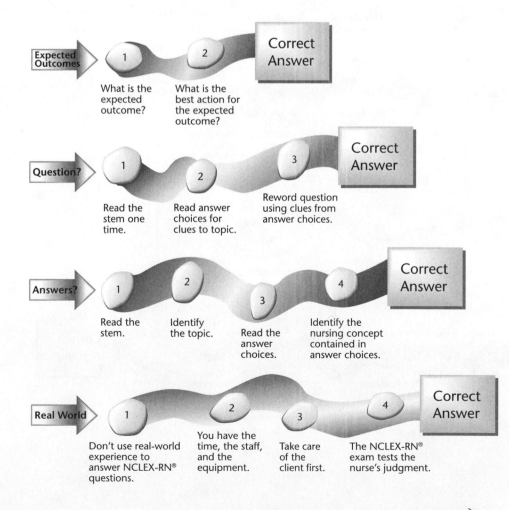

Expected Outcomes
1. What is the expected outcome?
2. What is the best action for the expected outcome?
→ Correct Answer

Question?
1. Read the stem one time.
2. Read answer choices for clues to topic.
3. Reword question using clues from answer choices.
→ Correct Answer

Answers?
1. Read the stem.
2. Identify the topic.
3. Read the answer choices.
4. Identify the nursing concept contained in answer choices.
→ Correct Answer

Real World
1. Don't use real-world experience to answer NCLEX-RN® questions.
2. You have the time, the staff, and the equipment.
3. Take care of the client first.
4. The NCLEX-RN® exam tests the nurse's judgment.
→ Correct Answer

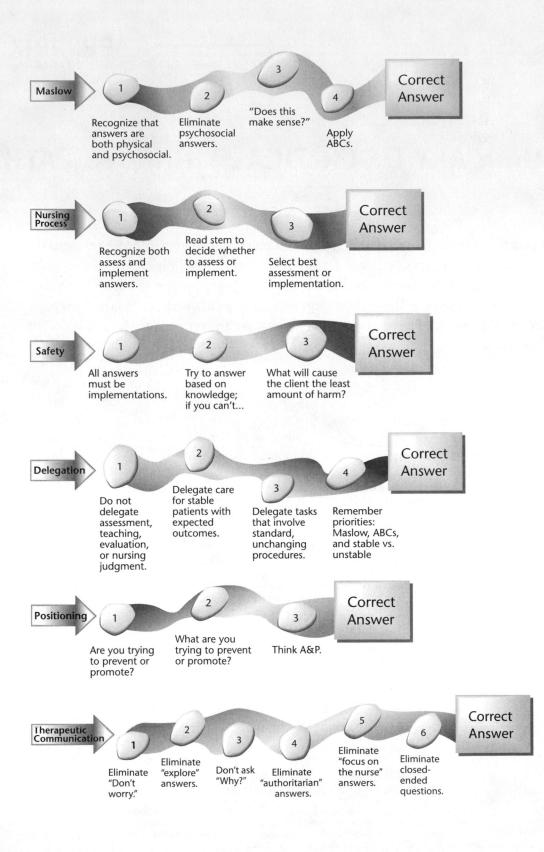

Maslow

1 — Recognize that answers are both physical and psychosocial.

2 — Eliminate psychosocial answers.

3 — "Does this make sense?"

4 — Apply ABCs.

Correct Answer

Nursing Process

1 — Recognize both assess and implement answers.

2 — Read stem to decide whether to assess or implement.

3 — Select best assessment or implementation.

Correct Answer

Safety

1 — All answers must be implementations.

2 — Try to answer based on knowledge; if you can't...

3 — What will cause the client the least amount of harm?

Correct Answer

Delegation

1 — Do not delegate assessment, teaching, evaluation, or nursing judgment.

2 — Delegate care for stable patients with expected outcomes.

3 — Delegate tasks that involve standard, unchanging procedures.

4 — Remember priorities: Maslow, ABCs, and stable vs. unstable

Correct Answer

Positioning

1 — Are you trying to prevent or promote?

2 — What are you trying to prevent or promote?

3 — Think A&P.

Correct Answer

Therapeutic Communication

1 — Eliminate "Don't worry."

2 — Eliminate "explore" answers.

3 — Don't ask "Why?"

4 — Eliminate "authoritarian" answers.

5 — Eliminate "focus on the nurse" answers.

6 — Eliminate closed-ended questions.

Correct Answer

NURSING TERMINOLOGY

abduction – movement away from the midline

abraded – scraped

acetonuria – acetone in the urine

adduction – movement toward the midline

afebrile – without fever

albuminuria – albumin in the urine

ambulatory – walking

amenorrhea – absence of menstruation

amnesia – loss of or defective memory

ankylosis – stiff joint

anorexia – loss of appetite

anuria – total suppression of urination

apnea – short periods when breathing has ceased

arthritis – inflammation of joint

asphyxia – suffocation

atrophy – wasting

auscultation, auscultate – to listen for sounds

bradycardia – heart rate lower than 60 beats per minute

Cheyne-Stokes respirations – increasing dyspnea with periods of apnea

choluria – bile in the urine

clonic tremor – shaking with intervals of rest

conjunctivitis – inflammation of conjunctiva

coryza – watery drainage from nose

cyanotic – bluish in color due to poor oxygenation

defecation – bowel movement

dental caries – decay of the teeth

dentures – false teeth

diarrhea – excessive or frequent defecation

diplopia – double vision

distended – appears swollen

diuresis – large amount of urine voided

dorsal recumbent – lying on back, knees flexed and apart

dysmenorrhea – painful menstruation

dyspnea – difficulty breathing

dysrhythmia, arrhythmia – abnormal heartbeat

dysuria – painful urination

edematous – puffy, swollen

emaciated – thin, underweight

emetic – agent given to produce vomiting

enuresis – bed-wetting

epistaxis – nosebleed

eructation – belching

erythema – redness

eupnea – normal breathing

excoriation – raw surface

exophthalmos – abnormal protrusion of eyeball

extension, extend – to straighten

fatigued – tired

feigned – pretended

fetid – foul

fixed – motionless

flaccid – soft, flabby

flatus, flatulence – gas in the digestive tract

flexion – bending

flushed – pink or hot

Fowler's position – semierect, knees flexed, head of bed elevated 45–60 degrees

gavage – forced feeding through a tube passed into the stomach

glossy – shiny

glycosuria – glucose in the urine

gustatory – dealing with taste

heliotherapy – using sunlight as a therapeutic agent

hematemesis – blood in vomitus

hematuria – blood in the urine

hemiplegia – paralysis of one side of the body

hemoglobinuria – hemoglobin in the urine

hemoptysis – spitting of blood

horizontal – flat

hydrotherapy – using water as a therapeutic agent

hyperpnea – rapid breathing

hypertonic – concentration greater than body fluids

hypotonic – concentration less than body fluids

infrequent – not often

insomnia – inability to sleep

instillation – pouring into a body cavity

intermittent – starting and stopping, not continuous

intradermal – within or through the skin

intramuscular – within or through the muscle

intraspinal – within or through the spinal canal

intravenous – within or through the vein

involuntary, incontinent – unable to control bladder or bowels

isotonic – having the same tonicity or concentration as body fluids

jackknife position – prone with hips over break in table and feet below level of head

jaundice – yellow color

knee-chest position – in face-down position resting on knees and chest

kyphosis – humpback, concavity of spine

labored – difficult, requires an effort

lacerated – torn, ragged edged

lateral position – on the side, knees flexed

lithotomy position – on the back, buttocks near edge of table, knees well flexed and separated

lochia – drainage from the vagina after delivery

lordosis – sway-back, convexity of spine

manipulation, manipulate – to handle

menopause – cessation of menstruation

menorrhagia – profuse menstruation

metrorrhagia – variable amount of uterine bleeding occurring frequently but at irregular intervals

moist – wet

monoplegia – paralysis of one limb

mucopurulent – drainage containing mucus and pus

mydriasis – dilation of pupil

myopia – nearsightedness

myosis – contraction of pupil

nausea – desire to vomit

necrosis – death of tissue

nocturia – frequent voiding at night

obese – overweight

objective – able to be documented by other than observation

oliguria – scant urination, less than 400 mL per 24 hours

orthopnea – inability to breathe or difficulty breathing while lying down

palliative – offering temporary relief

pallor – white

palpation, palpate – to feel with hands or fingers

paraplegia – paralysis of legs

paroxysm – spasm or convulsive seizure

paroxysmal – coming in seizures

pediculi – lice

pediculosis – lice infestation

percussion, percuss – to strike

persistent – lasting over a long time

petechia – small rupture of blood vessels

photophobia – sensitive to light

photosensitivity – skin reaction caused by exposure to sunlight

pigmented – containing color

polyuria – excessive voiding of urine

profuse, copious – large amount

projectile – ejected or projected some distance

pronation – turning downward

prone – on abdomen, face turned to one side

prophylactic – preventative

protruding – extending outward

pruritus – itching

ptosis – drooping eyelid

purulent drainage – drainage containing pus

pyrexia – elevated temperature

pyuria – pus in the urine

radiating – spreading to distant areas

radiotherapy – using x-ray or radium as a therapeutic agent

rales, crackles – abnormal breath sounds

rapid – quick

rotation – to move in circular pattern

sanguineous drainage – bloody drainage

scanty – small in amount

semi-Fowler's position – semi-erect, head of bed elevated 30–45 degrees

serous drainage – drainage of lymphatic fluid

Sims' position – on left side, left arm behind back, left leg slightly flexed, right leg slightly flexed

sprain – wrenching of a joint

stertorous – characterized by snoring

stethoscope – instrument used for auscultation

strabismus – squinting; misalignment of the eyes

stuporous – partially unconscious

subcutaneous – under the skin

subjective – observed

sudden onset – started all at once

superficial – on the surface only

supination – turning upward

suppurating – discharging pus

syncope – fainting

syndrome – group of symptoms

tachycardia – fast heartbeat, greater than 100 beats per minute

tenacious – tough and sticky

thready – barely perceptible

tonic tremor – continuous shaking

Trendelenburg position – flat on back with pelvis higher than head, foot of bed elevated 6 inches

tympanic – filled with gas

urticaria – hives or wheals, eruption on skin or mucous membranes

vertigo – dizziness

vesicle – fluid-filled blister

visual acuity – sharpness of vision

void, micturate – to urinate or pass urine

COMMON MEDICAL ABBREVIATIONS

ABC – airway, breathing, circulation

abd. – abdomen

ABG – arterial blood gas

ABO – system of classifying blood groups

ac – before meals

ACE – angiotensin-converting enzyme

ACS – acute compartment syndrome

ACTH – adrenocorticotrophic hormone

ad lib – freely, as desired

ADH – antidiuretic hormone

ADL – activities of daily living

AFP – alpha-fetoprotein

AIDS – acquired immunodeficiency syndrome

AKA – above-the-knee amputation

ALL – acute lymphocytic leukemia

ALP – alkaline phosphatase

ALS – amyotrophic lateral sclerosis

ALT – alkaline phosphatase (formerly SGPT)

AMI – antibody-mediated immunity

AML – acute myelogenous leukemia

amt. – amount

ANA – antinuclear antibody

ANS – autonomic nervous system

AP – anteroposterior

A&P – anterior and posterior

APC – atrial premature contraction

aq. – water

ARDS – adult respiratory distress syndrome

ASD – atrial septal defect

ASHD – atherosclerotic heart disease

AST – aspartate aminotransferase (formerly SGOT)

ATP – adenosine triphosphate

AV – atrioventricular

BCG – Bacille Calmette-Guerin

bid – two times a day

BKA – below-the-knee amputation

BLS – basic life support

BMR – basal metabolic rate

BP – blood pressure

BPH – benign prostatic hypertrophy

bpm – beats per minute

BPR – bathroom privileges

BSA – body surface area

BUN – blood urea nitrogen

C – centigrade, Celsius

$\bar{c}$ – with

Ca – calcium

CA – cancer

CABG – coronary artery bypass graft

CAD – coronary artery disease

CAL – chronic airflow limitations

CAPD – continuous ambulatory peritoneal dialysis

caps – capsules

CBC – complete blood count

CC – chief complaint

cc – cubic centimeter

CCU – coronary care unit, critical care unit

CDC – Centers for Disease Control and Prevention

CHF – congestive heart failure

CK – creatine kinase

Cl – chloride

CLL – chronic lymphocytic leukemia

cm – centimeter

CMV – cytomegalovirus

CNS – central nervous system

CO – carbon monoxide, cardiac output

CO2 – carbon dioxide

comp – compound

cont – continuous

COPD – chronic obstructive pulmonary disease

CP – cerebral palsy

CPAP – continuous positive airway pressure

CPK – creatine phosphokinase

CPR – cardiopulmonary resuscitation

CRP – C-reactive protein

C&S – culture and sensitivity

CSF – cerebrospinal fluid

CT – computerized tomography

CTD – connective tissue disease

CTS – carpal tunnel syndrome

cu – cubic

CVA – cerebrovascular accident or costovertebral angle

CVC – central venous catheter

CVP – central venous pressure

D&C – dilation and curettage

DC – discontinue

DCBE – double-contrast barium enema

DIC – disseminated intravascular coagulation

DIFF – differential blood count

dil. – dilute

DJD – degenerative joint disease

DKA – diabetic ketoacidosis

dL, dl – deciliter (100 mL)

DM – diabetes mellitus

DNA – deoxyribonucleic acid

DNR – do not resuscitate

DO – doctor of osteopathy

DOE – dyspnea on exertion

DPT – vaccine for diphtheria, pertussis, tetanus

Dr. – doctor

DRE – digital rectal exam

DVT – deep vein thrombosis

D/W – dextrose in water

Dx – diagnosis

ECF – extracellular fluid

ECG, EKG – electrocardiogram

ECT – electroconvulsive therapy

ED – emergency department

EEG – electroencephalogram

EMD – electromechanical dissociation

EMG – electromyography

ENT – ear, nose, and throat

ERCP – endoscopic retrograde cholangiopancreatography

ESR – erythrocyte sedimentation rate

ESRD – end-stage renal disease

ET – endotracheal tube

F – Fahrenheit

FBD – fibrocystic breast disease

FBS – fasting blood sugar

FDA – U.S. Food and Drug Administration

FFP – fresh frozen plasma

FHR – fetal heart rate

FHT – fetal heart tone

fl – fluid

FOBT – fecal occult blood test

4 × 4 – piece of gauze 4 inches by 4 inches; used for dressings

FSH – follicle-stimulating hormone

ft. – foot, feet (unit of measure)

FUO – fever of undetermined origin

g – gram

GB – gallbladder

GCS – Glasgow coma scale

GFR – glomerular filtration rate

GH – growth hormone

GI – gastrointestinal

gr – grain

gtt – drops

GU – genitourinary

GYN – gynecological

h, hrs – hour, hours

(H) – hypodermically

Hb, Hgb – hemoglobin

HCG – human chorionic gonadotropin

HCO_3 – bicarbonate

Hct – hematocrit

HD – hemodialysis

HDL – high-density lipoprotein

Hg – mercury

HGH – human growth hormone

HHNK – hyperglycemia hyperosmolar nonketotic coma

HIV – human immunodeficiency virus

HLA – human leukocyte antigen

H_2O – water

HR – heart rate

HSV – herpes simplex virus

HTN – hypertension

Hx – history

Hz – hertz (cycles/second)

IAPB – intra-aortic balloon pump

IBBP – intermittent positive pressure breathing

IBS – irritable bowel syndrome

ICF – intracellular fluid

ICP – intracranial pressure

ICS – intercostal space

ICU – intensive care unit

I&D – incision and drainage

IDDM – insulin-dependent diabetes mellitus

IgA – immunoglobulin A

IM – intramuscular

I&O – intake and output

IOP – increased intraocular pressure

IPG – impedance plethysmogram

IPPB – intermittent positive-pressure breathing

IUD – intrauterine device

IV – intravenous

IVC – intraventricular catheter

IVP – intravenous pyelogram or intravenous pyelography

JRA – juvenile rheumatoid arthritis

K^+ – potassium

kcal – kilocalorie (food calorie)

kg – kilogram

KO, KVO – keep vein open

KS – Kaposi's sarcoma

KUB – kidneys, ureters, bladder

L, l – liter

lab – laboratory

lb. – pound

LBBB – left bundle branch block

LDH – lactate dehydrogenase

LDL – low-density lipoprotein

LE – lupus erythematosus

LH – luteinizing hormone

liq – liquid

LLQ – left lower quadrant

LOC – level of consciousness

LP – lumbar puncture

LPN – licensed practical nurse

Lt, lt – left

LTC – long-term care

LUQ – left upper quadrant

LV – left ventricle

LVN – licensed vocational nurse

m – minum, meter, micron

MAO – monoamine oxidase inhibitor

MAST – military antishock trousers

mcg – microgram

MCH – mean corpuscular hemoglobin

MCV – mean corpuscular volume

MD – muscular dystrophy, medical doctor

MDI – metered dose inhaler

mEq – milliequivalent

mg – milligram

Mg – magnesium

MG – myasthenia gravis

MI – myocardial infarction

mL, ml – milliliter

mm – millimeter

MMR – vaccine for measles, mumps, rubella

MRI – magnetic resonance imaging

MS – multiple sclerosis

N – nitrogen, normal (strength of solution)

NIDDM – non–insulin dependent diabetes mellitus (type 2)

Na$^+$ – sodium

NaCl – sodium chloride

NANDA – North American Nursing Diagnosis Association

NG – nasogastric

NGT – nasogastric tube

NLN – National League for Nursing

noc – at night

NPO – nothing by mouth (nil per os)

NS – normal saline

NSAID – nonsteroidal anti-inflammatory drug

NSNA – National Student Nurses' Association

NST – non-stress test

O$_2$ – oxygen

OB-GYN – obstetrics and gynecology

OCT – oxytocin challenge test

OOB – out of bed

OPC – outpatient clinic

OR – operating room

$\overline{os}$ – by mouth

OSHA – Occupational Safety and Health Administration

OTC – over-the-counter (drug that can be obtained without a prescription)

oz. – ounce

$\overline{p}$ – with

P – pulse, pressure, phosphorus

PA Chest – posterior-anterior chest x-ray

PAC – premature atrial complexes

PaCO$_2$ – partial pressure of carbon dioxide in arterial blood

PaO$_2$ – partial pressure of oxygen in arterial blood

PAD – peripheral artery disease

Pap – Papanicolaou smear

pc – after meals

PCA – patient-controlled analgesia

pCO$_2$ – partial pressure of carbon dioxide

PCP – *Pneumocystis carinii* pneumonia

PD – peritoneal dialysis

PE – pulmonary embolism

PEEP – positive end-expiratory pressure

PERRLA – pupils equal, round, react to light and accommodation

PET – postural emission tomography

PFT – pulmonary function test

pH – hydrogen ion concentration

PICC – peripherally inserted central catheter

PID – pelvic inflammatory disease

PKD – polycystic disease

PKU – phenylketonuria

PMS – premenstrual syndrome

PND – paroxysmal nocturnal dyspnea

PO, po – by mouth

pO_2 – partial pressure of oxygen

PPD – positive purified protein derivative (of tuberculin)

PPE – personal protective equipment

PPN – partial parenteral nutrition

PRN, prn – as needed, whenever necessary

pro time – prothrombin time

PSA – prostate-specific antigen

psi – pounds per square inch

PSP – phenolsulfonphthalein

PT – physical therapy, prothrombin time

PTCA – percutaneous transluminal coronary angioplasty

PTH – parathyroid hormone

PTSD – post-traumatic stress disorder

PTT – partial thromboplastin time

PUD – peptic ulcer disease

PVC – premature ventricular contraction

q – every

QA – quality assurance

qd – once a day

qh – every hour

q 2 h – every two hours

q 4 h – every four hours

qid – four times a day

qs – quantity sufficient

R – rectal temperature, respirations, roentgen

RA – rheumatoid arthritis

RAI – radioactive iodine

RAIU – radioactive iodine uptake

RAS – reticular activating system

RBBB – right bundle branch block

RBC – red blood cell or red blood count

RCA – right coronary artery

RDA – recommended dietary allowance

resp – respirations

RF – rheumatic fever, rheumatoid factor

Rh – antigen on blood cell indicated by + or –

RIND – reversible ischemic neurologic deficit

RLQ – right lower quadrant

RN – registered nurse

RNA – ribonucleic acid

R/O, r/o – rule out, to exclude

ROM – range of motion (of joint)

Rt, rt – right

RUQ – right upper quadrant

Rx – prescription

$\bar{s}$ – without

S., Sig. – (Signa) to write on label

SA – sinoatrial node

SaO_2 – systemic arterial oxygen saturation (%)

sat sol – saturated solution

SBE – subacute bacterial endocarditis

SDA – same-day admission

SDS – same-day surgery

S/E – side effects

sed rate – sedimentation rate

SGOT – serum glutamic-oxaloacetic transaminase (see AST)

SGPT – serum glutamic-pyruvic transaminase (see ALT)

SI – International System of Units

SIADH – syndrome of inappropriate antidiuretic hormone

SIDS – sudden infant death syndrome

SL – sublingual

SLE – systemic lupus erythematosus

SMBG – self-monitoring blood glucose

SMR – submucous resection

SOB – shortness of breath

sol – solution

sp gr – specific gravity

spec. – specimen

s̄s̄ – one half

SS – soapsuds

S/S, s/s – signs and symptoms

SSKI – saturated solution of potassium iodide

stat – immediately

STD – sexually transmitted disease

subcut, SubQ – subcutaneous

sx – symptoms

Syr. – syrup

T – temperature, thoracic (followed by the number designating specific thoracic vertebra)

T&A – tonsillectomy and adenoidectomy

tabs – tablets

TB – tuberculosis

T&C – type and crossmatch

TED – antiembolitic stockings

temp – temperature

TENS – transcutaneous electrical nerve stimulation

TIA – transient ischemic attack

TIBC – total iron binding capacity

tid – three times a day

tinct, tr. – tincture

TLC – total lymphocyte count

TMJ – temporomandibular joint

TPA, t-pa – tissue plasminogen activator

TPN – total parenteral nutrition

TPR – temperature, pulse, respiration

TQM – total quality management

TSE – testicular self-examination

TSH – thyroid-stimulating hormone

tsp. – teaspoon

TSS – toxic shock syndrome

TURP – transurethral prostatectomy

UA – urinalysis

um – unit of measurement

ung – ointment

URI – upper respiratory tract infection

UTI – urinary tract infection

VAD – venous access device

VDRL – Venereal Disease Research Laboratory (test for syphilis)

VF, Vfib – ventricular fibrillation

VPC – ventricular premature complexes

VS, vs – vital signs

VSD – ventricular septal defect

VT – ventricular tachycardia

WBC – white blood cell or white blood count

WHO – World Health Organization

WNL – within normal limits

wt – weight

X PO – 10 grains per orem

STATE LICENSING REQUIREMENTS

Note: State licensing requirements may have changed after this book was published. Contact your state board of nursing for the latest information.

ALABAMA

Board of Nursing
RSA Plaza, Suite 250
770 Washington Avenue
Montgomery, AL 36104
Mailing address:
P.O. Box 303900
Montgomery, AL 36130-3900
Phone: (334) 293-5200
Fax: (334) 293-5201
Website: *www.abn.alabama.gov*

Temporary Permit: 90 days; $50

Licensure Fee/By Examination: $85

Licensure Fee/By Endorsement: $85, plus $3.50 transaction fee

NCLEX-RN® Test Fee: $200

Reexamination Limitations: Must wait 45 days; $85

License Renewal: December 31, every even year; $78.50 if renew by November 30; $203.50 if renew between December 1–December 31

CEU Requirements: 24 contact hours per biennial renewal period. Nurses licensed by examination are required to have four contact hours of board-provided continuing education for the first renewal (included in the total number of hours to be earned). MEDCEU contact hours are no longer accepted.

ALASKA

Board of Nursing
Robert B. Atwood Building
550 W. 7th Avenue, Suite 1500
Anchorage, AK 99501-3567
Phone: (907) 269-8161
Fax: (907) 269-8196
Website: *http://commerce.alaska.gov/dnn/cbpl/ ProfessionalLicensing/BoardofNursing.aspx*

Temporary Permit: Six months; $50

Licensure Fee/By Examination: $175 permanent license fee; $50 application fee, plus $59 fingerprint fee

Licensure Fee/By Endorsement: $175 permanent license fee; $50 application fee, plus $59 fingerprint fee

NCLEX-RN® Test Fee: $200

Reexamination Limitations: Must wait 45 days

License Renewal: November 30, every even year; $175

CEU Requirements: Method 1: Two of the three required for renewal: (1) 30 contact hours of CE, (2) 30 hours of uncompensated professional nursing activities, (3) 320 hours of employment as a registered nurse. Method 2: Completed a board-approved nursing refresher course. Method 3: Attained a degree or certificate in nursing, beyond the requirements of the original license, by successfully completing at least two required courses. Method 4: Successfully completed the National Council Licensing Examination. Licensees are subject to a random mandatory audit of continuing competency. Those selected for the audit will be notified in writing and given 30 days to submit proof of continuing competency claimed for the concluding licensing period.

ARIZONA

Board of Nursing
4747 N. 7th Street, Suite 200
Phoenix, AZ 85014-3655
Phone: (602) 771-7800
Fax: (602) 771-7888
Website: *www.azbn.gov*

Temporary Permit: Six months, must have passed the NCLEX exam; $50

Licensure Fee/By Examination: $300, plus $50 fingerprint fee

Licensure Fee/By Endorsement: $150, plus $50 fingerprint fee

NCLEX-RN® Test Fee: $200

Reexamination Limitations: Must wait 45 days; $100

License Renewal: April 1, every 4 years; $160

CEU Requirements: None

ARKANSAS

State Board of Nursing
University Tower Building
1123 South University, Suite 800
Little Rock, AR 72204-1619
Phone: (501) 686-2700
Fax: (501) 686-2714
Website: *www.arsbn.arkansas.gov*

Temporary Permit: 90 days or until receipt of examination results; $25

Licensure Fee/By Examination: $75, plus $38.50 for criminal background check

Licensure Fee/By Endorsement: $100, plus $38.50 for criminal background check

NCLEX-RN® Test Fee: $200

Reexamination Limitations: Must wait 45 days; $75

License Renewal: Birthday, every 2 years; $75

CEU Requirements: One of the following: (1) 15 contact hours, (2) certification/recertification during renewal period, or (3) completed a minimum of 1 college credit hour course in nursing with a grade of C or better during the licensure period.

CALIFORNIA

Board of Registered Nursing
1747 North Market Boulevard, Suite 150
Sacramento, CA 95834
Mailing address:
P.O. Box 944210
Sacramento, CA 94244-2100
Phone: (916) 322-3350
Fax: (916) 574-7697
Website: *www.rn.ca.gov*

Temporary Permit: Interim license pending results of first exam; 6 months if by endorsement; $50

Licensure Fee/By Examination: $150 application fee, plus $49 fingerprint fee

Licensure Fee/By Endorsement: $100, plus $49 fingerprint fee

NCLEX-RN® Test Fee: $200

Reexamination Limitations: Must wait 45 days; $150

License Renewal: Last day of the month following birth date, every 2 years; $140

CEU Requirements: 30 contact hours every 2 years, exempt for first 2 years following initial licensure

COLORADO

Board of Nursing
1560 Broadway, Suite 1350
Denver, CO 80202
Phone: (303) 894-2430
Fax: (303) 894-2821
Website: *www.dora.state.co.us/nursing*

Temporary Permit: Four months by endorsement only; fee is included in application fee

Licensure Fee/By Examination: $88 initial exam

Licensure Fee/By Endorsement: $43

NCLEX-RN® Test Fee: $200

Reexamination Limitations: May take 3 times within 3 years; if unsuccessful, must take refresher course

License Renewal: September 30, every 2 years; $109

CEU Requirements: None

CONNECTICUT

Board of Examiners for Nursing
Department of Public Health
RN Licensure
410 Capitol Avenue
MS# 13PHO
P.O. Box 340308
Hartford, CT 06134-0308
Phone: (860) 509-7603, Menu Option 2
Fax: (860) 509-8457
Website: *http://www.ct.gov/dph/cwp/view. asp?a=3143&q=388910*

Temporary Permit: 120 days by endorsement only, nonrenewable; must hold valid license in another state. Fee is included in application fee.

Licensure Fee/By Examination: $180

Licensure Fee/By Endorsement: $180

NCLEX-RN® Test Fee: $200

Reexamination Limitations: Must wait 45 days

License Renewal: Last day of birth month, every year; $100

CEU Requirements: None

DELAWARE

Division of Professional Regulation
Board of Nursing
861 Silver Lake Boulevard
Cannon Building, Suite 203
Dover, DE 19904
Phone: (302) 774-4500
Fax: (302) 739-2711
Website: *http://dpr.delaware.gov/boards/nursing*

Temporary Permit: Expires 90 days after graduation date, pending exam results; 90 days by endorsement; $35

Licensure Fee/By Examination: $124

Licensure Fee/By Endorsement: $124

NCLEX-RN® Test Fee: $200

Reexamination Limitations: Must wait 45 days; can retake for up to 2 years; $20

License Renewal: February 28, May 31, and September 30, every odd year; notified of amount of renewal fee at time of renewal

CEU Requirements: 30 contact hours every 2 years. Nurses licensed by exam are exempt from CE requirements for the first renewal after initial licensure. Minimum practice requirement of 1,000 hours in 5 years or 400 hours in 2 years.

DISTRICT OF COLUMBIA

Department of Health
Health Regulation & Licensing Administration
Board of Nursing
899 North Capitol Street NE, 1st Floor
Washington, DC 20002
Phone: (877) 672-2174
Fax: (202) 727-8471
Website: *http://doh.dc.gov/service/health-professionals*

Temporary Permit: Supervised letters of practice, 90 days, $32.50

Licensure Fee/By Examination: $187

Licensure Fee/By Endorsement: $230

NCLEX-RN® Test Fee: $200

Reexamination Limitations: Must wait 45 days; $85

License Renewal: June 30, even-numbered years; $145

CEU Requirements: 24 contact hours of CE in the licensee's current area of practice every 2 years.

FLORIDA

Board of Nursing
Medical Quality Assurance/Licensure Services
4052 Bald Cypress Way, BIN C02
Tallahassee, FL 32399-3251
Phone: (850) 245-4125
Fax: (850) 245-4172
Website: *www.doh.state.fl.us/mqa*

Temporary Permit: None

Licensure Fee/By Examination: $204 initial exam

Licensure Fee/By Endorsement: $218

NCLEX-RN® Test Fee: $200

Reexamination Limitations: Must wait 45 days; remedial training program is required after 3 attempts; $119

License Renewal: Biennially, various dates, $90

CEU Requirements: 24 contact hours every 2 years. One hour per month. Two hours in the prevention of medical errors; 1 hour in HIV (one time only); and 2 hours in domestic violence (every third renewal) by a provider approved by the state of Florida; proof of training in latter two prior to licensure. Nurses licensed by examination during the current renewal period are exempt from additional CE requirements for the first renewal period only.

Georgia

Board of Nursing
237 Coliseum Drive
Macon, GA 31217-3858
Phone: (478) 207-2440
Fax: (478) 207-1660
Website: *http://sos.georgia.gov/plb/rn*

Temporary Permit: None

Licensure Fee/By Examination: $40

Licensure Fee/By Endorsement: $60

NCLEX-RN® Test Fee: $200, plus $12 when registering by telephone

Reexamination Limitations: Must wait 45 days, must pass within 3 years of graduation; $40

License Renewal: January 31; $65

CEU Requirements: None

Hawaii

PVL/DCCA
Board of Nursing
P.O. Box 3469
Honolulu, HI 96801
Phone: (808) 586-3000
Fax: (808) 586-2689
Website: *http://hawaii.gov/dcca/pvl/boards/nursing*

Temporary Permit: By endorsement with employment verification

Licensure Fee/By Examination: $40

Licensure Fee/By Endorsement: $135 or $180, depending on the year license is issued. Noted on application information sheet.

NCLEX-RN® Test Fee: $200

Reexamination Limitations: Must wait 45 days

License Renewal: June 30, every odd year (deadline May 31); contact board for renewal fee

CEU Requirements: None

Idaho

Board of Nursing
280 North 8th Street, Suite 210
P.O. Box 83720
Boise, ID 83720-0061
Phone: (208) 334-3110
Fax: (208) 334-3262
Website: *http://ibn.idaho.gov*

Temporary Permit: 90 days by endorsement; $25

Licensure Fee/By Examination: $132, includes fingerprinting fee

Licensure Fee/By Endorsement: $152, includes fingerprinting fee

NCLEX-RN® Test Fee: $200

Reexamination Limitations: Must wait 45 days

License Renewal: August 31, every odd year; $90

CEU Requirements: None

Illinois

Board of Nursing
James R. Thompson Center
100 West Randolph Street, Suite 9-300
Chicago, IL 60601
Phone: (312) 814-2715
Fax: (312) 814-3145
Website: *http://www.idfpr.com/profs/info/Nursing.asp*

Temporary Permit: May practice as license-pending registered nurse under direct supervision for 3 months; 6 months by endorsement; $25

Licensure Fee/By Examination: $91

Licensure Fee/By Endorsement: $50

NCLEX-RN® Test Fee: $200

Reexamination Limitations: Must wait 45 days; must pass within 3 years from first writing to board

License Renewal: May 31, every even year; $30

CEU Requirements: 20 hours of CE every 2-year license renewal cycle

INDIANA

State Board of Nursing
Professional Licensing Agency
402 West Washington Street, Room W072
Indianapolis, IN 46204
Phone: (317) 234-2043
Fax: (317) 233-4236
Website: *www.in.gov/pla/nursing.htm*

Temporary Permit: 90 days if by endorsement; $10

Licensure Fee/By Examination: $50

Licensure Fee/By Endorsement: $50

NCLEX-RN® Test Fee: $200

Reexamination Limitations: Must wait 45 days

License Renewal: October 31, every odd year; $50

CEU Requirements: None

IOWA

Board of Nursing
RiverPoint Business Park
400 SW 8th Street, Suite B
Des Moines, IA 50309-4685
Phone: (515) 281-3255
Fax: (515) 281-4825
Website: *http://nursing.iowa.gov*

Temporary Permit: 30 days if by endorsement. Fee is included in application fee.

Licensure Fee/By Examination: $143

Licensure Fee/By Endorsement: $169

NCLEX-RN® Test Fee: $200

Reexamination Limitations: Must wait 45 days

License Renewal: 30 days prior to the 15th of month of birth, every 3 years; $99

CEU Requirements: 36 contact hours or 3.6 CEUs for renewal of a 3-year license. For renewal of license issued for less than 3 years, 24 contact hours or 2.4 CEUs every 3 years. It is also mandated that RNs who regularly examine, attend, counsel, or treat dependent adults or children in Iowa are required to complete training related to the identification and reporting of child/dependent adult abuse. The licensee is required to complete at least 2 hours of training every 5 years. The course must be approved by the Iowa Department of Public Health Abuse Education Review Panel. The board of nursing requires the licensee, at the time of renewal, to document completion of the training requirements. A list of approved courses is available at *www.idph.state. ia.us/bh/abuse_ed_review.asp*.

KANSAS

State Board of Nursing
Landon State Office Building
900 SW Jackson Street, Suite 1051
Topeka, KS 66612-1230
Phone: (785) 296-4929
Fax: (785) 296-3929
Website: *www.ksbn.org*

Temporary Permit: 120 days only by endorsement. Fee is included in application fee.

Licensure Fee/By Examination: $75

Licensure Fee/By Endorsement: $75

NCLEX-RN® Test Fee: $200

Reexamination Limitations: Must wait 45 days, can take unlimited number of times; after 2 years the applicant must provide an approved study plan.

License Renewal: Last day of birth month; odd years for those born in an odd-numbered year, even years for those born in an even-numbered year; $60

CEU Requirements: 30 contact hours every 2 years

KENTUCKY

Board of Nursing
312 Whittington Parkway, Suite 300
Louisville, KY 40222-5172
Phone: (502) 429-3300, (800) 305-2042
Fax: (502) 429-3311
Website: *www.kbn.ky.gov*

Temporary Permit: Six months or until applicant is unsuccessful on NCLEX-RN exam; 6 months by endorsement; fee included in application fee.

Licensure Fee/By Examination: $110, plus $40 if applying using paper application. Initial fingerprint card and fee of $16.50 must be mailed to the Kentucky State Police.

Licensure Fee/By Endorsement: $150; fingerprint fee, $16.50; additional $40 if applying using a paper application

NCLEX-RN® Test Fee: $200

Reexamination Limitations: Must wait 45 days, no limit on number of times can be taken

License Renewal: September 15–October 31, annually; $50 if online, $90 if paper renewal

CEU Requirements: 14 contact hours every year; 2 hours of mandatory AIDS CE approved by the Kentucky Cabinet for Health Services once every 10 years. A one-time, 3-hour domestic violence requirement must be completed within 3 years of the date of initial licensing. Pediatric Abusive Head Trauma CE is a one-time continuing education course of at least 1.5 hours covering the recognition and prevention of pediatric abusive head trauma; nurses have 3 years from the date of licensure to complete the course.

LOUISIANA

State Board of Nursing
17373 Perkins Road
Baton Rouge, LA 70810
Phone: (225) 755-7500
Fax: (225) 755-7584
Website: *www.lsbn.state.la.us*

Temporary Permit: Pending results of first exam; fee is included in application fee. If by endorsement, 90 days; $50.

Licensure Fee/By Examination: $100, plus $42.50 for criminal background check

Licensure Fee/By Endorsement: $100, plus $42.50 for criminal background check fee

NCLEX-RN® Test Fee: $200

Reexamination Limitations: Must wait 45 days; can take up to four times

License Renewal: December 31, every year; $80

CEU Requirements: For all RNs: 5, 10, or 15 contact hours every year, based on employment

MAINE

Board of Nursing
161 Capitol Street
P.O. Box 158 State House Station
Augusta, ME 04333
Phone: (207) 287-1133
Fax: (207) 287-1149

Website: www.maine.gov/boardofnursing

Temporary Permit: 90-day letter of endorsement. Fee is included in application fee.

Licensure Fee/By Examination: $75

Licensure Fee/By Endorsement: $75

NCLEX-RN® Test Fee: $200

Reexamination Limitations: Must wait 45 days

License Renewal: Birthday, every 2 years; $75

CEU Requirements: None

MARYLAND

Board of Nursing
4140 Patterson Avenue
Baltimore, MD 21215-2254
Phone: (410) 585-1900 or (888) 202-9861
Fax: (410) 358-3530
Website: *www.mbon.org*

Temporary Permit: 90 days by endorsement, not renewable; $40

Licensure Fee/By Examination: $100

Licensure Fee/By Endorsement: $100

NCLEX-RN® Test Fee: $200

Reexamination Limitations: Must wait 45 days

License Renewal: 28th day of month of birth, odd years for those born in an odd-numbered year, even years for those born in an even-numbered year; $69.

CEU Requirements: None

MASSACHUSETTS

Board of Registration in Nursing
239 Causeway Street, Suite 500
Boston, MA 02114
Phone: (617) 973-0900, (800) 414-0168
Fax: (617) 973-0984
Website: *www.mass.gov/dph/boards/rn*

Temporary Permit: Not granted

Licensure Fee/By Examination: $230

Licensure Fee/By Endorsement: $275

NCLEX-RN® Test Fee: $200

Reexamination Limitations: Must wait 45 days; re-exam costs $80 if taken within one year; after one year, $230

License Renewal: Birthday, every even year; $120.

CEU Requirements: 15 contact hours every 2 years

MICHIGAN

Department of Licensing and Regulatory Affairs
Bureau of Health Care Services
Board of Nursing
P.O. Box 30193
Lansing, MI 48909
Phone: (517) 335-0918
Fax: (517) 373-2179
Website: *www.michigan.gov/healthlicense*

Licensure Fee/By Examination: $54, plus $62.75 finger-printing fee

Licensure Fee/By Endorsement: $54, plus $62.75 fingerprinting fee

NCLEX-RN® Test Fee: $200

Reexamination Limitations: Must wait 45 days. Must pass within one year or 3 attempts. After 3 failures, must attend education program for approval to retest 3 more times.

License Renewal: First March 31 after initial licensure (may be 1 year or less), then March 31, every 2 years; $60

CEU Requirements: None for first-time renewal; 25 hours every 2 years; 1 hour in pain and symptom management.

MINNESOTA

Board of Nursing
2829 University Avenue SE #200
Minneapolis, MN 55414-3253
Phone: (612) 317-3000
Fax: (612) 617-2190
Website: *www.nursingboard.state.mn.us*

Temporary Permit: 60 days, license by exam; $60. One year if by endorsement, no fee.

Licensure Fee/By Examination: $105, plus $10.50 eLicensing surcharge

Licensure Fee/By Endorsement: $105, plus $10.50 eLicensing surcharge

NCLEX-RN® Test Fee: $200

Reexamination Limitations: Must wait 45 days; retake within 1 year or application becomes null; $60

License Renewal: Birth month, every 2 years; $93.50

CEU Requirements: 24 contact hours every 2 years

MISSISSIPPI

Board of Nursing
713 Pear Orchard Road, Suite 300
Ridgeland, MS 39157
(601) 957-6300
Fax: (601) 664-9304
Website: *www.msbn.ms.gov*

Temporary Permit: 90 days by endorsement; $25

Licensure Fee/By Examination: $100

Licensure Fee/By Endorsement: $100

NCLEX-RN® Test Fee: $200

Reexamination Limitations: Effective January 15, 2011, candidates may take the NCLEX examination a maximum of 6 times and within 2 years of graduation with at least 46 days between examinations; $100

License Renewal: October 1–December 31, every even year; $100

CEU Requirements: None

MISSOURI

Board of Nursing
3605 Missouri Boulevard
P.O. Box 656
Jefferson City, MO 65102-0656
Phone: (573) 751-0681
Fax: (573) 751-0075
Website: *www.pr.mo.gov/nursing.asp*

Temporary Permit: Six months, by endorsement only. Fee is included in application fee.

Licensure Fee/By Examination: $45 initial exam

Licensure Fee/By Endorsement: $51

NCLEX-RN® Test Fee: $200

Reexamination Limitations: Must wait 45 days; $40

License Renewal: April 30, every odd year; $50

CEU Requirements: None

Montana

Department of Labor and Industry
Board of Nursing
301 South Park, 4th Floor
P.O. Box 200513
Helena, MT 59620-0513
Phone: (406) 841-2202
Fax: (406) 841-2305
Website: *www.nurse.mt.gov*

Temporary Permit: 90 days; $25

Licensure Fee/By Examination: $100

Licensure Fee/By Endorsement: $200

NCLEX-RN® Test Fee: $200

Reexamination Limitations: Must wait 90 days, up to 5 attempts in 3 years. After failing twice, must present a plan of study to the board before next retake. If one doesn't pass within 3 years, must take Nursing Program before sixth retake.

License Renewal: December 31, every 2 years; $100

CEU Requirements: 24 contact hours every 2 years

Nebraska

Board of Nursing
DHHS, Public Health Licensure Unit
301 Centennial Mall South, 3rd Floor
P.O. Box 94986
Lincoln, NE 68509-4986
Phone: (402) 471-4376
Fax: (402) 471-1066
Website: *http://dhhs.ne.gov/publichealth/Pages/crl_nursing_nursingindex.aspx*

Temporary Permit: If by endorsement, 60 days or until the expiration date of the license from the other state, whichever occurs first. Fee is included in licensing fee.

Licensure Fee/By Examination: $123 generally; $30.75 for initial licensure in even years between May 1 and October 31 (because the license will be issued within 180 days of the renewal date)

Licensure Fee/By Endorsement: $123

NCLEX-RN® Test Fee: $200

Reexamination Limitations: Must wait 45 days

License Renewal: October 31, every even year; $123

CEU Requirements: 20 contact hours within the last renewal period, no more than 4 hours of which may be from CPR or BLS, and 10 of which must be peer reviewed and approved.

Nevada

Board of Nursing
5011 Meadowood Mall Way, Suite 300
Reno, NV 89502-6547
Phone: (775) 687-7700 or (888) 590-6726
Fax: (775) 687-7707
Website: *www.nevadanursingboard.org*

Temporary License: Six months, not renewable. Fee is included in application fee.

Licensure Fee/By Examination: $100, plus $51.25 fingerprinting fee

Licensure Fee/By Endorsement: $105, plus $51.25 fingerprinting fee

NCLEX-RN® Test Fee: $200

Reexamination Limitations: Must wait 45 days, up to three times, then only with remediation

License Renewal: Birthday, every 2 years; $100

CEU Requirements: 30 contact hours every 2 years at renewal. One-time requirement of 4 hours on bioterrorism. New grads may be exempt from CE requirements for their first renewal period.

New Hampshire

Board of Nursing
21 South Fruit Street, Suite 16
Concord, NH 03301-2431
Phone: (603) 271-2323
Fax: (603) 271-6605
Website: *www.state.nh.us/nursing*

Temporary Permit: Six months or until results of first exam are received and license is issued; $20

Licensure Fee/By Examination: $120, plus $51.50 for criminal record release authorization

Licensure Fee/By Endorsement: $120, plus $51.50 for criminal record release authorization

NCLEX-RN® Test Fee: $200

Reexamination Limitations: Must wait 45 days

License Renewal: Birthday, every 2 years; $100

CEU Requirements: 30 contact hours in 2 years immediately preceding license application including workshops, conferences, lectures or other education offerings designed to enhance nursing knowledge, judgment, and skills.

NEW JERSEY

Board of Nursing
P.O. Box 45010
124 Halsey Street, 6th Floor
Newark, NJ 07101
Phone: (973) 504-6430
Fax: (973) 648-3481
Website: *http://www.njconsumeraffairs.gov/nursing*

Temporary Permit: Not available

Licensure Fee/By Examination: $200, plus $25.30 for criminal history background check

Licensure Fee/By Endorsement: $200, plus $66.30 fingerprinting fee

NCLEX-RN® Test Fee: $200

Reexamination Limitations: Must wait 45 days; only with remediation after 3 attempts

License Renewal: May 31, every 2 years; $120

CEU Requirements: 30 contact hours every 2 years

NEW MEXICO

Board of Nursing
6301 Indian School Road NE, Suite 710
Albuquerque, NM 87110
Phone: (505) 841-8340
Fax: (505) 841-8347
Website: *nmbon.sks.com*

Temporary Permit: 24 weeks from graduation if application process is completed within 12 weeks of graduation; 6 months if by endorsement; $50. Must have NM employment verified.

Licensure Fee/By Examination: $110 initial exam, plus $44 for criminal background check

Licensure Fee/By Endorsement: $110, plus $44 for criminal background check

NCLEX-RN® Test Fee: $200

Reexamination Limitations: Every 45 days; $60; up to 4 times. If the candidate fails to pass the exam in 1 year, the candidate must resubmit an initial examination application to the Board with all required documentation and fees.

License Renewal: Every 2 years from date of issue; $93

CEU Requirements: 50 contact hours in the 2 years preceding renewal, including 15 in pharmacology and 5 in the area of practice.

NEW YORK

Board of Nursing
NYS Education Department
Office of the Professions
Division of Professional Licensing Services, Nurse
 Unit
89 Washington Avenue
2nd Floor West Wing
Albany, NY 12234-1000
Phone: (518) 474-3817, ext. 280
Fax: (518) 474-3398
Website: *www.op.nysed.gov/prof/nurse*

Temporary Permit: Must have completed all other requirements for licensure except the licensing examination. Valid for 1 year from date of issue or until 10 days after the applicant is notified of failure on the licensing examination, whichever occurs first. Graduates of New York state nursing programs may be employed without permit for 90 days immediately following graduation; $35.

Licensure Fee/By Examination: $143 (includes first license and 3-year registration)

Licensure Fee/By Endorsement: $143

NCLEX-RN® Test Fee: $200

Reexamination Limitations: Must wait 45 days

License Renewal: Every 3 years; $65

CEU Requirements: Three contact hours on infection control every 4 years; 2 contact hours on child abuse (one-time requirement for initial licensure)

NORTH CAROLINA

Board of Nursing
P.O. Box 2129
Raleigh, NC 27602-2129
Phone: (919) 782-3211
Fax: (919) 781-9461
Website: *www.ncbon.com*

Temporary Permit: None for new graduates. By endorsement: 6 months or until the endorsement is approved, whichever occurs first; not renewable. Fee is included in application fee.

Licensure Fee/By Examination: $75; plus $38 for criminal background check

Licensure Fee/By Endorsement: $150, plus $38 fingerprint fee

NCLEX-RN® Test Fee: $200

Reexamination Limitations: Must wait 45 days; $75

License Renewal: Month of birth, every 2 years; $92, plus $38 for criminal background check. The North Carolina Board of Nursing no longer accepts paper applications for renewal or reinstatement of RN and LPN licenses.

CEU Requirements: Various options to fulfill continuing competency requirement, including 30 contact hours of CE

NORTH DAKOTA

Board of Nursing
919 South 7th Street, Suite 504
Bismarck, ND 58504-5881
Phone: (701) 328-9777
Fax: (701) 328-9785
Website: *www.ndbon.org*

Temporary Permit: By endorsement: 90 days; fee is included in endorsement fee. By exam: 90 days after the date of issue or upon notification of exam results, whichever occurs first.

Licensure Fee/By Examination: $130, includes fee for criminal history record check

Licensure Fee/By Endorsement: $160, includes fee for criminal history record check

NCLEX-RN® Test Fee: $200

Reexamination Limitations: Must wait 45 days, up to five attempts in 3 years; $130

License Renewal: Online between October 1 and December 31, every other year; $120

CEU Requirements: Nursing practice for relicensure must meet or exceed 12 hours within preceding 2 years.

OHIO

Board of Nursing
17 South High Street, Suite 400
Columbus, OH 43215-7410
Phone: (614) 466-3947
Fax: (614) 466-0388
Website: *www.nursing.ohio.gov*

Temporary Permit: 180 days if by endorsement, not renewable. Fee is included in endorsement application fee. Written verification required.

Licensure Fee/By Examination: $75

Licensure Fee/By Endorsement: $75

NCLEX-RN® Test Fee: $200

Reexamination Limitations: Must wait 45 days; $75

License Renewal: June 30, every odd year; $65

CEU Requirements: 24 hours in a 2-year period, except in the case of first renewal after licensure by examination. One of 24 hours must pertain to Ohio law.

OKLAHOMA

Board of Nursing
2915 North Classen Boulevard, Suite 524
Oklahoma City, OK 73106
Phone: (405) 962-1800
Fax: (405) 962-1821
Website: *www.ok.gov/nursing*

Temporary Permit: 90 days if by endorsement; $10

Licensure Fee/By Examination: $85, plus $3.50 online application fee

Licensure Fee/By Endorsement: $85, plus $3.50 online application fee

NCLEX-RN® Test Fee: $200

Reexamination Limitations: Must wait 45 days; pass within 2 years; $85, plus $3.50 online application fee

License Renewal: Last day of birth month, every even year; $75

CEU Requirements: None; however, 24 contact hours in 2 years preceding renewal is one of the 5 renewal options

OREGON

Board of Nursing
17938 SW Upper Boones Ferry Road
Portland, OR 97224-7012
Phone: (971) 673-0685
Fax: (971) 673-0684
Website: *www.osbn.state.or.us*

Temporary Permit: None

Licensure Fee/By Examination: $160, plus $52 for criminal background check

Licensure Fee/By Endorsement: $195, plus $52 for criminal background check

NCLEX-RN® Test Fee: $200

Reexamination Limitations: Must wait 45 days, up to 3 years from the date of graduation; $25

License Renewal: Birthday, every 2 years; $150

CEU Requirements: One-time requirement of 7 hours of pain management-related CE. One hour must be a course provided by the Oregon Pain Management Commission.

PENNSYLVANIA

Board of Nursing
P.O. Box 2649
Harrisburg, PA 17105-2649
Phone: (717) 783-7142
Fax: (717) 783-0822
Website: *http://www.portal.state.pa.us/portal/server. pt/community/state_board_of_nursing/12515*

Temporary Permit: One year maximum; examination results preempt permit, $35

Licensure Fee/By Examination: $35 if educated in PA; $100 if educated out of state

Licensure Fee/By Endorsement: $100

NCLEX-RN® Test Fee: $200

Reexamination Limitations: Must wait 45 days, $30

License Renewal: Renewal date by license number every 2 years; $65

CEU Requirements: 30 hours in 2 years preceding renewal

RHODE ISLAND

Board of Nurse Registration and Nursing
   Education
Three Capitol Hill
Room 105
Providence, RI 02908-5097
Phone: (401) 222-5700
Fax: (401) 222-3352
Website: *www.health.ri.gov/for/nurses*

Temporary Permit: Pending results of first exam but no longer than 90 days after graduation. Not renewable. No fee.

Licensure Fee/By Examination: $135

Licensure Fee/By Endorsement: $135

NCLEX-RN® Test Fee: $200

Reexamination Limitations: Must wait 45 days; $130

License Renewal: Expires March 1, every 2 years—renew before February 15 by license number; $90

CEU Requirements: 10 contact hours in preceding 2 years

SOUTH CAROLINA

Board of Nursing
P.O. Box 12367
Columbia, SC 29211-2367
Phone: (803) 896-4550
Fax: (803) 896-4515
Website: *www.llr.state.sc.us/pol/nursing*

Temporary Permit: 90 days by endorsement only; $10

Licensure Fee/By Examination: $90 online, $115 in person

Licensure Fee/By Endorsement: $100 online, $125 in person

NCLEX-RN® Test Fee: $200

Reexamination Limitations: Must wait 45 days, up to 4 times in 1 year, then must remediate; $65

License Renewal: April 29, every year; $50

CEU Requirements: One of the following, every 2 years: (1) 30 CE contact hours, (2) maintenance of certification or recertification by a national certifying body, (3) completion of an academic program of study in nursing or a related field, or (4) verification of competency and number of hours practiced as evidenced by employer certification

South Dakota

Board of Nursing
4305 S. Louise Avenue, Suite 201
Sioux Falls, SD 57106-3115
Phone: (605) 362-2760
Fax: (605) 362-2768
Website: *www.doh.sd.gov/boards/nursing/*

Temporary Permit: 90 days or untill receipt of examination results; $25

Licensure Fee/By Examination: $100, plus $43.25 for criminal background check

Licensure Fee/By Endorsement: $100, plus $43.25 for criminal background check

NCLEX-RN® Test Fee: $200

Reexamination Limitations: Must wait 45 days, maximum of 4 times per year in 3 years, then must requalify; $100

License Renewal: Birthday, every 2 years; $90

CEU Requirements: Minimum practice requirement of 140 hours in any 12-month period during the past 6 years, or total of 480 hours during the past 6 years

Tennessee

Board of Nursing
Heritage Place, MetroCenter
227 French Landing, Suite 300
Nashville, TN 37243
Phone: (615) 532-5166
Fax: (615) 741-7899
Website: *http://health.state.tn.us/Boards/Nursing*

Temporary Permit: Six months if by endorsement; $25

Licensure Fee/By Examination: $90

Licensure Fee/By Endorsement: $105

NCLEX-RN® Test Fee: $200

Reexamination Limitations: Must wait 45 days, up to 3 years, then only with remediation; $100

License Renewal: Last day of month of birth, every 2 years; $65

CEU Requirements: Continued practice requirement over a 5-year period; plus continued competency demonstrated by documentation of 2 of 15 options

Texas

Board of Nursing
333 Guadalupe, Suite 3-460
Austin, TX 78701
Phone: (512) 305-7400
Fax: (512) 305-7401
Website: *www.bon.state.tx.us*

Temporary Permit: 120-day permits issued for completing a refresher course; no extensions; $15

Licensure Fee/By Examination: $139

Licensure Fee/By Endorsement: $200

NCLEX-RN® Test Fee: $200

Reexamination Limitations: Must wait 45 days; unlimited testing within 4 years of eligibility; $139 retake fee

License Renewal: Every even year for those born in even years, every odd year for those born in odd years (initial licensure period ranges from 6 months to 29 months depending on birth year); $73

CEU Requirements: 20 contact hours or achievement of an approved national nursing certification, every 2 years. Nurses licensed by exam or by endorsement are exempt from CE requirements for the first renewal after initial licensure.

Utah

Board of Nursing
Heber M. Wells Building, 4th Floor
160 East 300 South
Salt Lake City, UT 84111
Phone: (801) 530-6628
Fax: (801) 530-6511
Website: *www.dopl.utah.gov/licensing/nursing.html*

Temporary Permit: Four months; $50

Licensure Fee/By Examination: $100

Licensure Fee/By Endorsement: $100

NCLEX-RN® Test Fee: $200

Reexamination Limitations: Must wait 45 days

License Renewal: January 31, every odd year; $58

CEU Requirements: Must have (1) practiced not less than 400 hours during 2 years preceding application for renewal, or (2) have completed 30 contact hours, or (3) have practiced not less than 200 hours and completed 15 contact hours during 2 years preceding application for renewal.

VERMONT

Board of Nursing
90 Main Street, 3rd Floor
Montpelier, Vermont 05620-3402
Phone: (802) 828-2396
Fax: (802) 828-2484
Website: *www.vtprofessionals.org/opr1/nurses*

Temporary Permit: 90 days or upon results of exam, whichever comes first; $25

Licensure Fee/By Examination: $90

Licensure Fee/By Endorsement: $150

NCLEX-RN® Test Fee: $200

Reexamination Limitations: Must wait 45 days; various review requirements if 2–4 exam failures; if 5 exam failures, must contact Board of Nursing office; $30

License Renewal: March 31, every odd year; $95

CEU Requirements: Minimum practice requirement of 960 hours in 5 years or 400 hours in 2 years

VIRGINIA

Board of Nursing
Department of Health Professions
Perimeter Center
9960 Mayland Drive, Suite 300
Henrico, Virginia 23233-1463
Phone: (804) 367-4515
Fax: (804) 527-4455
Website: *www.dhp.virginia.gov/nursing*

Temporary Permit: 90 days pending results of exam; 30 days by endorsement, which may be extended at the discretion of the board

Licensure Fee/By Examination: $190

Licensure Fee/By Endorsement: $190

NCLEX-RN® Test Fee: $200

Reexamination Limitations: Must wait 45 days; $50

License Renewal: Last day of month of birth, every even year for those born in even years, every odd year for those born in odd years; $140

CEU Requirements: Beginning August 1, 2015, one of the following in the 2 years preceding renewal: (1) specialty certification, (2) 3 academic credit hours, (3) board-approved refresher course, (4) evidence-based practice project or study, (5) publication, (6) teaching 3 academic credit hours, (7) teaching 30 contact hours of continuing education, (8) 15 contact hours plus 640 hours practice, or (9) 30 contact hours

WASHINGTON

Nursing Care Quality Assurance Commission
310 Israel Road SE
P.O. Box 47864
Olympia, WA 98504-7864
Phone: (360) 236-4700
Fax: (360) 236-4738
Website: *http://www.doh.wa.gov/
   LicensesPermitsandCertificates/
   NursingCommission.aspx*

Temporary Permit: None

Licensure Fee/By Examination: $88

Licensure Fee/By Endorsement: $88

NCLEX-RN® Test Fee: $200

Reexamination Limitations: Must wait 45 days

License Renewal: Birthday, every year; $97

CEU Requirements: All registered nurses must document continuing competency. To comply, all licensed nurses must do the following every 3 years upon submission for renewal: collect documentation of 531 hours of active nursing practice within the previous 36-month review period; keep documentation to show completion of 45 hours of continuing education, self-assessment, and reflection (for personal use only); and attest to having met continuing competency requirements.

WEST VIRGINIA

Board of Examiners for Registered Professional
  Nurses
101 Dee Drive, Suite 102
Charleston, WV 25311-1620
Phone: (304) 558-3596
Fax: (304) 558-3666
Website: *www.wvrnboard.com*

Temporary Permit: 90 days from graduation date
pending results of first exam; 180 days if by endorsement; $10

Licensure Fee/By Examination: $51.50

Licensure Fee/By Endorsement: $60

NCLEX-RN® Test Fee: $200

Reexamination Limitations: Must wait 45 days; additional requirements are needed after 2 attempts

License Renewal: October 31, every year; $35

CEU Requirements: 12 contact hours every year

WISCONSIN

Department of Regulation and Licensing
1400 East Washington Avenue
Madison, WI 53703
Mailing Address: P.O. Box 8935
Madison, WI 53708-8935
Phone: (608) 266-2112
Fax: (608) 261-7083
Website: *http://dsps.wi.gov/Default.aspx?Page=*
  582ce3ce-0028-404c-9373-14bfd6cf17c8

Temporary Permit: 90 days pending results of exam;
90 days if by endorsement, non-renewable; $10

Licensure Fee/By Examination: $90

Licensure Fee/By Endorsement: $82

NCLEX-RN® Test Fee: $200

Reexamination Limitations: Must wait 45 days; $15

License Renewal: February 28 or 29, every even year;
$86, late fee $25

CEU Requirements: None

WYOMING

Board of Nursing
130 Hobbs Avenue, Suite B
Cheyenne, WY 82002
Phone: (307) 777-7601
Fax: (307) 777-3519
Website: *https://nursing-online.state.wy.us*

Temporary Permit: 90 days by endorsement or by
exam. Fee is included in application fee. Temporary
permit is not renewable.

Licensure Fee/By Examination: $190, plus $5 if by
credit card

Licensure Fee/By Endorsement: $195, plus $5 if by
credit card

NCLEX-RN® Test Fee: $200

Reexamination Limitations: Must wait 45 days, maximum of 10 times within 5 years of graduation; $195

License Renewal: December 31, every even year; $110

CEU Requirements: One of the following: 500 practice
hours or 20 RN continuing education hours in the
last 2 years; or 1,600 practice hours, refresher course,
specialty certification, or passing the NCLEX in the
last 5 years

PEARSON PROFESSIONAL CENTERS OFFERING NCLEX-RN® EXAMINATIONS

The following is a listing of some NCLEX-RN® examination sites. More sites may be available in your area. For more information, please visit the website of the National Council of State Boards of Nursing at *ncsbn.org*.

U.S. Examination Sites

ALABAMA

2 Chase Corporate Drive, Suite 20
Birmingham, AL 35244

401 Lee Street NE, Suite 602
Decatur, AL 35602

Carmel Plaza
2623 Montgomery Hwy., Suite 4
Dothan, AL 36303

Executive Center One
900 Western America Circle, Suite 212
Mobile, AL 36609

400 East Blvd., Suite 103
Montgomery, AL 36117

ALASKA

Denali Towers North Building
2550 Denali Street, Suite 511
Anchorage, AK 99503

AMERICAN SAMOA

Pago Plaza
PO Box AC, Suite 222
Pago Pago, AS 96799

ARIZONA

Portico Place, 2121 Building
2121 W. Chandler Blvd., Suite 209
Chandler, AZ 85224

2501 West Dunlap Avenue, Suite 260
Phoenix, AZ 85021

Merrill Lynch Building
5210 East Williams Circle, Suite 722
Tucson, AZ 85711

ARKANSAS

1401 S. Waldron Road, Suite 208
Fort Smith, AR 72903

Conway Building
10816 Executive Center Drive, Suite 209
Little Rock, AR 72211

Landmark Building
210 North State Line Avenue, Suite B100
Texarkana, AR 71854

CALIFORNIA

Anaheim Corporate Plaza
2190 Towne Centre Place, Suite 300
Anaheim, CA 92806

2001 Junipero Serra Blvd., Suite 530
Daly City, CA 94014

7555 N. Palm Avenue, Suite 205
Fresno, CA 93711

South Bay Centre
1515 West 190th Street, Suite 405
Gardena, CA 90248

23792 Rockfield Blvd., Suite 200
Lake Forest, CA 92630

1551 McCarthy Blvd., Suite 108
Milpitas, CA 95035

Transpacific Center
1000 Broadway, Suite 470
Oakland, CA 94607

Centrelake Plaza
3401 Centrelake Drive, Suite 675
Ontario, CA 91761

Union Bank Building
70 S. Lake Avenue, Suite 840
Pasadena, CA 91101

2190 Larkspur Lane, Suite 400
Redding, CA 96002

1690 Barton Road, Suite 102
Redlands, CA 92373

3010 Lava Ridge Court, Suite 170
Roseville, CA 95661

8950 Cal Center Drive
Building 1, Suite 215
Sacramento, CA 95826

Sunroad Financial Plaza
11770 Bernardo Plaza Court, Suite 463
San Diego, CA 92128

9619 Chesapeake Drive, Suite 208
San Diego, CA 92123

140 East Via Verde, Suite 110
San Dimas, CA 91773

201 Filbert Street, Suite 200
San Francisco, CA 94133-3238

570 Rancheros Drive, Suite 110
San Marcos, CA 92069

Gill Office Building
1010 South Broadway, Suite F
Santa Maria, CA 93454

5300 West Tulare Avenue, Suite 108
Visalia, CA 93277

Westlake Corporate Centre
875 S. Westlake Blvd., Suite 106
WestLake Village, CA 91361

COLORADO

The Triad
5660 Greenwood Plaza Blvd., Suite 510
Greenwood Village, CO 80111

University Center Professional Building
41 Montebello Road, Suite 312
Pueblo, CO 81001

9101 Harlan Street, Suite 220
Westminster, CO 80031

CONNECTICUT

Merritt on the River - North Tower
20 Glover Avenue, Suite 19
Norwalk, CT 06850

35 Thorpe Avenue, Suite 105
Wallingford, CT 06492

Putnam Park
100 Great Meadow Road, Suite 404
Wethersfield, CT 06109

DELAWARE

The Kays Building
1012 College Road, Suite 104
Dover, DE 19904

111 Continental Drive, Suite 109
Newark, DE 19713

DISTRICT OF COLUMBIA

1615 L Street NW, Suite 410
Washington, DC 20036

FLORIDA

Premier Point South
237 South Westmonte Drive, Suite 245
Altamonte Springs, FL 32714

1191 East Newport Center Drive, Suite PHA
3rd Floor, Penthouse A
Deerfield Beach, FL 33442

2815 NW 13 Street, Suite 101
Gainesville, FL 32609

Spring Lake Business Center
Building 3
8659 Baypine Road, Suite 305
Jacksonville, FL 32256

8615–8617 South Dixie Highway
Miami, FL 33143

1707 Orlando Central Parkway, Suite 300
Orlando, FL 32809

Royal Palm at Southpoint
1000 South Pine Island Road, Suite 260
Plantation, FL 33324

M & I Bank Building
1777 Tamiami Trail, Suite 508
Port Charlotte, FL 33948

Baypoint Commerce Center
877 Executive Center Drive, Suite 350
St. Petersburg, FL 33702

2286–2 Wednesday Street
Tallahassee, FL 32308

Sabal Business Center 5
3922 Coconut Palm Drive, Suite 101
Tampa, FL 33619

GEORGIA

2410 Westgate Drive, Suite 102
Albany, GA 31707

1117 Perimeter Center West, Suite 311 East
Atlanta, GA 30338

Augusta Riverfront Center
One 10th Street, Suite 640
Augusta, GA 30901

Lakeside Commons I Building
6055 Lakeside Commons Drive, Suite 110
Macon, GA 31210

Georgetown Center
785 King George Blvd., Suite C
Savannah, GA 31419

Overlook II Professional Building
239 Village Center Parkway, Suite 280
Stockbridge, GA 30281

GUAM

267 South Marine Drive, 2nd Floor, Suite 2E
Tamuning, GU 96913

HAWAII

1441 Kapiolani Blvd., Suite 204
Honolulu, HI 96814

IDAHO

9183 W. Black Eagle Drive
Boise, ID 83709

ILLINOIS

200 West Adams Street, Suite 1105
Chicago, IL 60606

103 Airway Drive, Suite 1
Marion, IL 62959

Norwoods Professional Building
4507 N. Sterling Avenue, Suite 302
Peoria, IL 61615

1827 Walden Office Square, Suite 540
Schaumburg, IL 60173

3000 Professional Drive, Lower Level, Suite C
Springfield, IL 62703

INDIANA

German American Bank Building
4424 Vogel Road, Suite 402
Evansville, IN 47715

Dupont Office Center Building 2
9921 Dupont Circle Drive West, Suite 140
Fort Wayne, IN 46825

2629 Waterfront Parkway East Drive, Suite 100
Indianapolis, IN 46214

The Pyramids at College Park
3500 DePauw Blvd., Bldg. 2, 8th Floor, Suite 2080
Indianapolis, IN 46268

Chase Bank/Everest College Building
8585 Broadway, Suite 745
Merrillville, IN 46410

630 Wabash Avenue, Suite 221
Terre Haute, IN 47807

IOWA

Wells Fargo Building
327 2nd Street, Suite 370
Coralville, IA 52241

Northwest Bank & Trust Company
100 East Kimberly Road, Suite 401
Davenport, IA 52806

4300 South Lakeport, Suite 204
Sioux City, IA 51106

Colony Park Office Building
3737 Woodland Avenue, 3rd Floor, Suite 340
West Des Moines, IA 50266

KANSAS

Hadley Center
205 E. 7th Street, Suite 237
Hays, KS 67601

Gage Center Office Suites
4125 SW Gage Center Drive, Suite 201
Topeka, KS 66604

Equity Financial Center
7701 E. Kellogg, 7th Floor, Suite 750
Wichita, KS 67207

KENTUCKY

2720 Old Rosebud Road, Suite 180
Lexington, KY 40509

1941 Bishop Lane, Suite 713
Louisville, KY 40218

LOUISIANA

Corporate Atrium Building
5555 Hilton Avenue, Suite 430
Baton Rouge, LA 70808

2800 Veterans Blvd., Suite 256
Metairie, LA 70002

Pierremont Office Park
920 Pierremont Road, Suite 212
Shreveport, LA 71106

MAINE

10 Ridgewood Drive, Suite 2
Bangor, ME 04401

201 Main Street, Suite 4A
Westbrook, ME 04092

MARYLAND

3108 Lord Baltimore Drive, Suite 103
Baltimore, MD 21244

Bethesda Towers
4350 East West Highway, Suite 525
Bethesda, MD 20814

9891 Broken Land Parkway, Suite 108
Columbia, MD 21046

1315 Mount Herman Road, Suite B
Salisbury, MD 21804

MASSACHUSETTS

Park Square
31 St. James Avenue, Suite 725
Boston, MA 02116

295 Devonshire Street, 2nd Floor
Boston, MA 02110

One Monarch Place
1414 Main Street, Suite 1110
Springfield, MA 01144

Reservoir Place
1601 Trapelo Road, Suite 203
Waltham, MA 02451

255 Park Avenue, 6th Floor, Suite 604
Worcester, MA 01609

MICHIGAN

Burlington Office Center I
325 E. Eisenhower Parkway, Suite 3A
Ann Arbor, MI 48108

Waters Building
161 Ottawa Avenue NW, Suite 307
Grand Rapids, MI 49503

3390 Pine Tree Road, Suite 101
Lansing, MI 48911

Rublein Building
290 Rublein Street, Suite B
Marquette, MI 49855

Travelers Tower I
26555 Evergreen Road, Suite 850
Southfield, MI 48076

City Center Building
888 W. Big Beaver Road, Suite 490
Troy, MI 48084

MINNESOTA

5601 Green Valley Drive, Suite 150
Bloomington, MN 55437

Triad Building
7101 Northland Circle, Suite 102
Brooklyn Park, MN 55428

Washington Drive Executive Center
3459 Washington Drive, Suite 107
Eagan, MN 55122-1347

North Shore Bank Place
4815 West Arrowhead Road, Suite 100
Hermantown, MN 55811

Greenview Office Building
1544 Greenview Drive SW, Suite 200
Rochester, MN 55902

MISSISSIPPI

1755 Lelia Drive, Suite 404
Jackson, MS 39216

431 W. Main Street, Suite 340
Tupelo, MS 38801

MISSOURI

Buttonwood Building
3610 Buttonwood Drive, Suite 102A
Columbia, MO 65201

Ward Parkway Corporate Centre
9200 Ward Parkway, Suite 101
Kansas City, MO 64114

Blue Ridge Tower
4240 Blue Ridge Blvd., Suite 705
Kansas City, MO 64133

2833 (A) East Battlefield, Suite 106
Springfield, MO 65804

Center Forty Building
1600 S. Brentwood Blvd., Suite 120
St. Louis, MO 63144

10805 Sunset Office Drive, Suite 402
St. Louis, MO 63127

MONTANA

Transwestern 1 Building
404 North 31st Street, Suite 230
Billings, MT 59101

Arcade Building
111 N. Last Chance Gulch, Suite 4K
Helena, MT 59601

NEBRASKA

44 Corporate Place Office Park
300 North 44th Street, Suite 104
Lincoln, NE 68503

Nebraskaland Bank Building
121 N. Dewey, Suite 212
North Platte, NE 69101

Omni Corporate Park
10832 Old Mill Road, Suite 4
Omaha, NE 68154

NEVADA

Tower Building
101 Convention Center Drive, Suite 330
Las Vegas, NV 89109

Corporate Point
5250 S. Virginia, Suite 301
Reno, NV 89502

NEW HAMPSHIRE

Capital Plaza
2 Capital Plaza, 3rd Floor
Concord, NH 03301

NEW JERSEY

1125 Atlantic Avenue, Suite 107
Atlantic City, NJ 08401

1099 Wall Street West, Suite 104
Lyndhurst, NJ 07071

100 Village Blvd., Suite 201
Princeton, NJ 08540

1543 State Route 27, Lower Level–Basement
Somerset, NJ 08873

NEW MEXICO

Bank of Albuquerque Building
2500 Louisiana Blvd. NE, Suite LL–1B
Albuquerque, NM 87110

NEW YORK

1365 Washington Ave., Suite 107
Albany, NY 12206

45 Main Street, Suite 706
Brooklyn, NY 11201

6700 Kirkville Road, Suite 204
East Syracuse, NY 13057

421–423 East Main Street, Suite 100
Endicott, NY 13760

2950 Express Drive South, Suite 145
Islandia, NY 11722

1979 Marcus Avenue, Suite 205
Lake Success, NY 11042

100 William Street, Suite 1200
New York, NY 10038

500 Fifth Avenue, Suite 3120
New York, NY 10110

9734 64th Road
Rego Park, NY 11374

The Design Center
3445 Winton Place Plaza, Suite 211
Rochester, NY 14623

Gardens Office I
1110 South Avenue, Suite 400
Staten Island, NY 10314

122 Business Park Drive, Suite 4
Utica, NY 13502

18564 US Route 11, Suite 7
Watertown, NY 13601

Cross West Office Center
399 Knollwood Road, Suite 218
White Plains, NY 10603

Centerpointe Corporate Park
325 Essjay Road, Suite 104
Williamsville, NY 14221

NORTH CAROLINA

One Town Square
One Town Square Blvd., Suite 350
Asheville, NC 28803-5007

4601 Charlotte Park Drive, Suite 340
Charlotte, NC 28217

Quorum Office Park
7520 East Independence Blvd., Suite 250
Charlotte, NC 28227

Meridian Corporate Center
2520 Meridian Parkway, Suite 475
Durham, NC 27713

1105 Corporate Drive, Suite B
Greenville, NC 27858

8024 Glenwood Avenue, Suite 107
Raleigh, NC 27612

Market Street Central
2709 Market Street, Suite 206
Wilmington, NC 28405

Stratford Oaks
514 S. Stratford Road
Knollwood Level, Suite 102
Winston-Salem, NC 27104

NORTH DAKOTA

Kirkwood Office Tower
919 S. 7th Street, Suite 400
Bismarck, ND 58504

3170 43rd Street South, Suite 102
Fargo, ND 58104

NORTHERN MARIANA ISLANDS

Del Sol Building
Suite 102, P.O. Box 505140
Saipan   96950

OHIO

Springside Center
231 Springside Drive, Suite 125
Akron, OH 44333

3201 Enterprise Parkway, Suite 10, Basement
Beachwood, OH 44122

355 E. Campus View Blvd., Suite 140
Columbus, OH 43235

OffiCenter 2
700 Taylor Road, Suite 180
Gahanna, OH 43230

4770 Duke Drive, Suite 385
Mason, OH 45040

Metro Woods Building
1789 Indian Wood Circle, Suite 120
Maumee, OH 43537

3033 Kettering Blvd., Suite 320
Moraine, OH 45439

2001 Crocker Road, Suite 350
Westlake, OH 44145

OKLAHOMA

Trails Office Park
3000 South Berry, Suite 200
Norman, OK 73072

5100 N. Brookline, Suite 282
Oklahoma City, OK 73112

7136 South Yale
Executive Center I, Suite 418
Tulsa, OK 74136

OREGON

Park Plaza West, Building 3
10700 SW Beaverton Hillsdale Hwy, Suite 595
Beaverton, OR 97005

3560 Excel Drive, Suite 105
Medford, OR 97504

Fox Tower
805 SW Broadway, Suite 420
Portland, OR 97205

The VA Outpatient Clinic Building
1660 Oak Street SE, Suite 250
Salem, OR 97301

PENNSYLVANIA

Commerce Corporate Center II
5100 W. Tilghman Street, Suite B-30
Allentown, PA 18104

Edgewood Place
3123 West 12th Street, Suite D
Erie, PA 16505

801 East Park Drive, Suite 101
Harrisburg, PA 17111

Pennsylvania Business Campus
110 Gibraltar Road, Suite 227
Horsham, PA 19044

205 Granite Run Drive, Suite 130
Lancaster, PA 17601

1800 John F Kennedy (JFK) Blvd., 10th Floor,
  Suite 1001
Philadelphia, PA 19103

Digital Place Office Complex
1500 Ardmore Blvd., Suite 401
Pittsburgh, PA 15221

2 Penn Center Blvd.
Penn Center Blvd. & Campbell's Run Road
Building 2, Suite 109
Pittsburgh, PA 15276

Stadium Office Park
330 Montage Mountain Road, Suite 102
Scranton, PA 18507

Valley Forge Office Center
530 E. Swedesford Road, Suite 109
Wayne, PA 19087

PUERTO RICO

Plaza Scotiabank
273 Ponce de Leon Avenue, Suite 501
San Juan, PR 00917

RHODE ISLAND

301 Metro Center Blvd., Suite 103
Warwick, RI 02886

SOUTH CAROLINA

Berkeley Building
200 Center Point Circle, Suite 350
Columbia, SC 29210

Halton Commons Office Park
301 Halton Road, Suite D1
Greenville, SC 29607

Rivergate Center II
4975 LaCross Road, Suite 255
North Charleston, SC 29406

SOUTH DAKOTA

VanBuskirk Office Building
5101 South Nevada Avenue, Suite 130
Sioux Falls, SD 57108

TENNESSEE

The Parklane Building
5200 Maryland Way, Suite 360
Brentwood, TN 37027

Franklin Building
5726 Marlin Road, Suite 310
Chattanooga, TN 37411

Sun Trust Bank Building
207 Mockingbird Lane, Suite 401
Johnson City, TN 37604

Keystone Center
135 Fox Road, Suite C
Knoxville, TN 37922

Lipscomb & Pitts Building
2670 Union Avenue, Suite 820
Memphis, TN 38112

6060 Poplar Avenue, Suite LL01
Memphis, TN 38119

Riverview Building
545 Mainstream Drive, Suite 410
Nashville, TN 37228

TEXAS

500 Chestnut Street, Suite 856
Abilene, TX 79602

1616 S. Kentucky, Suite C305
Amarillo, TX 79102

South Park One
1701 Directors Blvd., Suite 350
Austin, TX 78744

BBVA Compass Building
301 Congress Avenue, Suite 565
Austin, TX 78701

Prosperity Bank Building
6800 West Loop S., Suite 405
Bellaire, TX 77401

Corona South Building
4646 Corona Drive, Suite 175
Corpus Christi, TX 78411

12801 North Central Expressway, Suite 820
Dallas, TX 75243

4110 Rio Bravo Street, Suite 222
El Paso, TX 79902

14425 Torrey Chase Blvd., Suite 240
Houston, TX 77014

Gulf Freeway Building
8876 Gulf Freeway, Suite 220
Houston, TX 77017

500 Grapevine Highway, Suite 401
Hurst, TX 76054-2707

Wells Fargo Center
1500 Broadway Street, Suite 1113
Lubbock, TX 79401

3300 North A Street, Suite 228
Building 4
Midland, TX 79705-5457

Stonewater Tower West
6100 Bandera Road, Suite 407
San Antonio, TX 78238

10000 San Pedro, Suite 175
San Antonio, TX 78216

One America Center
909 East Southeast Loop 323, Suite 625
Tyler, TX 75701

Wells Fargo Bank Building
1105 Wooded Acres Drive, Suite 406
Waco, TX 76710

U.S. VIRGIN ISLANDS

Nisky Center, Suite 730 East Wing
St. Thomas, VI 00802

UTAH

1551 S. Renaissance Towne Drive, Suite 560
Bountiful, UT 84010

Draper Technology Center
11734 Election Road, Suite 180
Draper, UT 84020

Business Depot Ogden
1150 South Depot Drive, Suite 130
Ogden, UT 84404

VERMONT

30 Kimball, Suite 202
South Burlington, VT 05403

VIRGINIA

1900 N. Beauregard Street, Suite 12
Alexandria, VA 22311

1403 Greenbrier Parkway, Suite 530
Chesapeake, VA 23320

Graves Mill Office Park
424 Graves Mill Road, Suite 200-A
Lynchburg, VA 24502

825 Diligence Drive, Suite 120
Newport News, VA 23606

3900 Westerre Parkway, Suite 202
Richmond, VA 23233

Northpark Business Center
6701 Peters Creek Road, Suite 108
Roanoke, VA 24019

8391 Old Courthouse Road, Suite 201
Vienna, VA 22182

WASHINGTON

Oaksdale Center
1300 SW 7th Street, Suite 113
Renton, WA 98057

10700 Meridian Avenue North, Suite 407
Seattle, WA 98133

Mullan Centre
1410 N. Mullan Road, Suite 203
Spokane Valley, WA 99206

1701 Creekside Loop, Suite 110
Yakima, WA 98902

WEST VIRGINIA

BB&T Square
300 Summers Street, Suite 430
Charleston, WV 25301

The Jackson & Kelly Building
150 Clay Street, Suite 420
Morgantown, WV 26505

Wisconsin

Bishops Woods Centre
13555 Bishops Court, Suite L10
Brookfield, WI 53005

3610 Oakwood Mall Drive, Suite 102
Eau Claire, WI 54701

Johnson Bank Building
7500 Green Bay Road, Suite 311
Kenosha, WI 53142

Prairie Trail Office Suites II
8517 Excelsior Drive, Suite 202
Madison, WI 53717

735 N. Water Street, Suite 600
Milwaukee, WI 53202

Wyoming

Aspen Creek Building
800 Werner Court, Suite 310
Casper, WY 82601

INTERNATIONAL EXAMINATION SITES

AUSTRALIA

Level 6 , 287 Elizabeth Street
Sydney, New South Wales 2000

CANADA

HSBC Building
10055 106th Street NW, Suite 540
Edmonton, Alberta T5J 2Y2

Commerce Court Building
4190 Lougheed Hwy, Suite 103
Burnaby, British Columbia V5C 6A8

11 Holland Avenue, Suite 512
Ottawa, Ontario K1Y 4S1

1 Eva Road, Suite 400
Toronto, Ontario M9C 4Z5

21 St. Clair Avenue East, Suite 501
Toronto, Ontario M4T 1L9

7705 17th Avenue
Montreal, Quebec H2A 2S4

HONG KONG

Grand Millenium Plaza
Room 503, 5th Floor
181 Queen's Road, Central

INDIA

1-10-72/A/2, Pochampalli House, 3rd Floor
S P Road, Begumpet,
Hyderabad, Andhra Pradesh 500016

Yusuf Sarai Community Centre
4th Floor, Building 18, Ramnath House
New Delhi, Delhi 110049

45, 3rd Floor, Trade Center
Dickenson Road
Bangalore, Karnataka 560042

Building 9, 1st Floor
Solitaire Corporate Park, 167 Andheri
J B Nagar Link Rd., Chakala, Andheri (East)
Mumbai, Maharashtra 400093

6th Floor, Nelson Chambers, E Block,
115, Nelson Manickam Road,
Aminijikarai,
Chennai, Tamil Nadu 600 029

JAPAN

12F Osaka Dai-Ichi Seimei Bldg,
1-8-17 Umeda
Kita-ku
Osaka-shi, Osaka 530-0001

The Imperial Tower 18F
1-1-1, Uchisaiwai-cho,
Chiyoda-ku, TKY 100-0011

MEXICO

Industrial Atoto
Atlacomulco 500, 4th Floor
Naucalpan, Estado de Mexico 53519
Mexico City, Distrito Federal, 99999

PHILIPPINES

Trident Tower, 27th Floor
312 Senator Gil Puyat Avenue,
Makati City,
Manila 1227

TAIWAN

Hsin-Yi District
12F-3, No 163
Sec. 1 Keelung Road,
Union Century Building, 12F Room 3
Taipei City, 11070

UNITED KINGDOM

190 High Holborn
London WC1V 7BH

INDEX

G

gastrointestinal diagnostic tests, 243
general lead, using as therapeutic response, 95
general test-taking strategies, 21–29, 40–56
goals, 16
graphics questions, 30, 37, 442, 444
grief and loss, 182

H

hazardous and infectious materials, handling, 132–133
health and wellness, 157
Health Insurance Portability and Accountability Act (HIPAA), 109
health promotion and maintenance, 9–10, 149–174
    chapter quiz, 163–167
    chapter quiz answer and explanations, 168–174
    exam content related to, 149
    example of questions on, 10
    nursing actions included within, 9–10
    overview of category, 9–10
    percentage of questions on, 9, 149
health promotion/disease prevention, 157–158
    programs for, 158–159
health screening, 160
heart sounds, anatomical landmarks for, 33–34
heart disease prevention, 159
hemodynamics, 264
high-risk behaviors, 160
home safety, 133
hormone replacement therapy (HRT), 159
hot spot questions, 33–34
    answer choice, selecting and changing, 443
hygiene, personal, 207

I

IELTS® International, 455
ileostomy, 204
illness management, 264
imbalances, fluid and electrolyte, 263
immobility
    complications, 204–205
    interventions, 205

    main causes of, 204
immunizations, 159
implanted port, 224
implementation
    as part of nursing process, 15, 17, 75–76
    example of questions on, 17
    strategy, assessment vs., 75–79
incident/event/irregular occurrence/variance, reporting, 133
incorrect answer choices, eliminating, 43–47
infants, developmental stages and transitions, 154
infection control background, 130–131
infectious materials, handling *see* hazardous and infectious materials, handling
information technology, 114–115
informed consent, 114
inhaled medications, 226
injectable medications, 225–226
injury prevention *see* accident/injury prevention
integrated processes, 18–19
    caring, 19
    communication and documentation, 19
    teaching/learning principles
integumentary diagnostic tests, 243
intellectualization, as defense mechanism, 179
interactions *see* adverse effects/contraindications/side effects/interactions
interdisciplinary teams, collaboration with, 110
international administration, NCLEX-RN® exam, 453
international nurses
    abbreviations and, 468
    CGFNS® preparation, Kaplan programs for, 468–469
    Kaplan programs for, 468–470
    language, 467–468
    NCLEX-RN® essentials, 453–470
    NCLEX-RN® preparation, Kaplan programs for, 469
    nursing practice in United States, 455–456
    sample questions and answers for, 459–467
    U.S.-style nursing communication, 456–458
    vocabulary, 468
    work visas, 455
interventions
    behavioral, 177–178